HOW TO BEAT
THE HEART DISEASE EPIDEMIC
AMONG SOUTH ASIANS

Enas A. Enas, M.D., F.A.C.C.
with Sudesh Kannan, Ph.D

Advanced Heart Lipid Clinic
Downers Grove, IL

Printed in the United States of America

Book design by SUZETTE AYENSU

Heart Disease time line adapted from P. Libby, with permission © Lippincott, Williams & Wilkins.

Printed at Grace Printing, Chicago.

Library of Congress Control Number: 2005930287

ISBN Number: 0-9769953-0-1

This book is dedicated to

my father,

*the late **A. M. Enas**,*

who taught me early in life

that one must never stop learning

or stop sharing knowledge.

Dr. Enas Enas

my father,

*the late **N. R. Kannan**,*

who taught me through personal

example the power of knowledge

to improve one's life

Dr. Sudesh Kannan

CONTENTS

PREFACE

THERE IS A SILENT but deadly epidemic of heart disease raging on the Indian subcontinent—Bangladesh, India, Pakistan, and Sri Lanka—and people who emigrated from there. Why this killer epidemic is occurring, and what can be done about it, is what this book is about. It is a distillation of everything I have discovered in the past decade and a half about heart disease among people of South Asian Indian descent—and how to identify, prevent, control, and even reverse it.

In the early 1990s, when I began publishing articles in cardiology journals about heart disease among Indians, many in the medical community were skeptical that heart disease was any more prevalent among Indians than other populations. Through conducting autopsies and studying disease on the population level, pathologists and epidemiologists had known about these high rates for several decades. Internists, family practitioners, and even cardiologists, in contrast, were largely unaware of the epidemic.

Something was wrong. In response, I decided to set the story straight. For the past 15 years, I have maintained a laser-like focus on this tsunami of heart disease sweeping the Indian subcontinent, drawing attention to it through research, journal publishing, and about 100 speaking engagements a year. Gradually, medical professionals—both Indian and non-Indian—have become familiar with this massive problem. The public, however, still barely knows about it, including the Indian public.

This book is aimed at stemming and reversing the tide. In paper after paper, I have shown that the data are both undeniable and startling: For example, immigrants from the Indian subcontinent living in the US have a rate of premature heart disease *three to four* times higher than that of other Americans, regardless of gender or socioeconomic background. More recent studies suggest that heart disease rates among the more than a billion people living on the subcontinent, particularly in urban areas, are as high as, or higher than, the rates observed among Indians in the US. Researchers now conservatively estimate that at least **one out of ten** Indians suffers from heart disease.

One out of ten is simply an extraordinary figure. Morally and medically, it is also an unacceptable one. In the western world, incidence and death rates from cardiovascular disease continue to decline from their peak in the 1960s, because of lifestyle changes and improvements in treatment. In South Asia, by contrast, these rates are *rising*. According to data from the American Heart Association and the World Health Organization, in 1985 as many as 145 men per 100,000 and 126 women per 100,000 died from heart disease in India. By 2015, those numbers are expected to hit 295 for men and 239 for women—a doubling of rates over three decades, and this, despite the fact that a large proportion of Asian Indians are non-smoking vegetarians with *normal levels* of cholesterol, body weight, and blood pressure.

In 2002, by comparison, 170 American men per 100,000 and 131 women per 100,000 died from heart disease. If the current decline of 2% per year holds in the US, by 2015 the projected death rate from heart disease per 100,000 will be 128 men and 98 women. What makes heart disease among Indians so different? Here are six key features:

- **Prematurity** Heart attacks strike many Indians at a relatively young age (40-60 years). Many Indians know of fellow Indians who suffered their first attack when they were just 35 or even 25.

- **Severity** Among Indians, heart disease tends to be severe, malignant, and diffuse (spread out along an artery instead of in just one or two spots), making it hard to treat with bypass surgery or angioplasty. Many cases are simply inoperable. Even when successfully carried out, such procedures often serve only as temporary fixes. The underlying problem remains—the continuing buildup of plaque in the arteries. This means that, despite repeat surgeries and angioplasties, the blockages often return with a vengeance, leading to premature death.

- **Equally high rates among women** Until recently, heart disease was considered "a man's disease." Unlike in other ethnic groups, however, heart disease rates among Indian men and women are virtually identical, despite relatively low rates of smoking among Indian women.

- **High rates of heart disease despite low rates of the traditional risk factors** The prevalence of smoking, hypertension, high cholesterol, and obesity—the traditional heart disease risk factors—is similar or lower among Indians in the US compared to other Americans. Yet for any given level of cardiac risk factors, Indians are at about twice greater risk of developing heart disease.

- **Predilection for diabetes** Diabetes is 2-4 times more common among Indians in the US than other Americans. It occurs at a younger age, and even in the absence of obesity. Diabetes and heart disease appear to be strongly interactive among Indians—one leads to the other within a matter of 10-20 years.

- **A combination of genetic susceptibility and lifestyle factors** Indians seem to be more vulnerable to heart disease because of a genetic predisposition to abdominal obesity, high blood levels of a substance called lipoprotein(a), and a small-particle type of HDL (good) cholesterol that offers less protection against heart disease. These heredity-based risk factors magnify the harmful effects of lifestyle risk factors associated with physical inactivity, urban living, and a high-fat diet.

If you are Indian and are reading this, and holding your chest wondering "Oh my! I'm in trouble," I have good news for you. Heart disease is highly predictable, preventable, treatable and even reversible. We now have the technology, diagnostic tests, and medications to help you lower your risk factors substantially. While your genes may have loaded the gun, it is lifestyle choices that pull the trigger. Working with your doctor, you can significantly reduce your risk of heart disease through appropriate lifestyle changes and medications.

As advances in genetics and biotechnology usher in a new era of "personalized medicine" (*see* Chapter IV, Section 2, "Better Drugs, Better Prevention: The Promise of Personalized Medicine" box), we can look forward to a time when doctors will be able to offer their patients even more effective combinations of cardiovascular medications and risk-reduction strategies that are custom-tailored to each patient's unique individual genetic makeup. Yet even today, we have enough knowledge to reduce most people's heart disease risks to surprisingly low levels—*if only* more people would grasp the urgency of the need to do this, and translate that urgency into practical preventive action.

If I may offer you a brief but telling example. My co-author, Dr. Sudesh Kannan, had what many would consider a healthy lifestyle. He was predominantly vegetarian. He did not smoke. He exercised 20 minutes three times a week. He was not obese by traditional standards. So it came as a complete surprise when routine blood tests revealed that he had dyslipidemia, meaning that his blood lipids were gravely out of balance. He had low levels of HDL (good cholesterol) and high levels of LDL (bad cholesterol). His triglycerides, a marker for diabetes, were above 500 mg/dL—three times the normal level.

With the same perseverance that earned him a doctorate from the University of Virginia, Sudesh decided to attack dyslipidemia, researching it in books and medical papers and looking for advice not only on how to treat it but on how to manage it through a healthy diet and increased physical activity. Then in 1995 Sudesh's brother, a physician, sent him an article I had published in *Clinical Cardiology* (vol. 18, 1995) titled "Malignant Heart Disease in Young Indians."

That article, Sudesh says, marked a turning point in his life. Not only did he regain control over his cholesterol and triglyceride levels, but he went on to run three marathons and complete two 100-mile bike rides. Today, his energy level is astounding. I can unhesitatingly state that Sudesh's health is a testament to the proposition that small lifestyle changes can yield major rewards in quality of life. Consider this: In many ways, the human body is constantly trying to heal itself. From T-cells to homeostasis, it has a sophisticated array of self-corrective systems within it that are all designed to do one thing: keep the body in optimal health. Give it the right inputs of daily physical activity, plenty of water, and a healthy diet, and it will respond magnificently—often far better than any medication can get it to do.

Sudesh joined me to co-author this book because he is concerned about one thing: much of what I have uncovered and published in journals over the past 15 years, he says, still remains unknown to the average Indian, and even many physicians. Not only are the prevention and management strategies for Indian heart disease unfamiliar, but the dimensions of the problem itself have not been fully grasped. It remains under the radar. The Indian Ocean tsunami of December 26, 2004 that killed an estimated 290,000 people received extensive 24-hour international media coverage—as well it should. The response was magnificent and appreciated. To put it in perspective, however, heart disease kills more people in the nation of India alone than the tsunami did *every three months*. That fact does not even make it into the Health Section of most major newspapers, never mind primetime TV news. Yet every three months, more than 300,000 Indians slip away under the waves of coronary artery disease. Heart disease has indeed become the "Silent Scream" among South Asians—snuffing out lives by the thousands everyday while others go on with their lives, oblivious to the killer stalking the region.

In the Book of Hosea, God explains: "My people are destroyed from *lack of knowledge*" (4:6). After considering how dramatically his health had turned around—through the simple application of *knowledge* derived from sound research data—it was Sudesh who urged me to write a book that would send a clear message to Asian Indians at home and abroad, and the physicians who take care of them.

Over the past 15 years, I have presented and conducted more than 1,000 lectures and seminars to physicians in the US and India as well as Indians living in Chicago on the subject of heart disease. This book distils the extensive feedback I have received from my audiences and seminar participants into a set of practical preventive and treatment strategies. It is intended to serve as a quickly digestible companion to a more professional edition, *Heart Disease among South Asians: Unraveling the Mysteries, Debunking the Myths*, scheduled for release in 2006. That version will have substantially more references and research data than this one.

How the Book is Organized

The book's eight Chapters are grouped into three parts. *Part One*, **Understanding Your Situation**, presents fundamental concepts of heart disease with special focus on Indians. It highlights what makes heart disease different among Indians and summarizes some of the paradoxical relationships that exist between heart disease, risk factors, and different populations. *Part Two*, **Taking Action**, presents strategies for lifestyle improvements in an easy-to-understand format. *Part Three*, **Further Issues**, discusses in detail, the various medications for prevention and treatment of heart disease. Each of the eight Chapters is further divided into a handful of clear, self-contained subsections. Here is how the book is arranged:

▶ **Chapter I** introduces the basics of how atherosclerosis—the hardening and narrowing of arteries due to plaque—leads to heart disease and eventually heart attack. Section 1 would be particularly helpful for readers who need a basic understanding of heart disease and heart attack, as well as a simple introduction to the essential terminology of cardiology. The rest of Chapter I provides an overview of heart disease among Indians worldwide. It also highlights the unique features of heart disease among Indians, particularly its prematurity and malignant nature.

▶ **Chapter II** discusses the principles of heart disease prediction and the importance of such traditional risk factors as smoking, high cholesterol, high blood pressure, a sedentary lifestyle, and diabetes, and how diseases like high blood pressure interact with other risk factors to create secondary effects of their own. This Chapter should be helpful for both physicians and lay readers.

▶ Geared more toward healthcare professionals and advanced readers, **Chapter III** discusses more complex concepts of heart disease and emerging risk factors, such as C-Reactive protein, lipoprotein(a), homocysteine, abdominal obesity, and metabolic syndrome. Many of these novel risk factors are of prime importance to understandingand managing heart disease among the Indian population.

▸ **Chapter IV** unravels the causal factors underlying what I call the Indian Paradox, the high rate of premature, severe heart disease among Indians despite low rates of traditional risk factors. The Chapter examines the paradox of high-risk-factors, low heart-disease found in many other populations to show that there appear to be **tipping points** in the risk profile of an ethnic group, or for that matter an individual. Before this tipping point is reached, group members are well-protected from high rates of heart disease. But the addition of just one more elevated risk factor—less physical activity, for example, or a few extra pounds, or a major change in diet perhaps through immigration or urbanization-often begins to tip the scale, breaking down the protective shield and neutralizing the advantage they had enjoyed until then. This triggers the rapid acceleration of cardiovascular disease. Before the tipping point was reached, their genes seemed to protect them from the harmful effects of lifestyle risk factors. Once the tipping point is passed, however, any adverse effect created by a change in lifestyle becomes amplified, heightening the person's vulnerability to heart disease and hastening atherosclerosis.

As the Chapter goes on to show, precisely this seems to have occurred among Native Americans over the past century, among African Americans since the 1960s, particularly women, among Japanese and Chinese who have immigrated to the United States, and now, among people live on the Indian subcontinent or who trace their origins to it. Chapter IV also highlights the distinctive features of female heart disease, then draws attention to the important observation that heart disease begins during childhood. This makes it vital to initiate preventive strategies at a very young age. Based on extensive epidemiological data, this Chapter will be particularly helpful to physicians and advanced readers.

▸ **Chapter V**, together with VI and VII, forms a single organic unit that offers practical steps you can take toward healthy living. Chapter V presents strategies for preventing heart disease, including a balanced nutrition program and information on choosing good carbohydrates, good fats, and healthful cooking oils. A full section is devoted to the motivational issues that facilitate or impede your ability to initiate and sustain healthy lifestyle changes. Chapter V also devotes a section to the critical issue of designing a feasible and enjoyable physical activity program tailored to your needs, likes, and dislikes. This Chapter is targeted toward a general audience as well as physicians looking for more effective ways of presenting appropriate lifestyle strategies to their patients.

▸ **Chapter VI** outlines strategies for controlling various risks factors and diseases through both lifestyle changes and medication. It provides valuable information about managing high blood pressure, high cholesterol, low HDL, lipoprotein(a), triglycerides, diabetes, metabolic syndrome, and obesity. Individuals living with these conditions will find this Chapter particularly relevant, as would physicians seeking to treat Indian patients more aggressively for these disorders.

▸ **Chapter VII** offers several tools for diagnosing heart disease and assessing your risk before actual symptoms begin to occur. In addition to discussing interventions such as   coronary angioplasty and bypass surgery, the Chapter also provides cardiac patients with up-to-date information on living a healthy life after a heart attack. This Chapter is especially recommended to post-surgery patients and their families, as well as anyone concerned about their risk of a future heart attack. Physicians will also find that the Chapter goes to considerable technical depth in digesting and summarizing the latest studies.

▸ **Chapter VIII** discusses statins and niacin, two medications of central importance in preventing and treating heart disease. It also covers other medications and devices, including pacemakers and defibrillators. This Chapter will help you to understand the medications your doctor may prescribe for you—a highly important step because understanding correlates strongly with adherence to medication.

How can you get the most out of this book?

There are two main objectives: Part One will help you understand the threat that heart disease and its complications pose to South Asians in particular. Parts Two and Three will equip you with practical tools and options to help you create a comprehensive prevention strategy if you are Asian Indian or have Indian patients. After reading this book, you should be able to:

- **understand** the most common medical terms and concepts employed in discussing heart disease, allowing you to better interact with your doctor or with your Indian patients;

- **make** informed healthcare decisions that go beyond simply achieving conventional cut-points that may not be aggressive enough for your case;

- **grasp** in simple, clear English the latest scientific information about heart disease and its complications—including angina, heart attack, and sudden death;

- **comprehend** the key genetic and lifestyle factors that make South Asians especially vulnerable to cardiovascular disease, how these two types of factors interact, and what makes the combination of several risk factors multiplicative rather than merely additive; and

- **understand** what treatments are used after a major coronary event, the continuing risks that exist after coronary angioplasty, stent or bypass surgery, and how to manage these risks to reduce your chances of repeat procedures and further attacks.

Among the specific capabilities this book offers its readers are:

- **How to avoid a premature heart attack.** Discusses how to recognize several major risk factors that are particularly common among Indians, why it is vital to recognize them early, and how to manage them. Example: Blood tests exist today that can help you identify if you are at high risk for a heart attack at a young age.

- **How women can reduce their risk of heart disease.** Identifies several features of heart disease that tend to be unique to women, who often are under-diagnosed for heart disease.

- **How to prevent diabetes.** Shows you how you can combine appropriate physical activity with readily available components of the Indian diet with which you are already familiar to create lifestyle changes that will reduce your risk to diabetes.

- **How to familiarize yourself with non-traditional or emerging risk factors.** Identifies little-discussed, "emerging" risk factors that are especially common among Indians and put them at very high risk for heart disease. Some of these still unfamiliar factors can multiply by several times the risk of developing premature heart disease when more traditional risk factors are also present, because the two work together synergistically.

This book lends itself well both to a single read and in-depth study. In addition to a comprehensive **Glossary** at the end, each section of each Chapter ends with **Key Points** that summarize the information provided. For those interested in further exploration of particular issues, there is a list of references at the end of the book, along with significant technical details within the book to which you may want to refer back after a first reading. Through the use of side panels, boxes, and capsules, the book presents a lively account of the ins and outs of heart disease in a way that does not intimidate, confuse, or bore.

Finally, a note on the scientific foundation of the research summarized here. The information cited in this book derives from numerous studies involving thousands of patients over decades. The results of these studies form the basis of the advances in knowledge about heart disease presented in this book. Appendix B outlines many of these studies and concludes with a list of reports by various recommending agencies. Appendices C and D offer additional details about the Prudent Nutrition Program outlined in Chapter V.

Medical Terminology for Non-Medical People

Without sounding too technical, appropriate medical terms have been included so you can communicate more effectively with your physician. We have gone to great lengths to make these terms easily understandable even to a lay person with no medical background. Yet the book will be equally useful to healthcare professionals—family physicians, internists, nurses, dieticians, nutritionists, residents, and medical students—particularly those who provide care to people of Indian origin.

Although the book's focus is on heart disease in Indians, people of **other ethnicities** will also find it helpful, especially those with a family or personal history of premature heart disease, or who need repeat angioplasty or bypass surgery. Indeed, Chapter IV discusses half a dozen other ethnic groups and the genetic and lifestyle factors that predispose them to, or protect them from, heart disease.

A word about motivational issues: Unlike a crash diet before a wedding, lifestyle changes such as nutrition and exercise are best approached not as one-time events but as ongoing, lifelong practices. Yet how do you initiate, let alone sustain, a fundamental change in orientation over several years or even decades? To address this, I have included a section on motivation that offers pointers to help you overcome the most common psychological obstacles people face in internalizing a lifestyle change and making it a permanent feature of their daily life. If you start today, you can literally be physiologically younger next year: more healthy, more energetic, more fit, and at lower risk for cardiac disease and diabetes.

Indians and non-Indians in both the medical and non-medical communities must work together to make heart disease and diabetes among at-risk populations such as Indians more widely known, and ultimately more rare. My overriding goal in writing this book is to harness everything I know to help you gain greater control over your life and enhance its quality and length so you can realize the full productive potential within you. I hope you find it clear, informative, practical, and timely. Above all, remember: It is not what you know, but what you *do* with what you know that counts.

Good health, and best of luck!

Enas A. Enas, MD, F.A.C.C.
Lisle, Illinois
November, 2005

A Word about Terminology

Throughout this book, the term Indian refers to people who trace their origin to the Indian subcontinent—meaning Bangladesh, India, Pakistan, and Sri Lanka—including those who now live abroad but originate from one of these four countries. "Indian" in this context is ethnically interchangeable with "South Asian," "Indo-Asian," or "Asian Indian." The term thus excludes native Americans but includes more than people from the nation of India.

Measurement Units: As is conventional, blood glucose levels, triglyceride levels, and cholesterol levels are stated throughout this book in milligrams per deciliter (mg/dL). Blood pressure is stated in millimeters of mercury (mmHg).

CO-AUTHOR'S NOTE

IT IS AN HONOR AND A PRIVILEGE to coauthor this book with Dr. Enas, particularly because of the opportunity it opens up to share crucial information with millions of at-risk people—Indians and non-Indians alike—who have no medical background. This book is a tribute not only to the hundreds of lives Dr. Enas has saved as a cardiologist but the thousands he has changed, including my own, by giving patients and readers the knowledge tools they need to prevent or manage their heart disease.

Drawing on years of painstaking medical investigation, epidemiological research, personal observation, and clinical practice, Dr. Enas has condensed the most salient information and insights from his vast database of scientific knowledge to create this compendium of knowledge on how to win the war against premature, malignant heart disease. This book, in just a few hundred pages, is the "Cliff Notes" version of everything this man knows about fighting coronary artery disease among people with a nature-nurture risk profile that predisposes them to it. The section on the Prudent Nutrition Program, for example, is based on an article he published in 2003 which itself has nearly 400 references.

In western countries such as the United States, the tremendous strides made over the past three decades in identifying the risk factors of heart disease, and controlling them through medication and lifestyle modifications, have cut the incidence of heart attack by more than 50% among their populations. By contrast, measured in overall numbers, Indians have benefited little from these advances in detection, management, and prevention-whether they live in Asia or in the west. Heart disease, in fact, has become more widespread on the Indian subcontinent, not less.

This book, used well, could help reverse that trend. If you belong to an at-risk population such as Asian Indians-or if you simply have high risk factor levels as an individual, such as having blood relatives who have had heart disease-I urge you to take action to reduce your risks of heart disease and diabetes by reading this invaluable book. Speaking from personal knowledge, I promise you an eye-opening experience. When you are done, share it with friends, family, and colleagues. Let's work together to slay this monster in our midst.

Finally, Dr. Enas and I will appreciate any comments, questions, or suggestions you may have. We can be reached at book@cadiresearch.com, or mail us your correspondence at:

Dr. Enas A. Enas & Dr. Sudesh Kannan
CADI Research Foundation
1935 Green Trails Drive
Lisle, IL 60532

Sudesh Kannan, PhD
Chicago, Illinois

FOREWORD

I feel a special kinship to Asian Indians with heart disease because my father died of a heart attack at 47 and my brother, a vegetarian, had coronary bypass surgery at 44. My family and many Asian Indians most likely have one or more genes that predispose us to developing premature coronary artery disease. As a resident in Internal Medicine in the early 1980s, I was struck by the number of young Asian Indians that came in with premature heart disease. Later, as a cardiologist, I was introduced to Dr. Enas Enas, a fellow cardiologist who had also noticed this emerging phenomenon. Initially, a number of speculative explanations were suggested: perhaps it was the stress of recent immigration, or the notion that South Asians have congenitally small coronary arteries.

Not satisfied with any of these explanations, Dr. Enas launched the Coronary Artery Disease in Asian Indians (CADI) study to help unravel the mystery of premature heart disease in Asian Indians, utilizing Indian physicians living in the US as the first cohort for evaluation. The results of this study are now considered the basis for understanding the risk factors that lead to heart disease in Asian Indians.

Rather than high LDL cholesterol or cigarette smoking, which are the most common risk factors for the US population, it turned out that Asian Indians, at least those in the US, had low HDL, high triglycerides, high lipoprotein(a), and a marked predisposition toward metabolic syndrome, abdominal obesity, and diabetes. The entire US population is experiencing an epidemic of obesity and metabolic syndrome. For the Asian-Indian immigrant community, however, the harm caused by this epidemic is magnified at least three or four times because their genes seem to be less protective. As a cardiologist, I have witnessed the tragic consequences firsthand: a young physician, who recently emigrated from India with three small children, then suddenly died; or the female Asian Indian engineer who needed a coronary artery bypass at just 42.

Dr. Enas, who first sounded the alarm bell on this distressing epidemic through the CADI study, has worked tirelessly ever since then to educate physicians and the public about the true dimensions of this growing problem. With more than two decades of clinical practice and bench research to his name, Dr. Enas is a gifted cardiologist whose all-engrossing mission to expose the truth about Indian heart disease has led him to publish several dozen articles in major American, British and Indian cardiology journals since the early 90s. His research on heart disease among Indians has made him a valued speaker on the lecture circuit, where he has had opportunity to further sharpen his views and exchange insights with other leading experts at major scientific conventions.

Written with his colleague Sudesh Kannan, Ph.D., this book is a wonderful guide for helping Asian Indians and others to overcome their genetic predisposition toward heart disease through sound lifestyle advice and proper medical management. As a preventive cardiologist, I am optimistic that the incidence of coronary heart disease, a highly preventable disease, can be substantially reduced in the developing world, as it has in countries such as the United States.

A book of this breadth and trenchancy is a "must read" for all physicians who treat people from the Indian subcontinent. But it is not a guide for Asian Indians only. It is also for those of us who share these all-too-common genes that predispose some people to premature, malignant heart disease. Unless we take action, and take it soon, I fear that tragic consequences are inevitable. Dr. Enas's book provides more than a ray of hope against that possibility: it points out a strong, clear path that we can walk.

Michael Davidson, M.D., F.A.C.C.
Professor of Medicine and Pharmacology
Director of Preventive Cardiology and Atherosclerosis Research
Rush University Medical Center
Chicago, IL

FOREWORD

For more than a decade now, I have closely followed the pioneering research undertaken by Enas A. Enas, M.D., F.A.C.C. on heart disease among Indians. Like many others, who live on the Indian subcontinent, I am personally aware of the heartrending consequences of heart attack among young Indians.

Dr. Enas has contributed several articles on this subject for our newspaper, *India Tribune* that have been very well received by our readers. But newspapers, as you know, usually don't last more than a few days on the coffee table, if that, before they are unceremoniously replaced by latest ones. I was, therefore, delighted to learn that Dr. Enas had decided to put all of the latest scientific information in a book that can be understood by someone without any medical background. *How to Beat the Heart Disease Epidemic among South Asians: A Prevention and Management Guide for Asian Indians and Their Doctors* should become required reading for all South Asians: Indians, Pakistanis, Bangladeshis and Sri Lankans.

Research centers and public health bodies are learning that Indians and other South Asians are developing heart disease at a younger age than other populations, well before retirement age. The World Health Organization estimates that, in 1990 alone, 1.2 million people in India died from heart disease. It is projected that, by 2020, this number will have risen by 111%. This compares to just a 15% increase in the United States and a 77% rise in China. Compared to the US figure, the heart disease outlook in India is even worse than it appears because of the different demographics: India's population in 2020 will be much younger overall than that of the US, where medical advances and lifestyle changes are creating many octogenarians. One expects 80-something-year olds to have some heart disease. One does not expect a relatively young population with a median age under 40, such as in India, to *double* its heart disease rate in one single generation. Indeed, current projections suggest that, by 2020, India will have the greatest number of cardiovascular disease patients (heart attack and stroke) of any country in the world. This trend carries tragic personal, emotional, as well as economic implications for our country.

Dr. Enas says that there is a false conception that the problem is unique to immigrant Indians living overseas. While Indians, who live in the US, develop heart disease three to four times more frequently than white Americans, studies reveal that heart disease rates among Indians back home—especially those living in the subcontinent's cities—are as high as, or higher than, those of Indian immigrants overseas.

Considering the enormity of the problem we face, the appearance of Dr. Enas's book has elated my spirits. It is not only timely but also imperative. Despite all that has been said about heart disease in newspapers, despite all the specials on CNN and *20/20* and *48 Hours*, much of the medical and non-medical community still has not really focused its attention on the problem with the kind of urgency it truly deserves.

From its opening pages, *How to Beat the Heart Disease Epidemic among South Asians* reads like a thriller novel—fast, factual, and hard-hitting as it unearths the clues to this silent killer and leads the reader toward a clear solution supported by evidence. He writes as an insider who has lived in close proximity to an old enemy and has come to know its favorite tricks, hiding places, and *modus operandi.*

This extraordinary book does not simply tell you that heart disease is bad for you. Under the skillful guidance of its author, through his gift for identifying key issues and offering key insights into this complex topic, it shows you *why* heart disease is bad for you, how it can take over your life without your expecting it, and what steps you can take to keep it at bay.

Over several Chapters, Dr. Enas convincingly shows how heart disease risk factors and the complications they generate, including diabetes, hypertension, chronic kidney disease, silent inflammation and metabolic syndrome, have a multiplier effect on each other. They work together synergistically to accelerate coronary artery disease in vulnerable people. As study after study is presented, one begins to see a disease pattern emerging that crosses age, ethnic, and nationality boundaries and transcends gender and socioeconomic lines. The underlying message soon becomes clear: almost as certainly as the typhoon season arrives every year, a high combination of risk factors *will*—unless you are very lucky—lead to heart disease and to a coronary event at some point in your life, and the likelihood is greater if you are Indian. Exposing yourself year after year to the risk factors that lead to heart disease is like a lifetime of not brushing or flossing your teeth: sooner or later, extensive tooth and gum disease is virtually inevitable.

Clearly, if all it took for people to follow good medical advice were a few paragraphs such as these here, we would be well on our way to solving all the major epidemics of our day! But it takes more. One needs to be able to see the issue. *How to Beat the Heart Disease Epidemic among South Asians* explains cardiovascular disease from the perspective of an experienced cardiologist on a mission to expose the work of a killer that has been decimating communities around the world. His findings arise from a stupendous wealth of clinical observations, comparative research, journal reading, case studies, medical record examinations, and the invaluable anecdotal insights that one can glean only from countless conversations with real patients.

It is this impressive accumulation of evidence, related in clear, straightforward language, that, I believe, will convince the skeptical and compel the indifferent toward real change. As such, this book stands almost unique within the medical literature for the power of its message. Yet, its tone is not one of doom and gloom. On the contrary, the book's thesis centers on the premise that the majority of heart disease risk factors are modifiable and, thus, controllable. Those who start now stand an excellent chance of improving not only their own health outlook but also that of their children and other family members. To that effect, Dr. Enas emphasizes heart-healthy strategies that anyone can adopt, should adopt, and tell their family and friends about.

The issue we face is this: Everyone already knows that smoking, high blood pressure, and a high-fat, high-calorie diet are damaging to cardiovascular health. The real question is, how do we move from talk to walk, and from knowledge to action? What we need is a book that goes beyond the obvious and brings the reality of heart disease to readers in a fresh, clear and compelling way. This book does that.

I have no doubt that this valuable and highly informative book will become a reference book for medical students, a seminal resource for medical professions, and a valuable and much-consulted guide for the benefit of people from all walks of life and of all ethnicities.

J.V. Lakshmana Rao
Managing Editor, India Tribune
Chicago, IL

ACKNOWLEDGMENTS

Numerous individuals provided endless encouragement, input, help of various sorts, and constructive suggestions to enable the completion of this book, but special thanks are due the following:

Drs. Naras and Kusum Bhat, for editing the first draft and insisting that I write this version of the book before the professional edition.

My mentor Dr. Salim Yusuf, who provided invaluable guidance and support in the design, execution, and publication of the landmark CADI Heart Study. A co-author of many of my publications, he has been a marvelous source of inspiration and support.

Dr. Jeremiah Stamler, doyen of preventive cardiology, who helped in the design and completion of the CADI Study.

Dr. Thomas Pearson, for help with the CADI Study, particularly measurement of lipoprotein(a).

Dr. Michael Davidson, for his invaluable investigative instincts and insights in the initial stages of the Study.

Dr. Gundeep Singh and Dr. Neal Puthumana, who spent 1000s of hours with me writing, editing, and composing this book's Chapters.

Dr. Chacko Vinod, for helping me condense and assimilate vast amounts of research data into tables, graphs and figures, both for this book and for other research publications.

Mr. Lakshmana Rao, for his valuable editorial assistance, especially for making the book digestible for people without a medical background.

Manoj Enas, Beni Enas, and Yogesh Patel, for meticulously reviewing the book cover to cover.

Serge Nalva, for invaluable suggestions and editorial assistance that improved the clarity of the book.

Dr. C.S. Pitchumoni, for editorial assistance and his constant encouragement during my research.

My editor Franklyn Ayensu, for his many creative suggestions, for elevating the book to a higher standard of readability, and for polishing its language and presentation.

Carlos A. Irizarry for meticulous attention in typesetting.

And finally, my wife Mary Enas, for her constant support and her willingness to assume so many of my non-medical responsibilities, allowing me to focus on research and publishing.

Dr. Sudesh Kannan: My deepest thanks to my wife Akila Thyagarajan, who supported me indefatigably despite the considerable time I had to spend away from our family. As an individual with graduate degrees in Nutrition & Food Science, Akila contributed substantially to the nutrition sections of this book. An excellent cook, she has taught me that food can be both healthy *and* scrumptious. My brother, Dr. Suresh Kannan, and my sister-in-law Dr. Geetha Kannan continuously encouraged and supported me in this endeavor.

In addition, we would both like to acknowledge the contributions of the following people:

Dr. Rabindra Malhotra, Dr. Sunil Lulla, Dr. M.P. Ravindranathan, Anjali Kiran, Father Ignatius, Dr. George Thomas, Lora Lee Coulter, Dilip Gohil, Darshan Variyam, Dr. Roy Thomas, Dr. A. Senthil Kumar, Alex Siegman, Dr. Ram Thinakkal, Sanjay Dave, Dr. Adoor Amanulla, Kris Vijay, Narendra Bahalodker, Vini Chacko, and Dr. Paul Cherian.

Finally, we are both grateful to dozens upon dozens of other people in our lives—people who have encouraged us with their words, their wisdom, their personal examples, and their unspoken support to make this book a reality. Thank you, thank you!

COLOR PLATES

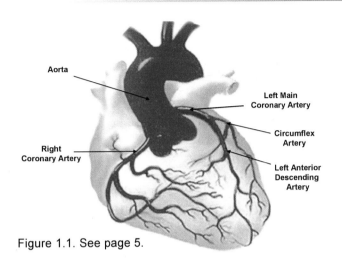

Figure 1.1. See page 5.

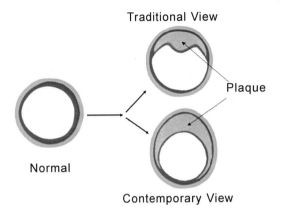

Traditional View

Plaque

Normal

Contemporary View

Figure 1.2. See page 7.

Glagov's coronary remodeling hypothesis

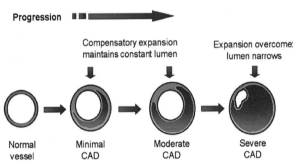

Progression

Compensatory expansion maintains constant lumen

Expansion overcome: lumen narrows

Normal vessel

Minimal CAD

Moderate CAD

Severe CAD

Figure 1.3. See page 8.

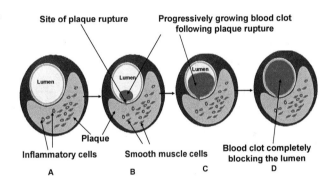

Site of plaque rupture

Progressively growing blood clot following plaque rupture

Lumen

Lumen

Lumen

Inflammatory cells

Plaque

Smooth muscle cells

Blood clot completely blocking the lumen

A   B   C   D

Figure 1.4. See page 8.

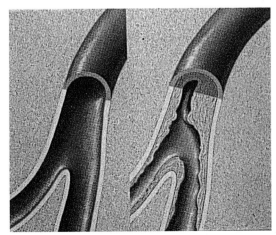

Figure 1.5. See page 10.

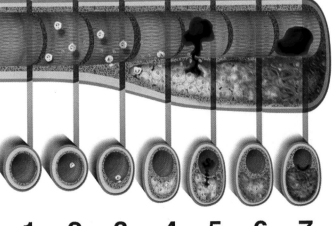

1   2   3   4   5   6   7

Figure 1.6. See page 10.

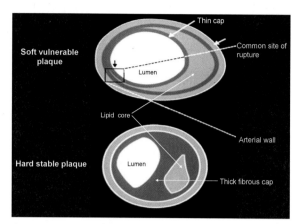

Figure 1.7. See page 11.

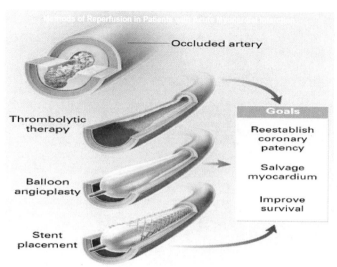

Figure 1.8. See page 22.

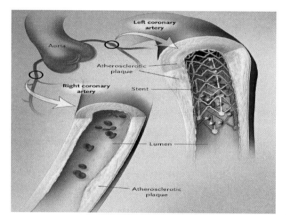

Figure 1.9. See page 22.

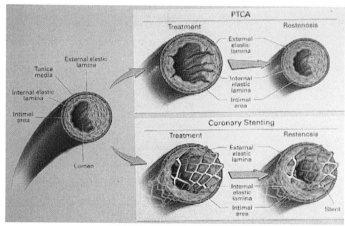

Figure 1.10. See page 23.

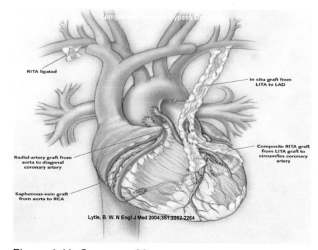

Figure 1.11. See page 23.

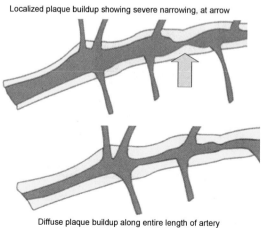

Figure 1.12. See page 23.

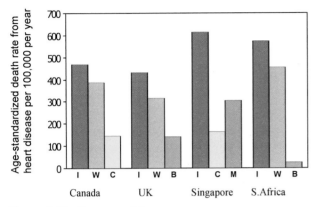

Figure 1.13. See page 24.

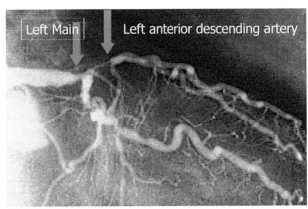

Figure 3.2. See page 85.

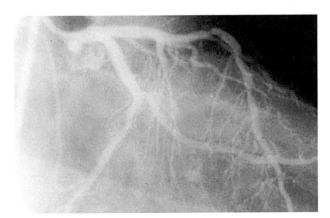

Figure 3.3. See page 85.

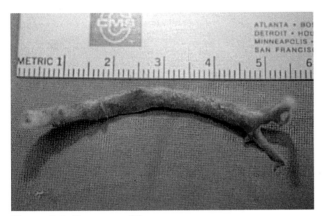

Figure 3.4. See page 92.

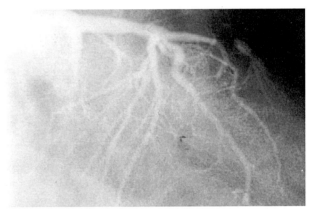

Figure 3.5. See page 92.

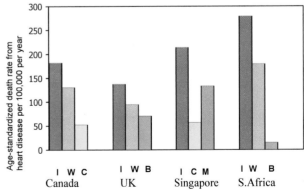

Figure 4.8. See page 143.

Figure 1.1. The arteries that supply the heart muscle. The left main coronary artery originates from the aorta and divides into the left anterior descending artery and the circumflex artery. These two arteries supply oxygen-rich blood to the all-important left ventricle (on the right side of the picture). The right coronary artery also branches off the aorta. It supplies blood to the right side of the heart.

Figure 1.2. Contemporary versus traditional views of how plaque forms. Until recently, it had been assumed that advanced plaque buildup always reduces the internal diameter of the artery by protruding into the artery in the form of a clearly visible plaque (upper image). Newer studies show that much of this plaque buildup occurs within the arterial wall itself, without protruding into the artery, and often without narrowing it or obstructing blood flow (lower image). The person experiences no chest pain, and therein lies the danger. Most often, the rupture of this soft, intra-wall plaque, not the hard large plaques that protrude into the artery channel, is what is responsible for a heart attack. Source: Glagov, S. Ref. 1.23.

Figure 1.3. Coronary artery showing plaque buildup. Stage 1, typical in young children, shows no buildup. Stage 2 shows mild buildup (the dark blue area). In Stage 3, moderate plaque buildup almost encircles the artery. Note that the plaque just thickens the wall. It has not yet narrowed the lumen because the artery expands (or "remodels" itself) to compensate. Absence of narrowing does not mean no plaque buildup. Only during Stage 4 does the lumen narrow. Stretched to its limit, compensatory expansion is no longer possible. Notice the dramatic change in lumen diameter between Stage 3 and Stage 4. Artery narrowing is one cause of a heart attack. The more common cause is plaque rupture and blood clot formation. Source: Glagov, S. Ref. 1.23. *Reproduced with permission©* Massachusetts Medical Society.

Figure 1.4. Coronary artery showing plaque rupturing and clot forming before a heart attack. In contrast with Figure 1.3, where plaque narrows the artery's lumen, causing chest pain, the more dangerous plaques are the inflamed ones that rupture without your knowing. A soft, lipid-rich plaque buried in the artery wall bursts and begins releasing its contents into the blood. This triggers the body's "damage control" response. Like fire fighters, platelets rush to the scene to form a clot to contain the damage. Without a blood thinner such as aspirin, the clot may grow (image 3), eventually blocking the entire lumen (image 4) and potential starving part of the heart muscle of blood, causing muscle cell death. Source: Libby, P. Ref. 1.33.

Figure 1.5. A healthy artery and a diseased artery with extensive plaque. The healthy artery's inner surface of (left) is completely smooth, and blood flow unhindered. Little sticks to it. The diseased artery's surface (right) is distorted, distended, and uneven from atherosclerosis caused by elevated risk factor levels. Endothelial dysfunction had organically altered the lining. The damaged, inflamed surface is pockmarked with hundreds of microscopic cracks where fat deposits can hide. The very biochemical structure of the lining has thus become less stable, more fragile, and more vulnerable to harboring plaques that can rupture. The difference between the healthy and unhealthy artery linings is similar to the difference between nonstick cookware and a pan roughened and caked with foods that have burned onto its inner surface, making it easier for more food to stick onto it.

Figure 1.6. Atherosclerosis timeline: How endothelial dysfunction progresses in an artery. The seven segments that make up this longitudinal section represent time periods, each with a corresponding cross-section, below (oval images). **Stage 1** A healthy child's artery, with a smooth surface that resists plaque formation. Little adheres to it. **Stage 2** In the presence of risk factors such as obesity, physical inactivity, and cholesterol, fatty streaks begin accumulating in the artery wall, typically between a person's fifth and ninth year. This changes the artery lining, "furring" it up and making it stickier. **Stages 3 and 4** As fat and cholesterol deposits continue to accumulate, the wall thickens and the lumen starts to shrink. Notice how much thicker the artery wall now is. **Stage 5** Plaque rupture. As lesion progresses, inflammation sets in and weakens the fibrous cap over the plaque, leading to rupture. This releases a Pandora's Box of highly thrombogenic materials directly into the blood, triggering the body's blood-clotting response to try to contain the damage. The clot (or thrombus) can become so big it blocks off the artery. **Stage 6** Blood clots lead to heart attacks if the balance between prothrombotic and fibrinolytic mechanisms in that area of the artery is unfavorable. If the balance is favorable, the clot becomes incorporated back into the plaque that burst. This can greatly enlarge the plaque and narrow the artery at that site. **Stage 7** Erosion. Occasionally, a blood clot can form without any plaque rupture, simply through surface erosion of the artery's endothelial layer (like scraping your skin). Source: Libby, S. Ref 1.33. *Reproduced with permission* © Lippincott, Williams & Wilkins.

Figure 1.7. How stable and vulnerable plaques differ. The vulnerable plaque (top) has a lot of cholesterol but very little calcium in its lipid pool, make it soft, like an egg yolk. It is also covered by only a thin cap that can easily burst, resulting in a heart attack. Such plaques tend to grow within the arterial wall itself, without narrowing the artery's internal diameter. By contrast, the stable plaque (bottom) is unlikely to burst because of its thick, tough fibrous cap and the small, relatively dry lipid (fatty) pool at its core. Inside it, there is a lot of calcium and fibrin, both of which are hard and tend not to become inflamed. Stable plaques can look impressively large on an angiogram, but they rarely break open and produce a heart attack. Their danger lies in sometimes growing large enough to restrict blood flow to the heart muscle, producing chest pain (stable angina). Source: Libby, P. Ref. 1.34.

Figure 1.8. Ways of reestablishing blood flow in a blocked coronary artery. Top sketch shows an artery completely blocked by a blood clot. Sketch 2: Clot is dissolved through thrombolytic (clot-busting) therapy. Sketch 3: Balloon angioplasty -- a tiny balloon is placed on the end of a catheter, a thin plastic tube, and pushed into an artery from the surface of the patient's skin. Guided into the heart and into blocked artery, the balloon is then inflated. Like a broom, it sweeps out the clot. Sketch 4: A wire mesh called a stent is placed inside the artery and opened up like an umbrella to reestablish coronary patency (meaning, reopen the artery). "Myocardium" refers to the heart muscle. Source: Lange, R. A. Ref. 1.32. *Reproduced with permission* © Massachusetts Medical Society.

Figure 1.9. Implanting a stent in a coronary artery to reopen it. Expanded views of the left and right coronary arteries. A stent, a small cage-like device made of wire mesh, has been inserted into the left coronary artery (on right side of figure) to reopen it after severe narrowing by plaque. The right coronary artery (on the left) has no stent and is beginning to close with plaque buildup. Although the latest stents release small quantities of a drug that helps prevent re-narrowing, re-narrowing often occurs if the patient does not make lifestyle changes. These include taking statins, ACE-inhibitors, and/or folate, controlling diabetes and hypertension through exercise, managing their weight, eating a healthier diet, and quitting smoking. Source: Hermann, H.C. Ref. 1.2. *Reproduced with permission* © Massachusetts Medical Society.

Figure 1.10. Renarrowing of an artery following angioplasty and stent. The image on left is an artery with a severely narrowed lumen. Top left: Balloon angioplasty (PTCA is short for percutaneous transluminal coronary angioplasty) was undertaken, and it tore and ruptured the plaque. Top right: Re-narrowing (restenosis) has occurred after the healing of the injury. Bottom left: A stent is put in place to restore openness to the artery. Bottom right: Re-narrowing has occurred following the placement of the stent, with newly built-up plaque seeping through the spaces in the stent. The recurrence of re-narrowing tells us that neither angioplasty nor stents are a 100% failsafe solution to atherosclerosis and heart disease. They work best when combined with concerted lifestyle modifications. Restenosis following the insertion of a stent is not related to high LDL cholesterol. It is common among people with low HDL, high lipoprotein(a), and diabetes, such as Indians (For more on this, see Chapter VII, Section 6.) Source: Bittl JA. Ref 1.8. *Reproduced with permission* © Massachusetts Medical Society.

Figure 1.11. A completed coronary artery bypass operation. The right coronary artery (red vessel on lower left side of image, abbreviated RCA) has been bypassed using a section of a vein from the patient's leg (thick blue vessel on left). One end is attached to the aorta, and the other to the right coronary artery. This reroutes blood around the blocked section of the right coronary artery. The left anterior descending artery (thick red vessel in center and on right side of image, abbreviated LAD) has also been bypassed using a section of the person's left inner thoracic artery (abbreviated LITA). Thoracic means chest. One end of the LITA is attached to the aorta, the other to the LAD. Also, on the extreme right of the image, a piece of the right inner thoracic artery (RITA) has been grafted onto the LITA that has itself just been grafted. (The yellow casing surrounding the LITA and RITA arteries is a healthy form of fat the body's organs need.) Source: Lytle, BW. Ref. 1.37. *Reproduced with permission* ©Massachusetts Medical Society.

Figure 1.12. Localized versus diffuse plaque buildup. The yellow represents plaque. The red is the lumen, where blood flows. Top sketch: The artery is severely narrowed but only at one site (see arrow). The overall buildup of plaque is relatively small. Localized buildup such as this is easily visible on an angiogram and ideally suited for balloon angioplasty or bypass surgery. For decades, this is how all severe atherosclerosis was depicted. Bottom sketch: Thick, diffuse plaque buildup along the entire length of the artery, but without localized narrowing. The overall amount of plaque is more than twice that in the top sketch, and the atherosclerosis here is much worse. The entire lumen is narrowed because of the extensive buildup. This is the kind of diffuse buildup — common among

Indians and people with type I malignant heart disease — that often makes for inoperable heart disease, because there is too much plaque to be pushed out by angioplasty, flattened with a stent, dissolved with thrombolytic therapy, or bypassed with surgery.

Figure 1.13. Age-standardized death rates from heart disease among Indian men per 100,000 per year compared to other ethnic groups in Canada, UK, Singapore and South Africa. Note that in each of these four countries, Indians have the highest mortality rates. (I= Indians, B=blacks, W=whites, C=Chinese, M= Malays). Source: Enas, EA. Ref. 1.16. *Reproduced with permission© British Journal of Diabetes & Vascular Disease.*

Figure 3.2. Coronary angiogram of Dr. Sudarshan Sadhasivam's coronary arteries. In an angiogram, a dye is injected into the arteries. The physician can see the dye only to the extent that the artery is not blocked. If you can see the dye, that is good news; if you cannot, that is bad news. The dye here showed up very faintly, revealing severe narrowing (75%) of Prof. Sadhasivam's left main coronary artery and almost total blockage (99% narrowing) of his left anterior descending artery. Blockage of these two arteries is associated with the highest risk of cardiac death. The dye in the third artery, the right coronary artery, could not be seen at all, meaning that this artery was completely blocked. (To understand why, see the next figure, 3.3). Note: A strong solid white image indicates a healthy arteri with out plaque.

Figure 3.3. An actual plaque removed from the right coronary artery of Dr. Sudarshan Sadhasivam. This unusually large plaque, more than two inches long and made up mainly of lipoprotein(a), was pulled out in a single piece from Prof. Sadhasivam's right coronary artery. Despite his strongly health-oriented lifestyle, this plaque had completely filled his right coronary artery. It attests to the danger that lipoprotein(a) poses to people with elevated levels of it, including millions of Indians.

Figure 3.4. Indians have small coronary arteries . . . The Myth. This angiogram of Dr. Peter Chacko's coronary arteries, at age 44, is the kind of evidence that keeps alive the myth that Indians have small coronaries. Compared to the angiogram in Figure 3.5 — also of Dr. Chacko's coronary arteries, but five years earlier — the arteries here appear positively minuscule. Actually, they are very large indeed, but extremely rapid plaque buildup during the five years prior to this angiogram had almost completely blocked all three of his major coronary arteries, making them appear almost invisible on an angiogram, and conveying the false impression that he and other Indians have tiny arteries. Figure 3.5 proves otherwise. In many healthcare systems, angiograms typically are done only when a person has advanced heart disease. Thus, the angiogram of Dr. Chacko's coronaries five years earlier (Fig. 3.5), before his heart disease became really severe and his coronary arteries narrowed, was a fortuitous occurrence.

Figure 3.5. Indians have small coronary arteries . . . The Facts. Dr. Peter Chacko's angiogram, at age 39, showing the true size of his large coronary arteries. Note that the angiogram here is at the same magnification as the one in Figure 3.4. During an angiogram, arteries are filled with a dye to enable visualization: strong, thick white lines indicate big, healthy arteries. Yet in the later angiogram of Figure 3.4, one can hardly see any of the three major arteries that, five years earlier, had showed up so boldly here — not because they are small, but because they are blocked. Fact: Indians' coronary arteries are neither smaller nor larger than anyone else's. But high levels of homocysteine, high lipoprotein(a), and low HDL constitute a disturbingly common triad of risk factors among Indians that often result in swift atherosclerotic progression, as indeed they did in the case of Dr. Chacko, and in the space of just five years.

Figure 4.8. Age-standardized death rates from heart disease among Indian women per 100,000 per year compared to other ethnic groups in Canada, UK, Singapore and South Africa. Note that in each of these four countries, Indians have the highest mortality rates. (I= Indians, B=blacks, W=whites, C=Chinese, M= Malays). Source: Enas, EA. Ref 4.21.

Part One

Understanding Your Situation

Chapter I

Grasping the Basics of Heart Disease

Section 1.1 of Chapter I, *Atherosclerosis, Heart Disease, and Heart Attack*, explains the development and progression of heart disease. you will learn why some people are more susceptible to heart disease than others, what plaque does in your arteries, how stress and other factors can trigger a heart attack, why it is unwise to wait for detectable symptoms before concluding that you may be vulnerable to having a heart attack, and how the atypical symptoms of many Indian heart attack victims put them at a disadvantage to prompt diagnosis. You will also learn about the similarities and differences between a stroke and a heart attack, the most common conditions, consequences, and complications of heart disease, how doctors diagnose them, and some of the procedures they use in treating heart disease and heart attacks. ◆

The next section, *Heart Disease among Indians Living Abroad*, builds up a systematic case by looking at the incidence and prevalence of heart disease, heart attacks, and cardiac mortality among populations of Indians living in many different countries, and comparing these rates to those of other groups living in the same countries. This section highlights particular studies such as the landmark CADI and Framingham studies. Since the environment in each of the countries examined is constant for all the populations who live there, the implication is strong that any differences in heart disease rates must be largely attributable to two things: either heredity differences that create different levels of vulnerability or protection among various groups, or variations in lifestyle such as diet, nutrition, and daily activity level. Indians appear to have both. ◆

Section 1.3, *An Epidemic on the Indian Subcontinent*, parallels Section 1.2 but focuses its lens on Indians on the subcontinent itself and wonders whether living in a developing-country environment has conferred any advantage on them regarding heart disease. Heart disease, after all, has often been considered a "rich man's disease," brought on by a sedentary lifestyle in front of a big-screen TV and a high-calorie diet rich in cakes, prime-cut meats, and other fatty foods. People in developing countries, who live a hardier, more active, and more abstemious life, were thought to be much less susceptible to cardiovascular disease. As you will learn from Section 1.3, today the actual truth appears to be quite different. Even rural Indians are fast catching up to the high rates of heart disease first observed among Indian emigrants living abroad. ◆

The final section of Chapter I, *Malignant Heart Disease in Young Indians*, looks more closely at three features that make heart disease in Indians particularly serious: it (a) occurs **early**, (b) hits **hard**, and (c) is found even in individuals with **few or none** of the standard, traditional risk factors. In addition to its extreme prematurity, severity, and weak association with traditional risk factors, Indian heart disease clinically speaking also tends to be diffuse—spread along multiple sites throughout the length a coronary artery, making treatment more difficult. In Chapter IV, we will look at possible reasons why heart disease among Indians tends to be so malignant. ◆

1.1 ▶ Atherosclerosis, Heart Disease, and Heart Attack

HEART DISEASE is responsible for more deaths and disability among Americans, both male and female, than any other killer, and it is quickly establishing itself as the leading cause of death and disability among Asian Indians as well. In 2002 more than one out of every three Americans (34.2%) had some form of cardiovascular disease, and almost one million (927,4000) died from heart disease, according to the American Heart Association. The most recent estimate for the direct and indirect cost of strokes and cardiovascular disease in the United States—counting hospitalization costs, medication, home health care, and lost productivity—is $393.5 billion a year. This is more than twice the total cost of all cancer and HIV cases combined.

Furthermore, the incidence of heart disease is spreading worldwide. For example, as Asian countries adopt a more sedentary westernized lifestyle, together with the high-fat, high-salt diet and processed foods that have come to be associated with technological affluence, researchers are noticing that "western" diseases are becoming more prevalent causes of death in Asia. In every region of the world except sub-Saharan Africa, noncommunicable diseases such as cardiovascular disease are quickly becoming the dominant causes of death and disability.

The first stages of heart disease begin in childhood, and it progresses silently for decades until, in millions of people, it results in a heart attack or even sudden death. The majority of deaths occur before the person even reaches the hospital. Most people do not worry about getting a heart attack if they do not have any chest pain. In reality, chest pain occurs only in a fraction of people who suffer a heart attack or sudden death. Managing a silent killer that often does not announce its intentions requires understanding what heart disease is, and what it does.

> **A Word about Terminology**
> Throughout this book, the term Indian refers to people, who trace their origin to the Indian subcontinent—meaning Bangladesh, India, Pakistan, and Sri Lanka—including those who now live abroad but originate from one of these four countries. "Indian" in this context is ethnically interchangeable with "South Asian," "Indo-Asian," or "Asian Indian." The term thus excludes native Americans but includes more than people from the nation of India.
>
> **Measurement Units:** As is conventional, blood glucose levels, triglyceride levels, and cholesterol levels are stated throughout this book in milligrams per deciliter (mg/dL). Blood pressure is stated in millimeters of mercury (mmHg).

THE VOCABULARY OF HEART DISEASE – A BASIC PRIMER

To do this, it would help if we first went over a few of the common terms doctors use to discuss it. Cardiovascular disease is really an umbrella term, a collection of interrelated disorders that affect your heart and/or your blood vessels. *Cardio* means heart; *vascular* refers to vessels. Your heart and vessels make up your **cardiovascular system**. The two are intimately connected. Heart disease is one form of cardiovascular disease, and coronary heart disease is the most frequently occurring form of serious heart disease. In fact, throughout this book, the term **heart disease** will be used to mean **coronary artery disease** (or CAD).

Although there are many kinds of heart disease—hypertension, for example—coronary artery disease is by far its most serious form.

Affecting 13 million Americans, CAD refers to diseases that affect the handful of arteries that supply blood to the heart. Symptoms of **angina** (or chest pain) occur when these arteries become narrowed and clogged, limiting blood flow to parts of the heart muscle. A **heart attack** occurs when the blood flow in a coronary artery is completely sealed off by a massive **blood clot**, depriving that part of the heart muscle of oxygen, blood and nutrients.

Blocked arteries can also lead to strokes or other **cerebrovascular** diseases (*cerebro* refers to brain). A stroke is really a "brain attack." Like a heart attack, it results from a major blockage of blood flow—this time, to the brain.

If CAD is the most serious kind of heart disease, **hypertension** (or high blood pressure) is the most common kind of cardiovascular disease as a whole, affecting more than 60 million Americans. Although hypertension is a disease of the blood *vessels*—it creates secondary disorders that can affect the heart or brain. It frequently leads to a stroke or to heart failure, although less often to a heart attack.

A Domino Effect
Your heart consists of three things: muscle, arteries, and valves. Each can become diseased, and the diseases of each can lead to disease in the other two. Your cardiovascular system is therefore a highly interactive system with backward and forward linkages. Disease in one part can ultimately trigger a domino effect.

Peripheral vascular disease When an artery that supplies vital nutrients to the heart is suddenly clogged, this can lead to a heart attack. If the artery is in the brain instead, a stroke may occur. If instead it is located in an arm or leg, peripheral vascular disease, or PVD, may result. Unless diagnosed early and treated, PVD can result in amputation. Other less common types of heart disease not discussed extensively in this book include valvular heart disease, congenital heart disease, and cardiomyopathy.

Now that we have developed a basic vocabulary of heart disease, it is time to open up a real heart and take a look inside. Here, then is Heart Anatomy 101.

DOWN IN THE ENGINE ROOM: THE HUMAN HEART

THE HEART is a muscular pump a little larger than your fist and weighing about half a pound. It pumps blood nonstop. Every 24 hours, an adult heart expands and contracts 100,000 times, pumping about 2,000 gallons of blood through the body's 60,000 miles of arteries and veins, the network of tubes that carry blood throughout the body. How does a vein differ from an artery? **Arteries** carry bright red, oxygen-rich blood from your heart to your body's organs. **Veins** bring dull-red, oxygen-depleted blood back to the heart. Veins, in a sense, are the giant transportation system bringing back tired workers at the end of the day to get cleaned up and revived for another day's work. But before your heart sends the blood back into your body for reuse, the right side of the heart sends it into the "workshop" for cleaning and filtration (in the lungs, kidneys, and liver) and re-oxygenation (in the lungs). This lung-kidney-liver workshop then sends the rejuvenated blood back to the heart for shipment out to the body. The entire thing works very well—so long as you do not have plaque and other diseases compromising the performance of these four vital organs: heart, lungs, kidneys, and liver.

What Factors Trigger Coronary Artery Disease?

You can develop heart disease through 1. genetic risk factors you inherited, 2. congenital defects of the heart that you were born with, or 3. unhealthy lifestyle choices that accelerate the progression of atherosclerosis and plaque formation.

You cannot do as much about the first two types of risk factors—genetic factors and congenital abnormalities—as you can about the third set, lifestyle choices, although even people with congenital abnormalities and genetically determined risk factors can now live near-normal lives for many decades, thanks to the tremendous effectiveness of the medications, medical treatments, and surgical procedures developed in the past 30 years to combat cardiovascular disease.

The most serious of the controllable (i.e., lifestyle) risks include:

- smoking
- obesity
- physical inactivity
- stressful emotions such as anger, hostility and depression
- failing to take your cholesterol-lowering and blood pressure medications
- failing to treat conditions that worsen heart disease, such as diabetes and metabolic syndrome
- eating foods high in saturated and trans fats, refined carbohydrates, cholesterol, and salt

These seven risks, taken together, constitute the most common and greatest controllable causes of coronary artery disease in all populations, including Indians.

To do this work, the heart has four chambers—two up, two down. The top two chambers, the right and left **atria**, are like your "Incoming Mail" boxes. They receive blood from the veins and send it down to the ventricles below. The lower two chambers, the right and left **ventricles**, are like "Outgoing Mail" boxes. They pump blood out. Atria above take in blood; ventricles below pump out blood.

Like a bicycle pump, each of the heart's four chambers has a one-way-only valve that lets blood flow in one direction only, forward. In short, your heart is made up of three things:

- **Muscle**, especially the powerful left ventricle
- **Arteries**, particularly the coronary arteries that supply the heart with oxygen and nutrients
- **Valves** that keep the blood moving in one direction

Over your lifetime, any or all of these three can become diseased or begin to fail. Diseases of the heart *muscle*, of the coronary *arteries*, or of the heart *valves* together make up what physicians collectively call **heart disease**. Now that we have looked briefly at the structure of the heart, let's look more closely at what causes it to become diseased. We will focus specifically on coronary artery disease.

> **The Circulatory Cycle**
> Tired blood carrying waste products from your body tissues enters the heart through the right atrium. It is sent down to the right ventricle, one of your heart's two powerful pumps. The right ventricle shoots it out to the lungs, for oxygenation and refreshing. It is then sent back to the left atrium. From there, the blood is sent down into the powerful left ventricle, which pumps it out into the body through the giant artery called the aorta. And the process starts all over again.

CORONARY ARTERIES: LIFELINES OF THE HEART

THE ABBREVIATION CAD, meaning Coronary Artery Disease, is often used in books and articles to refer to heart disease in general. Why? You can develop large, unstable plaques in any artery anywhere in your body, but it is when you develop them in your coronary arteries that you are in real trouble. The study of heart disease is, in large part, the study of what is happening in your **coronary arteries**. Turn your wrist over and look at the veins running just under the skin. The coronary arteries look like that. They wrap around the surface of the heart like delicate strings, running down the front, back, and sides of the heart muscle. You need to know what they are, what they do, and why it is important to keep them plaque-free. Here are the facts.

Although the heart pumps blood to the rest of the body, being an organ itself it too needs its own blood supply, just as workers in a food-processing factory need food themselves. This is the function of the coronary arteries. They supply blood and nutrients to the heart muscle itself. As the heart "exports" oxygen-rich blood to the body through the left ventricle—the heart's main pumping engine—it reserves some of this blood for its own private use by diverting some of it into the coronary arteries. As shown in **Color Plate 1.1.** *Major Coronary Arteries that Supply the Heart Muscle (page xvii)*, the two major coronary arteries—the left main coronary artery and the right coronary artery, colored red—branch off the aorta. The aorta, the largest blood vessel in the body, about the thickness of a garden hose, functions as the heart's main faucet. After coming off the aorta, the two coronary arteries

The left ventricle is the heart's Main Engine Room. It makes up more than two-thirds of the heart's entire muscle mass. Because it does so much work, it is particularly vulnerable to a heart attack.

> **Left main coronary, Left anterior descending, and Circumflex coronary.**
> Different segments of one coronary artery have different names. Why? After all, your body's arteries, beginning with the aorta down to your feet, are all interconnected. There is no point where one artery abruptly becomes a completely new, independent artery. Yet we cannot just call them all the same artery. Much the way a street name can change when it enters a new neighborhood, a coronary artery changes name depending on which portion of it we are talking about. It is simply an identification convention.

divide into smaller vessels that supply the heart muscle. When one of these huge coronary arteries becomes blocked by a very large plaque, or a plaque that ruptures and creates a large blood clot, it is not like your

What is Multi-Vessel Disease?

A person has **one-vessel coronary disease** when only one of their coronary arteries is severely narrowed or blocked. **Two-vessel** disease means two are blocked. You have **three-vessel** when all three are occluded. Generally, the larger the coronary artery, the greater its capability for triggering a heart attack, if it becomes blocked by plaque.

kitchen sink becoming clogged. It is more like an entire hydroelectric dam becoming blocked: The consequences to the heart are catastrophic. Yet in billions of people around the world, these arteries slowly start to become blocked and narrowed almost from birth. Identifying powerful but easy steps that can slow down this process is what much of this book is about.

Let's back up to the top, starting on the left side. The first inch or so of the left coronary artery is called the **left main coronary artery**. It is about as wide as a drinking straw. A heart attack resulting from a blockage of this segment of the artery is relatively rare (one out of every 50 attacks), but it carries the highest risk of death: 75% of heart attacks that result from a blockage of the left main artery are fatal. Most patients with left main coronary artery disease die suddenly without even having a heart attack.

Moving further down, the next segment of the left coronary artery is typically the **left anterior descending artery**—chillingly referred to as the "widow-maker" artery. It supplies most of the left ventricle, especially the frontal part (or anterior). When blockage of this artery results in an "anterior" heart attack, the likelihood of dying is twice as high as from heart attacks caused by blockages in other arteries.

Also branching off the left main coronary artery is the **circumflex artery**. It wraps around the left side of the heart and toward the back. It is typically small, but in a few individuals it may be as large as the left anterior descending artery. Blockage of this artery tends to result in a lateral (side) heart attack. A lateral heart attack is about half as likely to lead to death or to complications as an anterior (frontal) heart attack.

Now let's go to the right side of the heart. Like the left coronary artery, the **right coronary artery** originates from the aorta and supplies the right side of the heart muscle. Usually small, in some individuals it may be quite large. A blockage of this artery results in an inferior heart attack. ("Inferior" here does not mean worse. It just means lower. Anterior means front, posterior means back, and lateral refers to the sides of the heart).

If this sub-section has conveyed anything to you, it should be this: Do not let your coronary arteries become blocked, under any circumstances. Yet every year, tens of millions—including millions of Indians—succumb to this fate, partly because until recently we had not grasped atherosclerosis very well. In many communities around the world—even in the west—the partially erroneous traditional understanding of atherosclerosis continues to prevail. Let's see why this matters so much.

TWO VIEWS OF ATHEROSCLEROSIS

PLAQUE FORMATION, and the heart disease that results from it, is a highly deceptive process. The failure of medicine to understand it well until recently has led both doctors and their patients to under-appreciate, under-diagnose, and under-treat this serious disease. A decade or two ago, doctors thought heart attacks were caused mainly by the narrowing of arteries by accumulated plaque, because they were literally looking at heart attacks through the lens of angiograms, and arterial narrowing is what an angiogram can detect. More recent research has put the spotlight on what angiograms do not detect: plaques that are about to rupture.

Until recently, doctors thought heart attacks were caused mainly by narrowed arteries, because that is what angiograms detect. But arterial narrowing is not even half the story.

In fact, atherosclerosis can cause heart problems in two distinct ways: through the narrowing of an artery by a plaque that becomes too big, and through the rupture of an unstable plaque that, like an erupting volcano, bursts and releases substances that trigger the formation of a potentially life-threatening blood clot.

The old view was not altogether wrong, just incomplete. Arteries still do get narrowed, and people come to the hospital complaining of chest pain caused by exactly that. But, in fact, the great majority of heart attacks are caused by the *second* mechanism, plaque rupture. Let's look at this more closely.

The **traditional** view of atherosclerosis was that most major cardiac events such as heart attacks resulted from the narrowing of a coronary artery by a plaque that bulges out into the open channel of the artery, reducing its diameter and limiting or cutting off blood flow to some part of the heart muscle. This presents an incomplete, and in many ways inaccurate, picture. In what ways?

An atheroma is the collective term for all the unhealthy pieces of tissue, such as fatty streaks, that grow within the wall of an artery, beginning during your childhood, and ultimately turn into either stable or vulnerable plaques.

First, *take plaque shape:* As a plaque grows and thickens, we now know that it may not show any distinct bulging at all (**see Color Plate 1.2,** *Contemporary Versus Traditional Views of Plaque Shape, page xvii*). Many plaques do bulge out into the artery, but many do not. This makes them hard to detect even with advanced medical equipment. This can give the false impression that the person has only mild or even nonexistent atherosclerosis. Bulging, when it does happen, is merely the tip of an "iceberg" that has been building inside the artery wall for decades. In fact, plaque buildup does not begin to show through the lining of the artery until approximately 40% of the plaque's maximum size has already formed within the wall.

Second, *the developmental timeline:* The narrowing of an artery, and the bulging that some plaques show, both occur at a much later stage of atherosclerosis than was once thought. Arterial narrowing—and the chest pain that accompanies this—is actually the *very last stage* of atherosclerosis, when the disease is advanced. By the time you actually get chest pain from artery blockages, it is often already too late. We are now finding out that atherosclerosis is a slow, systematic process that *starts in childhood* and progresses silently for many decades, its pace determined by the number and severity of cardiovascular risk factors to which the person is exposed. Indeed, its foundations may even be laid during gestation: Studies show that atherosclerosis occurs more rapidly in children whose mothers had high levels of cholesterol while pregnant. Even teenagers and young adults may have varying stages of atherosclerosis, with fatty streaks

Plaque, Cholesterol, and Atherosclerosis
What causes blockages in an artery?
Blockages are caused by the buildup of plaque in the wall of an artery and along the artery's innermost lining, in a process known as atherosclerosis. Atherosclerosis, pronounced ath-ro-skluh-ROW-sis, is far and away the major (but not the only) cause of heart attack and stroke. It is a big word, but you need to know it because the chances are that it is taking place in your body even as you read this, and it often has fatal long-term consequences. From the Greek words athero (meaning paste) and sclerosis (hardness), atherosclerosis is probably as old as humankind itself and has been found even in the embalmed mummies of ancient Egyptian pharaohs. But only in the last few decades has plaque buildup established itself as the cause of more than 50% of all deaths in western countries.

What, exactly, is plaque? Plaque, which looks and feels a bit like pizza cheese, is a sticky paste made up of LDL cholesterol, lipoprotein(a), fat, blood platelets, calcium, waste products from cells, blood-clotting fibrin, and other blood substances that becomes deposited within the lining of an artery. LDL, which stands for **low-density lipoprotein**, is the bad kind of cholesterol. Atherosclerosis involves a complex interaction of processes in which LDL and lipoprotein(a) gradually oxidize—essentially, rust—to form fatty streaks, and ultimately a plaque with a cover over it. This oxidation cannot be reversed once it occurs, but having high levels of HDL (or good) cholesterol in your blood can prevent some of the oxidation of LDL into plaque. Plaque hardens and thickens the artery wall and—what is even more dangerous-leads to the possibility of the plaque bursting and causing a heart attack.

The roles of LDL and HDL cholesterol in heart disease are discussed at greater length in Chapter II. Meanwhile, here is a rule of thumb to help you remember which is good and which is bad: You want your **HDL** level to be **High**, and your **LDL** level to be **Low**.

and plaques in their arterial walls. In some people with multiple risk factors, atherosclerosis can become severe by their twenties or thirties.

> **Modus Operandi of a Silent Killer**
>
> If coronary arteries narrowed as soon as plaque started to build, many people would get chest pain in their 20s, call their doctor, and begin treatment and lifestyle modifications. Arterial narrowing would give them advanced warning in the form of chest pain that something was wrong.
>
> The danger of atherosclerosis is that, in the first several decades of your life, plaque does not narrow your arteries and cause pain. It tries to, but for several years your arteries expand in diameter to compensate for this narrowing, until they are stretched to their limit and can expand no more.
>
> There is worse: The large, hardened, highly visible plaques that narrow your arteries and generate chest pain are not the most dangerous plaques. The most dangerous are the soft inflamed plaques buried deep inside the artery wall that burst and trigger a heart attack, often without your feeling anything ahead of time.

Look at the sequence of images presented in **Color Plate 1.3**, *Cross-section of a Coronary Artery Showing Plaque Buildup, page xvii.* A normal, healthy artery (far left), for example in a young child, has a thin, elastic, flexible wall and looks whistle-clean, like a brand-new garden hose that has no buildup of mold, grime, or leaves inside it. As coronary artery disease progresses and clumps of fat and cholesterol thicken the artery wall, the artery (stage 2) expands to maintain its internal diameter, and it succeeds in doing this for several decades. It is only after the intra-wall plaque buildup has become extensive (stage 3)—and the artery has expanded as far as it can go—that the internal diameter of its passageway has no choice but begin to shrink with further plaque buildup. Stretched to its limit, the artery does not have very many options left. At that point, narrowing often occurs quickly and severely (stage 4).

Third, *causal effect:* A third way in which the traditional view of atherosclerosis was wrong is causal effect. Most heart attacks are not caused by arterial narrowing at all. The severe narrowing seen in stage 4 of Figure 1.3 typically leads to a type of recurrent chest pain called stable angina, not to a heart attack. In fact, more than two out of every three heart attacks result from a sudden blockage of coronary arteries that, *before the crisis, showed only mild or moderate atherosclerotic block-* age. The typical heart attack occurs in a coronary artery that had narrowed by only 20%. That means something other than arterial narrowing must be going on: that something is the rupture of an inflamed plaque that triggers the formation of a blood clot (*see* **Color Plate 1.4**, *Cross Section of a Coronary Artery Showing Plaque Rupture, page xvii*). We need to understand what this inflammation is, why inflamed plaques rupture, and how they cause heart attacks. Let's turn to that now.

Plaque rupture

> As recently as 2004, most artist illustrations of plaques in arteries still showed them as little bumps bulging out into the lumen. What was missing from these portrayals was *the main story*! Meaning, the thick, lipid-rich plaques that don't bulge into the artery at all, but instead change the very size and thickness of the artery wall itself, stretching the artery lining taut like the skin of an over-grilled sausage.
>
> In fact, a plaque can force an artery to enlargen to two or three times its usual diameter, creating weak thin walls that, like a balloon blown to its limit, may he-mor-rhage, quite often in the brain.

AS WE HAVE JUST SEEN, arterial narrowing, while serious, is not as critical an issue as plaque rupture. But why do plaques rupture at all? Doctors cannot say just by looking at a plaque whether it is the kind that will rupture. But we now know that an *inflamed* plaque is the most likely kind to rupture. We have seen that the traditional view of atherosclerosis was inaccurate on several fronts:

• The shape of plaques: Many do not bulge at all; they are buried deep within the wall of the artery

• The timeline of plaque formation and artery narrowing: Plaques form much earlier than was first thought, and narrowing occurs much later than was traditionally believed

• The cause of heart attacks: Plaque rupture, not arterial narrowing, causes most heart attacks

Inflammation: There is another way in which the old view was wrong. It portrayed atherosclerosis and plaque buildup as essentially a *physical* process: Arteries, physicians believed, narrow through the sheer accumulation of cholesterol-based lipids, similar to the way dirt gathers cumulatively on a car windshield. It was seen essentially as a mechanical process that results in a "plumbing" problem, like that of a clogged kitchen drain. Fatty deposits, doctors believed, steadily accumulate in a more or less linear way, eventually narrowing the artery if given enough time. If a blood clot then comes along, it may get stuck in the small opening of this narrowed artery, and you would be in trouble. Today, we know that plaque does not merely build up, layer after layer. Atherosclerosis chronically inflames the inner lining—or endothelium—of the artery, making it unstable and vulnerable to plaque eruptions. Just as neglected teeth and gums are not simply encrusted mechanically with plaque but become chronically inflamed and diseased, so do the inner surfaces of coronary arteries when people neglect their health.

In fact, the entire atherosclerotic process is inflammatory from beginning to end. It is inflammation that allows the lining of the artery, normally impermeable, to be penetrated by cholesterol-rich fatty streaks that become plaques. It is inflammation that causes the protective cap over a plaque to rupture, creating what is essentially an open sore that begins to spill its contents directly into the blood in the artery. And it is inflammation that often creates a massive blood clot at the site of the rupture, a clot that ultimately becomes the cause of the heart attack.

In short, atherosclerosis goes far beyond the mere accumulation of a thick layer of plaque. Indeed, when you compare the cross-section of a normal, healthy artery with that of an artery thickened by plaque, the contrast looks like the difference between the midsection of a 20-year-old gymnast with virtually zero body fat, versus the midsection of a 300-pound obese person. One is completely smooth and sleek; you could drop a bead of water on it and it would simply roll off smoothly with no interruption. By contrast, the inner walls of the artery thickened by plaque are distended, misshapen, and packed with fat. Their surfaces, damaged by years of atherosclerosis triggered by hypertension, smoking and cholesterol, look uneven and pock-

All of us have had a pimple at one time in our lives. The skin covering the pimple is often red, stretched, and inflamed, and is easily broken. A similar process occurs when a fat-filled plaque stretches the lining of an artery whose walls, over many years, have become thickened and weakened by layers of plaque. Eventually, like an inflamed pimple, the layers of covering tissue that keep the atheromic plaque from coming into direct contact with the blood stream are likely to rupture. In response, your body rushes platelets to the area to try to create a blood clot to cover over the open rupture. Although this clotting response is a protective response, this is the foundation of a heart attack. If the internal diameter of the artery is already narrow where the plaque is, the blood clot can block off blood flow, and heart muscle cells begin to die. A heart attack is the death of heart muscle.

Arterial Hardening versus Plaque Rupture

The traditional view of atherosclerosis presented it simply as the physical build-up of plaque on the lining of an artery, narrowing and hardening it. The emerging view centers on the role of soft, yolk-like plaques that become inflamed and rupture, stimulating a blood clot to form that can lead to a life-threatening heart attack if it becomes big enough to cut off blood supply to a part of the heart muscle.

The traditional model, however, was not entirely inaccurate. Before age 30 or thereabouts, plaque buildup is relatively mechanical and cumulative, and inflammation and rupture are less likely. Secondly, arterial hardening is real and harmful. Rupture is not the only danger. A healthy artery has highly elastic walls that expand easily to allow more blood to flow through when you suddenly need to run upstairs. A healthy coronary artery can expand to allow **five times** its normal volume of blood when needed. Hardened arteries cannot expand easily. If a plaque blocks or ruptures in a hardened artery, it is all the more difficult for the heart to get the oxygen it needs. The same plaque in a highly expandable coronary artery may not threaten the person's life. In short, recent research has focused on the role of plaque rupture, but arterial hardening still remains a real danger.

Plaque versus Clots: What Really Causes Heart Attacks?

Forty years ago, physicians believed that heart attacks were caused primarily by blood clots. Then we learned about plaque, and plaque formation became the lens through which we came to understand heart attack. Today, we have a more integrated view: we know that heart attacks typically involve both blood clots and plaque, and that the process is driven by inflammation.

The vast majority of heart attacks occur not because plaque chokes off one of your coronary arteries but because a soft, unstable, lipid-rich plaque-sometimes quite small-bursts and releases substances that stimulate your body to begin forming a blood clot at the site of the ruptured plaque. If this clot grows quickly, often without any pain warnings, it can induce a heart attack by preventing blood flow to a portion of your heart muscle and starving it of oxygen. Hard, stable plaques, by contrast, have little risk of rupturing. They can progressively narrow the channel of a coronary artery, but this is more likely to cause chest pain well before it causes a heart attack.

Not only are far more heart attacks caused by soft plaques that rupture, but these plaques often do not show up on an angiogram because they are buried smoothly inside the wall of the artery, like a coiled snake hidden in tall grass. The large, hard, visually noticeable plaques that show up impressively on an angiogram are not your greatest worry because they give advanced warning of their danger by causing chest pain when they narrow an artery. Silent, hidden soft plaques are the real landmines of heart disease.

marked with hundreds of microscopic cracks where fat deposits hide.

Frankly, an artery with substantial atherosclerosis looks like an accident waiting to happen—which is precisely what often happens. As shown in **Color Plate 1.5**, *Cross-section of a Healthy Artery and a Diseased Artery, page xvii*, the difference between a healthy and a diseased artery is not simply that the one with a lot of plaque is narrower. More than just narrowing, the second artery's lining has been organically changed: its very biochemical structure has become less stable, more fragile, more uneven, more inflamed, and more vulnerable to harboring soft plaques that may suddenly rupture.

This is a simplified account of what cardiologists call *endothelial dysfunction*—the set of damaging changes that can occur to the artery lining (*see* **Color Plate 1.6.** *Atherosclerosis Timeline Showing Progression of Endothelial Dysfunction, page xvii*). Caused by atherosclerosis, endothelial dysfunction makes your arteries more vulnerable to the conditions that lead to heart attacks.

Implications of our new understanding

OUR NEW UNDERSTANDING of atherosclerosis has important implications: First, it tells us that patients and doctors should not wait until a coronary angiogram shows severe arterial narrowing before taking heart disease seriously, because narrowing already suggests that the disease is advanced. As we saw earlier, in Figure 1.3, even seemingly healthy people with a normal amount of opening in their coronary arteries, and who have never had chest pain, may still have a dangerously large amount of plaque, putting them at high risk for a heart attack.

Second, we have now learned that doctors and patients must pay much more attention to how plaques develop and ways of reducing the chances of rupture. You need to change those lifestyle habits that accelerate plaque formation and plaque inflammation, even if there is no direct evidence that you have plaque in your arteries, because by the time you get that direct evidence, the disease is already far gone.

Third, we now know that it is short-sighted to focus primarily on the large plaques that may be highly visible on an angiogram, because plaque visibility has little to-do with how dangerous the plaque is. The most dangerous plaques are the soft, lipid-rich, inflamed plaques that are often buried, out of sight, inside the artery wall. The ones visible on the surface are, therefore, often just the tip of an iceberg. Most plaques are hidden deep within the artery wall, making them hard to detect even when using advanced medical equipment. This means you cannot rely on angiographic detection to tell you when to begin a preventive strategy.

Stable versus vulnerable plaques

Recent research, in short, has taught us that not all plaques are the same. Some are much more likely to rupture and lead to heart attacks, while othes are more stable. See **Color Plate 1.7**, *How stable and vulnerable plaques differ, page xviii.* The difference lies in their structure and content. These differences in structure and content have given rise to the term **vulnerable plaque**. Let's look at this a bit more closely.

Like a skin wound that forms a scab to protect it, or a corn on a toe, a plaque is covered by a hard fibrous cap which keeps its contents from coming into contact with the blood flowing through your artery. A stable plaque that is not likely to burst is one that has a thick, tough fibrous cap lying over it, and a small, relatively dry lipid (fatty) pool at its core. Inside it, there is a lot of calcium and fibrin, both of which are hard and tend not to become inflamed. Stable plaques can be large and look very impressive on a coronary angiogram, but they rarely break open and produce a heart attack. They become dangerous only when they grow large enough to restrict blood flow to the heart muscle, producing a form of chest pain called stable angina.

An unstable plaque, also called vulnerable plaque, is a totally different beast. Often smaller, this inflamed plaque has a thin, easily broken cap overlying a soft, large, yolk-like, lipid-rich pool at its core, with very few calcium deposits in the plaque to give it some firmness or toughness. In addition, it contains numerous inflamed cells, making it much more likely to rupture and release its contents directly into your bloodstream, creating a large blood clot. Vulnerable plaques have substances in them that make your blood excessively prone to clotting when the plaque's contents contaminate your bloodstream, causing blood platelets and other substances to clump together to form a life-threatening blood clot. In almost every case, heart attacks are caused by a soft, vulnerable plaque that ruptured and formed a clot.

The difference between the content of a stable plaque and that of an unstable plaque is like the difference between the yolk of a hard-boiled egg and that of a raw egg. Guess which one is more likely to break?

While hard plaques, once formed, cannot be regressed, the more dangerous soft plaques can. Medication called statins draw cholesterol out of soft plaques, making them smaller, harder, and more stable. Hard plaques, by contrast, are like plaque that forms on teeth, which needs to be scraped off with a hard instrument. A hard plaque that becomes too large must be physically flattened through a procedure such as balloon angioplasty.

Vulnerable blood

Just as some plaques are more vulnerable to fissuring, some people's blood is also more vulnerable to clotting, and thus more likely to lead to heart attack than that of others. What creates vulnerable blood? The causes include smoking, low levels of HDL, and high levels of lipoprotein(a), homocysteine, fibrinogen and triglycerides. (We will discuss these in greater depth in later Chapters.) All of these can contribute to making your blood more likely to clot excessively.

Inflammation of the Artery is an Active Process

Atherosclerosis is not just the passive buildup of plaque, and plaque is not just grime, like dirt on your body after a game of soccer. Plaque is a sign of active damage. The fatty streaks that represent the first signs of plaque indicate that there is inflammation present in the artery wall. Without this inflammation, cholesterol-rich fat cannot breach and penetrate the inner lining of the artery wall and become buried inside it. In fact, when your body detects that plaque is starting to form in your arteries, your immune system sends white blood cells to the site where the plaque is accumulating to try and repair the damage and heal the inflammation.

In a sense, having plaque is like having a constant fever running through your arteries. It signals that atherosclerosis has damaged the inner lining of your arteries—the **endothelium**. Just as the skin of a chameleon continually adapts to light conditions and other cues in its environment, the endothelium is a sensitive, "active" layer of cells that is constantly sensing, assessing, and rapidly responding to small changes and stimuli in the blood that flows over it. Secondly, a healthy endothelium is "watertight": it is impenetrable to substances in the blood. Hypertension, diabetes, smoking, and other factors that promote atherosclerosis (a) reduce the ability of the endothelial surface to adapt to change, (b) weaken its ability to prevent unwanted blood clots, and (c) damage the endothelium by making it easy for LDL cholesterol to penetrate it and become buried within the arterial wall as plaque. In short, atherosclerosis creates a **diseased lining** that can no longer fight effectively to protect you from cardiovascular complications.

Plaque Remains Silent for Decades

Almost everyone knows of a friend or relative who felt a twinge of pain and went to the hospital, only to be told that their illness was so advanced that it was inoperable, or would require years of treatment. Early and mid-stage atherosclerosis falls in the category of **"silent"** disease. The human body frequently uses **pain** to signal the presence of disease, but this is not the case in early- and midstage atherosclerosis. Even in a modern hospital, plaque can be hard to detect unless it is advanced, because for decades it builds up without showing through the artery's lining in a distinct bulge. The artery lining looks smooth.

Yet, like a volcanic mountain rumbling far beneath the surface, soft buried plaque can be very active. It can suddenly erupt, spewing its contents directly into the artery and triggering the formation of a potentially dangerous blood clot. Researchers discovered that many people in their teens and 20s have atherosclerosis not through doctors performing diagnostic tests and finding the plaque, but through performing autopsies on young people who had died in accidents and examining their blood vessels. Pathology, not angiography, is what told doctors that millions of young people have significant atherosclerosis. But "pathology," by definition, means it is too late! You need to discover it earlier than that. How? Not by waiting for chest pain to signal its presence, but by assessing your own personal risk factors and taking aggressive, proactive, preventive action.

Consider that, for about two-thirds of men and about half of women in the US, heart disease is like high blood pressure. It is painless. The first sign they receive of their heart disease is often the last: a heart attack or sudden death. In fact, although the typical heart attack occurs in a coronary artery with only 20% narrowing, a treadmill stress test detects heart disease only when one or more of the person's arteries is narrowed by 75% or greater.

The reason aspirin can help to prevent a heart attack is that it makes blood less vulnerable. Conversely, Merck & Co.'s worldwide withdrawal in 2004 of its anti-inflammatory arthritis drug Vioxx in response to a public health advisory issued by the U.S. Food and Drug Administration was based on indications that Vioxx increases the risk of a heart attack by making blood more vulnerable.

Half a century ago, doctors considered the major cause of heart attacks to be coronary thrombosis—the simple blockage of a coronary artery by a blood clot. Today, we know that most heart attacks are caused by a combination of plaque-formation (atherosclerosis) and blood clots (thrombosis), particularly among people who have vulnerable blood along with a large number of vulnerable plaques. Plaque is the number-one enemy, but clots play a role in the final stage. The good news is that, through lifestyle choices, you can reduce the vulnerability of both your blood and your plaques, as well as keep the number of plaques you develop to a minimum.

Vulnerable heart

Just as some blood and some plaques are more vulnerable than others, some hearts are more vulnerable. A vulnerable heart is one that has been damaged by a heart attack or other causes, which render it unusually susceptible to fatal conditions such as ventricular tachycardia (a form of arrhythmia) or to ventricular fibrillation that can result in cardiac arrest or sudden death. (These conditions will be discussed shortly). A person, who has survived a heart attack or cardiac arrest, is generally considered to have a vulnerable heart. Surviving a major coronary event is clearly wonderful news, but the point is that it is far better not to have had such an event at all in the first place, because that very history places you at greater future risk. Like a bone that has been broken before, a post-coronary event heart may never quite fully regain its earlier robustness.

Vulnerable patient

We are now recognizing that there is a category of patients, who should be referred to as vulnerable patients. The combination of vulnerable plaque, vulnerable blood, endothelial dysfunction, and a vulnerable heart makes for a *vulnerable patient* who is at high risk of a heart attack or stroke. Fortunately, cardiologists recognize such patients relatively easily from their medical history and appropriate tests. Through assessing a patient's cardiovascular risk factors, physicians can identify vulnerable patients who are likely to have numerous vulnerable plaques and/or vulnerable blood. The challenge now is for doctors to be able to identify vulnerable patients earlier and more easily, and for patients to be able to recognize the presence of hereditary and lifestyle factors that may be heightening their vulnerability to coronary artery disease, putting them at risk for a tragic event down the road.

It is important to note the progressive nature of heart attacks. A heart attack tends to predispose you to sustaining another, often more severe, heart attack—partly because the underlying causes that triggered the first attack (for example, dyslipidemia) may be unchanged, and partly because the heart attack itself can weaken your heart and cause further complications, including making the patient less likely to be physically active. In addition, as mentioned, much of the plaque that is the basis of most heart attacks grows within the wall of the coronary artery itself rather than on the inside lining of the artery, especially during the early stages of atherosclerosis. Unlike large, on-the-surface plaques, this intra-wall plaque cannot be physically flattened through interventions like angioplasty. It can, therefore, lay a foundation for a series of cardiac events later in your life. Fortunately, these vulnerable plaques are the ones that respond most dramatically to cholesterol-modifying therapy.

The role of stressful emotions

Plaque: Size is Not What Matters
In the traditional view, large plaques are the cause of both angina and heart attacks. In the contemporary view, large plaques cause a gradual onset of stable angina in a patient, for example, during exercise; but what causes heart attacks is inflamed plaques, whether large or small. Size is not the relevant factor. Inner composition is. Many dangerous, inflamed plaques are so small they do not even show up on an angiogram. A coronary angiogram cannot tell which plaques are vulnerable to rupture. They can only tell which ones are becoming so large than they may cause angina.

What actually triggers a heart attack? Why does it occur today instead of next week? The underlying cause, of course, is heart disease. In a more immediate sense, however, heart attacks are like angina often set off by emotional stress, anger, extreme excitement, or a sudden burst of physical exertion, particularly by a normally inactive person. Emotional stress, such as heated disputes at work or at home, great fear, or mental stress generated by tight deadlines at work, increases blood pressure and releases stress hormones, particularly in women. In one heart attack study, more than half of the respondents said they had been very upset or stressed in the 24 hours preceding their attack. Anger is particularly deadly: The risk of a heart attack is particularly high up to two hours following an angry outburst. Although it is impossible to avoid all emotional stress, we can reduce our risk of heart attack by learning to better cope with stress and mastering techniques that allow it to drain away.

Sudden vigorous exercise in an inactive person also raises the risk that a plaque will burst and produce a heart attack. Inactive people concerned about heart attacks should avoid vigorous exercise until they consult

Is heart disease a degenerative disorder?

Quite likely your initial response to this question was yes, but the answer actually is no. Heart disease is often chronic and progressive, but it is not accurate to describe it as a degenerative disease. Here is the difference: Degenerative diseases, such as cataracts or arthritis, get worse simply as a result of the aging process. Although there may be a few things one can do to slow down their rate, on the whole, there isn't much one can do. They worsen naturally over time.

Heart disease, by contrast, does not have to get worse over time. It is not inevitable. You do not get heart disease simply because you are growing old. The fact is that you can be 90 years old and not have plaque in your coronary arteries. It does not get there simply because you became old. The process of atherosclerosis is an active, dynamic process that results in part from specific, intentional choices a person makes or fails to make. And that is the difference.

True, some of your chance of developing heart disease may depend on your ethnic group and the genetic profile you inherited. Nevertheless, like type 2 diabetes or obesity, heart disease is highly controllable, even reversible. Much depends on you. This is why it is improper to think of cardiovascular disease as a degenerative disease. It is largely a disease of choice—and choice depends on knowledge.

their physician, especially in very cold weather, which can place further stress on the heart. When you do begin to exercise, start gradually so as not to shock your system.

HEART DISEASE AND ITS CONSEQUENCES

Does Exercise Thwart or Trigger Heart Attacks?

Okay, this is a bit of a trick question. The answer is, *both*. The cardioprotective benefits of regular exercise far outweigh its risks. Among its benefits—too many to list here—it lowers blood triglyceride levels, boosts HDL levels, lowers blood pressure, helps control body weight, improves the heart's ejection fraction, keeps your coronary and other arteries elastic, and improves cardio-respiratory fitness. Those who exercise regularly at moderate intensities for long periods of time (such as marathon runners) have the lowest rate of heart disease - less than one-fourth that of sedentary individuals.

Nevertheless, there are a few cautions: A recent study suggests that people who rarely exercise are nearly seven times more likely than those who regularly exercise to have a heart attack, if they engage in sudden vigorous activity. In other words, bursts of physical activity after years of inactivity carry risks. **Second**, in rare cases—as in the famous instance of Dr. James Fixx (*see below*)—exercise may precipitate a heart attack in an athlete who already has heart disease (in Fixx's case, possibly hypertrophic cardiomyopathy) or who has several very serious risk factors for heart disease (again, like Fixx).

Finally, exercise can prevent you from realizing that you have coronary disease because, for any given level of coronary disease, angina is delayed in people who exercise, since their fit heart compensates for the blockages. None of this, however, should deter you from regular physical activity. The unfortunate Dr. Fixx, for one, may have died much earlier had he not exercised so much. Get going!

HEART DISEASE can have many consequences. We will look at seven major ones: Cardiac arrest, sudden death, stable angina, unstable angina, heart attack, heart failure, and silent ischemia.

A central question in the detection, management and treatment of heart disease is: How do you discover it when there are no obvious symptoms? A stress test on a treadmill in a cardiologist's office can be a great detection tool, but there is an erroneous impression that a stress test that turns up negative (meaning normal) means you are off the hook.

Not necessarily. It simply may be that your heart disease is not sufficiently advanced for it to have been noticeable in the test. Fairly advanced coronary disease is relatively easy to detect—either through a stress test or the chest pain that the disease itself generates. In contrast, less advanced disease—for example, 50% blockage of the artery rather than 75%—is a greater challenge. This is why it pays to understand the different forms that heart disease can take and be able to read the initial symptoms in order to distinguish them from one another. With the heart, time often is of the essence.

a. Cardiac arrest

Cardiac arrest, an abrupt loss of heart function in which the heart suddenly stops pumping, is one of the dreaded complications of heart disease. It can occur unexpectedly, with or without a heart attack. If the person is not resuscitated immediately, it can lead to sudden death within an hour of any symptoms. It is believed that Terri Schiavo, who spent the final 15 years of her life in what many experts considered a persistent vegetative state before her feeding tube was removed in March 2005, suffered severe brain damage from cerebral hypoxia caused by cardiac arrest. Cardiac arrest can have several immediate causes, including:

- ventricular tachycardia (or rapid irregular heart beat)
- ventricular fibrillation (or rapid chaotic unproductive heart beats)
- asystole (or absence of detectable electrical activity in the heart)
- or all three

Usually, cardiac arrest starts as ventricular tachycardia and quickly advances to ventricular fibrillation, which compels the heart to stop pumping blood. Ventricular fibrillation can occur in people without a heart attack, including even young athletes. Cardiac arrest caused by ventricular tachycardia and/or fibrillation can be reversed if the victim is treated with an electric shock within seven to ten minutes after onset. Every additional minute spent without defibrillation reduces a victim's survival chances by 7-10%.

Cardiac arrest caused by asystole, or complete stoppage of the heartbeat, is more serious. One's survival chances are low. All untreated ventricular tachycardia and ventricular fibrillation eventually result in asystole.

Finally, a small number of cardiac arrests are caused by extreme slowing of the heart. If you suspect a cardiac arrest, call 911 and begin cardiopulmonary resuscitation (CPR) immediately. Table 1.1 gives the warning signs of cardiac arrest and how to distinguish it from common fainting.

> **Consequences of Heart Disease**
> Heart diseases such as atherosclerosis can lead to
> • Cardiac arrest
> • Sudden death
> • Stable angina
> • Acute coronary syndrome (unstable angina)
> • Heart attack
> • Silent heart disease and silent ischemia
> • Heart failure

b. Sudden death

The most frightening of all the consequences of heart disease is the prospect of dying suddenly with no warning. This indeed is what happened to James Fixx, the famous author of the runaway bestseller *The Complete Book of Running*, who collapsed suddenly on July 21, 1984 and died, just one minute after setting a regional master's record in a 3000-meter run. His story suggests that regular exercise, although extremely important, cannot by itself guarantee you protection from serious heart disease. Fixx, it turns out, had several risk factors: He had markedly elevated cholesterol and his father had died from a heart attack at 43. A former two-packs-a-day smoker, who was 60 pounds overweight when he started exercising regularly, Fixx's autopsy showed two severely occluded coronary arteries (one at 80%, the other near-total), and also suggested that he may have had hypertrophic cardiomyopathy. He may also have had warning signs that he ignored. Had he not lost 60 pounds and become a runner, Fixx may well have died earlier.

Table 1.1. Signs of Cardiac Arrest

Signs	Actions to confirm cardiac arrest
Sudden loss of responsiveness; no spontaneous movement	No response to gentle shaking
No normal breathing	The victim does not take a normal breath when you check for several seconds
No circulation	No palpable pulse

The important thing to bear in mind is that heart disease often kills without giving any advance warning symptoms at all. That is why aggressive prevention is so important. For about 30% of people with heart disease, sudden death with no chest pain whatsoever is the first and last symptom of heart disease they ever face. Sudden death is nevertheless extremely uncommon in people with relatively normal-functioning hearts. As in the case of James Fixx, it is generally the result of disease accelerated by risk factors such as smoking, family history, and abdominal obesity, which is a risk factor even in someone whose body weight and BMI (or body mass index) are normal. Every year, some 250,000 Americans die from sudden death without ever being hospitalized for heart disease, and about two-thirds of all deaths from heart disease occur before the person reaches the hospital, even in major metropolitan centers. Owing to advances in nationwide efforts at prevention and treatment of heart disease in the US, the rates of sudden and non-sudden deaths have decreased more than 50% over the past half century, but there is as yet no evident decline among people living on the Indian subcontinent.

> **Think Prevention, not Treatment**
> While many more Americans could benefit from a heart transplant than currently do, only about 2,000 hearts become available each year and there are long waiting lines. Bypass surgeries, stents, and coronary angioplasties, though less rare than transplants, are also very expensive. This means keeping your heart healthy rather than replacing it or repairing it is the real answer. Prevention rather than treatment is the key to cardiovascular health.

c. Stable angina

Angina pectoris, often simply called angina, refers to pain or discomfort in the chest that may radiate down your arm or into your jaw and typically lasts 2-15 minutes. Angina occurs when one or more of the coronary arteries that supply the heart muscle with blood and oxygen becomes severely narrowed through plaque buildup (atherosclerosis), depriving the heart muscle of oxygen-rich blood. The result is pain. It is important not to rely on the onset of angina as the first warning sign to adopt a heart-healthy lifestyle. Rather, it indicates the presence of a disease that is already advanced and the evident failure of whatever medical treatment you were receiving.

Health Smart Tips
It is important not to see angina as the first warning to begin making heart-healthy choices. Rather, it uually represents the failure of medical therapy to prevent and detect disease that is now already quite advanced.

In contrast to unstable angina, which is worse, stable angina is a chronic condition; unstable angina is an acute condition that is closer to a full-blown heart attack. Stable angina is usually brought on by the physical stress of exercise (fast walking, climbing stairs, mowing lawn, sex) or by emotional stress (anger, excitement, fright), and stops with rest. Pain occurs when the heart needs more oxygen than your clogged coronary arteries can supply. This temporary imbalance between supply and demand, which can be seen on an electrocardiogram (ECG or EKG), is called **ischemia** (pronounced *is-KEEM-yuh*). Angina is your body alerting you that ischemia is occurring.

If your coronary artery disease worsens, then as time goes by your angina will occur with less and less physical exertion because your heart's ability to receive oxygen through your narrowed coronary arteries is decreasing.

What are the signs of stable angina? Most people describe the discomfort as a feeling of pressure, tightness, or heaviness in the center or left side of their chest area. Some describe it as a "crushing of the chest," "as if an elephant stepped on my chest," or "a truck sitting on my chest." The discomfort often radiates into the left arm, jaw, or upper back. Occasionally, and particularly in women, the discomfort is felt only in one of these other areas, without any discomfort in the chest. Chest discomfort is usually accompanied by shortness of breath or sweating and is typically brought on by moderate-to-severe physical activity.

What should you do? Resting relieves the pain by decreasing the heart's oxygen demand; taking **nitroglycerine** also relieves the pain, by dilating the coronary arteries and thereby increasing oxygen supply (see Chapter VIII, Section 3).

Note, however, that although chest pain has become one of the most common reasons for emergency room visits among middle-aged men and women in the US, *not all chest pain is angina.* Diseases of the lung, stomach, esophagus, and chest wall muscle can all cause chest pain. For example, a "pins and needles" type of chest pain is usually not due to heart disease. Cardiologists use the presence or absence of risk factors to differentiate cardiac chest pain from non-cardiac. It is, nevertheless, better to be over-cautious than under-cautious, and take all chest pain seriously.

From the earlier discussion of the stages of atherosclerosis, it should be clear that, although angina may be your first clue that you have heart disease, developing angina actually signifies a state of atherosclerosis that is already advanced, because the kind of significant artery narrowing that causes chest pain does not typically occur until decades of heart disease. Chest pain that is caused by CAD should, therefore, be considered a very loud—and belated—cry for help from your coronary arteries.

d. Unstable angina (Acute Coronary Syndrome)

Like stable angina, unstable anginal pain is caused by partially blocked coronary arteries, but it is more severe and occurs at random and without warning, often when you are merely resting. It lasts longer than stable angina, is less responsive to medication, and happens more often. Unstable angina usually advances to a heart attack unless the person receives appropriate treatment. Unlike in a full-blown heart attack, however, blood tests after unstable angina typically show no evidence of actual heart muscle damage. Occasionally, a coronary spasm, in which the arterial walls temporarily contract, can lead to unstable angina. This is particularly common at rest but it can also be brought on by exposure to cold weather.

Unstable angina is one *type* of Acute Coronary Syndrome (or ACS, for short). The other is heart attack. In fact, the term "unstable angina" is rapidly disappearing in favor of ACS. The diagnosis of ACS, and which type you have, is decided only after several days of monitoring, blood tests, and ECGs. Because a heart attack often passes through several different phases in a 24- to 48-hour period, it can take two to three days of looking at your ECG wave tracings to be able to tell what kind of ACS you may be having.

e. Heart attack (myocardial infarction)

If unstable angina is more serious than stable angina, heart attack is worse still. The medical term for a heart attack is myocardial infarction, or MI. An MI occurs (usually in the left ventricle) when one of the coronary arteries that supply the heart muscle with blood and oxygen becomes completely blocked with a blood clot, usually one that formed after the rupture of a soft, fatty plaque. In much the way that brain damage often occurs, this prolonged deprivation of oxygen causes permanent, irreversible damage to the heart muscle, resulting in scar tissue and compromising the heart's ability to contract. By contrast, stable angina (unlike heart attack) is caused not by a blood clot following plaque rupture but by the gradual narrowing of the coronary artery as a result of increasing plaque buildup.

Unlike stable angina, and even more than unstable angina, the pain of a heart attack usually lasts more than 15 minutes and does not go away with rest. Immediate treatment—for example, when the attack occurs at a hospital—can often stop it from continuing to develop, thereby minimizing heart muscle damage in patients in the middle of an acute heart attack. Immediate treatment usually involves emergency angioplasty and/or clot-busting therapy, but heart muscle cannot be salvaged if the person *reaches the hospital too late* or the hospital does not have the right facilities.

Angina's Loud Cry
In September 2004, former US president Bill Clinton, then 58, underwent a four-hour quadruple coronary artery bypass surgery at New York—Presbyterian Hospital. Happily, the surgery was successful and uneventful. Recall, however, that six months earlier, Clinton had started experiencing chest pain typical of stable angina, but this was somehow ignored, as is often the case with most of us. Angina's loud cry needs to be headed with great urgency, because once you "hear" it, it is almost beginning to get too late.

f. Heart failure

The term "heart failure" can be misleading: it does not mean your heart has stopped. It means it can no longer pump effectively. It has varying degrees of severity. Heart failure may result from several things: a large heart attack, several minor and often unrecognized heart attacks, or other causes such as high blood pressure, obesity, diabetes, and viral infection. While a heart attack develops suddenly and dramatically, over a matter of a few minutes, heart failure develops gradually over years.

The most common symptoms of heart failure are shortness of breath, swollen feet and legs, a buildup of fluid in the lungs, and fatigue. Those with advanced heart failure are often bedridden and get short of breath even walking to the bathroom. The outlook for people with severe heart failure is no better than those with cancer: 50% die within five years. The incidence of heart failure in the US has risen dramatically. Currently, five million Americans have heart failure, and one million new cases are added every year. It is now the most common cause of hospitalization in elderly patients because many more people are surviving their heart attacks through medical intervention, but are not recovering fully. Fortunately, heart failure is often a treatable and thus reversible condition.

How does a heart attack lead to heart failure? Although former president Bill Clinton had scar tissue successfully removed from his lung and chest cavity in March 2005, removing scar tissue from the heart itself cannot be done. For the millions who suffer heart attacks every year, the cells in the oxygen-starved part of the heart muscle die and form tough scar tissue that can no longer work like healthy heart cells. This scar tissue gets incorporated into the heart itself. Many heart attack survivors, therefore, develop heart failure. Over time, the heart's walls grow thin and floppy, and the heart ceases to pump effectively.

What Exactly is an ECG, and What Do Those Spikes Mean?

An electrocardiogram, or EKG or ECG for short, is a recording of the tiny electric current produced by the heart. An ECG is the line that goes "flat" when someone dies on a TV program like ER. The test is done using electrodes attached to your chest and plugged into an ECG machine that translates your heart's electric impulses into line tracings on paper. By analyzing the pattern of spikes and dips (called waves) produced by your heart, a doctor can tell if there is any damage as a result of a heart attack, if your heart is beating abnormally (arrhythmia), or if there is any disease in the heart muscle. Cardiologists use the letters P-Q-R-S-T to describe the different parts of an ECG tracing. Each spike or dip has its own letter. So you might hear your cardiologist talking about the "ST segment," or "the QRS complex," or the P wave. Each has a meaning. For example, the P wave represents the electrical activity in your two atria. The Q, R, and S waves display the electrical activity in your ventricles. A heart attack will often produce an elevation of the **ST segment**.

g. Silent heart disease and silent ischemia

Not only can a heart attack be silent (meaning painless), but the heart disease that leads to it also usually progresses silently for several decades. Chest pain develops only when heart disease is far advanced. This means that waiting for chest pain before one begins to take a proactive approach to heart disease is as flawed a strategy as waiting for labor pain to discover that you are pregnant and need to begin prenatal care.

In addition, there is no clear correlation between severity of heart disease and its symptoms. You may have severe heart disease that is depriving your heart muscle of oxygen, yet experience few or no symptoms. This is called **silent ischemia,** which, as we saw in the paragraphs on angina, means the insufficient supply of blood to a bodily organ. Even though it may go away after exercise, ischemia indicates that some of the living muscle tissue of your heart is highly vulnerable to a heart attack in the not-too-distant future because one or more of your arteries has narrowed severely. The risk of having a heart attack when you have silent ischemia is as high as when you have symptoms of angina. In fact, silent ischemia accounts for more than half of all coronary angioplasties and bypass surgeries done in the US.

How do you know if you have silent ischemia? Silent ischemia can be detected from the way your ECG (or EKG) readout looks during an exercise treadmill stress test, commonly done in the offices of most cardiologists and many physicians in the US. It can also be detected by your wearing a 24-hour heart ECG monitor called a Holter monitor, which looks like a large Walkman. These diagnostic techniques are discussed more extensively in Section 3 of Chapter VII, but let's look briefly at what an ECG, or electrocardiogram, is.

Electrocardiograms (ECGs)

The death of heart muscle cells caused by a heart attack or by ischemia releases high levels of certain enzymes and proteins, such as troponin, which can be detected by testing the person's blood. The greater the damage, the higher the troponin levels. Depending on the shape of your **ECG tracings**, cardiologists classify heart attacks as:

- Heart attacks with ST-segment elevation, or
- Heart attacks without ST-segment elevation

The first results in much greater damage to the heart. (Cardiologists once distinguished the two kinds as Q-wave heart attacks and non-Q-wave.) All these special words—Q-wave, ST-segment—refer to particular telltale changes that show up on your ECG tracing if you have a heart attack. Typically, elderly people have a non-ST-segment elevation (mild) heart attack, often followed by an ST-segment elevation (major) heart attack within a few weeks or months. By contrast, younger and middle-aged people typically have ST-segment elevation (major) heart attacks when they do have an attack.

MORE ON HEART ATTACKS

The warning signs of a heart attack

BECAUSE WE LIKE TO LOOK on the bright side, we often play down the warning signs of an impending heart attack. Yet each year 1.1 million Americans suffer a heart attack; one-third do not survive. What are the signs of a heart attack? It is not always easy to know if you are having one. Typically, however, as with angina, you may experience heavy pressure or pain in the chest, with the discomfort possibly radiating down your left arm or up toward your jaw. Sometimes the discomfort may be confined to these regions only without acompanying chest pain. Unlike angina, the symptoms tend to be more severe, last longer, and resist improvement even with rest. You may experience nausea, vomiting, shortness of breath, weakness, dizziness, fainting, or profuse sweating. Victims often get a sense of impending doom.

Ignorance Is Not Always Bliss
One in four heart attack victims, it is estimated, do not realize they have had an attack until later, when they have an electrocardiogram for unrelated reasons and discover it. Despite the lack of pain, the damage produced by a silent heart attack is still very real, and can predispose you to further heart attacks.

Monday mornings and heart attack
Heart attacks are more likely between 6:00 a.m. and 10:00 a.m., when your blood pressure is the highest, and more common on Mondays, possibly because of the stress of returning to work.

Never dismiss heart attack symptoms as "probably just some indigestion or heartburn." It is far better to raise a false alarm than to succumb to a real one. If you suspect that you or someone near you is having a heart attack, take immediate action. Chew or crush and swallow a regular 325mg dose of aspirin and call 911 and your doctor. Even though early arrival to the emergency room markedly increases your chances of survival, you are nevertheless strongly advised *not to drive yourself* to the hospital, nor allow anyone other than a trained medic team to drive you to the hospital. A cardiac arrest in the car may be more than the unprepared driver can handle, and could reduce his as well as your chances of survival.

Another factor that makes the detection of heart attacks tricky especially among Indians is that many Indian heart attack victims have **atypical symptoms** that are hard to recognize and thus can lead to critical lost time in obtaining treatment. If mortality rates among Indians are to fall, emergency staff and physicians must more easily recognize the atypical symptoms Indians often have.

The severity of a heart attack

Because the major coronary arteries supply so much of the heart muscle, a blockage of one or more of these arteries can wreak havoc. It is, therefore, critical to do everything you can to keep your coronary arteries healthy and in full flow. Nevertheless, when a critical artery is blocked, other arteries can often pick up the slack and do double-duty, preventing serious consequences, at least for a while. More muscle is damaged when these collateral arteries, the ones that could have provided alternate blood routes, are also diseased and blocked, as often occurs in patients, who are having a second or a third heart attack. Put simply, when the "reserve team" is also sick, your chances of survival are lessened and complications tend to be more numerous.

Surviving a heart attack, therefore, depends not only on how diseased the blocked artery is, but also how many arteries in total are blocked, and the severity of the blockages. Usually your prognosis (the medical term for your chances of getting better) is good when only one coronary artery is involved, bad with two, and worst when all three major coronary arteries are severely narrowed.

Silent heart attack

Although severe chest pain is the hallmark of a heart attack, an attack can also occur with little or no chest pain. As stated earlier, in 20-30% of all heart attacks, there is no serious chest pain. These patients may often mistake their mild discomfort for an upset stomach, heartburn, or indigestion and take a couple of antacid tablets. Others who have a high threshold for pain may not realize that their pain is particularly serious. It is estimated that as many as one in four heart attack victims did not know they have had a heart attack until they go in for an ECG for unrelated reasons. Almost half of diabetic patients, and many women, do not get typical chest pains while having a heart attack. Some may have atypical symptoms such as shortness of breath, abnormal heart beat, nausea, extreme fatigue, or profuse sweating. Many diabetics have nerve damage that reduces their sense of pain in the chest and heart. A patient's long-term outlook after a silent heart attack is no different than that of someone who has had typical chest pain.

> **Some Warning Signs of a Stroke**
> - Sudden numbness or weakness felt in the face, arm, or leg, especially on one side of the body
> - Sudden confusion, trouble speaking, or understanding speech
> - Sudden trouble seeing in one or both eyes
> - Sudden trouble walking, dizziness, or loss of balance or coordination
> - Sudden severe headache with no obvious cause

STROKES VERSUS HEART ATTACKS

IT HAS BEEN SAID that stroke and heart disease are "first cousins with common grandparents." Those common grandparents are their risk factors. Nevertheless, risk factors affect the two slightly differently. In contrast to a heart attack, uncontrolled high blood pressure is by far the strongest predictor of stroke. For heart attack, it is cholesterol and plaque. Yet the similarities are also distinct: In a heart attack, clogged coronary arteries choke off the supply of oxygen and blood to the heart muscle, and the affected heart muscle dies. In a stroke, the same process occurs in the brain. In fact, many cardiologists have begun to refer to strokes as *brain attacks* because of the similarity in terms of oxygen deprivation.

The *symptoms* of a stroke, however, are quite different. Most heart attacks are accompanied by severe crushing chest pain (although a minority of them are painless). In contrast, the majority of strokes cause no pain. Some strokes can be quite small. Multiple small strokes can lead to dementia, which expresses itself as forgetfulness and difficulty engaging in basic thinking.

The risk of having a stroke doubles during each decade of life after age 55, and two-thirds of all strokes occur in people over age 65. A stroke is often preceded by a Transient Ischemic Attack (TIA) or a **mini-stroke.** The main difference between a mini-stroke and a stroke is that the symptoms of a mini-stroke disappear within a few minutes to a few hours, whereas in a stroke they persist and are often accompanied by disability. Three out of 100 mini-strokes will lead to a major stroke within 30 days, and seven out of 100 mini-strokes will lead to a stroke within a year.

> **Heart Attack and Stroke**
> Many people believe heart attacks are less disabling than strokes, but one often leads to the other. About 40% of people who survive a heart attack eventually develop a stroke, resulting in paralysis and disability; and about 80% of people who get a stroke do not die from it instead they die from a heart attack later on. The links between the two diseases underscore their common foundation: both heart attacks and strokes are cardiovascular diseases, although strokes are triggered more by high blood pressure, and heart attacks are triggered more by cholesterol-based atherosclerosis. In both cases, a healthy diet, weight control, and daily physical activity greatly reduce the probability.

What exactly causes a stroke? There are two major causes, and in each case, part of your brain tissue dies:

i. Ischemic strokes (80% of all strokes) are caused by inadequate blood supply to the brain, and are more common among whites

ii. Hemorrhagic strokes (20% of all strokes) are caused by an artery in the brain bursting and leaking blood uncontrollably. They are more common among blacks and Asians, and more lethal than ischemic strokes

Ischemic strokes occur when a blood clot blocks an artery and chokes off blood supply, as in a heart attack. Hemorrhagic strokes occur when an artery supplying the brain ruptures, like a water pipe, usually because of excessively high blood pressure inside it. Blood then leaks uncontrollably into the brain tissue, going where it should not. One might loosely say that, hemorrhagic strokes are caused by *too much* blood, while ischemic strokes are caused by *not enough* blood and oxygen getting to the brain. Of note, a hemorrhagic stroke is believed to have claimed the life of the Franklin Delano Roosevelt, the 32nd president of the United States. Although strokes more often lead to disability than death, for many patients, living with a severe stroke is worse than death.

In 1990 half a million people in India died from stroke, a number projected to more than double by 2020. Alarmingly, approximately 12% of these strokes occurred in people younger than 40. Yet a 2005 hospital-based study of 942 subjects at Christian Medical College in India, a major medical center located in the Punjab region, found that 45% of them did not know the brain was the organ affected in a stroke, and 33% were unable to describe a single warning symptom of stroke.

THREE OTHER CARDIAC CONDITIONS

■ **Arrhythmia:** Arrhythmia is a disturbance in the electrical activity of the heart that creates abnormalities in heart rate and rhythm. During arrhythmia, the heart may beat too slowly, too rapidly, or both, meaning irregularly. Some arrhythmias like ventricular fibrillation and tachycardia can be life-threatening. Some experience arrhythmia as a skipping or fluttering sensation in the chest; others complain of "racing" of the heart. It can cause chest pain, shortness of breath, light-headedness, or no symptoms. Let's look at one particular type of arrhythmia.

■ **Atrial fibrillation:** The most common arrhythmia is atrial fibrillation, a condition that afflicts more than six million mainly elderly Americans. In atrial fibrillation, the upper chambers of the heart (the atria, singular: atrium) fail to contract effectively or in coordination with each other. They are out of sync with each other. The condition is usually treated with medications. Left untreated, this arrhythmia can lead to heart failure or stroke. Patients with atrial fibrillation are five times more likely to get a stroke. The prevalence of atrial fibrillation doubles every 10 years starting at age 65. That means, for example, that 75-year-olds are twice as likely to have atrial fibrillation as 65-year-olds. Atrial fibrillation often has no symptoms, but other people experience very high heart rates. They may express it in phrases like "My heart was beating out of my chest."

A typical adult's resting heart rate falls somewhere between 50 and 75. In very challenging atrial fibrillation patients whose heart rates exceed 200 beats a minute and who are not responding to medication, surgery may be performed. In a novel procedure, surgeons cut a shallow maze-like pattern into the surface of the heart's upper chambers, the atria, forcing the heart muscle to develop scar tissue. Since scar tissue does not carry electrical impulses, this prevents the erratic electrical signaling that produces atrial fibrillation. A recent approach that is non-invasive yet yields similar results uses high-intensity ultrasound to create the same kind of non-electrical scar tissue.

> **Automatic External Defibrillators**
> The benefit of placing automatic external defibrillators (AEDs) in stressful public places such as airports and offices, where cardiac arrests are frequent, has been documented. Easy to use, they have saved lives even when used by persons with no prior experience. AEDs are now FDA-approved for home use, and you can buy one, such as the Philips HeartStart Home Defibrillator, for about $1,500. However, because it is less likely that a cardiac arrest will be witnessed at home, you should consider whether that money may be better spent on other preventive and therapeutic strategies.

■ **Cardiomyopathy:** So far, we have looked primarily at coronary heart disease—which refers to conditions caused mainly by plaque in coronary arteries blocking the flow of blood to the heart. Cardiomyopathy, by contrast, refers to the severe weakening of the heart muscle itself, not the coronary vessels, so that the heart can no longer pump strongly. The most common type is dilated cardiomyopathy

(DCM), typically caused by end-stage heart disease that enlarges the heart, making it unable to pump well. Sudden death is common among cardiomyopathy patients, and some of them benefit from an implanted cardioverter defibrillator (see Chapter VIII, Section 3). Unlike most coronary heart disease, cardiomyopathy is inoperable. Unlike other muscles in the body, heart muscle tends not to heal itself. Cardiomyopathy, therefore, almost always leads to heart failure.

COMMONLY USED TERMS IN HEART DISEASE

• **Cardiac catheterization:** A catheter is a very thin, long, flexible tube. In a cardiac catheterization, a catheter is inserted into a blood vessel and slowly advanced, like a feeding tube, toward the heart from the surface of the patient's skin. It is done for both diagnostic and treatment purposes. General anesthesia is not needed, but the physician typically numbs the area before inserting the catheter and gives the patient a mild sedative. The patient does not ordinarily feel the movement of the catheter within his or her blood vessels.

• **Coronary angiogram:** A coronary angiogram is essentially an x-ray of a coronary artery to check for any plaque that may have narrowed or blocked the vessel. Angiograms have been the gold standard for the diagnosis of heart disease for decades. An easily detectable dye is injected into the artery through a catheter, and the physician uses x-ray equipment to follow the dye as it flows through the artery.

• **Coronary angioplasty:** Often, a coronary angioplasty (or simply, balloon angioplasty) is done on a patient who has substantial blockage of his or her coronary arteries but whose heart disease is not so severe as to require full-scale bypass surgery. A special catheter with a small balloon at the tip is used to open up the diseased artery without entailing actual surgery. The catheter is pushed into the artery and the balloon is then inflated. This stretches the artery and flattens and often ruptures the plaque that was preventing the blood from flowing.

• **Coronary atherectomy:** Atherectomy is a procedure in which a catheter that has a special grinding device at one end is used to clear away plaque in a blocked artery, much like a chain might be used to unclog a blocked kitchen drain. It is done to improve blood supply to the heart without surgery.

• **Coronary stent**: A stent (**see Color Plate 1.8**, *Methods of Opening Up and Re-establishing Blood Flow in coronary arteries following a Heart Attack, page xviii*) is a small tubular device that is permanently placed in an artery to keep it propped open, often following an angioplasty. The major advantage of a stent over just simple balloon angioplasty is that a stent can reduce the rate of restenosis (re-blockage of arteries caused by the buildup of new tissue) by up to 50%. Drug-eluting (meaning drug-releasing) stents are a new advance that have now reduced the restenosis rate by more than 90% (see Chapter VII, Section 6).

• **Coronary artery bypass surgery:** Coronary artery bypass graft surgery, often rather irreverently referred to as CABG (pronounced "cabbage"), is a life-saving procedure in many patients with severe heart disease such as left main coronary artery disease or triple-vessel disease (**Color Plate 1.9.** *page xviii*), *A Coronary Artery Bypass Operation*). It is called a bypass because, just as in road construction work when traffic has to be rerouted, the surgeon reroutes or "bypasses" blood flow *around* the clogged portion of the artery to restore supply to areas of heart muscle that were in danger of starving from lack of oxygen (see Chapter VII, Section 5).

• **Coronary event:** In principle, a coronary event (or cardiac event) can be any episode that declares the presence of complications from heart disease. In practice, the term is reserved for major episodes. This could be acute stable or unstable angina, or the onset of a clinical crisis such as a heart attack, or sudden cardiac death, or a medical intervention such as angioplasty, stenting, or bypass surgery. As discussed earlier, heart disease progresses silently for many decades before announcing itself in a major coronary event.

• **Coronary interventions:** A coronary intervention is any procedure performed on a severely narrowed coronary artery to improve blood supply. This includes Coronary Artery Bypass Grafting (CABG) surgery, coronary angioplasty and coronary stenting. **Color Plate 1.10.** *page xviii* shows the placement of a coronary stent in the left coronary artery, **Color Plate 1.11.** *page xviii* shows restenosis of the arteries through the metallic stent. Patients with diffuse disease, where there is plaque buildup on the entire artery are not suitable for coronary interventions (**Color Plate 1.12.** *page xviii*). These topics are discussed in detail in subsequent Chapters.

KEY · POINTS · IN · A · NUTSHELL

♥ Cardiovascular disease begins in childhood and progresses silently for many decades.

♥ Atherosclerosis (or plaque buildup) does not result in narrowing of the artery until very late in the disease process.

♥ Heart disease is not an unavoidable degenerative disease that is found in all elderly people; it is actively promoted by a combination of genetic factors and lifestyle choices.

♥ The various risk factors such as smoking and high cholesterol damage the artery lining in a process called endothelial dysfunction. This lays a foundation for future heart attacks or other cardiac complications.

♥ The mechanical view of plaque formation as a kind of "junk" that builds up layer after layer and clogs up an artery like a kitchen drain distorts the truth. The current view is that the composition of the plaque is more important than size of the plaque.

♥ Most heart attacks are caused not by an artery narrowing due to the buildup of hard, large plaques detectable on an angiogram, but by a blood clot that forms after the rupture of a soft, inflamed, lipid-rich plaque, often quite small.

♥ No correlation exists between the severity of heart disease and its symptoms. Very severe heart disease may have few or no readily identifiable symptoms.

♥ Heart disease gives advanced warning in the form of chest pain (angina) only one-third of the time. Most of the time, it manifests as a heart attack or sudden death without warning.

♥ Don't wait for the onset of chest pain to begin a heart-healthy lifestyle. Angina rather indicates that your heart disease is already far along, because arterial narrowing does not begin until atherosclerosis is advanced.

♥ Half of all sudden deaths occur in people with no known heart disease history, and two-thirds occur before the person reaches the hospital, even in major metropolitan centers.

1.2 ▶ Heart Disease among Indians Living Abroad

Some 20 million Indians live outside India, nearly 1.7 million of them in the US (census data from 2000). Disconcertingly, the heart disease rate among America's Indian immigrants is three to four times higher than that of the general population. Equally troubling, these high rates are observed even among health-oriented Indians, including vegetarians and physicians. Over the past half century, similarly high rates have been found among Indians in Canada, Fiji, Kenya, Malaysia, Mauritius, Qatar, Singapore, South Africa, Tanzania, Trinidad, and Uganda. This section summarizes the most recent data on the magnitude and seriousness of heart disease among Indians worldwide.

> **Did you know...**
> *According to the 2000 US Census, the average per capita income of Indians in the US is $60,093, compared to the US average of $38,885 and Indian average of $534.*

The most accurate way to do this is to compare mortality rates, hospitalization rates, incidence rates, and prevalence data. These are the most commonly used measures of the impact of heart disease on a population. To better appreciate the material below, it is important that you first grasp what terms like prevalence and incidence mean. For a fuller review, read *Appendix A: Measuring the Impact of Heart Disease*, at the end of this book. Meanwhile, here is a quick summary of the terms we will be employing:

- The **prevalence** of a disease is the proportion of a population who have that disease at any given time. It offers a "snapshot" of the total number of people who currently have that disease, regardless of when they first developed it.

- The **incidence rate** of a disease, in contrast to prevalence, is the number of *new* cases diagnosed each year or over a given period of time. Incidence is, therefore, a rate, while prevalence is a stock. If incidence is like the rate at which water is entering a bathtub from a faucet, prevalence is the total amount of water currently in the bathtub. A **high-incidence, low-prevalence disease** would be a seasonal disease such as the flu. Many new cases emerge each year particularly in winter

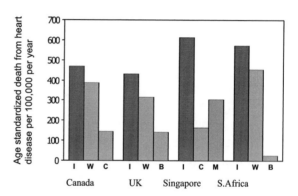

Figure 1.13.. **Age-standardized death rates from heart disease among Indian men per 100,000 per year compared to other ethnic groups in Canada, UK, Singapore and South Africa.** Note that in each of these four countries, Indians have the highest mortality rates. (I= Indians, B=blacks, W=whites, C=Chinese, M= Malays) Source. Enas, EA. Ref 1.16. *Reproduced with permission © British Journal of Diabetes & Vascular Disease.*

(giving it a high incidence), but it has a low prevalence (total number) because people recover from it quickly. On average, not many people have the flu at any point. In contrast, a **low-incidence, high-prevalence disease** might be heart disease or diabetes. Such chronic, life-long illnesses tend to have a low annual incidence, but over time they acquire high prevalence.

> Although Indians are the highest socioeconomic group in the US, and one of the best educated, the Kaiser Study found that the hospitalization rate for heart disease among its Indian patients was **four times** that of its non-Indian patients.

- The **hospitalization** rate, or number of new admissions, is a rough surrogate for the incidence rate. Like airline flight manifests, it is relatively easy for hospitals to total up how many people they admitted in a year with a particular disease because they keep careful year-round records.

- The **mortality** rate, or **death** rate, of a disease is the estimated proportion of the population who have died from it over a period of time, for example, the past year.

Let's step back for a moment. The overall point to bear in mind here is that, no matter which measure one uses to assess heart disease rates worldwide, the evidence consistently shows that Indians have the highest or among the highest rates of heart disease—regardless of what region they live in, their socioeconomic background, their religion, or their gender. To put it bluntly: the Indian community, including those living abroad, is at very high risk of heart disease (Figure 1.13).

HEART DISEASE RATES: HIGH NO MATTER HOW YOU SLICE IT

Indians in the United States

Upon initial reflection, one would not expect Indians in the US to be more susceptible to heart disease than any other group. For one thing, many are vegetarians. For another, a large percentage of them are highly educated professionals, and heart disease is very much a disease that reflects lifestyle choices. Highly educated groups—physicians, for example—tend to take aggressive steps to modify their lifestyle and bring their heart disease rates down. Indians have a higher socioeconomic status than any other ethnic group in the US, including whites. Although they comprise only 0.3% of the US population, Indians make up 5% of its physician population and 10% of cardiologists. As of 2000, Indians in the US included 50,000 engineers, 45,000 Ph Ds, 40,000 physicians and 10,000 medical students and medical residents. Their level of professional attainment makes it all the more surprising that they would have such high levels of heart disease.

*The heart disease rate in the Physicians Health Study was **one-third** that of the general US population. In the CADI Study, it was **four times** that of the US population.*

The reasons for this are considered at length in Chapter IV, particularly Section 1, *Cracking the Indian Paradox*. Our present concern here is to document the full picture with evidence that goes beyond the merely anecdotal.

The Kaiser Study Although national data on heart disease incidence in Indians are unavailable in the US, one major health maintenance organization (HMO), Kaiser Permanente, has conducted a comprehensive and revealing study using its very extensive patient population base. A key finding of the Kaiser Study was that the hospitalization rate for heart disease among Indian patients was *four times* higher than the rest of its patient population, especially for coronary angioplasty and bypass surgery (Figure 1.14) This finding is all the more alarming because Kaiser Permanente is a conservative HMO that subjects only the most deserving cases to such expensive procedures. Over-diagnosis and over-treatment tend to be rare in managed care. This means that the Indians, who were hospitalized for heart procedures, truly urgently needed them. To put it mildly, that their hospitalization rate is four times higher is a cause for concern .

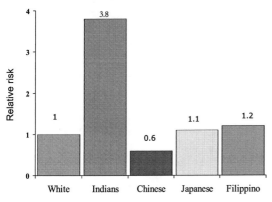

Figure 1.14. Relative rates of hospitalization for heart disease among Kaiser Permanente patients in California. Note that Indians are hospitalized for heart disease nearly four times more often than whites, and more than six times more often than Chinese. Other Asian Americans have rates similar to whites. Source: Klatsky, AL. Ref. 1.29.

Although the CADI study participants were mostly physicians, the study was more representative than it sounds because they came from different parts of India and settled in different parts of the US. Also, a third of them were not physicians at all but their spouses. The group was thus demographically representative of Indian physicians in the US, and perhaps of Indian professional families, if not quite of the overall Indian population.

The Coronary Artery Disease in Indians (CADI) Study

The Coronary Artery Disease in Indians Study—or CADI Study, for short—was the first systematic investigation of heart disease among people of Indian origin.

Commissioned by the American Association of Physicians of Indian Origin (AAPI) and conducted between 1990 and 1993, I was its principal investigator. Right off the bat, one distinctive feature of it was that virtually every other previous study had included Indians from various backgrounds. Statistical diversity is normally a good thing, but in these studies this often meant an *overrepresentation* of participants from lower socioeconomic backgrounds and hence a potential skewing of the heart disease data.

*For the same degree of atherosclerosis, Indian Canadians have **twice** the heart disease rate of whites, while Chinese Canadians have **half** the rate.*

The CADI Study, for the first time, showed that the high risk of heart disease among Indians *applied just as much* to highly educated physicians, including cardiologists, who were knowledgeable about the traditional risk factors for heart disease. That was the true surprise, and the startling finding, of the study. It discovered that, despite an extremely low prevalence of standard risk factors among its 1,700 participants, about 10% of these Indian doctors had documented heart disease.

In the 1970s and early 80s, deaths from heart disease decreased in the UK for other ethnic groups but increased for Indians, especially Indian women. In a country such as the UK with such high rates of heart disease among the general population, studies show that Indians there have even higher rates.

The CADI Study was also particularly significant because it was a methodologically rigorous project that reached its conclusions cautiously and conservatively. Indeed, it may actually have *underestimated* rather than overestimating heart disease prevalence among Indians.

One particularly disturbing figure emerged when the CADI data were compared to data from the landmark Framingham Offspring Study (see Appendix B). The age-adjusted prevalence of heart disease for men in the 30-69 age group in the Framingham Study was **25** per 1000. It was **100** in the CADI Study. In other words, Indian physicians were *four times* more likely to develop heart disease than whites (see Figure 1.14). Strikingly, this rate was identical to the four-fold higher rate of hospitalization observed among Indians in California in the Kaiser Permanente study, mentioned above (see Figure 1.13).

Other findings: Little difference in heart disease rates was found among the approximately one-third of participants who were the spouses of physicians (primarily husbands of women doctors). They, too, had high rates. Second, the rates did not vary significantly between vegetarians and non-vegetarians, nor between people from different Indian states (although a trend toward a higher rate was observed among physicians originally from Kerala). Finally, unlike other studies, the CADI Study did not find high rates of heart disease among Indian women. This, however, was attributed to the young age of the women participants as well as their small number, which made the sample size more vulnerable to statistical error.

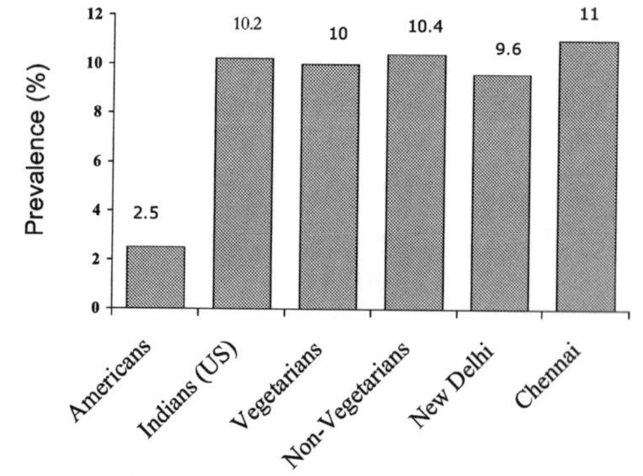

The main point, however, should not be lost: The CADI study focused on physicians—cardiologists, internists, family practitioners—who were aware of the risk factors of heart disease and were, on the whole, doing the best they could to live a healthy lifestyle in terms of diet, exercise, weight management, and so on. With the exception of diabetes, they had an unusually low prevalence of standard risk factors. (These factors are discussed in Chapter II)

Differences in heart disease rates frequently disappear when studies are adjusted for socioeconomic sta-

Figure 1.15. Prevalence of heart disease among non-Indian Americans compared to Indians in the US in the CADI Study (second column), were four times as likely to develop heart disease as non-Indian Americans, followed in the Framingham Offspring Study (first column). In comparison to Column 1, the great similarity of heart disease prevalence found in Columns 3 and 4 (vegetarians and non-vegetarians in the CADI Study, respectively) and in Columns 5 and 6 (Indians living in New Delhi and in Chennai, in two different regions of India) strongly suggests that Indians have a genetic predisposition toward heart disease that transcends both geographical region and nutritional choices. Source: Enas, EA. Ref. 1.16. *Reproduced with permission © British Journal of Diabetes & Vascular Disease.*

tus, so the results of the CADI Study were also compared with the Physicians Health Study. This was another long-term study involving more than 22,000 healthy male American physicians who, like the CADI doctors, were very well-informed about the dangers of heart disease and the benefits of prevention. The heart attack rate in the Physicians Health Study was *one-third* that of the overall US population—what one would expect for such a strongly health-oriented group. In the CADI Study, by contrast, the heart attack rate was *four times* that of the overall US population.

*In one study, heart disease rates in South African Indians were nearly **30 times** higher than among South African blacks.*

Whichever way one looks at it, the high rates of heart disease among Indian physicians contrasts sharply not only with the very low rates found in the Physicians Health Study but with the rates among Americans in general. The CADI Study raised the larger question: Why? Because of this, it became a stimulus for further investigative study in the US, in India, and in other countries.

Indians in Canada

The rates of cardiovascular diseases and cancer vary markedly among various ethnic groups in Canada. white Canadians have high death rates from both cancer and heart disease, whereas Canadians of Indian descent have high death rates from heart disease and lower death rates from cancer (see Figure 1.13. Chinese Canadians, by contrast, have low death rates from heart disease but high death rates from cancer. The SHARE Study (see Appendix B), on the other hand, showed that Indians had the highest prevalence of heart disease (11%), similar to that found in the CADI Study. The prevalence was double that of whites (5%) and five times higher than for Chinese (2%).

Heart disease rates have fallen in Canada over the last two decades, but the decline has been slowest among Indians. For the same degree of atherosclerosis (plaque buildup), Indian Canadians have double the heart disease rate of whites, while Chinese Canadians have half the rate of whites. These wide variations in heart disease rates in a study controlled for atherosclerosis levels raise the possibility that, at least for heart disease, different risk factors and protective factors exist among Canadians from different ethnic groups, and that these factors promote or counter the effects of atherosclerosis to varying degrees.

Indians in the United Kingdom

Death rates from heart disease in the UK are among the highest in the world, next only to the countries of the former Soviet Union. This is consistent with the high rates of standard heart disease risk factors found there, and the relatively modest level of intervention of these risk factors. Yet, even in a country with such high heart disease rates among the general population, studies show that Indians living in the UK have even higher rates. For example, they have substantially higher heart disease mortality rates than whites, while blacks and Chinese have substantially lower rates than whites (Figuer 1.13). In one study, the death rate from

How the CADI Study was Conducted: A Rigorous Methodology

About 8% of the participants had at some point in their lives had a heart attack or angina (chest pain due to heart disease). Another set of the participants had had coronary angioplasty, stent, or bypass surgery. By adding up the two categories, the study estimated that the prevalence of heart disease among Indians-the percentage of Indians alive with heart disease-was 10%.

This figure is fairly conservative because of the methodological rigor of the study and its selection criteria. First, only individuals with "hard" evidence of heart disease-such as a heart attack, or severe blockages detectable on a coronary angiogram-were included. People, who had simply had some chest pain but without a confirming abnormal coronary angiogram, were not included. More than 90% of the participants had had their heart disease documented by a coronary angiogram. For the few whose diagnosis of heart disease had not been confirmed by an angiogram, an electrocardiogram had been used. However, because an electrocardiogram was not done for all participants, there could have been an additional number of participants who had silent heart disease which was not detected.

Finally, only physicians healthy enough to travel to the AAPI conventions were included. In short, the Study was accurate, conservative, and methodologically rigorous. Given that they were virtually all physicians, the prevalence of heart disease among Indians is probably even higher than the Study found.

heart disease among Indians was 55% higher than the national average. The differences in heart disease rates were even higher at younger ages—230% higher in Indians younger than 40, compared to whites of the same age, and 313% higher in Indians younger than 30 compared to whites of the same age. It was similarly found that Indians developed their first heart attack at a much younger age, resulting in earlier death. Even Indian doctors die *15 years earlier* than their white colleagues in the UK.

Using data from 1970 to 1972 and 1979 to 1983, the heart disease mortality rate decreased in both men and women in the UK—for example, it decreased by a total of 8% for Western European, American, and Caribbean men during those years—but it increased 6% among Indian men and, even more strikingly, 13% among Indian women. In another study, Indians were twice as likely to be admitted to hospital with a heart attack, and twice as likely to die over the subsequent six months, than white patients. On a brighter note, Indians have the lowest rates of cancer in the United Kingdom. Their high risk of heart disease, however, parallels that of Indians elsewhere.

On the Indian subcontinent itself, important differences exist among Bangladeshis, Pakistanis, Sri Lankans, and national Indians in cardiac mortality and in the prevalence of cardiac risk factors. For example, in one study, deaths from heart disease were 47% higher among Bangladeshis, 42% higher among Pakistanis, and 37% higher among Indians than whites. It is noted that the Indians in the study had slightly higher overall socio-economic status than the Pakistanis and Bangladeshis, which is an important predictor of heart disease (see Chapter III, Section 1), although the direction of its influence depends partly on the stage of development.

These mortality rate differences track traditional risk factor differences. For example, Bangladeshis, who had the highest mortality rates, also tended to have the highest risk factors, particularly men: They had high rates of smoking (57%), the highest concentrations of triglycerides (180 mg/dL), high blood glucose levels (119 mg/dL), and the lowest levels of HDL or good cholesterol (38 mg/dL). They also had the highest rates of diabetes (27%), but the lowest blood pressure levels. Shortness of height is associated with a higher risk of heart attack (see Chapter III, Section 1), and Bangladeshis were the shortest: men were on average 5 feet 4.5 inches tall, versus 5 feet 7 inches for Indians and 5 feet 8.5 inches for whites. These data underscore the fact that the importance of the standard risk factors cannot be ignored (see Chapter IV, Section 1).

Indians in Singapore and Malaysia

Indians make up 7% of Singapore's population. Of these, 80% originate from South India and Sri Lanka. The first report of high levels of heart disease among Singaporean Indians was published in 1959. Based on nearly 10,000 post-mortem studies, the report showed that Indian Singaporeans had seven times the heart disease rate of Chinese Singaporeans. Subsequent studies over the past four decades have shown that Indians are three to four times more likely to have heart attacks than Chinese Singaporeans. This 300-400% difference in heart disease rates between Chinese and Indian Singaporeans even as far back as four decades ago is the first indication that Indians may be genetically predisposed toward heart disease.

There is, however, an even more telling statistic. Over the past 25 years, harmful changes in lifestyle and environment—including higher rates of smoking, greater obesity, more fattening diets, and a more sedentary lifestyle—have doubled the death rates from heart attacks in Singapore. (Little of this increase in mortality rates can be attributed to genetic changes, which take place over a much longer time frame.) What is significant is that the 300% difference in heart disease rates between Chinese and Indian Singaporeans has not narrowed over this 25-year period. The mortality rates have doubled for *both* Indians and Chinese. One would have expected to see somewhat of a convergence. After all, it is highly unlikely that Indians gained twice the weight as Chinese, smoked twice as many more cigarettes, and ate twice as much more fat.

Yet the data show that the increase in risk factor levels from adverse changes in lifestyle has been similar in Chinese and Indians. These data suggest fairly convincingly that harmful changes in lifestyle related to **affluence, urbanization, and sedentary living** have had a greater net adverse effect on Indians than on Chinese. In all likelihood, the adverse lifestyle changes that have taken place in Singapore have magnified the harmful effects of preexisting genetically inherited risk factors. The most recent data (from 2002) indicate that the incidence of heart attacks, and death rate from heart attacks, is more than three times higher among Indian men than Chinese, and twice as high among Indian women. Similar trends have been observed in Malaysia. In a study of patients who had a heart attack before 40, 56% were Indians, even though Indians comprise only 10% of the Malaysian population.

Indians in Fiji and Mauritius

Indians in Fiji have high rates of diabetes and heart disease and very high mortality rates from these two conditions. Indians with diabetes also have a higher risk of heart disease than the Melanesians, the Fiji natives. For example, compared to people without diabetes, the relative risk of developing heart disease among diabetics is four times higher in Indians compared to only two times higher in Melanesians.

The 1.2 million people who live on the island of Mauritius, in the Indian Ocean, are approximately 70% Indians, 28% Creole, and 2% Chinese. Death rates from heart disease and stroke for the overall population are among the highest recorded in the world (18% in men and 33% in women). However, among them, the Chinese have the lowest and the Indians have the highest rates of heart disease. There has been a substantial rise in obesity in Mauritius. This could further increase the rates of diabetes and heart disease. (The way diabetes and heart disease interrelate is discussed in Chapter II, Section 7.)

Indians in the Middle East

In the Middle East, once again, one finds that heart disease is more common among Indians and occurs at a much lower age than in the native Arab population. In a study of more than 2,500 patients with documented heart attacks, 71% of all patients 40 years old or younger were Indians, even though Indians make up only 5% of the general population. Most Arabs who had heart attacks were significantly older.

Indians in South Africa and Uganda

In the 1970s, South Africans had high rates of heart disease, with whites having the highest rates in the world. Indians, however, have now surpassed this, with particularly high rates at younger ages. Although the overall rates have been declining in South Africa, the reduction has been much slower among Indians. Heart disease among Indians in South Africa is both premature and severe. A recent study in South Africa found three-vessel disease (significant narrowing of all three of the big coronary arteries) in 52% of the patients who had a heart attack before age 45. This high prevalence of multi-vessel disease in young Indians is consistent with studies conducted on Indians in other parts of the world (see section 4).

Risk factors: One study found a substantial difference in fat intake between Indians and blacks. Fat made up 40% of the daily calorie intake of Indians, compared to just 15% for blacks. Furthermore, the major source of dietary fat for blacks was peanuts, in contrast to cottonseed oil and *ghee* (clarified butter) for Indians. Ghee, although tasty, is one of the most cholesterol-laden foods in the world, three times worse than regular butter. (See Chapter V, Section 4, which discusses good and bad oils.) The available data suggest that South African blacks may be protected against heart disease through diet and other factors. For example, heart disease rates were nearly 30 times lower in South African blacks than Indians. In Uganda, heart disease was determined as the major cause of death (43%) among Indians even as early as 1959.

Indians in the Caribbean

The relative risk of hospital admissions for heart attack as compared with white men was 50% in Caribbean men but 200% for Indians. A major survey in Trinidad, the St. James Survey (see appendix B) followed nearly 2,000 adults who had been free of heart disease for 10 years for the development of new heart disease. The relative risk of having a first major coronary event (heart attack, death etc) among Indians was twice that of whites and seven times higher than for people of other ethnic origins, after adjusting for differences in age.

The data from the UK, Trinidad, Uganda, and South Africa suggests very low rates of heart disease in blacks despite a high prevalence of hypertension and stroke. In most of the countries of the Caribbean, heart disease rates among Indians are more than double those of blacks. Since the environment is the same, this suggests that the variation is attributable to either genetics or differences in lifestyle, activity level, body weight, and diet.

Indians and stroke

Conflicting reports have been published on stroke rates among Indians living abroad, with most countries—Canada, for example—reporting no higher rates. However, the stroke rates among Indians in Singapore are similar to those of the Chinese, who are known to have the highest rates of stroke. Data from the UK also show that stroke rates for Indians are very high and fall between the rates for whites and blacks. This is not surprising since heart disease and stroke share common risk factors.

KEY · POINTS · IN · A · NUTSHELL

- ♥ The rate of heart disease among Indians is two to four times higher than people of other ethnic origin.
- ♥ Evidence from multiple countries and regions of the world consistently shows that Indians have the highest or among the highest rates of heart disease, regardless of their religion, gender, or socioeconomic background.
- ♥ High rates of heart disease have been observed among Indians living in the US, Canada, Singapore, the UK, South Africa, Middle East, Trinidad, Mauritius, Fiji, Kenya, and many other countries.
- ♥ Since the environment in each of these countries is the same for Indians as for other populations who live there, the variation must be attributable either to genetics or to differences in lifestyle, activity level, body weight, and diet.
- ♥ Vegetarian and non-vegetarian Indians have similarly high rates of heart disease.
- ♥ Stroke rates have been reported to be high among Indians in the UK and Singapore, but not especially high in other countries.

1.3 ▶ An Epidemic on the Indian Subcontinent

In the preceding section, we saw that in numerous countries around the world, Indian immigrants have either the highest, or close to the highest, rates of heart disease of any ethnic group—regardless of their gender, religious practice, social class, or economic status. But what about Indians "at home"? This section examines heart disease on the Indian subcontinent itself, home to approximately 1.5 billion people—a billion in India, half a billion in Bangladesh, Pakistan, and Sri Lanka.

Heart disease has often been considered an "affluent person's disease"—an illness associated with easy living, a sedentary lifestyle, and a high-calorie diet rich in cakes, prime-cut meats, and other fattening foods. People in developing countries, who tend to live hardy, frugal lives, are thought to have a low susceptibility to the cardiovascular illnesses of the rich. Africans, for example, have little heart disease.

But not so with Indians. Researchers are discovering that heart disease rates on the Indian subcontinent have all but caught up with the high rates observed among Indians living abroad. For example, a major study found that the prevalence of heart disease in New Delhi and Chennai, both in India, was 10% and 11% respectively—slightly higher than the 10% rate among the Indian participants in the American-based CADI Study (*see the preceding section*). Over the past three decades, heart disease rates in the nation of India have **doubled** in rural areas and **tripled** in urban areas. In Bangladesh, Pakistan, and Sri Lanka, the rates are similar to India's, with urban

In the past three decades, heart disease rates have doubled in rural areas of India, and tripled in its urban areas.

By 2020, according to the WHO the number of Indian citizens dying each year from heart disease will exceed 2.4 million, more than twice the number in 1990. One of every four cardiac patients in the world will be Indian.

areas generally showing double the rates in rural areas. There is, in short, an epidemic of heart disease currently sweeping the Indian subcontinent.

Although national or regional data are generally unavailable on the incidence and mortality rates of diseases in India, there are telling indications from individual studies. For example, at Christian Medical College Hospital in Vellore, a major tertiary medical center, heart disease rates have steadily and dramatically increased over three decades—from 4% of all medical admissions in 1960, to about 33% in 1989. Studies from other parts of India also suggest an epidemic is underway. The World Health Organization estimates that, in 1990, 1.2 million Indians died from heart disease and predicts that this number will *more than double* by 2020, giving India the greatest cardiovascular disease burden of any nation by that year. In the same 30-year period, the death rate from heart disease will rise by just 15% in the US. By 2010, the WHO states, 100 million Indians will have heart disease. In fact, *more than 25%* of all cardiac patients in the world will be Indian.

By comparison, 13 million Americans, out of about 296 million, are currently estimated to have heart disease—a proportion only half that of the estimate among Indians. If the comparison looks even worse when age-adjusted: a much larger proportion of Indians who have heart disease are younger than 70. By contrast, many of the 13 million Americans with heart disease are well past retirement age, which is when one would expect more people to have heart disease.

Rural versus Urban

Equally disturbing is the trend pattern created by modernization: Despite higher rates of smoking in rural India, the heart disease rate among rural dwellers is about half that among urban Indians. City-dwelling Indians have traded in the cleaner air, lower-fat diet, and natural physical exercise of rural areas for an urban life marked by greater pollution, richer food, sedentary desk jobs, and home lives spent in front of the TV. In the last three decades, heart disease rates in urban India, particularly in south India, have risen by more than three times, from 3% to 11%. The state of Kerala, for example, has a prevalence of 13% in urban areas, compared to 7% in rural Kerala.

Some studies show that heart disease rates are highest in Sikhs and lowest in Muslims and Hindus, and that Sikhs have the highest prevalence of diabetes, obesity and hypertension, but the lowest smoking rates (reflecting a religious prohibition). A 2005 study found a high prevalence of hypertension, diabetes, obesity, particularly abdominal obesity, lipid abnormalities and metabolic syndrome in the Punjabi Bhatia community in North India. Let's turn to the other countries that make up the Indian subcontinent.

Heart Disease in Bangladesh, Pakistan and Sri Lanka
Data show that heart disease in Bangladesh, Pakistan and Sri Lanka is widespread, premature, and severe. A 2005 study found that one in four Pakistani adults above age 40 has heart disease. It frequently occurs as multi-vessel disease and at multiple sites along an artery, and often leads to heart attacks that strike in the absence of the usual warning signs. It is associated with high levels of smoking, diabetes, abdominal obesity, physical inactivity, and hypertension, along with low levels of awareness about heart disease risks. Other risk factors in these countries include high levels of cholesterol, low HDL, elevated blood sugar, inadequate screening, low socioeconomic status, and an unhealthy diet marked by overconsumption of deep-fried foods and saturated fat from ghee, coconut oil, coconut milk, and coconut pulp.

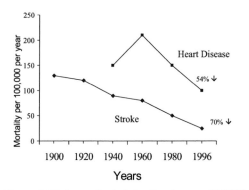

Figure 1.16. Age-adjusted death rates per 100,000 per year for heart disease and stroke in the US, from 1900 to 1996. Mortality rates have declined substantially for both stroke and heart disease because of a nationwide decrease in risk factor levels and improvements in treatment. The same is not true in many developing countries, as Figure 1.17. Source: CDC 1999.

Bangladesh

Heart disease is not only widespread in Bangladesh but often premature and severe. In one study, multi-vessel disease (the severe narrowing of two or more coronary arteries) was present in 54% of people younger than 45 (average

age was 34 years) and in 74% of people older than 55 years. In addition, like Indians and Pakistanis, Bangladeshi patients with heart attacks do not have the typical symptoms of severe crushing chest pain. This absence of the usual warning signs may lead to delays in rushing the patient to the hospital.

Pakistan

As in India, a recent survey undertaken in Karachi, Pakistan, showed high levels of heart disease risk factors: hypertension (39%), obesity (52%), sedentary life style (65%), and diabetes (15%). In addition, awareness of cardiac risk factors was low. A study of medical students in Pakistan also showed a high prevalence of cardiac risk factors, such as unhealthy diet and physical inactivity, low awareness, and inadequate screening practices. The results underscore the urgent need to promote preventive knowledge and practices among medical students as well as the general population. A new generation of prevention-oriented physicians who can counsel patients would go a long way to slow down and reverse these trends.

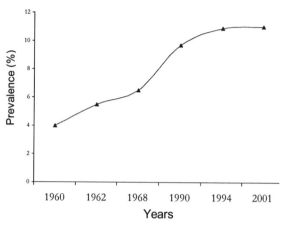

Figure 1.17 The prevalence of heart disease in India, 1960 to 2001. Note that the prevalence (meaning the percentage) of Indians who have heart disease has risen 300% over the past 40 years. Source: Krishnaswami, S. Ref.1.30. *Reproduced with permission© Indian Heart Journal.*

Heart disease among the younger adults is common in Pakistan. In a study of nearly 1,000 patients who had had a first heart attack, 16% were younger than 45. Among the important predictors of premature heart disease in Pakistan were smoking, *ghee* intake, elevated levels of blood sugar, high cholesterol, low socioeconomic status, and a family history of heart disease. For the first time in a study, **parental consanguinity** (marriage between first cousins or close relatives) was found to be a strong predictor of heart disease, perhaps for genetic reasons. Intermarriage is still common in many communities and regions of India and Pakistan and may be another risk factor to be concerned about.

Sri Lanka

Between 1980 and 1988, heart disease mortality rates doubled in Sri Lanka. The prevalence of heart disease was 10%, similar to that of India. The prevalence of risk factors was also high in Sri Lanka. For example, more than half (58%) of those surveyed smoked. On average, HDL (good cholesterol) levels were also low at 38 mg/dL. Finally, more *than 80%* of the fat consumed in Sri Lanka is saturated fat from coconut oil, coconut milk, and coconut pulp.

Contrasting heart disease trends in the US and India

In 1968, heart disease rates were virtually identical in India and the US. As mentioned earlier, in the last 30 years, the age-adjusted heart disease mortality rate has fallen 60% in the US, and similar declines have been observed in other developed countries, such as Finland, Canada, Australia, and Japan. In sharp contrast to these declines, however, heart disease rates in India have *tripled* during this same period. Thus, within the space of a single generation, heart disease rates in India have gone from virtually identical to that of Americans to **four times higher**.

Does a vegetarian diet protect Indians from heart disease as it does other ethnic groups of the world? No. It could if it were done right, but the potential effects are countered by unhealthy additions to the Indian vegetarian diet.

In one sense, heart disease in India appears to be following a similar developmental pattern as the sequence observed in the US, where high rates first appeared in urban and affluent populations, and only later in poorer and rural populations. Unlike in most western countries in the past three decades, however, where death rates from heart attack have declined sharply, it remains high in India—twice what they are in the US, for instance. A study undertaken at the Christian Medical College in Vellore involving 1,320 patients admitted with full-fledged heart attacks analyzed death rates among these patients during their hospital stay and within 30 days of discharge. A large fraction (83%) received lifesaving thrombolytic therapy to dissolve the offending blood clot in the coronary artery. Yet, 17% died in-hospital, double that of US hospitals (8-9%). The findings are significant because the study was undertaken at a major medical college. In small, community hospitals in India, patient care is likely to be inferior and corresponding death rates even higher.

Does a vegetarian diet protect Indians?

The short answer to this question is, not really. Unlike in other populations, vegetarianism offers little protection against heart disease among Indians because Indian vegetarians tend to avoid fish (which is highly cardioprotective when it contains omega-3 fats) and to eat a lot of saturated dairy fat, trans fats, and high glycemic carbohydrates. (For a fuller discussion of this, which I have called "contaminated vegetarianism," see Chapter IV, Section 1, under "Common myths and misconceptions about heart disease among Indians.") The data bear this up: Virtually no Muslim Indians are vegetarians, and at least 60% of the Hindu Indians are vegetarians. Since heart disease rates tend to be much lower among vegetarians than among non-vegetarians worldwide, one might expect the rates among the Hindus to be lower. Yet, the exact opposite is true: several studies have found that the almost entirely non-vegetarian Muslims had lower rates. Overall nearly 50% of Indians are vegetarians, but heart disease rates among them are as high as for Indian non-vegetarians.

These data underscore the general finding, when a large number of studies are examined, that heart disease rates among Indians often tend not to correlate with their levels of the standard risk factors. Low levels of conventional risk factors do not appear to shield Indians from heart disease. On the other hand, high levels of these risk factors are just as harmful to them as they are to people of other ethnicities, if not more.

Indian women

Like Indian men, Indian women the world over have very high rates of heart disease. In fact, the excess level of heart disease in Indians over that of other populations is even greater in women than in men. Chapter IV, Section 3 takes this up in greater detail.

KEY · POINTS · IN · A · NUTSHELL

- ♥ Heart disease rates continue to increase on the Indian subcontinent and are now as high there as in Indians living in other parts of the world.
- ♥ The rates are as high in Pakistan, Bangladesh, and Sri Lanka as they are in India.
- ♥ A 2005 study found that one in four Pakistani adults above age 40 has heart disease.
- ♥ Although heart disease rates were virtually identical in India and the US 30 years ago, they are currently **four times** higher in India.
- ♥ This marked difference is due to a more than 50% decrease in heart disease in the US and a more than 200% increase in India.
- ♥ In the past three decades, heart disease rates in India have **doubled** in rural areas and risen **three-fold** in urban areas. Urban rates now generally run twice as high as rural rates.

1.4 ▶ Malignant Heart Disease in Young Indians

ONE NIGHT in March 1971, Jagdish, a young Indian physician interning at one of Chicago's major teaching hospitals, was taken to the Emergency Room (ER) complaining of chest pain. Given how young he was—he was 25—he was sent home after a few tests and a brief examination. Over the next few days, he returned twice more with the same complaint. Each time, he was discharged after a relatively cursory examination. His youth, and his apparent condition—some sort of cardiac event—were at odds with each other. On his fourth visit to the ER in five days, Jagdish was diagnosed with an acute heart attack and admitted. Over the years, however, the treatment and management of his heart disease were insufficiently aggressive, again perhaps because of his young age. Fifteen years after that heart attack in 1971, Jagdish suddenly died while awaiting a heart transplant.

Compared to whites in the study, the Indians were younger and smoked less and fewer had hypertension. Yet their heart disease was more severe, diffuse, and more likely to be multi-vessel.

How Young is Young?

Premature heart disease is heart disease that occurs *before you start getting old*. It is defined as heart disease diagnosed under the age of 55 years in men and under 65 years for women. **Extremely premature** heart disease is heart disease that occurs *in the young*—most often defined in someone under 45 or under 40. In this book, it is defined as under 45.

In 1972, barely a year after Jagdish had first come to the ER with chest pain, my beeper went off in the middle of the night, summoning me to the Cardiac Care Unit (CCU) of the same hospital to take over another physician's shift. Ravi, a 26-year-old first-year medical resident on duty in the CCU, once again Indian, had been admitted in the same unit following a heart attack. Not long thereafter, a *third* Indian, a 39-year-old engineer, was rushed in after suffering a massive heart attack that had severely damaged the heart muscle. Tests showed that Patel's heart disease was so far advanced that it was inoperable. He died five years later.

And this was all in one Chicago-area hospital over a 15 or 16 month period. The stories admittedly are anecdotal, but telling. Coronary heart disease among Indians **strikes early, strikes hard, and strikes unexpectedly.** In Section 2, we looked at the high rates of premature, severe, malignant heart disease among Indian immigrants in many different countries. In Section 3, we discovered strong parallels to this among Indians on the Indian subcontinent itself. Chapter IV, Section 1 attempts to explain this epidemic and why it has taken the particular contours it has taken. The current section moves the discussion forward by examining three cardinal features that make heart disease in Indians truly distinctive, and to some degree even unique:

- Its extreme prematurity (as all three cases, above, indicate)
- Its severity and extensiveness (as indicated in the third case)
- Its occurrence in persons with *few or no* major traditional risk factors

Let's look at the first: prematurity.

I. PREMATURITY: INDIAN HEART DISEASE STRIKES EARLY

Advanced heart disease is generally more common among older people. Heart disease is described as premature when a man under 55, or a woman under 65, suffers of one or more coronary events—such as a heart attack, death, coronary angioplasty, or bypass surgery. Like most heart disease, premature heart disease is caused by atherosclerosis (the hardening and narrowing of the arteries), which begins early in life. In the case of premature heart disease, however, the process accelerates and progresses much more rapidly.

On average, Indians develop heart disease about *10 years earlier* than other populations, and young Indians often have heart disease as severe as older Indians. Alarmingly, even Indian doctors, who know about the dangers of heart disease and the importance of prevention, on an average *die 15 years earlier* than non-Indian doctors in the UK. In the west (the US and Europe together), 15% of men and 12% of women who die from heart disease die before reaching 65. In India, the figure is 35%—more than double the figure for Europeans and Americans. Still, heart disease *is* the most common cause of premature death in both Europe and the US, but it is primarily a disease of senior citizens, with more than 60% of heart attacks and bypass surgeries in the US occurring in people older than 65 years of age. The median age of a first heart attack among Europeans is 59 years, and 60 years among Chinese. Among people from the Indian subcontinent, it is 50 years—fully 10 years earlier.

Table 1.2. Three Types of Heart Disease

Classification	Characteristics
Type I: extremely premature, malignant heart disease	Typical age of onset: Younger than 45 years of age Develops in the presence or absence of traditional risk factors Triggered by high levels of emerging risk factors Highly prevalent on Indian subcontinent and among people of Indian descent living in other countries Severe atherosclerosis and narrowing, with diffuse, multi-site distribution of plaque all along several coronary arteries
Type II: standard heart disease	Typical age of onset: Older than 65 years of age Triggered by high levels of traditional risk factors Patients typically have low levels of the emerging risk factors Prevalent in most parts of the world and in most sub-populations. Wide range of severity of atherosclerosis, from mild to very severe.
Type III: a mixed type	Typical age of onset: Between 45 and 65 years of age Triggered by moderate levels of emerging risk factors, such as Lp(a), along with varying levels of traditional risk factors

Classifying heart disease among Indians

Another way to grasp just how premature and malignant Indian heart disease can be is to place heart disease within a classification system. Like diabetes, heart disease can be classified into two fundamental types—I and II. With heart disease, there is a third category, type III, which is a composite mix of the first two. The numerical breakdown of heart disease around the world into the three types has not been studied well thus far. Indians, however, may have a predominance of type I. Approximately 35-40% of Indians with heart disease have type I disease compared to 5-10% among other populations.

Like Type 1 diabetes, which develops very early in a person's life and is not triggered by lifestyle choices the way type II diabetes is, type I heart disease similarly occurs in the young—defined as persons younger than 45. Hence its name, extremely premature malignant heart disease. Again, like type 1 diabetes, it is not triggered by lifestyle choices or by high levels of the traditional heart disease risk factors, such as smoking, obesity, hypertension, inactivity, or a diet too rich in saturated fat and cholesterol—although the presence of these factors certainly makes type I worse.

The key fact about type I heart disease is that it can develop in the presence or absence of high levels of the traditional risk factors. In fact, among Indians, it typically develops in their absence, because Indians tend to have rates of smoking, general obesity, high blood pressure, and high cholesterol that are similar to or lower than, for example, whites. Indians who develop Type 1 heart disease, however, tend to have a family history of premature heart disease, along with multiple emerging risk factors (*see* Chapter III). Indians, as we have seen previously, also have a higher prevalence of diabetes, metabolic syndrome, abdominal obesity, and low levels of HDL. Of this, diabetes and metabolic syndrome may well account for perhaps one quarter to one third of heart disease among Indians.

In Type 1 disease, there is usually severe narrowing of multiple arteries, often at multiple sites on the same artery. A study in the United Kingdom found four Indians, who had suffered a heart attack between 18 and 22 years of age—either an extraordinary coincidence or yet another

Table 1.3. Age-specific death rates from heart diseaseIn the UK in Indians and in the general population (1988-1992), per 100,000 people per year

Age	Men		Women	
	General population	Indian	General population	Indian
20-39	7	15	1	1
40-49	74	133	12	16
50-59	295	442	72	101
60-69	869	1059	331	450

Note that more than twice as many Indian men die from heart disease at young ages. Indian women also consistently have higher rates at older ages. Source: Balrajan, R. Ref. 1.05.

manifestation of the uniquely high prevalence of extremely premature heart disease among Indians worldwide. No members of other ethnic groups were found to have suffered a heart attack at such a young age.

Diffuse *heart disease means that the buildup of plaque has spread all along the coronary artery, occurring at multiple sites instead of just one or two specific locations where the artery is narrowed or thickened by plaque.*

(Revisit, also, the three anecdotes with which this section began.) Table 1.3, summarizes the death rates from heart disease among Indians compared to whites at different ages.

A British study found that the rate of first heart attacks among Indian men under the age of 40 was *10 times* that for whites of a similar age. Similar findings were observed in Malaysia and Qatar. In Malaysia, Indians, who make up less than 10% of the general population, accounted for 56% of heart attacks in people younger than 40. In Qatar, where Indians are again less than 10% of the population, the figure was 71%. A Singapore study found that 10 times as many Indian men under 30 died from heart disease as Chinese men of the same age. Other studies in the UK have shown a death rate from heart disease among under-30 Indians two to three times higher than for whites, but only 50% higher in the 60-69 age range. In short, the excess risk of heart disease among Indians over and above the rates found in others is most pronounced at younger ages. This gap decreases with advancing age, partly explained by the fact that many Indians who would have died from heart disease after age 60 have already died by then.

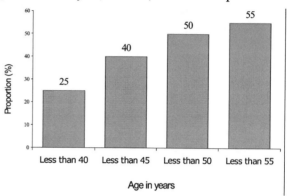

Figure 1.18 The percentage of first heart attacks among Indians that occur before a particular age. The leftmost column, for example, tells us that, of all the Indians who sustain a first heart attack, about 25% suffer this at an age younger than 40. In western countries, only about 5% of first heart attacks occur in people younger than 40. Source: Enas, EA. Ref. 1.07.

From the heart attack registries of Western countries, we can estimate that only 2% to 6% of all heart attacks are sustained by individuals younger than 40, compared to about 25% of heart attacks in India. Studies undertaken at Calicut Medical College in Kerala, India showed that, from 1971 to 1991, the rate of first heart attacks among patients younger than 40 increased **20-fold**. In 1971, for example, one in more than 80 heart attack patients at Calicut was under 40, compared to **one in every four** in 1991. Similar observations have been made at other medical institutions in Kerala and in other states in India.

II. SEVERITY: INDIAN HEART DISEASE STRIKES HARD

Causes of Inoperable Heart Disease
- Severe diffuse disease involving the entire artery
- Total occlusion (obstruction) of several coronary arteries
- Severe muscle damage leading to an ejection fraction less than 25%
- Inadequate healthcare facilities or other issues of affordability leading to late detection of heart disease

Let's now look at the second trait of Indian heart disease: its severity. Any way you examine it, heart disease among Indians strikes hard when it occurs. Severe heart disease is virtually non-existent among young Asians except on the Indian subcontinent; and in other populations, young heart attack patients have either a normal coronary angiogram or single-vessel disease. Approximately 75% of Indians who have had coronary angiograms showed severe narrowing of two or more of their coronary arteries. In all populations, severe heart disease tends to result in a massive heart attack, with a greater propensity for death, disability, and heart failure, which means the heart has lost some of its blood-pumping ability perhaps because of damage to the heart muscle.

In another indication of Indian heart disease severity, a British study found that, among patients with acute heart attack, Indians suffered a higher rate of cardiac arrest before reaching the hospital than patients from other ethnic groups. Among those Indians who survived the crisis and hospitalization, the death rates were twice as high over the ensuing six months, compared to other groups. This was true despite the fact that these Indians were on average younger and smoked less than the other heart attack patients in the study. They had equal access to medical care and there was no difference in medical management compared to whites.

The CADI study subjects did everything right, yet developed high rates of heart disease. This points to a genetic component to Indian heart disease, in addition to the environmental and nutritional factors.

Several Canadian studies have shown heart disease of greater severity among Indians than Native Canadians and Chinese. Additionally, Indian women in Canada undergoing coronary angiograms are twice as likely to have left-main or three-vessel heart disease than white women. This results in a higher rate of referral for bypass surgery. Compared to whites, Indians in Canada who suffer a heart attack also have higher rates of in-hospital mortality, and a greater need for bypass surgery. In one study, compared to other groups, Indians were five times more likely to die or to experience a recurrent heart attack within one year, despite a three-fold higher rate of bypass surgery.

Severe heart disease is also associated with a high rate of death, following bypass surgery (see Chapter VII, Section 5). In a Canadian study of nearly 3,000 patients undergoing coronary angiograms, 15% were Indians, although Indians make up only 2% of the Canadian population. In addition, compared to whites, these Indians were younger, smoked less, and fewer had hypertension; yet their heart disease was more severe, diffuse, and more likely to be multi-vessel.

The major determinants of heart disease severity are diabetes, low HDL, a high total cholesterol to HDL ratio, and high levels of Lp(a). Indians may be the only population with an excess of all four.

Inoperable heart disease

Although severe disease may mandate the need for bypass surgery, very severe and diffuse disease makes it difficult and sometimes impossible to operate (**see Color Plate 1.12** *Localized versus diffuse plaque buildup*). In addition, coronary angiograms and bypass surgery are in any case performed less frequently in many countries than in the US. Even in highly industrialized western countries

What is Severity, How Do You Measure It, and Why Does It Matter?

The **severity** of heart disease is an important indicator of a patient's chances of future health. In clinical practice, the two main factors used in measuring it are (i) the number of arteries that show narrowing, and (ii) the amount of narrowing as determined by a coronary angiogram. The distribution of plaque along the artery is another factor. Plaque buildup that is diffuse—meaning that it affects the entire, or almost the entire, length of the artery, rather than just one localized area—is regarded as more severe. Indians show severity on all of these dimensions, often presenting at the hospital with multi-vessel, diffuse and even inoperable heart disease.

Another criterion of severity is post-procedure outcomes. Severe heart disease leads to poorer outcomes. The more severe the disease, the greater the need for bypass surgery, angioplasty, or other procedures, and the more likely it is that there will be complications following the procedure. The likelihood of a recurrence—for example, of heart attack-is also higher. In a 15-year follow-up study of heart attack survivors who had their first attack when they were on average 48 years old, those with three-vessel disease were three times more likely to have one or more additional heart attacks, and eight times less likely to have an event-free survival compared with those with only single-vessel disease.

How do you measure or confirm severity? Angiograms are widely used to reveal the extent of heart disease, but an angiogram may appear normal unless the disease is already advanced. This is especially true in the case of many Indians who have diffuse, spread-out plaque build-up that is not visibly concentrated at any one point (**see Color Plate 1.12**). Ultimately, however, nothing beats a postmortem autopsy as the most accurate way of ascertaining severity. In fact, it was a definitive study of 9,568 autopsies undertaken in Singapore between 1950 and 1954 that conclusively showed, for the very first time in history, that Indians do have high rates of severe premature heart disease. Heart disease is not an abstract concept; pathologists and medical examiners can see it with their own eyes. That Singapore study showed a rate of coronary atherosclerosis seven times higher in Indians than in Chinese, as well as more severe disease.

such as Canada or the UK (both of which have national health insurance programs), the wait period to see a cardiologist can be very long; and compared to the practice in the United States both countries are less

> **Ejection fraction** is a measure of how much blood your heart can pump out with each heartbeat, versus how much it leaves behind. It measures your heart's pumping power. If your heart's ejection fraction is too low, the surgeon may consider it too risky to perform bypass surgery on you.

aggressive in doing angiograms. This sometimes means that, by the time a patient gets an angiogram, there is a greater chance that their heart disease has become advanced, particularly if, like Indians, they are already predisposed to having severe heart disease. A study in Birmingham, UK, for example, found a disproportionate number of Indians with advanced inoperable disease. Upon follow-up, it was found that four times as many Indians with inoperable heart disease died from heart disease as whites.

Another reason why your heart disease may be considered inoperable is if your heart is not pumping powerfully enough, perhaps because of damage to the heart muscle. If you have what is known as a low **ejection fraction** (less than 25%), you will usually not be accepted as a candidate for bypass surgery. Ejection fraction measures how hard the heart can pump. It is the percentage of blood your heart can pump out of the left ventricle, versus how much is left behind in the ventricle after the heartbeat. A healthy left ventricle pumps out at least 55% of the blood in it with each beat, yielding an ejection fraction of more than 55%.

Bypass surgery can be performed but it may provide little benefit if the muscle supplied by the arteries is significantly damaged. In addition, the likelihood of death during or following surgery (perioperative mortality) may be unacceptably high. Total occlusion is rarely seen in whites but not uncommon in Indians.

III. FEW OR NO TRADITIONAL RISK FACTORS: INDIAN HEART DISEASE STRIKES UNEXPECTEDLY

A major puzzle is that, with the exception of diabetes, the prematurity, severity, and high rates of heart disease found among Indians are not accompanied by particularly high rates of traditional risk factors. This was especially clear among the Indians in the CADI Study (*see also section 2*). The prevalence of high cholesterol, hypertension, and tobacco use among Indians is similar to or lower than that among whites and other populations. In fact, in the CADI study, the rates of smoking and obesity among Indians were below 5%, compared to above 25% for whites, as shown in Figure 1.19. The high rate of heart disease in the presence of low rates of traditional cardiac risk factors is called the "Indian

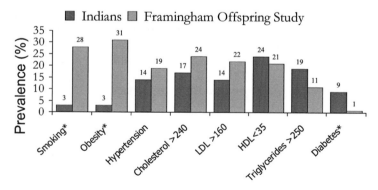

Figure 1.19. Differences in the prevalence of risk factors between Indian participants in the CADI Study and Americans in the Framingham Offspring Study. Compared to Framingham participants, the prevalence of standard risk factors such as smoking, obesity and high blood pressure among the Indians in CADI Study was far lower. The prevalence of high total cholesterol and high LDL was also quite a bit less among the Indians. Indians did have a greater prevalence of diabetes, however, as well as a greater prevalence of high triglyceride levels. Source: Enas, EA. Ref. 1.13.

Paradox" and is explained in detailed in Chapter IV Section 1.

The results of the CADI Study are particularly significant in framing the puzzle of why Indians develop severe heart disease even when they have low rates of obesity, smoking, and high blood pressure. The CADI subjects did everything right: Half were vegetarians; all of them ate a diet low in saturated fats and exercised an average of 134 minutes a week—at a time when the level of exercising recommended by health authorities was only 60 minutes a week. Despite all this, we found high levels of heart disease. (Although the CADI subjects, like other Indians generally, did have higher rates of diabetes, that alone was insufficient to explain their higher rates of heart disease, particularly given the low prevalence of other traditional risk factors among them.) The study's findings, therefore, point strongly to a genetic component, underscoring the need to keep searching for non-traditional risk factors that may be responsible for this anomaly.

In all populations, including Indians, the major factors that determine how severe your heart disease will be are diabetes, high levels of lipoprotein(a), low levels of HDL cholesterol, and a high ratio of total cholesterol to HDL. Indians, it appears, may be the only population with an excess of all four of the above-mentioned factors associated with severity. (For further details, see Chapter II, Sections 3, 4, and 7, and Chapter III, Section 10.) These four factors—diabetes, high Lp(a), low HDL, and high total cholesterol to HDL—may account for almost all of the greater severity of heart disease we see among Indians (see Chapter IV, Section 1).

Premature, severe heart disease often causes death or disability in the prime of life. When a person develops severe heart disease before the age of 40 and dies from it, never having made their full contribution to society, and often leaving behind a young dependent spouse and young children, the consequences can be truly tragic. Early testing, aggressive treatment, and diligent management of risk factors through lifestyle alterations is imperative among Indians to reduce the devastating economic, emotional, and social consequences to the individual and society that premature, severe, malignant heart disease currently poses to Indians everywhere.

> **Did you know...**
> Some traditional risk factors, such as high blood pressure and high total cholesterol, does not strongly correlate by themself with the severity of heart disease. Smoking, paradoxically, is usually associated with less severe heart disease, because smokers get heart attacks on average 10 years earlier than non-smokers.

KEY · POINTS · IN · A · NUTSHELL

♥ Coronary heart disease among Indians strikes early, strikes hard, and strikes unexpectedly.

♥ Heart disease among young Indians (young defined as under 45) is often severe and diffuse, and it follows a malignant course that may be classified as Type I heart disease.

♥ Indians typically develop a heart attack 10 years earlier than other populations.

♥ Young Indians have a much higher risk of heart attack than similarly aged people in other populations.

♥ Approximately one-third of all first heart attacks among Indians occur in Indians younger than 45, and their heart disease is often comparable in severity to that of older Indians.

♥ Serious forms of coronary artery disease, especially left main coronary artery disease and three-vessel disease are twice as common among Indians as in whites, and even more common among Indian women.

♥ Diabetes only partially explains the prematurity and severity of Indian heart disease. In addition to traditional risk factors such as diabetes (see Chapter II, section 6), Indians have high levels of newly discovered "emerging" risk factors such as homocysteine, CRP and LP(a). Together, these constitute the most likely cause of the prematurity and severity of heart disease among Indians.

Chapter II

Heart Disease: Far More Predictable than You Think

Section 1, **Predicting Heart Disease**, presents a broad outline of the Framingham Heart Study model for predicting heart disease. A brief tutorial on type of risks – relative, absolute and population-attributable, is provided. The section also discusses aspects of underestimation of the risk of heart disease in Indians using standard prediction models. ◆

Many of the cardiovascular risk factors such as high cholesterol, high blood pressure can often be modified. Such risk factors are called modifiable risk factors. Section 2, **Introducing the Traditional Risk Factors**, discusses important non-modifiable and modifiable risk factors for heart disease. The multiplicative effects of multiple cardiac risk factors are highlighted. ◆

The third section, **Cholesterol: The Arch-Villain of Atherosclerosis,** outlines the most important modifiable cardiac risk factor for preventing and managing heart disease. Indians tend to have cholesterol levels comparable to that of whites but the attendant risk for heart disease at a given level is at least twice that of the whites. This section also discusses why cholesterol levels among Indians should be lower than in other populations and also the importance of non-HDL cholesterol. ◆

Section 4, **HDL: Body Armor against Heart Disease**, explains the importance of HDL – the good cholesterol and its inverse relationship with severity of heart disease, need for bypass surgery and restenosis following angioplasty and bypass surgery. Nearly half of Indian men and nearly two-thirds of Indian women have low HDL. The importance of various ratios such as triglycerides to HDL ratio is also discussed. ◆

Section 5, **High Blood Pressure: The Silent Killer**, discusses the crucial role of this risk factor in stroke and heart disease and its multiplicative effects with other risk factors such as high cholesterol, triglycerides, low HDL and smoking. Current understanding on white coat hypertension and prehypertension are also discussed. ◆

The Diabetes Epidemic among Indians, the sixth section, guides the reader through the high prevalence of diabetes among Indians and its direct impact on increased cardiac risk. Indians develop diabetes 10-15 years earlier than other populations and at a lower body weight (20-30 lbs lower). Dramatic increases in diabetes rates in rural and urban India are also highlighted. The role of improper diet and a sedentary lifestyle as important causes of diabetes is explained. ◆

The last section, **How Diabetes Links to Heart Disease**, highlights the close link between diabetes and heart disease. Two-thirds of diabetics die from heart disease. The high rates of complications following angioplasty and cardiac bypass surgery especially among diabetic women are discussed. The greater risk of heart attack, heart failure, kidney failure, stroke and death among diabetic patients are examined. ◆

2.1 ▶ Predicting Heart Diseases

Heart disease is now the most predictable of all chronic diseases. Although it often does not announce itself until it is too late, your chance of having a heart attack and its telltales signs can be detected well in advance of actual danger. Yet, in approximately one out of every three people with heart disease, sudden death—which kills a quarter of a million Americans a year—is their first, last, and only symptom. The unexpected death in June 2002 of **Darryl Kyle**, the 33-year-old star baseball pitcher for the St. Louis Cardinals, reminds us all that even top athletes are not immune from sudden death. Kyle's autopsy showed that two of his three coronary arteries were 80% to 90% narrowed, meaning almost entirely blocked. But it need not have been this way, because before someone actually dies from heart disease, many things have to happen. Put another way, many ducks—in the form of risk factors and lifestyle choices—have to line up just right for you to have a heart attack or sudden death.

The fact is that heart disease is a multi-factorial disease that affects genetically susceptible individuals. There are many things you can do to find out if you are at risk; if you are, to reduce the chances that those risk factors will conspire to lead to tragedy. This Chapter discusses how heart disease is predicted, what the risk factor numbers mean for you, and how to interpret the risk guidelines depending on which ethnic group you are a member of.. You will learn about **the Framingham Risk Score**—the yardstick for predicting the risk of getting a first heart attack—and why this assessment tool may actually underestimate risk among Indians. You will also come to understand why the chances of developing heart disease varies among different populations and ethnic groups, even when they have the same level of traditional risk factors.

> ### A Word about Terminology
> Throughout this book, the term Indian refers to people, who trace their origin to the Indian subcontinent—meaning Bangladesh, India, Pakistan, and Sri Lanka—including those who now live abroad but originate from one of these four countries. "Indian" in this context is ethnically interchangeable with "South Asian," "Indo-Asian," or "Asian Indian." The term thus excludes native Americans but includes more than people from the nation of India.
>
> **Measurement Units:** As is conventional, blood glucose levels, triglyceride levels, and cholesterol levels are stated throughout this book in milligrams per deciliter (mg/dL). Blood pressure is stated in millimeters of mercury (mmHg).

> ### Did You Know...
> The risk factors that influence the likelihood that you will get a stroke, or that you will develop heart disease, are essentially the same. That is why this book uses the phrases "cardiovascular risk factors" and "cardiac risk factors" interchangeably.

Cardiovascular risk factors

A risk factor is any bodily condition or personal behavior that increases the chance of your developing some particular disease. The concept of a cardiovascular risk factor—things that increase your odds of developing heart disease or a stroke, or both—was developed from the Framingham Heart Study nearly 40 years ago. This landmark study initially identified three major cardiac risk factors: high cholesterol, high blood pressure, and smoking. Since then, the medical community has refined its understanding of cardiac risk even further, and other epidemiological studies in the US and Europe have now identified several traditional and nontraditional risk factors. The greater the number or the severity of your risk factors, the more likely it is that you will develop cardiovascular disease. Although scientists have identified more than 300 risk factors, there is no need to panic: You only need to know fewer than a dozen of them to live a healthful life! Essentially, there are just a handful of critical lifestyle choices to which you need to pay particularly careful attention to sharply cut down your chances of developing cardiovascular disease.

Continuous spectrum of risk

In earlier years, the medical-scientific community thought of most risk factors in **either/or** terms: Either you have it, or you don't. Either your blood pressure is too high, or it isn't. In other words, the medical community had relatively rigid cut-off points. If you are below, good; if you are above, bad. Risk factors, in other words, were regarded like pregnancy: You either are, or are not.

That thinking has changed, and it is extremely important that you see this. Today, virtually all risk factors are considered to exist **on a continuous spectrum**, with no sharp, rigid difference between present and absent. Thus, high levels of a particular risk factor such as cholesterol, blood sugar, or blood pressure means you are at greater risk for heart disease; but *equally importantly*, your having moderately high or even lower levels of risk factors, *does not mean you are off the hook*.

Furthermore, the cut-off points for many important risk factors have changed in the past few decades. For the most part, what used to be considered safe just 50 years ago is often now considered high. For example, a systolic blood pressure of 240—President Franklin Delano Roosevelt's blood pressure—was considered relatively acceptable back in the 1930s. Today, the optimum systolic blood pressure has been revised downward to less than 120 mm Hg. "120 over 80," until recently regarded as the optimum systolic-diastolic blood pressure has been drummed into the heads of many health-conscious people. But even those figures are now being revised downward further, to 115 over 75.

The idea behind the *continuous spectrum* understanding of a risk factor is that your blood pressure does not have to be 180 over 110 for your body to be developing the conditions that may lead to a coronary event or a stroke. Even at 120 over 80, you may slowly be moving toward heart disease, just not as quickly as if your blood pressure were 180 over 110. But the movement is not zero, which is why 115 over 75 may in fact be better.

In short, we do not suddenly start developing heart disease once we hit a magic number. We start sliding toward it almost the moment we are born, and the key to living a long, healthy life is to begin retarding your progress toward heart disease by minimizing *all* of your risk factors, bringing them down to the lowest possible levels that you can manage. Consider this: many people, perhaps most people, are **less healthy than they look on the surface.** One simply is unable to see the cardiovascular diseases that may claim them in 10, 20, or 30 years. There is no videotape that shows you the future end results of their present choices. Like a person falling off a cliff who has not hit the ground yet, one can feel perfectly fine—until the truth emerges and calamity hits.

To gain a better understanding of cardiac risk, let's look at a few of the most important concepts that physicians and scientists use in discussing issues in this area, starting with three kinds of risk. Absolute risk, relative risk, and population-attributable risk are three different measures of risk doctors use to describe the risk faced by an individual or a population group. Of these, absolute and population-attributable risk are particularly important.

> **Did you know...**
> European guidelines for predicting different people's risk of getting heart disease consider only cardiac death. They do not include heart attack in their risk assessment. European guidelines may, therefore, significantly underestimate the burden of heart disease and, in short, paint a slightly rosier picture.

Absolute risk

Your absolute risk for developing heart disease is the likelihood of your experiencing a cardiac event, such as a heart attack, heart failure, sudden death, or a procedure such as a coronary angioplasty or bypass surgery. Because your chances of contracting an illness is greater over a greater period of time and less over a shorter period, both American and European guidelines, as a matter of convention, use a 10-year period to express absolute risk. Thus, we might say: "Mr. A has a 10% absolute risk (that is, one out of ten chance) of developing heart disease over the next 10 years." It is important to bear in mind that absolute risk of heart disease among different populations may vary according to the presence, severity, and number of risk factors, because these factors affect different ethnic groups differently. The same risk factor can create different levels of absolute risk in different ethnic groups. For example, blacks tend to have higher blood pressure than whites, yet even at **identical levels of blood pressure, blacks still have double the rate of stroke** whites do. Similarly, at identical levels of cholesterol, the risk of a heart attack among Japanese is five times lower than that of Americans.

Relative risk

By contrast, your **relative risk** of developing heart disease is what your level of risk is *as compared to* (or relative to) members of another group. It is a comparative concept. For example: Mr. A who has a cholesterol level of 120, has a one in 200 chance of developing heart disease within 10 years. His absolute risk is therefore 1/200, or 0.5%. His office supervisor, Mrs. B, whose cholesterol level is 220, has a one in 20 chance, or an absolute risk of 5% (1/20). Mrs. B's husband, Mr. C, whose cholesterol level is 320, has a one in two chance of developing heart disease, or an absolute risk of 50%.

If Mr. C reduced his cholesterol to that of Mrs. B, he would achieve a reduction in relative risk of 90%: (50-5)/50. Similarly, if Mrs. B reduced hers to that of Mr. A, she would achieve a 90% relative risk reduction (5-0.5)/5. Notice this, however: *Although the reduction in relative risk is the same in both cases, the reduction in absolute risk is very large for Mr. C*, and not so much for Mrs. B (45% versus 4.5%)

In short, your *relative* risk from a particular risk factor may be 10 times higher than someone else's, but what matters the most is your *absolute* risk. Compared to Mrs. B, Mr.C has a 10-fold greater absolute risk to develop heart disease (50% versus 5%). Similarly, Mrs. B has an absolute risk 10-fold greater than Mr. A to develop heart disease (5% versus 0.5%). But Mr. C needs to worry much more about *his* 10-fold figure than Mrs. B has to worry about hers. Relative risk, in short, *does not tell* the full story. It needs to be interpreted alongside absolute risk. That is the lesson.

Let's take another example: The *relative* risk of developing heart disease from eating Transylvanian Dark Chocolate may be 20 times higher for people who eat it than for those who do not. But if the *absolute* risk of developing heart disease from eating this extremely rare chocolate is only 0.00005 percent, then it does not matter much if your relative risk of developing heart disease from eating it is 20 times higher than someone who does not. Medical phrases such as "20-fold" sound big and frightening—and sometimes they ought to be—but 20 times 0.0001 percent is still very small. When you read that your relative risk of developing heart disease from engaging in some behavior is "four-fold higher," than those who do not, remember to look at the underlying absolute risk. If that risk is already large, then four-fold is very serious. But if it is very small, then four-fold takes on a different meaning. That was Mrs. B's situation: She had a relative risk "10-fold" higher than Mr. A but it was 10 times greater than a risk level that was very small (0.5%).

Let me give you another example. Your relative risk of dying in a plane crash, if you fly from New York to California and back is double the risk of someone who flies only from New York to California. But is double the relative risk a good reason not to fly back home? No, because the underlying absolute risk of dying in a plane crash at all is quite small one chance per million for a flight from New York to California and 2 chances per million when you fly back. So although one doubles one's absolute risk in taking the return leg of your flight, few people worry about that, since the absolute risk remains very small.

Population-attributable risk

Population-attributable risk is a measure of risk that tries to capture the distinction between the individual as a *single* person, and the individual as a member of his or her population *group*. In other words, it draws our attention to the difference between, on the one hand, the risk an individual faces if he or she participates in a certain activity—for example, smoking—(which could be **very high**) and, on the other hand, the risk this individual's *entire population* group faces, taking into account whether or not they even participate in that activity (which could be **very low**).

An example would help to make this clear: Few Indian women smoke. However, an Indian woman, who *does* smoke, has a very high (individual) risk of heart attack, two to five times higher than a non-smoking Indian woman. On the other hand, since very few Indian women do, in fact, smoke, the *population-attributable* risk of sustaining a heart attack from smoking among Indian women is on the whole very low, even though the risk of getting a heart attack for the individual Indian woman who does smoke is very high. In contrast, the population-attributable risk of heart disease from smoking is very high among Indian men because at least one-third of Indian men (other than physicians) do smoke. Thus, population-attributable risk conveys the importance of a given risk factor in an entire population.

Take another example: On the individual level, the risk of being injured by going hang-gliding in a hurricane is extremely high (*if* you do in fact go); but the *population-attributable risk* of being injured while hang-gliding in a hurricane is, mercifully, extremely low, because few members of any population would be foolhardy enough to do such a thing. Population-attributable risk takes into account the actual practice of an entire group or population.

It is time now to see how these concepts are used in practice. In 2004, Dr. Salim Yusuf, director of the Population Research Institute at Canada's McMaster University and a world-renowned Indian cardiologist-scientist, reported on the results of the INTER-HEART Study, the largest-ever heart attack study undertaken. Involving more than 29,000 people from 52 countries, this multi-center, international study has identified **nine controllable risk factors** that account for more than nine out of ten of the heart attacks seen worldwide. What is particularly interesting is that these nine factors strongly predict heart attacks for every ethnic group in every part of the world. They are "universal." In order of importance, the nine risk factors are:

Table 2.1. Population-attributable risk for different risk factors for a first heart attack in the INTERHEART Study

	Relative risk	Population-attributable risk
Contributing factors		
Abnormally high cholesterol ratio	three-fold	+49%
Tobacco use	three-fold	+36%
Psychosocial factors (stress and depression)	three-fold	+33%
Abdominal obesity	two-fold	+20%
High blood pressure	two-fold	+18%
Diabetes	three-fold	+10%
Protective factors		
Regular physical activity	–	-12%
High fruit and vegetable intake	–	-14%
Alcohol in moderation	–	-7%

Source: Yusuf, S. Ref. 2.60.

1. An elevated cholesterol ratio—specifically high Apo B combined with low Apo A
2. Smoking
3. Diabetes
4. Hypertension
5. Abdominal obesity (that is, obesity around the stomach area)
6. Psychosocial factors (meaning stress and depression)
7. Failure to eat vegetables and fruits everyday
8. Failure to exercise regularly
9. Failure to drink small amounts of alcohol

Some of the key results of the INTERHEART Study summarized in Table 2.1 illustrates the importance of population-attributable risk. For both diabetes and abnormally high bad cholesterol levels (high LDL, low HDL), the *relative risk* for getting a heart attack is three-fold—meaning that it is three times what it is for those who do not have elevated cholesterol ratio or diabetes. However, the *population-attributable risk* for abnormal cholesterol ratio is 49%, but only 10% for diabetes, because although both are detrimental to your health, more people have abnormal cholesterol ratio than diabetes, so you are more likely to be one of them. Elevated bad cholesterol is more "prevalent." This is why it explains almost half of all heart attacks (49%), but diabetes explains only 10%. This five-fold difference in population-attributable risk is due to the differences in prevalence of these two risk factors. The prevalence of diabetes worldwide is only 5% compared to 50% for out-of-balance cholesterol (**dyslipidemia**). This is discussed in subsequent sections.

The good news: The INTERHEART study also found three *protective* factors: Liberal consumption of fruits and vegetables, regular physical activity, and alcohol consumption in **small amounts.** The relative importance of various risk factors is discussed in subsequent sections.

The Framingham Risk Score

The Framingham Risk Score is the Mother of all Risk Prediction Models. For example, the National cholesterol Education Program (NCEP) treatment guidelines for *people without heart disease* are based on the absolute risk calculated from the Framingham Risk Score. (People with heart disease and/or diabetes are already at very high risk and require the most aggressive treatment available. Therefore, the Framingham Risk Score is not applicable for these high-risk people.)

> **What does the INTER-HEART Study Tell Us?**
>
> Number one on the list of the nine controllable risk factors identified in the INTERHEART Study is elevated cholesterol levels. It can explain about *half* of all heart attacks. Cholesterol, smoking, diabetes, high blood pressure, obesity around the stomach area, and psychosocial factors such as stress and depression all play a key role in heart attacks. A person with all nine risk factors is about *130 times more likely* to get a heart attack than someone with none of them.

In assessing someone's risk for heart disease, the Framingham Risk Score takes into consideration factors such as your age, gender, whether you smoke, blood pressure, cholesterol levels, and HDL levels, and then predicts the likelihood that you will experience a coronary event over the next 10 years (See Chapter VII section 1). There is a striking disparity between the relatively low levels of 10-year risk and the much higher levels of lifetime risk given in the Framingham Risk Score. In reality, a low 10-year risk does not mean a low lifetime risk. For example, Framingham men in the lowest tertile (bottom one-third) of risk scores at 50 years of age had a 10-year cumulative risk of only four in 100, but had a *lifetime* risk of 50 in 100. Similarly, women in the lowest tertile had a 10-year cumulative risk of just two in 100, but a *lifetime* risk of 25 in 100.

In one sense, these data suggest that a 10-year risk prediction markedly underestimates the lifetime risk and underscores the need for continued vigilance for all individuals, including those who have been identified as "low risk" for heart disease. In another sense, what these data tell us is that, even if risky choices do not get to you in ten years, they eventually will. Even those that the Framingham Risk Score assess to be at low risk in the medium term (ten years) may be at considerable risk when you look further down the road.

Underestimation and overestimation of risk in different populations

No disease prediction model applies equally well to all populations. For example, heart disease predictions made using the American-based Framingham Risk Score apply more accurately to Americans than to Europeans. This is because, for any given level of traditional risk factors, the absolute mortality rate from heart disease varies from population to population. Some groups are more susceptible to heart disease, all other things being equal. For example, at identical ages and levels of smoking and blood pressure, the 10-year risk of a heart attack in a Southern European man with a cholesterol level of 240 mg/dL is similar to that of a Northern European man with cholesterol of just 160 mg/dL, and that of an American man with a cholesterol a level of 200 mg/dL. No single risk prediction model, however, can take all of these regional differences into account. For that reason, predictions based on the Framingham Risk Score, for example, overestimate the heart disease risk among Southern European (by about 50 %) and underestimate the risk in Northern Europeans (also by about 50 %). In reality, the absolute risk of a heart attack is three times higher among Northern Europeans than among Southern Europeans (Finns versus the French, for example) (see Chapter IV, Section 1).

In short, using the Framingham Risk Score to predict the absolute risk of heart disease in non-American populations such as those living in other countries is likely to lead to some significant errors. Similarly, studies in the UK show that, although prediction models developed there are fairly accurate in predicting cardiac risk in the overall population, these British models nevertheless overestimate the risk in blacks and Chinese, and underestimate the risk in Indians, Pakistanis and Bangladeshis.

Figure 2.1. shows the disparity between the actual standardized death rates from heart disease in Indians, Chinese, blacks and whites in the UK, and the death rates predicted by as widely used British model. While the model is accurate for British whites, the predicted rate for Indians, for example, is substantially lower than the actual rate. Because of such regional and ethnic variations, Europeans on the Continent have also developed their own model of risk prediction, called the Systematic Coronary Risk Evaluation (SCORE) Project.

Underestimation of risk in Indians

Given identical levels of risk factors, the absolute risk of heart disease in Japanese and Chinese is less than a third that of Americans and Europeans. The Framingham Risk Score predicts cardiac risk accurately in whites and blacks living in the US, but when applied to Chinese, Japanese, Hispanics, and Native Americans it overestimates their risk. A 2004 study found that the Framingham Risk Score, applied to Chinese living in China, overestimates their risk of heart disease by nearly 300%. The study found, however, that the model can really be recalibrated (modified) for application to the Chinese population using data derived from the Chinese population itself. This may be equally true for the Indian population and for other ethnic groups as well.

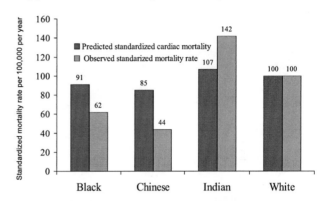

As stated earlier, the **British Prediction Model** underestimates cardiac risk among Indians. An ongoing prospective British study after a seven-year follow-up reported that the heart disease death rate among Indians is more than double as among whites—much higher than the British Prediction Model predicts. The researchers had made careful

Figure 2.1. Predicted and actual standardized death rates from heart disease in the UK among Indians and other selected populations. The model accurately predicts death rate for whites—the observed and predicted rates are identical—but it underestimates the death rate among Indians living in Britain, and overestimates it for blacks and Chinese. 100 is chosen as the standard death rate. Source: Quirke, TP. Ref. 2.43.

statistical adjustments for differences in cholesterol level, hypertension, smoking, diabetes, triglycerides, and abdominal obesity. What makes this data so powerful is that the British have some of the highest rates of death from heart disease.

Another British study found that traditional risk factors accurately predict the risk of heart disease among whites whereas the risk in Indians was 79% greater than predicted. It is advisable to multiply by a **factor of two** for Indians when the reader uses the American or European Prediction Models. My approach for risk estimation in Indians is outlined in Chapter VII section 1.

Until recently, there was no validated prediction model available that accurately predicts the cardiac risk in Indians. A new prediction model with adjustments to Framingham Risk Score has been published in 2005. According to this model adding 108 mg to the cholesterol level, or 50 to systolic blood pressure or 10 to age may provide a better estimate for predicting heart disease among Indians (see Chapter VII, Section 1). It appears that the cardiac risk among Indians with a total cholesterol of **160 mg/dL is similar to whites with total cholesterol 260 mg/dL.** Since the cardiac risk is higher in Indians than in whites, the cholesterol recommendations for Indians have to be more **stringent than for all** other populations.

Now that you have a basic understanding of the risk and risk factors, we will explore cholesterol, the most important risk factor for heart disease, in the next section.

KEY · POINTS · IN · A · NUTSHELL

- ♥ Heart disease has now become the most predictable of all chronic diseases.
- ♥ At a given level of traditional risk factors, heart disease rates vary by two- to three-fold among different populations.
- ♥ The Framingham Risk Score (FRS) is used to determine when to begin treatment for high cholesterol and the target level to be achieved in people without heart disease.
- ♥ The FRS accurately predicts the risk of a heart attack for both blacks and whites.
- ♥ The FRS overestimates the risk in Chinese, Japanese, Hispanics, Native Americans, and Southern Europeans.
- ♥ The FRS underestimates the risk of heart disease by a factor of two or more in Indians.
- ♥ The risk of heart disease among Indians with cholesterol of 160 mg/dL may be as high as Americans and Europeans with a cholesterol level of 260 mg/dL.

2.2 ▶ Introducing the Traditional Risk factors

As discussed in Section 1, cardiovascular risk factors raise the risk of developing coronary events such as a heart attack or stroke. These risk factors can be broadly classified as modifiable and non-modifiable. Non-modifiable are those over which we have no control, such as gender, advancing age, family history, and ethnicity. A prior history of heart attack is also a non-modifiable risk factor. By contrast, modifiable risk factors such as smoking, high cholesterol, obesity, lack of exercise, and high blood pressure, are those we can control through lifestyle changes and/or medications in order to reduce our risk of sudden death, heart attack, and stroke. Any given individual may have several of these risk factors or none. This Chapter discusses the importance of various modifiable risk factors (which can be improved by lifestyle changes or medication – such as high blood lipids and smoking) and non modifiable risk factors (age, gender, race, family history), with a focus on the Indian population.

Heart disease is uncommon before age 40, except among Indians. The risk of heart disease doubles every decade of a person's life. The risk of a coronary event in a 60-year-old with a cholesterol level of 160 mg/dL is similar to that of a 40-year-old with a cholesterol level of 320. Similarly, the risk of a coronary event in a 60-year-old with a systolic blood pressure reading of 120 mmHg is similar to that of a 40-year-old with a systolic pressure of 180. In the US and most other western countries, 75 to 85% of heart attack deaths occur after the age of 65. However, about 25% of heart attacks in Indians occur under the age of 40, and 55% occur under the age of 55. As discussed in previous Chapter 1 **section 4** the risk of a heart attack before age 40 is 5 to 10 times higher among Indians than in other populations.

Gender

For every woman who experiences a heart attack before 40, 10 such men have heart attacks. Men are more likely than women to get heart disease before age 55. Women lag behind men 10 years for developing heart disease and 20 years before developing a heart attack. However, the risk of

Table 2.2. Major risk factors for heart disease

Non-modifiable risk factors	Modifiable risk factors
1. Age 2. Gender 3. Family history of early heart attack, stroke, or death 4. Ethnicity (Asian Indian) 5. Prior heart disease including angioplasty, stent, and bypass surgery	1. High cholesterol 2. Low HDL 3. High blood pressure 4. Cigarette smoking or tobacco use 5. Diabetes

heart disease sky-rockets in women after the age of 50 (or following menopause) and by age 75 reaches that of men. In fact, in total, more women die from heart disease than men because of their higher life expectancy (see Chapter IV section 3). The risk of heart disease is particularly high and accelerated among women who undergo premature menopause.

Family history of early heart disease

The best way to prevent heart disease is to *choose your parents wisely*. However, I am yet to meet someone who has actually managed to do this. An individual is considered to have a family history of heart disease if the person's father or a brother is diagnosed with heart disease (heart attack, sudden death, coronary angioplasty, bypass surgery, and so on) before age 55, or in the person's mother or sister before age 65. Heart disease that occurs in relatives past these ages is not regarded as a family history of heart disease for the purposes of risk assessment. A family history of premature heart attack is equivalent to having a systolic blood pressure of 170 mm Hg, a total cholesterol level of more than 315 mg/dL, or an HDL level of less than 30 mg/dL, or smoking two packs of cigarettes a day. Persons with a family history of heart disease have a two- to four-fold higher risk of developing heart disease at a young age. Children of parents, who died before the age of 50 from heart disease, have a three- to six-fold risk of the same unless the underlying familial risk factors are identified and treated appropriately.

> Contrary to one would expect, men with low testosterone levels have a higher risk of heart disease than those with normal levels. These data suggest that normal testosterone levels may offer protection against the development of atherosclerosis in middle-aged men.

Sibling history of premature heart disease, particularly in a younger sibling, is an even stronger risk factor than parental history of premature heart disease. This is also true if the younger brother or sister has had coronary angioplasty or bypass surgery. The risk increases eight-to 15-fold in identical twins (monozygotic) if one twin died of heart disease at an early age. In a study of 8,549 asymptomatic adults, a family history of premature heart disease highly correlated with calcified plaques in the coronary arteries (see Chapter VII, Section 3) indicating asymptomatic heart disease. The risk is markedly increased in those, who also have metabolic syndrome, in addition to a sibling history of premature heart disease.

Although a family history itself is a non-modifiable risk factor, most people with a family history of heart disease have one or more modifiable risk factors. It is vitally important to identify and treat these modifiable risk factors early and aggressively. Furthermore, those with a family history of premature heart disease have a five to 10-fold higher rates of genetic risk factors, such as high levels of *lipoprotein(a)* and in many cases, *homocysteine* (see Chapter III Section 3 and 4). Many of the genetic risk factors *can be controlled* with appropriate treatment (see Chapter VI Section 5).

A family history of longevity is also important for precisely the opposite reasons to a family history of heart disease. Siblings of centenarians (persons who are older than 100) have an eight-to 17-fold higher probability of also living that long. Offspring of centenarians may inherit significantly better health, with 50% lower prevalence of risk factors.

Ethnicity

Heart disease rates, particularly death, vary more by than 10-fold among people of various ethnic origins. In general, Asians such as Chinese, Filipinos, and Japanese have the lowest rates of heart disease, but very high rates of stroke. Blacks (*except African Americans*) in general have very low rates of heart disease. African Americans have similar rates of heart disease as whites but greater rates of death and stroke. (See Chapter IV for an explanation of this.)

Prior heart disease

People, who have had a heart attack remain at high risk of repeat heart attack, and an annual death rate of 5-15%. The risk is increased to as high as 25-fold in whom LDL and HDL levels are not brought under control.

Major modifiable risk factors

A risk factor is considered major when its prevalence is high, testing is standardized, and effective treatment that reduces the risk is widely available. The major modifiable risk factors can predict not only a heart attack but also stroke, diabetes, and peripheral vascular disease. It is estimated that more than 90% of the people with heart disease and more than 50% of those without heart disease have at least one of the major modifiable risk factors.

Table 2.3. Prevalence of heart disease and stroke in the US by age and gender

	Heart disease		Stroke	
	Men %	Women %	Men %	Women %
45-54	3	2	1	2
55-64	12	4	3	3
65-74	12	6	6	6
75+	17	10	12	12

Source: American Heart Association. Ref.1.1

Smoking

India is the third-largest producer of tobacco after China and the US. Smoking is the single most important preventable cause of death worldwide, killing 440,000 smokers and 53,000 of their non-smoking loved ones (from passive, second-hand smoking) annually in the US alone. These rates may be several times higher in India. Smoking rates in the US have fallen to a historic low of 22% in 2004 (men 25% and women 20%). Within professions, smoking is lowest among American physicians (2%) and nurses (13%) compared to 24% in the general population. This is not the case for physicians in other countries. For example one in five Chinese and Japanese physicians is a smoker.

Smoking rates decline with age from 29% before age 25 to 9% above age 65, a welcome trend that may be partially due to death at young ages among heavy smokers. In general, a person, who smokes, dies 20 years earlier than a non-smoker. Because few young people get heart attacks, the relative risk of getting a heart attack if you are a smoker, compared to your non-smoking friends, is highest in younger age groups - usually five-fold in those below 40 years of age. By comparison, smokers older than 65 are "only" about twice as likely to get a heart attack as non-smokers in their age group. That is not because it is safer to smoke at 65 than at 40, but because more non-smoking 65-year-olds get heart attacks than non-smoking 40-year-olds. Cigarette smoking is also the strongest risk factor for *sudden cardiac death* – the risk is two to four times greater than that of nonsmokers.

> **Did you know ...**
> The traditional cardiac risk factors that occur in midlife are also associated with *Alzheimer's disease* and dementia in late life. The risk is increased by 25% in those with high blood pressure or smoking and 50% in those with high cholesterol or diabetes. The risk is more than doubled in those having all four of these risk factors.

Smoking damages the cardiovascular system in both the short and the long term. The short-term effect is reversible and is related to the formation of blood clots and constriction of blood vessels caused by nicotine. The long-term cumulative effect of smoking is the acceleration of plaque build-up in the arteries, which occurs in proportion to **"pack-years"** of smoking. Pack-years are defined as the years you smoke times the number of packs smoked a day. For example, a person smoking two packs a day for 20 years (2 x 20) and another person smoking one pack a day for 40 years (1 x 40) have identical pack-year (40 pack-years).

Smoking takes it toll in other ways. Recent studies have shown that HDL levels are about 5mg/dL lower among smokers and *3mg/dL lower* among children of smokers. In addition, smoking is a powerful predictor of lung cancer and chronic lung disease, as well as 25 other chronic conditions. Recent studies have shown that smoking is an important cause of metabolic syndrome and diabetes.

While smoking is uncommon among Indian women (less than 10%), it is common among Indian men (more than 30%), and there is a smoking trend beginning among young women in major Indian cities. Currently, the annual smoking tobacco-related death toll in India is estimated at 800,000. However, both nonsmoking men and women may suffer from the effects of passive (secondhand) smoking if they spend significant time in smoking environments.

A smoker is considered a former smoker after one year of abstinence. Yet, the benefits on the cardiovascular system after smoking cessation are fast (one day after quitting there is an improvement in heart rate).

Beedi (unfiltered, hand-rolled mini-cigarettes) are more popular in India than conventional cigarettes, especially among the working class. Contrary to belief, beedies are just as bad for you as regular cigarettes. Studies among Indians have shown a six-fold higher risk of heart attack among Indians who smoke 20 cigarettes or beedies a day, compared to Indian non-smokers.

Smokeless tobacco, also called snuff or "spit" tobacco has been tied to oral cancer and dental problems such as receding gum lines and bad breath. In 1986, the US Surgeon General concluded that smokeless tobacco is not a safe alternative to cigarettes or cigars. A 2005 study of young male volunteers showed harmful cardiovascular effects of smokeless tobacco. When the men chewed smokeless tobacco, their hearts beat faster, increasing by an average of 16 beats per minute. Their blood pressure also rose by 10mm Hg, and their adrenaline—also called epinephrine—went up by 50%, indicating *heightened physiological stress.*

A 1991 survey on tobacco use prevalence in Sri Lanka found that 38% of men and 1% of women smoke. The 2000 Sri Lankan national survey found that smoking has decreased to 24% of men, but increased to 6% in women. In most of Asia and the Indian subcontinent, a decrease in smoking in men is being counterbalanced by an increase in smoking in women and warrants aggressive public health measures.

> **The "Smoker's Paradox"**
> A person who smokes gets a heart attack 10 years earlier than a nonsmoker. A smoker is also at a very high risk of dying before reaching the hospital. Paradoxically, those who make it to the hospital alive have a better survival rate and long-term health than a non-smoker, if he or she quits the habit permanently. This "Smoker's Paradox," is due to a smaller plaque burden and generally the younger age of the smoker at the time of the heart attack.

Hypertension (high blood pressure)

High blood pressure is the most common cardiovascular disease, affecting over 65 million Americans (30 million men and 35 million women). Annually, it directly causes 50,000 deaths and contributes indirectly to another 250,000 deaths. High blood pressure is a ubiquitous and powerful risk factor for stroke, heart failure, kidney failure, and heart attack (see Section 5).

Diabetes

Diabetes is now considered more than just a risk factor for heart disease; it is now regarded as a heart disease equivalent. This means that diabetic patients, male or female, should be treated aggressively just as though they had heart disease—with multiple medications including aspirin, statins, or beta-blockers. Diabetes is found in 24% of white and 36% of black heart attack victims. This figure is likely to be closer to 50% among Indians. This topic is discussed in Sections 6 and 7.

High cholesterol

High cholesterol alone is a sufficient risk factor in many heart attacks. It can, by itself, lead to a heart attack even if you do not have any other risk factors. People with very high cholesterol levels (500 to 1000 mg/dL due to genetic abnormalities) often develop heart disease in early adulthood (twenties and thirties) and sometimes as early as childhood, even in the absence of other risk factors. Besides being sufficient in itself as a risk, high total and high bad cholesterol is also a **necessary risk factor** in all heart attacks. Individuals and populations with low cholesterol levels (less than 100 mg/dL) have very low rates of heart disease even when other coronary risk factors such as smoking, hypertension, and diabetes are present. Cholesterol is, therefore, now considered the most important risk factor for heart disease (see Section 3).

Multiple risk factors: a mutually synergistic effect

Risk factors for heart disease seldom occur in isolation. Instead, they are found clustered together, working in tandem. Multiple risk factors are the norm rather than the exception, and they tend to have a synergistic effect on each other, reinforcing one another. In the latest (2003) Behavior Risk Factor Surveillance system

(BRFSS) of more than 250,000 Americans, 30% reported no major risk factors, 33% had one, and 37% had two or more major risk factors for heart disease (see Appendix B). The prevalence of multiple risk factors was highest in blacks (49%) and Native Americans (47%), and lowest among Asians (26%). Those with low income (less than $10,000) had nearly twice the rate of multiple risk factors (53% versus 29%) of the high-income group (more than $50,000). Hawaii had the lowest (27%) and Kentucky the highest (46%) rate of multiple risk factors.

Tid bits
Cholesterol levels are on average about 4 mg/dL higher during winter than summer, probably due to a phenomenon called hemoconcentration, in which our blood gets slightly thicker as the climate gets colder.

In general, cardiovascular risk is elevated two-fold when the abnormality in the risk factor is mild, three-fold when the abnormality is moderate, and four-fold when the abnormality is severe. For example, a blood pressure of 120-140 may be considered mild abnormality, 140-160 may be considered moderate and more than 160 is considered a severe abnormality. When two or more risk factors are present, the risk is multiplicative, not additive. For example, very high blood pressure confers about a four-fold risk of heart disease, so does high cholesterol. However, a person with very high blood pressure as well as cholesterol has a 16-fold risk (i.e., 4 x 4) not an eight-fold risk (i.e., 4 + 4) of developing heart disease, compared to someone with optimal levels of blood pressure and cholesterol.

In the INTERHEART Study, the combination of smoking, diabetes and high blood pressure had 16 times the risk of a heart attack as compared to those with none of these risk factors. The addition of high LDL and low HDL increased the risk by 32 times. The addition of obesity to the above five increased the risk to 64 times.

Approximately 50% of patients treated for hypertension have dyslipidemia. Hypertensive patients on treatment who have diabetes or develop diabetes have a three-fold increased risk of developing heart disease, compared to those hypertensive patients who remained diabetes-free.

All conventional risk factors are associated with a significant risk of heart disease in Indians, as is true in all other populations. However, compared with whites, Indians have a lower prevalence of traditional risk factors (high blood pressure, high cholesterol, obesity, and smoking). The low prevalence of traditional risk factors among Indians is counterbalanced by a high prevalence of newly emerging risk factors, such as abdominal obesity, prediabetes, metabolic syndrome, high homocysteine and high lipoprotein(a) levels. These topics are discussed in Chapter III. In the next section, we will therefore take a closer look at cholesterol, the number-one risk factor for heart disease.

KEY · POINTS · IN · A · NUTSHELL

- ♥ Tobacco use, high blood pressure, high cholesterol, and low HDL are the major traditional risk factors for heart disease.
- ♥ Smokers get heart attacks 10 years earlier than nonsmokers.
- ♥ Smoking reduces one's life expectancy by 20 years.
- ♥ Traditional risk factors explain most of the risk of heart disease in older people, but less so in younger individuals.
- ♥ When two or more risk factors are present, the risk is multiplicative, not additive. For example, cardiac risk rises 16-fold when two severe risk factors are present that would each contribute only a four-fold increase on its own.
- ♥ Risk factors tend to travel together as friends: Having multiple cardiac risk factors is more common than having just one.
- ♥ A family history of premature heart disease is a strong indicator of genetic factors which predispose one to developing premature heart disease.

♥ Premature heart disease in a sibling is an even stronger risk factor than parental or grand-parental history.

♥ Diabetes is now considered more than a risk factor: it has been upgraded to a heart disease risk-equivalent.

2.3 ▶ Cholesterol: The Arch-villain of Atherosclerosis

Differences in cholesterol levels best explain international differences in heart disease rates except for the *rates in India, France, and Finland.* Many people consider cholesterol levels below 200 mg/dL to be a desirable and acceptable level and fail to recognize that, for example, one-third all heart attacks among Americans and one-half of heart attacks among Indians occur at these levels of cholesterol. Total cholesterol consists of HDL, the good cholesterol, LDL or bad cholesterol, and VLDL or ugly cholesterol. Whereas LDL and VLDL produce plaque build-up and heart disease, HDL actually removes cholesterol from the plaque and protects against heart disease. The non-HDL cholesterol contains LDL, VLDL, IDL and lipoprotein(a) and is a better predictor of cardiovascular risk than either LDL or total cholesterol level. This Chapter addresses the crucial role of total cholesterol, LDL, and non-HDL cholesterol in heart disease.

Cholesterol level is the central component of dyslipidemia, which refers to all the abnormalities that involve cholesterol and triglycerides, which are transported in the blood as HDL, LDL, and VLDL. Lipoprotein(a) and IDL are other important lipoproteins and are discussed in Chapters III and VII. Cholesterol is a soft, waxy substance found in the bloodstream and in every cell of the human body. A small amount of cholesterol is necessary for the healthy functioning of the cells, the formation of cell membranes (outer coats), and the production of bile acids that digest food. The liver produces all the cholesterol the body needs?in fact, three times the amount of cholesterol consumed in a normal diet per day. Many foods, particularly animal foods and saturated fats, can raise cholesterol to dangerous levels, resulting in heart disease and stroke.

Dyslipidemia (pronounced disslippy DEEMyuh) means your lipids are out of balance and not working properly. The prefix "dys" just means not working properly, as in the word dysfunctional. Your lipids are your HDL cholesterol, LDL cholesterol, and triglycerides. You need to have the right balance of HDL, LDL and triglycerides in order not to trigger plaque formation in your blood vessels.

Cholesterol and heart disease

The explosive increase in the knowledge of the crucial role of cholesterol in heart disease began with studies of heart attacks in two small children: a six-year-old boy and his eight-year-old sister, neither of whom had any risk factors other than a cholesterol level of more than 500 mg/dL. Michael Brown and Joseph Goldstein were awarded the Nobel Prize in Medicine in 1985 for unraveling the genetic basis of elevated cholesterol among these children. Although the early focus was on genetic forms of dyslipidemia with which one is born, research has now shifted to mass dyslipidemia promoted by an unhealthy lifestyle. Pioneering research by Ancel "Mr. Cholesterol" Keys, who passed away at age 100, and Dr. Jeremiah Stamler, still going strong at age 85, popularized the link between heart disease and elevated cholesterol levels resulting from an unhealthy lifestyle. Current evidence shows that more than 90% of the elevated cholesterol seen in people with and without heart disease is due to lifestyle factors, particularly a diet rich in **calories and saturated fat.**

It is estimated that a 10% reduction in cholesterol level in the entire nation, achievable through dietary modification, would result in a 30% reduction of heart disease. In fact, over the past three decades the US has indeed achieved such a reduction in cholesterol, from 230 to 200 mg/dL, a change which is responsible for about one-third of the reduction in heart disease rates in the US.

Cholesterol levels in young childhood predict development of heart disease in midlife. The relationship between cholesterol levels and heart attacks is present at all ages, but is strongest in people below 40 years old. In a 25-year long-term study of 11,017 men aged 18 to 39 years, those with cholesterol levels above 280 had a 16-fold increase in heart disease deaths compared to those with a level of below 160. (See Figure 2.2 *Age adjusted death rate as function of cholesterol levels*). The risk of death in young adults doubles with every 40 mg/dL increase in total cholesterol levels, beginning with 160 mg/dL in the US and 120 mg/dL in China. A long-term study of more than 3,000 Finnish businessmen 30 to 40 years old who were followed for 39 years showed that a low cholesterol level in midlife not only predicted survival but also a better quality of life in old age.

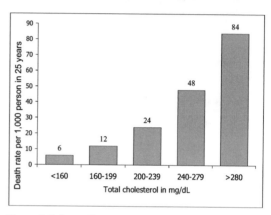

Figure 2.2. **Age adjusted death rate per 1,000 as a function of cholesterol levels in people below 40 years of age.** Note that the death rate doubles for every 40 points increase in cholesterol level, beginning with 160 mg/dL. The age adjustment is performed by making a correction for the fact that death rates increase naturally with age. Source: Stamler, J. Ref. 2.49.

Ethnic differences in cholesterol levels

Average total cholesterol levels vary markedly among different populations. In sub-Saharan Africa and rural China, the average cholesterol levels are as low as 80 mg/dL. In the Seven Countries Study (in the 1970s, see Appendix B), cholesterol levels in Japan were found to range from 125 to 225, compared to 200 to 350 in Northern Europe and in the US. The prevalence of high cholesterol (more than 250 mg/dL) was 7% in Japan, 39% in the US, and 56% in Finland. The most important finding of the study was that the absolute risk of heart disease varied five-fold among these countries and correlated directly with differences in cholesterol level. No other risk factors explained the differences in heart disease rates. Even today, populations with low cholesterol levels, such as the Japanese, Chinese, Koreans and blacks (except in African-Americans) have very low rates of heart disease, despite having some of the highest rates of smoking and high blood pressure.

> **Did you know...**
> The risk of heart attack with among Northern Europeans with the cholesterol of 240, is higher than Southern Europeans with the a cholesterol level of 320. Like wise, the risk of a heart attack among Indians with a cholesterol of 240 is higher than American with a cholesterol of 320.

Ethnic differences in cardiac risk from high cholesterol

The *absolute* risk of heart disease from high cholesterol varies *five-fold among* populations—that is, for a given level of cholesterol, different populations have different absolute risk. For any given level of cholesterol, Chinese, Japanese and French have a lower risk of heart disease than Americans and Northern Europeans. For example, at a cholesterol level of 200, the absolute risk of heart disease is 30% higher among Northern Europeans, but 300% lower among Japanese in comparison to the Americans. Recent studies (2004) have also shown that at identical levels of risk factors and cholesterol levels, the risk of heart disease among Chinese is only one-third that of Americans. However, the *relative* risk of heart disease from high cholesterol is very similar in different populations—meaning that a similar increase in cholesterol level, results in a similar increase in the risk of heart disease, regardless of their ethnicity. Currently, about 20% of Americans have cholesterol levels more than 240 mg/dL in contrast to below 5% among the Chinese.

Even today, populations with low cholesterol levels—including Japanese, Chinese, Koreans and blacks except African-Americans— have very low rates of heart disease, even when they have some of the highest rates of smoking and high blood pressure.

Cholesterol levels among Indians

Total cholesterol levels among Indians, in general, are lower than those of the whites, but substantially higher than those of other Asians, such as Japanese and

Chinese. Total cholesterol levels in the UK are high by international standards (240 in the UK versus 200 in the US). In the UK, the total cholesterol levels among Indians are lower than those among the whites (215 versus 240). In contrast, in the US, the mean cholesterol level among Indian men is similar to that for White men, but it is higher in Indian women.

The average cholesterol level in urban India has increased by 30 mg/dL in the past 30 years, from 170 to 200. During the same period, the cholesterol level in the US decreased by 30 mg/dL from 230 to 200. As a result, cholesterol levels in India are now similar to that of the US. There are some regional differences: cholesterol levels are considerably higher in the state of Kerala where the mean level is about 230, compared to 200 in Rajasthan. Also 32% of people in Kerala had cholesterol measuring more than 240 mg/dL, compared to 18% in the US. This is also true among doctors in Kerala.

Table 2.4. Heart attack and/or deaths per 1000 over 10 years, among high-risk European men with high blood pressure and smoking

		Heart attack or death per 10 years	
	Total cholesterol	Southern Europe	Northern Europe
Age 40	160 mg per dL	29	51
	240 mg per dL	48	84
	320 mg per dL	77	135
Age 60	160 mg per dL	87	193
	240 mg per dL	137	288
	320 mg per dL	288	407

Source: Menotti, A. Ref. 2.36. The risk of heart attack with amoung Northen Europeans with a cholesterol of 240 is higher than Southern Europeans with the a cholesterol level of 320.

Low cholesterol does not produce cancer

Many people fear that cholesterol that is too low can lead to cancer. Nothing could be further from the truth. It is well-known that many cancers cause unintentional weight loss, but planned healthy weight loss does not produce cancer. Similarly, undetected cancer is an important cause of low cholesterol, but it does not work the other way round: low cholesterol never produces cancer. If, however, your cholesterol levels drop dramatically without specific interventions, you should immediately contact your physician and get evaluated for cancer. In my practice, I have seen several individuals, including physicians, who had an unexplained drop in blood cholesterol level, and all were found to have cancer. The cholesterol levels usually rebound upon successful treatment and remission of the cancer. To summarize: low cholesterol may *indicate* the presence of cancer. Lowering your cholesterol level, however, never *produces* cancer.

High, desirable, and optimum cholesterol levels

There is a direct relationship between blood cholesterol level and heart disease that is graded and continuous - the higher the cholesterol level, the more likely it is that one will develop heart disease. However, to separate abnormal levels requiring medical attention and treatment from low-risk categories, medical authorities have established some "cut points": For most of the 20th century, 330 mg/dL was considered normal or acceptable. In 1987, the Adult Treatment Panel of the NIH National Cholesterol Education Program (NCEP ATP I) lowered the cut point for high cholesterol from 330 to 240. A cholesterol level of 200 to 239 was defined as borderline high, and below 200 as desirable. Since 1987, however, many people, including physicians, have neglected to pay attention to three succeeding NCEP ATP guidelines. These guidelines have brought the optimum LDL level to as low as 40 mg/dL (to be explained shortly), which corresponds to a total cholesterol less than 120 mg per dL. Taken together, these guidelines have reduced the cut-points for high cholesterol by more than 200 points (from 330 to below 120) in less than 20 years. They may very well go lower in the future.

Did you know...
At any given level of cholesterol, Indians have at least double the rate of heart disease compared to whites. This appears to be due to low levels of HDL, high levels lipoprotein(a) and other lipoprotein abnormalities commonly found in this population. A 2005 British study found that **adding 108 to the cholesterol** value obtained from the blood test may provide a better estimate for heart disease risk among Indians in that country.

Although total cholesterol below 200 mg per dL is still considered desirable by many, as 30% of heart attacks among Americans and 50% of heart attacks occur among Indians who have this level. Furthermore, this value is too high for many Americans, such as those with diabetes and/or heart disease, as explained above. This is certainly true for the vast majority of Indians, with or without diabetes or heart disease, even though many Indians take comfort when their total cholesterol level is below 200, feeling that they are in the safe zone. No one should take comfort in having cholesterol below 200, any more than they should feel complacent about a systolic blood pressure below 200 or a blood sugar below 200 mg/dL. The 2004 NCEP Guidelines have set optimum LDL at 40 mg/dL. An LDL 40 corresponds to a total cholesterol of 120. Currently, no one is required to keep the LDL this low, but people with heart disease and diabetes should maintain an LDL below 70, which corresponds to a cholesterol level below 150 mg/dL. The real risk of heart disease is reflected more in the levels of LDL and non-HDL cholesterol than total cholesterol.

Lipoproteins: The Good, the Bad, and the Ugly

Not all cholesterol is created equal. Studies over the past 20 years have clearly confirmed that cholesterol contains both atherogenic (bad) LDL and anti-atherogenic (good) HDL. The risk of heart disease comes from high levels of atherogenic lipoproteins. HDL actually protects you from heart disease. The challenge Mother Nature faces everyday is to send fat through blood; the two are mutually repellant, like oil and water. Blood is water-based; fat is essentially oil. The solution to this challenge is to "package" the fat in tiny "suitcases" called lipoproteins, which are tiny particles containing cholesterol, triglycerides, and proteins that allow fat to be carried around in the blood. There are several types of **lipoproteins,** specifically:

> **Did you know…**
> Cholesterol is a necessary and sufficient risk factor for heart disease. Necessary – because people do not get heart attack without some elevation in cholesterol level. Sufficient – because people get heart attack, even in the absence of other risk factors, when its levels are markedly elevated.

• High-density lipoprotein (HDL) cholesterol or "**good cholesterol**" (see section 4).
• Low-density lipoprotein (LDL) cholesterol or "**bad cholesterol**"
• Very low density lipoprotein (VLDL) cholesterol or "**ugly cholesterol**" (See Chapter VI, Section 4).

LDL cholesterol

Although earlier studies looked at the association of cholesterol with heart disease, the risk of developing heart disease is primarily borne by LDL cholesterol, which is the true cholesterol villain that clogs up the arteries and the most important determinant of heart disease the world over. For the sake of simplicity, the term LDL is used to reflect LDL cholesterol. LDL usually accounts for 60% of your total cholesterol.

The amount of LDL required for cellular functions is just 2.5 mg/dL in a cell, and possibly 25 mg/dL in blood. Clearly, millions of people have far more than that. It is this excess amount that is associated with the development of plaques, resulting in heart attack, stroke, and other coronary diseases. We are not born with high LDL. Newborns all over the world have an LDL below 40 mg/dL, but our LDL levels rise gradually in childhood depending primarily on how much saturated fat we eat. Once the LDL level exceeds 50 mg/dL, it begins to be deposited inside the coronary arteries and other arteries, laying a foundation for future heart disease. Oxidation of LDL is a necessary step before it can initiate plaque build-up. Antioxidants present in fresh fruit and vegetables but not antioxidant vitamin supplements, can prevent the oxidation of LDL and plaque buildup. (See Chapter VIII section 3).

Patients with genetic forms of high cholesterol maintaining and LDL 500 to 1,000 mg/dL have been documented to have suffered a heart attack as early as **18 months of age.**

LDL subclasses

LDL particles can now be fractionated into large, small, and intermediate-sized particles. Although high triglycerides per se are not atherogenic—that is, bad for you—elevated triglycerides makes the LDL smaller, denser, and therefore more dangerous (see Chapter VII Section 2).

Non-HDL cholesterol—a better risk predictor than LDL

Non-HDL cholesterol is obtained by subtracting the protective HDL from total cholesterol. Non-HDL cholesterol level, therefore, reflects the total burden of atherogenic (bad) lipoproteins, including lipoprotein(a), LDL, and VLDL. Furthermore, non-HDL cholesterol assessment is inexpensive, readily available, and does not require a fasting lipid profile. This topic is discussed in greater detail in Section 4. The interrelationship between cholesterol, triglycerides, HDL, LDL, VLDL, and non-HDL cholesterol is as follows:

Total cholesterol = VLDL+LDL+HDL
Non-HDL cholesterol = VLDL+LDL (i.e., everything except the HDL)
LDL= Total cholesterol – (VLDL + HDL)

> **Tid bits**
> Every 100 mg/dL increase in triglycerides results in a 20 mg/dL decrease in LDL, leading to a substantial underestimation of risk. The non-HDL cholesterol reflects the true risk in people with high triglycerides.

Both VLDL and LDL are calculated and not directly measured. Only total cholesterol and HDL are directly measured. VLDL is calculated as 20% of triglycerides (when triglycerides are below 400 mg/dL). As the triglycerides level increases, the VLDL level increases with a corresponding decrease in LDL levels. For example, every 100 mg/dL increase in triglycerides results in a 20 mg/dL increase in VLDL, with a corresponding 20 mg per dL decrease in LDL. In other words, high levels of triglycerides artificially lower your LDL readings, leading to a substantial underestimation of your heart disease risk.

This artificial lowering of LDL gives a false sense of security to both patients and doctors. This problem is particularly important for many Indians who have high triglyceride levels. The true risk is reflected in non-HDL cholesterol. A non-HDL cholesterol of less than 100 mg/dL would correspond to an LDL of less than 70. This would be considered a reasonable goal for Indians who are wants to prevent a second heart attack. (See Chapter V Sections 1 for detailed discussion). A non-HDL cholesterol of less than 130 can be recommended for Indians without heart disease or diabetes.

KEY · POINTS · IN · A · NUTSHELL

- ♥ Differences in cholesterol levels best explain the differences in heart disease rates that we see among most countries, except rates in India, France, and Finland.
- ♥ The likelihood of dying from heart disease in young people doubles with every 40 points increase in total cholesterol.
- ♥ Cholesterol levels among Indians are generally similar to whites, but are higher than for other Asians.
- ♥ For any given level of cholesterol, the risk of heart disease among Indians appears to be double that of other populations taken together.
- ♥ This means that the optimal level of cholesterol among Indians—the amount of cholesterol that is safe for them—is lower than for other populations.
- ♥ For example, Indians with a cholesterol level of 200 are about as likely to get a heart attack as whites with a cholesterol level of 300.
- ♥ The optimum level of LDL is 40 mg/dL; this corresponds to a total cholesterol level of 110 to 120.
- ♥ While no one is required to maintain an LDL of 40 mg/dL, an LDL below 70 mg/dL and non-HDL cholesterol less than 100 mg/dL is recommended for high risk people such as those with heart disease and diabetes.
- ♥ Non-HDL cholesterol greater than 100 mg/dL may be a better predictor of cardiac risk among Indians than an LDL cholesterol of more than 70.
- ♥ Having low levels of cholesterol does not make you get cancer, but a precipitous drop in your cholesterol level may indicate its presence.

2.4 ► HDL: The Body Armor Against Heart Disease

"It is much healthier for you to have low levels of total cholesterol in your blood." True or false? The answer is, it depends—on what that total cholesterol is made up of, and what the internal ratios of its components are. Any knowledgeable cardiologist would almost always take high total cholesterol and high HDL over low total cholesterol and low HDL. Why is that? You will learn the answer to that in this section.

HDL cholesterol, or simply HDL, is called "good" cholesterol because having a high level of it protects against the possibility of heart disease and heart attack. HDL carries excess cholesterol from the inner linings of your artery walls to the liver, where it is broken down and flushed out of your body. The more HDL you have, the more effectively it does this janitorial work. By removing the excess cholesterol, high HDL levels slow down plaque build-up and can even reverse it. Other benefits of high HDL include protection against inflammation, excessive blood clot formation, and **LDL oxidation** (which is a crucial step in the formation of plaque). In the Framingham Heart Study (see Appendix B), the HDL levels among the participants had the strongest relationship to the prevalence of heart disease in them, compared to all the other lipoproteins. In other words, having a high level of good cholesterol seems even more important than having low LDL (the bad cholesterol). Furthermore, having an HDL level that is too low is more common than having LDL that is too high. Low HDL is as important a risk factor as high LDL in every population. Among Indians, low HDL is if anything even more critical than for other populations. This section discusses the important role of low HDL in the presence and severity of heart disease, particularly among the Indian population.

The amount of junk in your house depends on two things—or more precisely, two rates: How fast it accumulates, and how quickly it is taken out. When the first rate is greater than the second, junk builds. Similarly, the development of plaque in your arteries depends not only on the rate at which LDL is entering the arterial wall, but also on the rate at which it is removed from the arterial wall. When the incoming cholesterol exceeds the outgoing cholesterol, the cholesterol is retained and the plaque grows. The quantity and the quality of your HDL determine how quickly cholesterol is taken out of your arteries, whereas your LDL level determines how quickly plaque buildup occurs. The two rates together determine whether you will experience plaque regression (good health) or plaque progression (danger); see Chapter VII Section 7).

The magnitude of risk of heart disease from low HDL is greater than that from high LDL, and twice as high as the risk of developing heart disease from high blood pressure. Cardiac risk increases four-fold with low HDL, compared to two-fold with hypertension. The risk is particularly high when the two conditions coexist. For example, among patients with high blood pressure, the risk of developing a heart attack is six-fold when their HDL is below 43 mg/dL, compared to two-fold when their HDL is above 43 (see section 5). Similarly, the risk from low HDL is further increased when high triglycerides and/or high cholesterol are present.

Low HDL and heart attack

High LDL levels are more important for the early development of atherosclerosis, whereas low HDL is more important in eventually producing coronary events such as heart attacks and death. In the Physicians Health Study (appendix A), among men with total cholesterol below 212, the risk of a first heart attack increased three-fold when their HDL was below 47, compared to those with HDL above 47. Japanese have low levels of total

The dangers of low HDL
• Premature heart attack and stroke.
• Rapid progression of atherosclerosis.
• Increased risk of recurrent heart attack and stroke.
• Increased risk of cardiovascular death.
• Increased risk of left main and three-vessel disease, necessitating coronary bypass surgery.
• Increased risk of restenosis following coronary angioplasty and stent.
• Increased risk of heart attack and death following bypass surgery.

cholesterol and high levels of HDL, which also means that their total cholesterol to HDL (TC/HDL) ratio is low. In a large Japanese study involving nearly 6,500 middle-aged men with average total cholesterol of 200, the risk of a first heart attack was four-fold higher in those with low HDL (below 48) than in persons with high HDL (above 65). Recurrent coronary events are nearly twice as common in patients with low HDL as in those with normal HDL. In one study, 75% of those with low HDL had coronary events compared to 45% with normal HDL. In the Framingham Heart Study, those with HDL below 40 had the highest risk of heart attack, irrespective of their total cholesterol level (*see* Figure **2.3**.) Conversely those who had HDL above 60 had the lowest risk of heart disease even when cholesterol level was high.

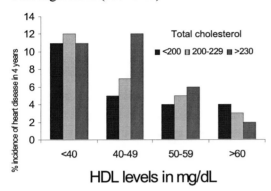

Figure 2.3. Incidence of heart attack as a function of total cholesterol (TC) and HDL in the Framingham Heart Study. Note that people with HDL below 40 mg/dL had the highest rate of disease, regardless of their total cholesterol level. Such low levels of HDL are particularly common among Indians and contribute to their high rates of heart disease. Source: Castelli, WP. Ref. 2.09. *Reproduced with permission©* American Medical Association.

In the Heart Protection Study (see Appendix B), the risk of a heart attack in people with HDL below 35 was higher than those with LDL above 135. In general, a 10 mg/dL decrease in HDL raises cardiac risk by the same amount as a 30 mg/dL increase in LDL. For example, a 10% decrease in HDL level leads to a 30-40% increase in the risk of developing and dying from heart disease, compared to only a 10% increase in risk for a 10% increase in LDL. Low HDL is also a strong predictor of recurrent events. The dangers of low HDL are summarized in the box.

HDL and longevity

Approximately 25% of the variation in the human lifespan is inheritable and HDL is one of those markers. HDL is truly the "elixir of life" and high levels of it are generally associated with exceptional longevity. Having high HDL is as good as having a grandmother overseeing the growth and nutrition of the g randchildren. In the Lipid Research Clinic Follow-up Study (See Appendix B), a 1 mg/dL increase in HDL was associated with a decrease in cardiovascular death of 4% in men and 5% in women over the five-year period. Furthermore, among men who also had heart disease at the beginning of the study, the risk of cardiac mortality was six-fold higher among those with HDL below 35, compared to those with HDL above 45.

Low, high and optimum HDL

An HDL less than 40 is considered low by National Cholesterol Education Program (NCEP) Guidelines (see Appendix B). However, the desirable level may be much higher in both men and women. In the Framingham Heart Study, the optimum HDL was 65; people with this level and above had the lowest risk of heart disease. The risk increased two-fold at HDL below 45 mg/dL and four-fold at HDL below 25.

Gender and ethnic differences in HDL

Is very high HDL good for you?
High HDL is highly protective against heart disease in people who exercise regularly such as marathon runners. In some populations, however especially in the people of Japanese origin very high HDL (75 to 100) is associated with less protection and even higher risk. This paradox has been attributed to their having a dysfunctional kind of HDL that may be the result of mutations in certain genes (the CETP gene).

The mean level of HDL cholesterol for American adults is 51 mg/dL with significant differences by gender and ethnicity. HDL levels remain the same in men throughout life but decrease in women after menopause. In general, HDL levels are about 10 mg/dL higher in women than in men, except for Indians among whom HDL levels are low in both men and women. HDL *below 50* is considered low in women, compared to *below 40* in men. Although HDL above 60 is considered high in both men and women, approximately 20% of the women who have heart attacks have HDL levels above 60. This clearly indicate that the optimal protective level of HDL may be much higher in women. The ARIC study (see Appendix B) showed a five-fold risk of heart attack among women with HDL below 40, compared to women with HDL above 80. (*See* Figure 2.4. *Rising risk of heart disease with decreasing HDL levels in women*).

HDL levels are 20 points higher in Japanese and 10 points higher in blacks than whites. In Turkish people, HDL levels are 10-15mg/dL lower than those of Europeans and Americans. HDL below 40 is found in 75% of men and 50% of women in Turkey.

Indians and dysfunctional HDL

HDL levels are approximately 10 points lower among Indians than whites. Approximately half of Indian men and two-thirds of Indian women have low HDL. Low HDL is three times more common among Indian women than women of any other ethnic origins in the US. Indians also have qualitative abnormalities of HDL that make their HDL less protective against heart disease. For example, at a given level of HDL, Indians have much smaller amounts of the cardioprotective large HDL and more of the less-cardioprotective small HDL particles. In addition to this skewed mix of large and small, the overall HDL particle size is unusually small and thus provides less cardiac protection, even when the person's HDL levels are not low (see Chapter VII Section 2). Approximately 60% of men and 40% of women with heart disease have low HDL values.

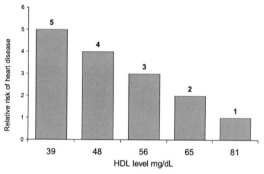

Figure 2.4. **Rising risk of heart disease with decreasing HDL levels in women.** Note the five-fold difference in risk in women with HDL 39, compared to those with HDL 81. Source: Sharrett, AR. Ref. 2.48. *Reproduced with permission*© Lippincott Williams & Willkins.

Low HDL is more common than high LDL

Among patients with premature heart disease, low HDL appears to be two to three times more common than high LDL. Among the 8,500 patients with heart disease screened for the VA HIT Study (see Appendix B), 63% had HDL below 40, compared to 13% with LDL above 160. In another study, 80% of women with heart disease had HDL below 45. Thus, depending on the gender and the particular cut-points used, low HDL may be present in more than half the patients with heart disease. The prevalence of low HDL is as high as *75 %* among people with heart disease and desirable cholesterol (below 200).

> **Did you know...**
> The risk of heart disease is twice as high among people with LDL of 100 but HDL of only 25 compared to those with LDL of 220 and HDL of 80.

Isolated low HDL refers to a situation in which low HDL is accompanied by normal levels of total cholesterol and triglycerides. Most people, and even some physicians, fail to realize the heightened risk of heart disease with isolated low HDL. An example will make this clear: The risk of heart disease is twice as high among people with LDL of 100 but HDL of only 25, compared to those with LDL of 220 and HDL of 80. The second group has much higher total cholesterol, but because their HDL is four times as high, they are at much lower risk. The risk is particularly high among diabetics and women.

Low HDL and severity of heart disease

Most patients and doctors fail to recognize the importance of low HDL particularity when the LDL level is low. Low HDL levels correlate highly with severity and extent of plaque burden irrespective of the LDL levels. The severity of disease in persons with low LDL and low HDL is *similar* to those who have high LDL and high HDL. In one study, the severity of heart disease was similar among those with LDL below 110 mg per dL and HDL below 30 mg per dL compared to those with LDL above 160 mg per dL and HDL above 45 mg per dL. Low HDL is also related to plaque progression, and the number of heart attacks.

Low HDL and the need for coronary angioplasty and bypass surgery

Although high LDL is strongly related to development of heart disease, it is not related to development of restenosis following coronary angioplasty or bypass surgery. In sharp contrast, low HDL is a *strong predictor* of the total number of diseased coronary arteries. In one study, the risk of three-vessel disease increased progressively with decreasing levels of HDL. Low HDL is a powerful predictor of both triple-vessel disease and left main coronary disease that require bypass surgery and may account for the high rate of left main and three-vessel disease observed in Indians. Low HDL levels correlate highly with the development of atherosclerosis in the bypass graft and with long-term survival. In one study, the 10-year survival rate following bypass surgery was less than half (38% versus 89%) in those with HDL above 39, compared with HDL below 39.

Low HDL is a powerful predictor of **restenosis** (renarrowing of a coronary artery) following coronary angioplasty, leading to repeat angioplasty or bypass surgery. In one study, the restenosis rate was nearly four times higher (64% versus 17%) in patients with HDL below 40 than in those with HDL above 40. The risk is markedly increased when lipoprotein(a) is elevated (see Chapter III Section 1).

Low HDL and stroke

Low HDL is a strong predictor of carotid stenosis (the narrowing by plaque of the carotid artery that supplies blood to the brain) as well as stroke. In one study, four times as many people with HDL below 40 had carotid stenosis as those with HDL above 58. In a 2005 study involving more than 7,500 people, a low HDL was a stronger predictor of stroke than high LDL. Each 10-point increase in HDL conferred a 14% reduction in stroke risk. It appears that the risk of stroke attributed to LDL may depend on the patient's HDL level.

Low HDL and metabolic syndrome

Low HDL is not only a component but also a strong predictor of metabolic syndrome .The other components of metabolic syndrome are elevated triglycerides, prediabetes, pre-hypertension and abdominal obesity (see Chapter III Section7).

Ratios involving HDL

The protective effects of high HDL as well as the magnifying effects of low HDL on total cholesterol, triglycerides, and lipoprotein(a) are reflected in various ratios. When your blood test results come back from the lab, it contains all the necessary information to calculate the various ratios. These ratios help determine how protective your HDL is against the harmful influence of high total cholesterol, high triglycerides, and high lipoprotein(a), or alternatively, how ineffective your low HDL level is against these other lipoproteins.

Even when all your other lipoprotein levels are normal, having low HDL confers a high risk of heart disease, because what doctors focus on is not just the absolute amount of any lipoprotein but rather the comparative ratio of your HDL level to the others. All the most clinically useful ratios therefore employ HDL in the denominator: In other words, we talk about your total cholesterol to HDL ratio, your triglyceride to HDL ratio, and your lipoprotein(a) to HDL ratio. The amount of HDL you have is ultimately what we compare all your other lipoproteins to.

> **Did you know...**
> The TC/HDL ratio captures the increased risk of heart disease from high cholesterol and low HDL. Many experts consider TC/HDL ratio to be a better predictor of heart disease than high LDL particularly in people whose cholesterol is below 240. A high TC/HDL ratio is more common among Indians than other populations and helps identify more high risk Indians for aggressive management of cardiac risk factors.

The total cholesterol to HDL ratio

This ratio allows identification of individuals with low total cholesterol and low LDL, who are at high risk because of low HDL. This ratio tells you about the opposing effects of total cholesterol and HDL. Total cholesterol/HDL ratio is a **stronger predictor** of heart disease than total cholesterol or HDL alone particularly among those with cholesterol below 240 (most Indians). The TC/HDL ratio is closely related to the presence, extent, and severity of heart disease, especially in those without high total cholesterol. The severity of heart disease is particularly high when the TC/HDL ratio is elevated.

At any given TC/HDL ratio, cardiac risk is greater in women than men. The 2004 Canadian guidelines for the treatment of cholesterol have incorporated TC/HDL ratio in their risk prediction model. The US Guidelines have not incorporated this TC/HDL ratio but incorporates both total cholesterol and HDL in the Framingham Risk Prediction Model. A TC/HDL ratio of below three is optimum, four may be considered acceptable. A TC/HDL ratio *above five* can identify those who are at high risk. Most Americans who have had a heart attack have a ratio of five or more. A TC/HDL ratio over six signifies very high risk, particularly when your total cholesterol level is in the 140-240 range. This level of risk is similar to that of people with a cholesterol of 360 and HDL of 60. The average TC/HDL ratio is 4.5 in the US a ratio that is associated with a three-fold rise in the risk of heart attack among diabetic patients who have low LDL, and a four-fold rise among diabetics who have high LDL levels.

Table 2.5. The cardiovascular risk according to total cholesterol /HDL ratio

TC/HDL ratio	Risk	Risk of heart Comments
Less than 3	Optimum	Typically seen in Western but not Indian vegetarians. Usual ratio of marathon runners and word class athletes
Less than 4	Acceptable	Typically seen among Chinese, Japanese and blacks; typical ratio among white women
4 to 6	Two-fold	Average ratio at the time of heart attack among Americans. Typically found among Indians without heart disease. Three-fold risk in people with diabetes and low HDL. Four-fold risk in people with diabetes and high LDL
6 to 8	Four-fold	Typical ratio among Indians with heart disease or diabetes
More than 8	Six-fold	Typical ratio among Indians with heart disease and diabetes

Although total cholesterol levels among Indians are similar to or lower than whites, more than half of Indians have a high TC/HDL ratio. In the CADI study of Indian physicians a TC/HDL ratio above five was four times more common among them than high LDL. For example, a TC/HDL ratio above five was found in 60% of the Indian physicians, but only 14% had an LDL above 160. Another study of young Indian physicians (medical residents) showed an average TC/HDL ratio of 5.5, versus 4.6 in White physicians. Thus, a high TC/HDL ratio is more common among Indians and helps identify more high-risk Indians for aggressive management. TC/HDL ratio is consistently high in Indians than other populations in several countries.

Among the various clinical trials, which tested the benefit of lowering LDL with statin medications, changes in TC/HDL ratio was a better predictor of benefit from this treatment than changes in either LDL or HDL levels by themselves. In many of these statin trials, participants who had low HDL levels experienced greater benefits than those who had higher HDL levels.

Table 2.6. total cholesterol /HDL ratio by Ethnicity in the US, UK, and India

		Men	women
UK	whites	4.2	3.5
	blacks	3.5	3.3
	Chinese	4.0	3.3
	Indian	4.2	3.5
	Pakistan	4.7	4.8
	Bangladeshi	4.8	4.8
US	whites	4.4	3.7
	blacks	3.8	3.5
	Hispanics	4.3	3.8
	Indians	6.2	5.8
	Indian Physicians	5.2	5.0
India	All	4.9	4.9

The triglyceride to HDL ratio—the poor man's test for small dense LDL

As we have already discussed earlier, small dense LDL is more harmful, and small HDL is less protective against heart disease than its larger counterparts. Usually expensive tests are used to determine the size of these particles. However, the triglyceride/HDL ratio, a good predictor of small dense HDL can be obtained from a simple and inexpensive lipid profile without any additional cost. A ratio of more than three, especially when accompanied by triglycerides above 130 mg/dL, signifies the presence of small dense LDL, which is associated with a three-fold relative risk of heart disease at all levels of LDL. Conditions that produce small dense LDL, such as high triglycerides, also produce small dense HDL. This ratio has also been found to be a strong predictor of heart-attack in a Harvard study. Individuals with high triglycerides by HDL ratio derive maximal benefit from exercise and lifestyle changes, even when they are not overweight.

The lipoprotein(a) to HDL ratio

In the FATS study (see Appendix B), the ratio of lipoprotein(a) to HDL was the strongest predictor of the severity of heart disease as well as of the progression of heart disease in patients who were being treated aggressively with multiple medications. This ratio may prove to be a very important predictor of heart attack among young Indians.

KEY · POINTS · IN · A · NUTSHELL

- ♥ Low HDL is defined as a level below 40 mg/dL in men and below 50 in women.
- ♥ Low HDL confers a two to three-fold high risk of heart attack, even in the absence of elevated total cholesterol level.
- ♥ Low HDL is two to three times more common than high LDL in people with premature heart disease.
- ♥ Among people with heart disease, low HDL is found in half of all patients and three-fourth of those with cholesterol below 200 mg/dL.
- ♥ A 10-point decrease in HDL has the same effect on cardiac risk as a 30-point increase in LDL.
- ♥ Low HDL correlates strongly with the severity of heart disease, the need for bypass surgery, and restenosis following angioplasty and bypass surgery.
- ♥ Approximately half of Indian men and two-thirds of Indian women have low HDL.
- ♥ Indians also have qualitative abnormalities of HDL (small-size HDL) that make their HDL less protective against heart disease.
- ♥ The optimum HDL appears to be at least 20 mg/dL higher than the currently prescribed cut-points, particularly among Indians.
- ♥ A high TC/HDL ratio is three to four times more common than high LDL among Indians and help identify high-risk Indians.

2.5 ▶ High Blood Pressure – The Silent Killer

High blood pressure is literally the force exerted as blood pumps into the arteries through the circulatory system and as the arteries resist the flow of blood. Like the water pressure exerted against the wall of a garden hose connected to a sprinkler system, which consists of one or two pulses a second with a rest period in between, your blood pressure is really made up of two different numbers: The higher number, or the systolic pressure, is the maximal pressure exerted against the arterial wall when your left ventricle contracts and fills your arteries with blood. The lower number, or the diastolic pressure, measures the blood pressure in between beats, when the left ventricle relaxes for a moment in order to refill with blood. The lifetime risk of developing hypertension at some point is more than 90%.

Hypertension is the medical term for high blood pressure. An optimum blood pressure **level is less than 120/80 mm Hg**; a blood pressure of 120-139 systolic or 80-89 diastolic is called prehypertension (see Table 2.6). Above 140 systolic or 90 diastolic, you have hypertension. Two in three Americans have either prehypertension or hypertension, making it the most common cardiovascular disease. High blood pressure, all by itself, does not often cause a heart attack. The risk of a heart attack among people with hypertension increases markedly when other cardiac risk factors, such as high triglycerides, high LDL and low HDL (that are very common in Indians).

The lifetime risk of developing hypertension at some point is more than 90%.

The lifetime risk of developing hypertension at some point is more than 90%. The risk of heart disease and stroke doubles with every 20-point increase in systolic pressure. The overall cardiac risk, compared to those with normal blood pressure, is two to four-fold, depending on the person's gender and number of other factors such as

Did You Know...
Beginning at a level of 115/75 mm Hg, every 20 point rise in systolic pressure is associated with a doubling of the risk for heart disease and stroke. It has been estimated that lowering everyone's systolic blood pressure to below 155 would reduce heart attacks by 50% and strokes by 60% and prevent seven million deaths annually worldwide.

cholesterol and smoking. It used to be thought that a high diastolic pressure (when the heart is relatively speaking at rest) was worse than a high systolic pressure (when the heart is working to pump out blood), because a high diastolic means that your heart is not resting well in between beats. In recent years, however, the emphasis has shifted from diastolic to systolic blood pressure, particularly in those older than 50. Approximately 30% of Indians and Americans have high blood pressure. This section reviews the importance of hypertension as a powerful cardiovascular risk factor. In this section, you will learn about optimum blood pressure, prehypertension, hypertension, white coat hypertension, ambulatory blood pressure monitoring, as well as the ethnic and in international differences in hypertension rates.

Hypertension is strongly related to stroke, heart failure and kidney failure but only weakly related to heart attack, in the absence of other risk factors. In addition, hypertension is also related to early-onset senility and dementia. Dementia results in forgetfulness, and the memory loss, commonly seen among older people is often due to multiple mini-strokes precipitated in part by high blood pressure. Kidney disease leading to dialysis is another dreaded complication of hypertension. In some individuals, kidney disease may, indeed, be the cause of high blood pressure. Of note, in more than 95% of cases, the cause of high blood pressure is unknown.

Optimum and high blood pressure

There has been a progressive lowering of the cut-point for the definition of hypertension. In the 1940s, President Franklin Delano Roosevelt had a blood pressure of 240/140, with kidney failure, heart failure, and multiple mini-strokes. Yet his blood pressure was considered "normal" and acceptable to many of the nation's foremost physicians who were treating him.

Prehypertension is defined as a systolic blood pressure between 120 to 139 mm Hg or a diastolic blood pressure between 80 to 89, or both. Approximately one-third of all adult Americans (65 million) have prehypertension, and another 65 million have hypertension. Patients with prehypertension are at twice the risk to develop hypertension and triple the risk of a heart attack as those with healthy blood pressure. Prehypertension is also associated with double the risk of stroke compared to those with normal blood pressure. The risk is double in blacks compared to whites at any given level of blood pressure. People with prehypertension requires health-promoting lifestyle modifications to prevent the development of true hypertension and cardiovascular complications.

High blood pressure seldom occurs in isolation and often tends to cluster with metabolic syndrome (See Chapter III, Section 7) and diabetes. This is particularly true for Indians. The risk from hypertension is magnified several fold in persons with diabetes, heart disease, and kidney disease, high triglycerides, and/or low HDL (See Table 2.8).

White coat hypertension

"White coat hypertension" refers to the temporary hypertension some people experience when their blood pressure is about to be taken at the doctor's office and they see the doctor's "white coat." Ironically, slim people who eat healthy food tend to have white-coat hypertension more often. Contrary to common belief, white coat hypertension is not entirely a harmless phenomenon. Newer research suggests that it may be an early indicator of cardiovascular disease. **Ambulatory**

Table 2.7 Classification of blood pressure

	Systoic (mm Hg)		Diastolic (mm Hg)
Normal	below 120	and	below 80
Prehypertension	120 to 139	or	80 to 89
Stage I hypertension	140 to 159	or	90 to 99
Stage II hypertension	Above 160	or	above 100

Note. Proactive action at the prehypertension stage can prevent the onset of hypertension and its complications.
Source: Chobanian, AV. Ref. 2.11.

blood pressure monitoring records the blood pressure for 24 hours, similar to 24-hour ECG monitoring. It is used to distinguish between white coat and true hypertension. A blood pressure above 135/85 on ambulatory monitoring (at home) is considered high, as opposed to above 140/90 in the clinic or hospital. Normally, blood pressure is 10 points lower during sleep than when awake. A smaller than normal fall during sleep is associated with a greater risk of stroke.

Table 2.8. Relative risk of a heart attack by blood pressure high triglycerides and low HDL

	Relative risk	
	Normal blood pressure	High blood pressure
Normal triglycerides	1	2
High triglycerides	3	4
Normal HDL	1	2
Low HDL	4	6

Source: Gaziano, JM. Ref..2.18.

Gender differences in high blood pressure

Over a 30-year period from ages 25 and 55, your blood pressure increases by about 16 points systolic and by nine points diastolic. The number of men with hypertension peaks between ages 45 and 54 and declines progressively thereafter. In contrast, the number of women with hypertension increases progressively with age. More women than men have hypertension—35 million versus 30 million men. The gender difference is even higher among those above 65 years (17 million women versus 10 million men). Most of the persons with hypertension (81%) are above 45 years of age.

Ethnic differences in high blood pressure

Table 2.9. Gender differences in the prevalence of high blood pressure by age in the US

	Men %	women
20-34	11	6
35-44	21	18
45-54	34	34
55-64	47	56
65-74	61	74
75+	69	83

Source: American Heart Association. Ref.1.01.

Hypertension is the most common cardiovascular disease, affecting 26% of the population worldwide. After many years of declining, incidence of hypertension has increased in the US - two million new cases of hypertension are diagnosed each year in the US alone. Between 1990 and 2000, the prevalence of hypertension increased from 23% to 30%. These trends are associated with increasing obesity and an aging population. The national goal (Healthy People 2010) calls for a reduction in the prevalence of hypertension from 30% to 16% by 2010. The number of Americans with high blood pressure has increased from 50 million to 65 million. (This increase was four-fold higher than population growth and reflects a true increase).

Hypertension rates vary by ethnicity, with blacks having the highest (41%), Hispanics the least (25%), with whites on the lower end (27%). Nearly one in two blacks over age 50 has hypertension. Hypertension is also more severe, malignant, and resistant to treatment in blacks. The prevalence of hypertension is 60% higher in European countries than in the US or Canada. Average blood pressure is about 10 points higher in European countries (136/83) than North America (127/77). This difference in blood pressure between Americans and Europeans are evident even among younger persons (35-39 years old) in whom treatment of hypertension is uncommon. This finding indicates that the difference in blood pressure between these countries are not due to differences in treatment.

Hypertension among Indians

Hypertension rates among overseas Indians are similar to or lower than those of whites in most countries. However, in the UK, prevalence of hypertension in Indians is two-fold higher than in whites and almost as high as in blacks. Indians in the UK also have higher morbidity and mortality from hypertension than whites, but lower than in blacks.

Hypertension is present in 25% of adults in urban India and 10% in rural India with wide regional differences (Table 2.9. In a study of 10,215 school children five to 14 years old in Delhi, the prevalence of hypertension was 12% in boys and 11% in girls. Hypertension control in India remains low,

Table 2.10 Prevalence of high blood pressure in different parts of India

City	Men	Women
Jaipur urban (1995)	30 %	33 %
Jaipur urban (2002)	36 %	37 %
Mumbai urban (1999)	44 %	45 %
Mumbai (executives 2000)	27 %	28 %
Thiruvananthapuram urban (2000)	31 %	36 %
Rajasthan rural (1994)	24%	7 %
Haryana (rural 1999)	5 %	5 %

Source: Gupta, R. Ref. 2.23.

as is true of much of the world. Most studies report that fewer than 10% of Indians with hypertension are taking steps to control their high blood pressure.

The next section will focus on the epidemic of diabetes with special attention to Indians. Diabetes is not only common, but intimately linked to heart disease.

KEY · POINTS · IN · A · NUTSHELL

- ♥ The optimum blood pressure level is below 120/80 mm Hg.
- ♥ Prehypertension is defined as a blood pressure of 120-139 systolic or 80-89 diastolic.
- ♥ Hypertension is defined as blood pressure above 140 mm Hg systolic or above 90 mm Hg diastolic.
- ♥ The lifetime risk of developing hypertension is above 90%.
- ♥ Blood pressure increases on an average of 16 points systolic from ages 25 to 55.
- ♥ The risk of heart disease and stroke doubles with every 20-point increase in systolic pressure.
- ♥ About 30% of Indians worldwide have hypertension, a rate similar to that of Americans.
- ♥ The cardiac risk from hypertension is markedly increased with the presence of other risk factors such as high cholesterol, high triglycerides, low HDL, smoking, and diabetes.

2.6 ▶ The Diabetes Epidemic among Indians

Diabetes is a chronic, incurable disease characterized by elevated blood sugar and lipids and an extremely high risk for heart disease and its complications. The link between diabetes and heart disease is so strong that some expert even refers to diabetes as heart disease with an accompanying elevated blood sugar level. Diabetes is the single most important metabolic disease, able to affect virtually every organ system in the body. Never have doctors known so much about how to prevent and control diabetes, yet an epidemic of diabetes is still currently raging. According to the most recent data, 6% of the US population, or 18 million Americans, have diabetes. Of these, five million—nearly one-third—are unaware that they even have the disease. Every year, one million Americans are newly diagnosed with diabetes; another 400,000 develop the condition for the first time but go undiagnosed. Thus, nearly half of patients with diabetes remain undiagnosed until they develop serious and irreversible damage to vital organs.

The Diabetes Equation

Abdominal Obesity

+ Sedentary Lifestyle

+ Over-consumption of white rice, white flour, sugar, & other refined carbohydrates

= High probability of developing diabetes

= Accelerated heart disease

If you are an American born in 2000, your lifetime risk for developing diabetes is now estimated to be more than one in three. If you are Indian, that risk appears to be at least one in two. Compared to other populations, diabetes is two to three times more common among Indians: one out of every three already has diabetes or prediabetes. Indians develop diabetes approximately 10 to 15 years earlier than other people and at a body weight 20 to 30 pounds less than whites. Abdominal obesity, a sedentary lifestyle, and excessive consumption of refined carbohydrates such as white flour and white sugar are the most important contributors. This section highlights the importance of diabetes as a major contributor to the excess burden of heart disease among Indians.

More than 90% of diabetes cases are Type 2 diabetes (to be discussed shortly). Unless otherwise specified, the term diabetes as used in this book refers to Type 2 diabetes. Diabetes requires lifelong monitoring and treatment to prevent complications and maintain quality and length of life. The elevated level of sugar in the blood results from your body's inability to properly regulate the production or use of insulin. In other words, diabetes is the result of defects in insulin secretion, insulin action, or both. The full name is diabetes mellitus, which literally means "sweet urine" in Latin. Elevated levels of blood glucose lead to its spillage into the urine, which makes it sweet. Indeed, in medieval India and other countries, tasting the patient's urine was the primary means of diagnosing diabetes. The severity of the diabetes was sometimes determined by counting the number of ants that gravitated toward the sweet urine.

Normally, blood glucose levels are maintained within a narrow range by two hormones, insulin and glucagon, both produced by the pancreas (an organ embedded deep in the abdomen, behind the stomach). After eating a hot fudge sundae, or any meal that has any carbohydrates in it, specialized cells called beta cells produce insulin which brings the level of sugar in the blood back to normal by breaking down the sugar. Glucagon, on the other hand, is produced by alpha cells to increase blood sugar levels and prevent it from falling dangerously low. Thus, the pancreas needs to be functioning properly to avoid either high or low blood sugar levels. Compared with non-diabetics, people with diabetes have a heightened risk for cardiac and non-cardiac complications, as shown in the box.

Let us briefly look at one of these complications. **Kidney damage** is one such dreaded complication. The risk of kidney damage increases in proportion to how long you have had your diabetes and is particularly common among those who have had it for 10 years or more. Diabetes is responsible for more than 50% of cases in which people with end-stage renal disease are on dialysis. A urine test for protein (microalbumin) can identify if you are at risk of kidney damage.

The price of diabetes

Diabetes is a medically expensive disease, partly because it has so many complications. The majority of diabetics, for example, are obese. Additionally, most diabetics have hypertension and/or dyslipidemia, each necessitating two or more medications. More than half of all diabetics are on at least three medications, and nearly one-third of diabetics are on at least five medications. Glucose monitoring and insulin therapy are also expensive. The overall medical cost of a diabetic patient is five times higher than a nondiabetic person.

Predicting diabetes

The causes of diabetes vary according to the type of diabetes, but several modifiable and non-modifiable risk factors for diabetes have been identified (Table 2.10). Lack of physical activity is one of the strongest predictors of diabetes. Both leisure-time and occupational physical activities have a protective role against diabetes (see Chapter VIII Section 8).

Diabetes and its Complications

Compared to being non-diabetic, the relative risk of developing a range of complications after becoming diabetic is very high. Here are some of the most common cardiac and non-cardiac complications:

- Two to four times more likely to have a heart attack
- Twice as likely to suffer a stroke
- Four times more likely to develop heart failure
- 17 times more likely to develop kidney disease
- 25 times more likely to develop blindness
- 300 to 400 times more likely to undergo amputation

Glycemic load

A high **glycemic load** refers to consumption of large quantities of sugar and other refined carbohydrates (discussed in greater detail in Chapter V Section 5). A growing body of evidence suggests that a high glycemic load increases several risks, including obesity, glucose intolerance, diabetes, dyslipidemia, and heart disease. Since about the 1950s, a sharp increase in consumption of refined carbohydrates, together with a decrease in fiber intake, has contributed to the epidemic of diabetes in the US. Not only did the per capita use of sweeteners increase 86% between 1909 and 1997, but also the type of sweeteners has changed dramatically. Corn syrup sweeteners, which were almost nonexistent at the turn of the last century, now comprise more than 20% of the total daily carbohydrate intake of Americans, and 10% of their total daily energy intake.

Table 2.11. Risk factors for diabetes

Modifiable lifestyle factors	Non-modifiable factors
• Obesity, particularly abdominal obesity • Prediabetes • High glycemic load • High saturated fat intake • High intake of trans fats • Physical inactivity • Metabolic syndrome • Hypertension • Urban lifestyle • Cigarette smoking	• Advancing age • Family history of diabetes • Spouse with diabetes • Delivery of a large baby (above eight pounds) • Polycystic Ovarian Syndrome • Non-White ethnicity, particularly Indian ethnicity

Soft drinks

In one study, women who consumed one or more sugar soft drinks (about 150 calories) gained significant weight and had a higher risk of developing diabetes. The researchers propose that it is both the high glycemic index of these beverages, as well as the weight gain that results from such high-calorie intake, that increases the risk of diabetes. Furthermore, soft drink consumption appears to be a marker for a more generally unhealthy lifestyle, with a higher likelihood of being sedentary, smoking, and eating a calorie-dense, fiber-poor diet. The implications of this study are tremendous and support the need to restrict the consumption of sugar-loaded soft drinks as well as encourage people, particularly younger people, to adopt increasingly healthier lifestyle choices.

Types of Diabetes

Type 1 diabetes

Type 1 diabetes, previously called juvenile diabetes or insulin-dependent diabetes, tends to strike during childhood. In Type 1 diabetes, the patient's pancreas produces absolutely no insulin. Type 1 sufferers therefore require multiple daily injections of insulin to survive. This condition is less associated with lifestyle changes.

Table 2.12. Different Types of diabetes

Types	Key aspects
Type 1	Typically diagnosed in children and thin adults. There is total destruction of beta cells, which cease insulin secretion
Type 2	Accounts for more than 90% of all diabetes. The primary defect is insulin resistance of the body's cells. To compensate, the pancreas secretes more and more insulin. There is galloping atherosclerosis and dyslipidemia up to 20 years before the person's blood sugar becomes elevated, which occurs with the beginning of beta cell failure. Type 2 diabetes is often caused by and responds to, lifestyle changes.
Type 2 in children and young adults	Almost unknown until 20 years ago, the incidence of Type 2 diabetes in children has risen 10-fold in the past decade. It now accounts for 10% of all diabetes in children and adolescents. Girls are twice as likely than boys to develop this condition.
Gestational	Diabetes is diagnosed during pregnancy. These women have a 5% chance of getting diabetes every subsequent year.
Pre-diabetes	Before people develop Type 2 diabetes, they almost always have "prediabetes" —blood glucose levels that are higher than normal (100 to 125 mg per dL) but not yet high enough to be diagnosed as full-blown diabetes.

Type 2 diabetes

Type 2, or adult-onset, diabetes is an effect of improper insulin usage, not production. The primary problem is the inability of the body's cells (primarily muscle and fat) to properly utilize insulin to break down sugar in the blood after a meal. This condition is known as *"insulin resistance."* As insulin resistance increases, the pancreas responds by producing more and more insulin for several decades to compensate for the insulin resistance of the body's cells and to keep the blood sugar from rising. Some Type 2 diabetics may have five to 10 times higher insulin levels than normal persons. This results in high triglycerides, low HDL, and galloping atherosclerosis. The risk of death is increased with increasing duration of diabetes; after 25 years, the risk is increased eight-fold among those with diabetes alone and 20-fold among those with diabetes and heart disease. Because of the overwhelming importance of this topic, an entire section is specifically allocated to it (see section 7).

Type 2 diabetes in children and young adults

The process of developing diabetes can begin even before you were born. The risk of developing diabetes at a young age increases exponentially when the following four factors are present - a low birth weight, childhood obesity, sedentary lifestyle and poor nutrition. Babies born to mothers who had gestational diabetes are prone to getting diabetes as a younger adult as well. These children have a greater decrease in insulin production capacity rather than increased insulin resistance.

Prediabetes

A meta-analysis of patient data has shown that the continuous relationship between blood sugar level and cardiovascular risk beginning with a blood sugar as low as 70 mg/dL, well below the range observed in diabetes or prediabetes.

According to 2004 estimates, 44 million Americans (30% of the population and 40% of those above 65 years) have prediabetes. What is it? Before people develop Type 2 diabetes, they almost always have "pre-diabetes." People with prediabetes have blood sugar levels higher than normal, but not yet high enough to be diagnosed as diabetes. Patients with prediabetes either have fasting glucose values from 100 to 125 mg/dL, or have glucose values from 140 to 199 mg/dL, measured two hours after a 75g glucose challenge test. The former is called impaired fasting glucose; the latter is called impaired glucose tolerance and is more common than the former.

Long-term damage to the body, especially the heart and circulatory system, begins during this long prediabetic stage, which usually lasts 10 to 20 years. Elevated fasting blood sugar, (usually obtained as part of routine blood tests such as a metabolic profile) predicts development of Type 2 diabetes. A metanalysis of patient data has shown that the continuous relationship between blood sugar level and cardiovascular risk beginning with a blood sugar as low as 70 mg/dL- well below the range observed in diabetes or prediabetes.

In the general American population, prediabetes usually develops between the ages of 40 and 60 years. The percentage of patients with prediabetes in whom overt diabetes develops is about 5% per year. In the Hispanic population, prediabetes typically develops earlier, between the ages of 20 and 30 years, and progresses to diabetes at a rate of 15% per year. The rate of progression from prediabetes to diabetes among Indians is not known, but likely to be similar to or higher than that of Hispanics. By making appropriate and intensive changes in lifestyle, you can prevent or delay the progression from prediabetes to diabetes by 60%.

Table 2.13. Age-adjusted prevalence of diagnosed diabetes in the US by ethnicity

	Men %	women
whites	6	5
blacks	10	13
Hispanics	10	11

Source: American Heart Association. Ref. 1.01.

Gestational diabetes

Gestational diabetes refers to *elevated blood sugar* diagnosed for the first time during pregnancy. Like heart disease, there is a correlation between diabetes and waist girth. Women whose waist size is above 32" have a three-to five-fold risk of developing gestational diabetes, which is associated with a high risk of complications, such as miscarriage and congenital abnormalities. In a European study involving more than 600,000 pregnant women, Indian women had a two-fold higher rate of diabetes before pregnancy and seven-fold higher rate of gestational diabetes, compared to other populations. Diabetes among them was associated with greater complications, including a three-fold higher risk of pre-term delivery. Women with gestational diabetes have a 50% risk of becoming diabetic within the next five to ten years (5% increased risk per year).

Diagnosis of diabetes

The three classic symptoms of diabetes are *polyuria* or too much urination, *polydipsia* or extreme thirst leading to excessive drinking of fluids, and *polyphagia,* or constant hunger leading to overeating. Currently, there is no justification to wait until all three symptoms develop to test for diabetes. Diagnosis of diabetes generally requires two blood glucose determinations on two different days. Fasting values of 126 mg/dL or above, and casual (random) values of 200 mg/dL or above, indicate diabetes. Efforts are currently underway to lower these cut-points to above 115 and above 180, respectively.

Diabetes among Indians

The propensity of diabetes in Indians abroad was first observed among Indians living in Fiji, Mauritius, US, Canada, Trinidad, Singapore and South Africa. The prevalence of diabetes among Indians in the US, UK and South Africa is as high as 16%. In one study in the UK, diabetes was found in 23% of Pakistanis, 26% of Bangladeshis, and 15% of Indians, compared to 5% in the white population. The prevalence of diabetes is particularly high after age 55 among Indians (See Table 2.14.) During the 1980s in the UK, mortality attributed to diabetes increased 23% among men, but 36% among men from the Indian subcontinent. The corresponding figures for women were 17% and 24%, respectively. Non-diabetic Indians have higher fasting blood glucose and AIC (a measure of the average blood sugar over the preceding three to four months) than whites after adjustment for cardiovascular risk factors, even when they are not known to be diabetic. This might suggest a higher proportion of prediabetics as well as undiagnosed diabetes.

Indians in Canada have higher rates of diabetes than the general population. In Singapore, about 15% of Indian adults have diabetes and another 15%

Table 2.14. The prevalence of diabetes in UK by ethnicity

	Men All ages	Men 55+	Women All ages	Women 55+
General population (%)	3	7	3	5
Indian (%)	10	19	7	15
Pakistani (%)	18	39	14	28
Bangladeshi (%)	19	31	15	26
Chinese (%)	5	16	5	12

Source: Heartstats.org. Ref. 2.25.

have prediabetes. Indians with diabetes are less prone to hypertension and renal complications than diabetic Chinese, but their risk of heart disease is substantially higher. A striking feature of diabetes among Indians is its lower age of onset. Indians develop diabetes 10-15 years earlier than other populations and the difference in diabetes rates is highest in those younger than 50. Diabetes is becoming increasingly common among affluent overweight children in India as a result of increasing obesity and a sedentary style. The highest risk is among children who were born small but who became fat by age eight. However, the tendency for diabetes is seen in Indian children even in the absence of obesity.

Table 2.15. Projected growth of diabetic population from 2000 to 2030 in millions

Countries	2000	2030
India	32	79
China	21	42
United States	18	30
Indonesia	8	21
Pakistan	5	14
Japan	7	9
Bangladesh	3	11

Source: Wild, S. Ref. 2.56.

The prevalence of diabetes in adults worldwide was estimated to be 4% in 2000, and is expected to rise to 5% by the year 2030. However, a 10-fold difference in prevalence from country to country is observed. Currently, the prevalence of diabetes varies from 2% in China to above 10% in Egypt, Fiji, and Ukraine.

Diabetes in India

A striking feature of diabetes among Indians is its lower age of onset. Indians develop diabetes 10-15 years earlier than other populations.

The prevalence of diabetes and prediabetes is among the highest in Indians. A recent large study involving 5,288 men and 5,928 women from six cities in India covering all regions of the country showed an age-standardized prevalence of diabetes of 12%. There has been a three-fold increase in the prevalence of diabetes (5% to 15%) and an eight-fold rise in prediabetes (2% to 17%) in South India in the last two decades. More importantly, about 50% of diabetes cases remain undiagnosed. India has the highest total number of diabetic patients and the number is expected to be nearly double that of Chinese and triple that of the US by 2030 (Table 2.15)

Too much food, or not enough activity?

Table 2.16. Increasing prevalence of diabetes and prediabetes in South India

	1984	1989	1995	2000
Prediabetes	2	8	12	17
Diabetes	5	8	9	14
Prediabetes and diabetes combined	7	16	21	31

Source : Ramachandran, A. 2.44.

Similar to heart disease, the rates of diabetes are lowest in rural regions, intermediate in suburban areas, and highest in urban metropolitan areas. The prevalence of diabetes is much higher in the cities, where the excess appears to be related more to lack of physical activity than to a change in the diet pattern. In urban areas of Kerala, for example, the overall prevalence of diabetes among people aged 30 to 64 was found to be 14%. It appears that even a minor imbalance between energy intake and output results in preferential accumulation of abdominal fat among Indians. Diet is also important, but less so than accumulation of visceral fat.

However, despite their more sedentary lifestyle compared to their rural-dwelling peers, the urban poor in the developing world, particularly India, have a lower prevalence of diabetes than the urban poor in developed

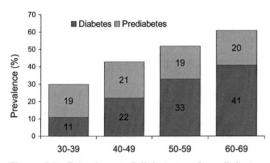

Figure 2.5. :Prevalence of diabetes and prediabetes among Indian men at different age groups. Note the four-fold increase in diabetes between age below 40 and above 60. Source: Qiao, Q. Ref. 2.42.

societies. These urban poor, nevertheless, have higher rates of complications of diabetes possibly due to lack of access to medical care. The prevalence of diabetes and prediabetes have increased steadily since 1984 (Table 2.15) The prevalence of prediabetes is particularly high at young ages among Indians. The high rate of prediabetes in India is alarming, since most people with prediabetes eventually turn diabetic.

Recently the prevalence of diabetes and prediabetes in more than 24,000 people in four Asian countries including 9848 Indians was reported. The prevalence of diabetes among Indians increased with age from 11% for people in the 30-39 age range to 42% for 60-69 year olds (see Figure 2.6) The prevalence of diabetes was higher among Indians than Chinese and Japanese at every age groups. It was nearly double among Indians younger than 40, more than double among Indians 40 to 60 and triple after age 60. (Figure 2.7.) The high prevalence of diabetes among young Indians (e.g., those in the 30-39 age group) underscores the need for testing Indians earlier than the usual recommendation of waiting until after age 45.

The overall prevalence of diabetes among urban Indians varies 15-20%. It is estimated that an additional 15-20 of the population may have prediabetes. Studies among Indians have shown that the rates of impaired glucose is double that of impaired fasting glucose . As a result , prediabetes and diabetes may underestimated among Indians if only fasting glucose is used. Overall it is likely that *every third urban-dwelling Indian* has diabetes or is likely to develop it soon. A summary estimate from several studies shows a three to four-fold

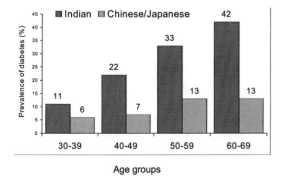

Figure 2.6. Differences in the prevalence of diabetes between Indians and Chinese and Japanese grouped together at different age groups. Source: Qiao, Q. Ref. 2.42.

higher prevalence of diabetes among Indians worldwide than whites, Chinese and Japanese.

In rural Pakistan, the overall prevalence of diabetes and prediabetes was 11% and 9%. Advanced age, positive family history of diabetes and obesity were associated with higher rates of diabetes. The prevalence of Type 2 diabetes in Bangladesh was 4% and prediabetes was 13% in rural areas in a 2003 study. People with higher family incomes had a significantly higher prevalence of diabetes (6% versus 3%) and prediabetes (16% versus 11%) than those with lower income. This pattern is also observed in India and Pakistan, and is in sharp contrast to people in western countries where people with a high socioeconomic status have a lower rate of diabetes.

Diabetes among abdominally obese, but normal weight Indians

Obesity is by far the strongest predictor of diabetes in genetically susceptible individuals, but not all populations are equally susceptible. Alan Cherrington, President of the American Diabetic Association, attended a conference on diabetes in India in 2004, where he was particularly struck by the low rates of obesity among Indian diabetic patients. In response, he stated," Much can be learned about the genetic predisposition to diabetes by studying diabetic patients in India … Current solutions to the problem of diabetes in India may differ from the prototype in the US and Europe."

> The prevalence of diabetes is three to four times higher among Indians in the top 20% of waist girth than among those in the lowest 20%. In contrast, the prevalence of diabetes is only twice as high among those in the top 20% of obesity (measured as high BMI) than those in the lowest 20% of BMI body fat range.

Indians develop diabetes at a body weight 20-30 pounds lower than whites. Fewer than 30% of diabetics in India are obese (using the conventional cut-point of a BMI above 30) compared to above 80% in the western world. Most Indians are relatively slim but heavy around their midsection, and this is a far more telling risk factor than general obesity in all populations (see Chapter III, Section 6). However, among Indians, abdominal obesity is an even more powerful risk factor than usual because Indians develop diabetes with even a mild degree of abdominal obesity (measured as waist girth). This is because of a background of heightened genetic susceptibility. The prevalence of diabetes is three to four times higher among Indians in the top 20% of waist girth than among those in the lowest 20%. In contrast, the prevalence of diabetes is only twice as high among those in the top 20% of obesity (measured as high BMI) than those in the lowest 20% of BMI.

Despite their lower body weight and younger age, Indians with diabetes have a higher prevalence of heart disease, unlike other Asian diabetics, who have a lower rate of heart disease than whites. The epidemic of heart disease among Indians is being driven partly by the combined effect of multiple risk factors in which abdominal obesity, insulin resistance, high glycemic load from overly processed foods, and physical inactivity play important roles to increase Indians' susceptibility to diabetes which, in turn, raises their susceptibility to heart disease.

KEY · POINTS · IN · A · NUTSHELL

- ♥ Diabetes is two to four times more common among Indians than other populations.
- ♥ One in three Indians has diabetes or prediabetes; this increases to one in two after age 50.
- ♥ Nearly half of all diabetes among Indians remain undiagnosed compared to one in three among Americans
- ♥ Indians develop diabetes earlier (10 to 15 years) and at a lower body weight (20-30 pounds lower) than other populations.
- ♥ Abdominal obesity, a sedentary lifestyle, and high glycemic load are the important contributors to diabetes among Indians.
- ♥ The overall medical cost of a diabetic patient is five times higher than a nondiabetic person.
- ♥ The cardiovascular risk starts with blood sugar level as low as 70 mg/dl and increases progressively as the person goes through prediabetes and diabetes.
- ♥ People with diabetes have two-to four-fold risk of having and dying from heart attack.
- ♥ The prevalence of diabetes has doubled in rural India and tripled in urban India over the past three decades.
- ♥ From 2000 to 2030, the diabetic population in India is projected to increase from 32 million to 79 million.

2.7 ► How Diabetes Links to Heart Disease

A person who has already had a heart attack has a three to five-fold higher risk of subsequent heart attack in the next five years than a person without heart disease. Diabetes is now considered a **heart disease risk-equivalent,** meaning that the risk of a diabetic patient with no symptoms of heart disease experiencing a major coronary event is as high as that of a patient who has already had one heart attack and no diabetes. Yet two out of three diabetics **are unaware** of their heightened risk of heart disease. The truth is that diabetes accelerates atherosclerosis, leading to a three-to six-fold increased risk of heart attack, stroke, amputation of limbs, or even death compared to non-diabetics. Additionally, diabetes and heart disease share common risk factors, including a diet high in saturated fat, physical inactivity, and dyslipidemia (abnormal lipids). This means that many of the same risk factors that promote heart disease also promote diabetes.

Some people develop diabetes first, followed by heart disease 10 to 20 years later; others develop heart disease first followed by diabetes in one or two decades. The risk of developing heart disease is increased **10-20 years before** diabetes is formally diagnosed, especially in women. Nearly one in five asymptomatic diabetic patients have severe heart disease requiring bypass surgery. Furthermore, like many heart attack victims who have advanced coronary disease, diabetics have a poor success rate and survival rate following angioplasty and bypass surgery. Since one leads to the other in virtually all cases, heart disease and diabetes can almost be considered two sides of the same coin. This section highlights the intimate links between diabetes and heart disease.

The crucial link between heart disease and diabetes

People with diabetes suffer heart attacks on average 10 years earlier than those without it; fully two-thirds or more will die from it. Because diabetes accelerates atherosclerosis, heart disease in diabetics is often more severe, aggressive, and extensive. Symptoms of heart disease may not be present in diabetics for many years, and approximately 25 to 50% of diabetics who have heart disease have silent heart attacks. Strokes are two to three times more common in people with diabetes than in those without it; heart failure is similarly three to eight times more common. The increased risk of heart disease is particularly high at young ages. Compared to people without diabetes, the prevalence of heart disease among persons with diabetes is:

- 14-fold higher in those below 45 years
- Three-fold higher in those 45 to 64 years
- Two-fold higher in those older than 65

Diabetic patients develop more severe and aggressive atherosclerosis at a young age. This results in larger heart attacks, as well as greater morbidity and mortality. In the most recent National Health Interview Survey (see Appendix B), diabetic Americans were five times more likely to have heart disease and stroke than Americans without diabetes. See box below.

Heart disease in diabetes: The ticking clock concept

A person may begin to develop heart disease many years before their diabetes is diagnosed. The sequence in which heart disease and diabetes

Crucial links between heart disease and diabetes

- Heart disease accounts for three-fourths of all hospitalizations deaths among diabetics.
- Two-thirds of diabetics are unaware of the excess risk of heart disease.
- Of the patients with heart disease, one-third has known diabetes and another one-third will have prediabetes or diabetes upon testing.
- Diabetes confers a two to eight-fold higher risk of heart attack and cardiac death; the risk of cardiac death rises 10 to 30-fold among women who have had diabetes for more than 15 years.
- Diabetics have more diffuse, multi-vessel and inoperable heart disease.
- Diabetics have poor outcome after coronary bypass surgery, angioplasty, and stenting.
- Diabetics have increased risk of recurrent heart attacks and out-of-hospital deaths.
- Short-term and long-term survival following a heart attack is poor among diabetics.
- Diabetics have a four-fold risk of heart failure and three-fold greater risk of fatal stroke.

develop was examined in the landmark Nurses Health Study, involving 117,000 healthy, non-diabetic female nurses and followed from 1976 to 1996. A total of 1,508 women had been diagnosed with diabetes at the beginning of the study. Over more than two million women-years of follow-up, 5,894 of the women developed diabetes, 1,556 women developed heart attack, and 1,405 developed strokes. Compared to women in the study, who remained free of diabetes and heart disease the entire 20 years, the risk of developing heart disease among those eventually diagnosed with diabetes was two-fold higher 15 years before they were diagnosed with diabetes. The risk was four times higher 0-10 years before being diagnosed with diabetes. *See* Figure 2.7.

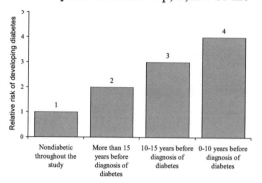

Figure 2.7. Relative risk of developing heart disease before diabetes is diagnosed. Note that, compared to a non-diabetic, the risk that a diabetic will be diagnosed with heart disease is twice as high 15 years before he or she is actually diagnosed, and four times as high 10 years before diabetes is diagnosed. Source: Hu, FB. Ref. 2.28. *Reproduced with permission* © The American Diabetes Association.

A diet high in saturated fat, a sedentary lifestyle, and atherogenic dyslipidemia are common risk factors for both conditions and possibly explain this phenomenon. The high risk of developing heart disease during the prolonged prediabetic phase can be identified by testing for dyslipidemia, metabolic syndrome, and prediabetes. One or more of these conditions are usually present 10 to 20 years before diabetes is formally diagnosed.

A Brief Primer on Terms Atherogenic (pronounced ath-row-JEN-ik) essentially means tending to trigger the buildup of plaque in your artery walls. The suffix "-genic" just means tending to create, as in the word carcinogenic (tending to cause cancer). Anything that is atherogenic tends to promote plaque, and thus atherosclerosis. Thus, for example, obesity and a diet high in cholesterol and saturated fat are atherogenic. **Dyslipidemia** means your lipids are out of balance and not working properly. The prefix "-dys" just means not working properly, as in the word dysfunctional. Your lipids are your HDL cholesterol, LDL cholesterol, and VLDL (triglycerides). You need to have the right balance of these in order not to trigger plaque.

Atherogenic dyslipidemia consists of high levels of non-HDL cholesterol, high triglyceride levels, low HDL cholesterol levels, and a preponderance of small-particle, dense LDL cholesterol. As your blood sugar increases, atherogenic dyslipidemia becomes diabetic dyslipidemia. To a greater degree than just high LDL levels alone, atherogenic dyslipidemia and diabetic dyslipidemia account for the high rates of heart disease and heart attacks before and after the diagnosis of diabetes.

Diabetes among heart disease patients

Diabetes is present in one third of patients with heart disease. Of those two- thirds without known diabetes, half have diabetes or prediabetes when tested. Thus diabetes and/or prediabetes are found in up to two-thirds of patients with heart disease *who are tested*, even in the absence of any diabetic symptoms. Diabetes is also strongly related to stroke. This is also true for people who have had a stroke. A 2004 study of stroke patients found diabetes in 24% and prediabetes in 28%, *upon testing*, although none of them were known to be diabetic prior to stroke. Unfortunately, most of these diabetics and pre-diabetics remain *undiagnosed*. These data show the intimate relationship between diabetes , heart disease and stroke and underscore the need for testing these patients for diabetes without waiting for symptoms.

People with diabetes suffer heart attacks on average 10 years earlier than those without it; fully two-thirds or more will die from it.

Greater cardiac risk among diabetic women

Diabetes leads to a higher risk of developing heart attack in women than in men. Although women are in general at a lower risk of developing heart disease as compared to men, diabetes *cancels* the protective effects of women's estrogens and removes the usual gender difference in the prevalence of heart disease. It is worth noting that, before menopause, women without diabetes have less than a 20% risk of developing heart attack compared to men. A study by Finnish researchers followed 845 diabetics and 1,296 nondiabetics for 13 years. All were between the ages of 45 and 65 and had no evidence of heart disease at the beginning of the study. After adjusting for age and all other risk factors, the risk of a heart attack was 14 times greater among the diabetic women, but only three times higher among the diabetic men, as compared to the nondiabetic group. The risk of a heart attack in a 45-year-old diabetic woman is almost as high as for a diabetic man of the same age. (See Chapter IV Section 3). Furthermore, following a heart attack, diabetic women have double the rate of recurrence and less survival than men. Diabetes increases the risk of heart failure eight-fold in women compared to four-fold in men (see Table 2.17).

> **Did You Know..**
> The risk of death is increased with increasing duration of diabetes. After 15 years, the risk is increased nine-fold among those with diabetes alone and 30-fold among those with diabetes and heart disease.

Diabetes is particularly common in women with premature heart disease. In fact, diabetes is three times more common in *Indian women* than in *Indian men* with premature heart disease. Compared to nondiabetic women, diabetic women have a substantially greater degree of dyslipidemia (higher total cholesterol, higher triglycerides, and lower HDL). This explains the higher risk and worse outcome of heart disease in women with diabetes.

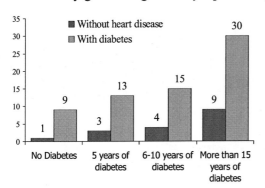

Figure 2.8. How the duration of diabetes and presence of heart disease in women affect the relative risk of dying from heart disease. Source: HU, FB. Ref. 2.29.

Diabetes and cardiac death

People with diabetes not only have a very high risk of developing heart disease, but also the highest risk of dying from it. Cardiovascular disease accounts for four out of five deaths in people with diabetes. The risk of cardiac death is markedly increased with the duration of a persons diabetes. Among women who have had diabetes for more than 15 years, the risk of cardiac death rises nine-fold in the absence of heart disease, but 30-fold if heart disease is also present (See Figure 2.8.) The corresponding numbers for men are four-fold and 14-fold, respectively.

Another study, which examined the relative risk of dying from heart disease among nearly 10,000 Europeans followed for 10 years, found that compared with those who never had diabetes or heart disease, the risk of cardiac death rose two-fold with angina, three-fold with diabetes, four-fold with a heart attack, and eight-fold when both diabetes and heart disease were present.

Impact of diabetes on angioplasty and bypass surgery

Diabetics account for 25-30% of patients undergoing a first coronary angioplasty/stent or bypass surgery, and 40% of those undergoing a repeat procedure. Despite recent therapeutic advances, such as new antiplatelet treatments and drug-eluting (drug-releasing) stents, outcomes for diabetic patients after angioplasty and stent are still significantly worse than for non-diabetics. The initial success rates in opening the coronary blockages in diabetics are similar to those observed in nondiabetics. However, diabetic patients have a higher rate of restenosis, recurrent heart attack, and/or death after coronary angioplasty and bypass surgery. In one long-term follow-up study of patients who had undergone

Table 2.17. Gender differences in the impact of diabetes on heart disease and its complications

	Women	Men
Excess risk of heart attack	five-fold	three-fold
Risk of dying from first heart attack	seven-fold	four-fold
Excess risk of heart failure	eight-fold	four-fold
One year mortality following a heart attack	44%	37%
Average time for recurrent heart attack or death	five years	eight years

angioplasty, diabetic patients had 50% lower event-free survival (36% versus 53%), 50% higher rates of heart attacks (29% versus 18%), and double the rate of death (36% versus 18%) compared to nondiabetic patients, The complication rates are even higher among diabetic women. A recent large study reported the impact of diabetes on 4,284 patients who had had coronary angioplasty and bypass surgery and were followed for three years. The diabetics among them had a 46% higher mortality compared to the nondiabetics (13% versus 8%), despite the frequent use of stents.

In a recent (2004) pooled analysis of several studies, diabetes was found to be the strongest clinical predictor of restenosis, with a 50% increased risk of repeat coronary interventions within one year. The rates of restenosis vary from 47% to 62% in diabetic patients, nearly double that of nondiabetic patients. Among diabetics, poor blood sugar control is the strongest predictor of need for revascularization.

Several studies have shown that diabetic patients undergoing coronary bypass surgery have a 50% lower death rate within five to seven years, compared to angioplasty/stent. The survival for diabetics is even better with bypass surgery that uses an internal mammary artery (located inside the chest wall). Diabetic patients undergoing bypass surgery have twice the operative mortality of nondiabetic patients. In other words, diabetes is not only associated with poor short-term and long-term survival, but also poor functional recovery after a bypass surgery.

Diabetes and silent heart disease

Many diabetic patients have extremely high rates of severe heart disease that require bypass surgery, even in the absence of symptoms. There is a clear need for early detection of heart disease in patients with diabetes. A stress test using imaging techniques appears to be well-suited to diabetics who may have heart diseases. In a 2005 study involving more than 1,400 diabetic patients without known heart disease, an abnormal stress imaging scan (which offers objective evidence of heart disease) was present in 58%. Strikingly, approximately 12-15% of asymptomatic diabetic patients had severe heart disease requiring bypass surgery. These patients with high-risk scans had a high annual mortality rate (6%). These findings underscore the importance of identifying such asymptomatic but high-risk individuals and treating them aggressivelyDiabetes and heart disease are inextricably intertwined; one tends to lead to the other within 10 to 20 years.

KEY · POINTS · IN · A · NUTSHELL

♥ Diabetes and heart disease are inextricably intertwined; one tends to lead to the other within 10 to 20 years.

♥ A diet high in saturated fat, a sedentary lifestyle, and atherogenic dyslipidemia are common risk factors for both heart disease and diabetes.

♥ Diabetics have a three- to six-fold greater risk of heart attack, heart failure, kidney failure, stroke, and death.

♥ The risk of heart disease begins as early as 20 years before diabetes is diagnosed; it is already up to four-fold, 10 years before diabetes is detected.

♥ Nearly one in six asymptomatic diabetic patients has severe heart disease requiring bypass surgery.

♥ The risk of death is increased with increasing duration of diabetes; after 15 years, the risk is increased nine-fold among those with diabetes alone and 30-fold among those with diabetes and heart disease.

♥ Diabetes poses a greater risk of heart disease to women, so much so that men and women with diabetes have similar rates of heart attack.

♥ Complications from diabetes are much more common and dangerous in women than in men.

♥ Diabetics have poor success and survival rates following angioplasty and bypass surgery.

♥ Two out of three diabetics are unaware of their excess risk of heart disease and its potential complications.

Chapter III

Newly Emerging Risk Factors

Section 1, **Emerging Risk Factors and Risk Markers**, discusses some of the latest research on new risk factors for heart disease. Risk markers such as erectile dysfunction and chronic kidney disease help identify people at high risk of heart disease. The section sets the foundation for discussion of key emerging cardiac risk factors for Indians. ◆

Section 2, **L-P-Little-a: The Deadliest Cholesterol of All**, outlines the genetic basis for prematurity and severity of heart disease among Indians. The multiplicative effect of lipoprotein(a) excess on low HDL, high LDL and high homocysteine is highlighted. The role of lipoprotein(a) excess in the restenosis of coronary arteries after coronary angioplasty, stent and bypass surgery in Indians is discussed. ◆

The third section, **Homocysteine: The Quasi-Cholesterol**, describes the role of high levels of homocysteine in the heightened risk of heart attack in Indians. The role of nutritional factors responsible for these high levels in Indians is highlighted. This section also discusses some safe and inexpensive prescription medicines that can lower homocysteine effectively. ◆

Section 4, **C-Reactive Protein: A Sign of Silent Inflammation**, explains how the levels of this protein in the blood indicates the degree of inflammation. High levels of CRP often correlate with risk of first and recurrent heart attacks and other complications. Brief description of the specific test (high sensitivity CRP) and some strategies for management are given. ◆

Section 5, **Obesity: The Large Price of a Sedentary Lifestyle**, describes the effect of obesity on dyslipidemia, hypertension and diabetes. For a given weight and Body Mass Index (BMI), Asians tend to have higher amount of body fat. This section highlights the difference in criteria for obesity between Asians and non-Asians. Various formulae and tables for calculating BMI are also outlined. ◆

Abdominal Obesity: The Shape of Cardiac Risk, the sixth section, guides the reader through cut-points for waist size for Indian men and women. It discusses why the fat stored in our belly area is more biologically active and harmful than fat in other parts of the body. An unhealthy abdominal girth is common even among Indians with "normal" weight and BMI. ◆

Section 7, **Metabolic Syndrome: The Ticking Time Bomb**, highlights how mildly abnormal levels of several common disorders, namely blood pressure, HDL, abdominal obesity, triglycerides and blood sugar can team up and cause diabetes and heart attack. While metabolic syndrome is on the rise among the Americans, it is increasing at an alarming rate among Indians. ◆

3.1 ▶ Emerging Risk Factors and Risk Markers

Until very recently, the research and treatment of heart disease has focused primarily on the traditional risk factors, which we have discussed in previous sections. However, many heart attacks, particularly premature heart attacks, cannot be traced back to these traditional or so-called standard risk factors. In particular, we now know that certain populations may be genetically more susceptible to heart disease because of the influence of new unfamiliar factors. These new factors, called emerging risk factors, may be genetic, nutritional, or environmental, and may be as important as traditional risk factors in certain populations, such as Indians. It is now believed that these new risk factors can explain most of the risk of heart disease that cannot be explained by the traditional risk factors.

> **A Word about Terminology**
> Throughout this book, the term Indian refers to people, who trace their origin to the Indian subcontinent—meaning Bangladesh, India, Pakistan, and Sri Lanka—including those who now live abroad but originate from one of these four countries. "Indian" in this context is ethnically interchangeable with "South Asian," "Indo-Asian," or "Asian Indian." The term thus excludes native Americans but includes more than people from the nation of India.
>
> **Measurement Units:** As is conventional, blood glucose levels, triglyceride levels, and cholesterol levels are stated throughout this book in milligrams per deciliter (mg/dL). Blood pressure is stated in millimeters of mercury (mmHg).

More than 300 emerging risk factors have been identified. Although more attention gets paid to the detrimental ones, there are also protective factors—such as regular physical activity and diet rich in fruits and vegetables—the absence of which may increase the risk of heart disease.

Then there are the risk markers such as peripheral vascular disease, or erectile dysfunction. They do not, by themselves, increase your risk of heart disease in a causal way, but the presence of one or more these is a strong indicator of heart disease. In other words, they function like red flags that help identify the disease. Many of these emerging factors are of great importance to Indians, irrespective of whether or not traditional risk factors are present. This section discusses many of the emerging risk factors and risk markers. As the box below shows, the emerging risk factors can be classified as *conditional, predisposing, or other*.

Conditional risk factors accelerate the development of heart disease in individuals who also have traditional risk factors. *Predisposing factors* increase one's susceptibility to other risk factors. A conditional factor is one that *worsens in effect* when you have traditional risk factors, whereas a predisposing factor is one that *worsens the effect* of traditional factors. For example, elevated lipoprotein(a), a conditional factor, markedly increases the risk of heart disease in individuals who also have high LDL and low HDL, both of which are traditional risk factors. By contrast, physical inactivity and being overweight, which are predisposing factors, markedly increase one's susceptibility to developing diabetes and hypertension, which in turn can lead to heart disease. Other categories include low birth weight, recurrent miscarriages, elevated uric acid, etc.

Emerging risk factors and risk markers.			
Conditional factors	**Predisposing factors**	**Other factors**	**Risk markers**
Elevated lipoprotein(a) Elevated homocysteine Elevated CRP Elevated triglycerides Elevated fibrinogen Small dense LDL	Physical inactivity Overweight and obesity Family history of early-onset heart disease Socioeconomic factors Hostility or rage Depression	Prediabetes Elevated uric acid Air pollution Recurrent miscarriages Short height Low birth weight	Erectile dysfunction Baldness Chronic kidney disease Peripheral vascular disease (PVD) Snoring

Endothelial dysfunction

In addition, all of these risk factors can produce something called endothelial dysfunction, which is not itself a risk factor, but plays a crucial role in the development of heart disease. Endothelium is the inner lining of a blood vessel. Endothelial dysfunction means the endothelium is not working well. This inner blood vessel lining produces several substances which control blood flow, blood clotting, and inflammation. For example, a blood vessel relaxes (open more widely) or constricts (closes down) because of signals from its endothelium. When the endothelium becomes dysfunctional due to the presence of risk factors, it can—like a malfunctioning computer—send signals that constrict the vessel and restrict blood flow to certain organs, even without the artery being clogged by a plaque or blood clot. Endothelial dysfunction is, therefore, the *earliest stage of atherosclerosis*, and occurs before the development of plaque.

The coexistence of two emerging risk factors in particular—lipoprotein(a) and homocysteine—is very common among Indians. It is associated with 30-fold increase in the person's relative risk of heart disease, compared to a 32-fold increase when all five traditional risk factors—smoking, diabetes, hypertension, high cholesterol, and low HDL—are present.

The degree of endothelial dysfunction in a person's vessels generally correlates well with the number and severity of his or her risk factors. Because all of the risk factors can produce endothelial dysfunction, it represents the cumulative effect of all cardiac risk factors on the blood vessels (though certain genetic factors may also contribute to it). Finally, the extent of endothelial dysfunction depends not only on the cumulative effect of risk factors, but also on the absence of protective factors such as regular exercise and the consumption of fruits, vegetables, and small amounts of alcohol.

Among the emerging risk factors, lipoprotein(a) and homocysteine are conditional factors of huge significance to Indians. Elevated levels of lipoprotein(a), discussed in Chapter III, Section 3, provide a *genetic susceptibility* to early heart disease. Homocysteine excess, discussed in Chapter III, Section 4, is unusually common among Indians and is likely related to dietary habits and *cooking practices* rather than genetic factors. The coexistence of these two risk factors is very common among Indians and is associated with a 30-fold increase in the person's relative risk of heart disease, compared to only a 20-fold increase when all five traditional risk factors (smoking, diabetes, hypertension, high cholesterol, and low HDL) are present.

Physical inactivity and fitness

In the US 40% of the population do not have enough physical activity. This figure may be higher among most Indians. In the UK, Physical inactivity is double among South Asians. Physical inactivity is a powerful predisposing risk factor, similar in magnitude to high cholesterol and smoking. In one landmark study of nearly 22,000 men who were followed for 30 years, low fitness was associated with a higher risk for death (52%) than even high cholesterol (34%) or high blood pressure (34 %). The risk of death in a low-fitness person without any other risk factors was actually found to be higher than that of a high-fitness person who had two or three standard risk factors (see Figure 3.1).

Urbanization within India, and emigration to the US and other western countries, are associated with decreased daily physical activity. This has resulted in an ever-increasing population of sedentary individuals who are at high risk of developing obesity, metabolic syndrome, diabetes, and heart disease.

Physical activity correlates directly with fitness. A person is generally considered fit if he can perform physical activity equivalent to at least seven METs (metabolic equivalent) without symptoms. A MET is the amount of oxygen a person consumes while at rest and is usually defined as 3.5 mL per kg per min (See Chapter V, section 8). This corresponds to walking six minutes on a treadmill (using the Bruce protocol – See Chapter VII, Section 3).

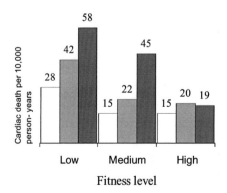

Figure 3.1. How fitness influences death rate per 10,000 person-years. Note that people with the lowest fitness levels have a higher rate of death than even persons with two or three risk factors who stay physically fit. Source: Blair, SN. Ref. 3.07 *Reproduced with permission* © American Medical Association.

Fitness and fatness

Cardio-respiratory fitness and amount of body fat are both related to health. Recent studies indicate that the health benefits of being lean are limited to fit men, and being fit may reduce the hazards of obesity. In the same long-term study, lean unfit men had double the risk of death as compared to men who were obese but fit. For example, unfit men with small waists (below 87 cm) had a greater risk of mortality of any cause, than did fit men with large waists (above 99 cm). Figure 3.1 shows the importance of low physical fitness resulting from low physical activity in comparison to traditional risk factors, such as smoking, high blood pressure, and high cholesterol. Among people with no risk factors, the risk of death per 10,000 person-years was 28 for low-fitness persons compared to 15 for people with a high fitness level. More importantly, the risk of death was 50% higher in low-fit people with no risk factors than in high-fit persons with two or three risk factors (28 versus 19). Naturally, low-fit persons with multiple risk factors had the highest risk of death of all (58 per 10,000).

Widened pulse pressure

The difference between systolic (upper reading) and diastolic blood pressure (lower reading) is called pulse pressure. Normal pulse pressure is 40mm Hg or less (for example, 120 minus 80). High pulse pressure (above 40 mm Hg) indicates stiffness of the arteries. High pulse pressure is a powerful predictor of stroke, heart attack, and heart failure, even when the blood pressure levels are within the normal range. A 10mm Hg rise in pulse pressure over normal has been associated with a 12% increase in heart attack and a 14% increase in heart failure. Risk is particularly high in the elderly, who often have low diastolic blood pressure and hence a broader contrast between diastolic and systolic.

Prediabetes (high normal fasting blood sugar)

The level of blood sugar level now considered normal has been reduced from 110 mg/dL to 100 mg/dL. Blood sugar levels between 100 and 126 mg/dL are considered prediabetes and are associated with greatly increased cardiac risk. Hemoglobin A1C level is a measure of a person's average blood sugar over a three-month period and is an independent risk factor for cardiovascular disease, regardless of the person's diabetes status. A hemoglobin A1C level less than 7% was previously considered normal and acceptable even among diabetics. A recent European study among non-diabetics showed a continuously increasing risk of heart disease as hemoglobin A1C level increased from 5% to 7% (see also Chapter VI, Section 8).

Elevated fibrinogen

This blood protein is involved in blood clotting. A high level of fibrinogen is associated with larger blood clots and a higher risk of heart disease. Indians have high levels compared with other populations. Niacin lowers fibrinogen, whereas fibrates elevate it.

Elevated uric acid

Elevated uric acid in the blood is usually associated with **gout** – a painful condition typically affecting the foot. Recent studies have shown that elevated uric acid level is not only a cardiac risk factor, but also a strong predictor of death from heart disease. Uric acid levels are elevated in people with obesity, chronic kidney disease, high levels of triglycerides and low HDL levels. Among people with high blood pressure, elevated uric acid is associated with increased risk for atherosclerosis, microalbuminuria (an early indicator of kidney damage), and left ventricular hypertrophy (enlargement of the heart predisposing it to heart failure). Certain lipid medications, such as fenofibrate (Tricor) and atorvastatin (Lipitor), lower uric acid levels.

Microalbuminuria

Normally functioning kidneys do not allow proteins to be lost in urine. Microalbuminuria (small amounts of protein in urine) is common in people with diabetes or hypertension. It is an early indicator of endothelial dysfunction and damage to blood vessels throughout the body. In a British study of 22,368 men who were followed for six years, the relative risk of a heart attack was double among those with microalbuminuria, and triple among those with macroalbuminuria (large amounts of protein in urine).

The prevalence of microalbuminuria is high in people with the metabolic syndrome. It is not only a kidney problem but is also a powerful predictor of cardiovascular risk. Only about 20-25% of patients with microalbuminuria live long enough to reach end-stage kidney disease?75-80 % die earlier from heart attack and stroke.

Chronic Kidney Disease (CKD)

Kidney damage usually goes unnoticed until it is too late. By the time symptoms such as weight loss, fatigue, and generalized itching appear, the disease is far advanced, requiring dialysis. An elevated level of blood creatinine (above 1.5 mg/dL in men and above 1.3 mg/dL in women) is an early sign of CKD. Creatinine is a waste product that comes from the wear and tear of muscles. A weakened or damaged kidney fails to remove all of it. Elevated creatinine is a measure of the kidneys' glomerular filtration rate (GFR), a calculation based on creatinine level. Normal GFR is above 120 mL/min.

> A patient with even mild to moderate chronic kidney disease is more like to die from cardiovascular disease than by developing end-stage kidney disdase that leads to dialysis.

A low GFR (below 90 mL/min) not only signifies kidney damage, but also a high risk of heart disease and stroke. In fact the risk of heart disease is so high that chronic kidney disease has recently been designated as a heart disease risk-equivalent, similar to diabetes. In addition, rates of complications following coronary angiogram, angioplasty and bypass surgery are markedly elevated in patients with CKD. Patients with mild to moderate CKD are more like to die from cardiovascular disease than from developing end-stage kidney disease, leading to dialysis. Anemia (low blood count) is another early indicator of kidney disease as well as the risk of death. A two gm drop from 14 to 12 gm is accompanied by a 25% increase in death within a few years.

Psychosocial factors

Several psychosocial factors have been associated with coronary events (heart attack, sudden death, and so on). These factors may literally indicate a crucial link between the head and the heart. Psychosocial factors fall into two broad categories: emotional factors and chronic stressors. Emotional factors include depression, anger, and hostility. Chronic stressors include lack of social support, low socioeconomic status, work stress, marital stress and caregiver stress. Depression is associated with a poor outcome following a heart attack and bypass surgery. In the INTERHEART Study (see Appendix A), nearly one-third of the heart attacks could be explained by psychosocial factors (meaning that the population-attributable risk was 30%). The magnitude of risk for heart attack for people with psychosocial stress was similar to that of people with hypertension and abdominal obesity, but less than that of smokers. Let us consider specific psychosocial factors.

Hostility and unexpressed anger are associated with a five-fold increase in heart attack and other coronary events. Hostility is also a predictor of death from heart disease among high-risk men. Among those who develop a heart attack, hostility is associated with a five-fold risk of death. Hostility is an important risk factor for premature heart disease and is three to four times more common in young patients who have had heart attacks (below 45 years of age) than in older patients. Young patients with hostility have an increased prevalence of several risk factors, including obesity, hypertension, and dyslipidemia. Persons with hostility also have increased catecholamine and enhanced platelet reactivity, resulting in *vulnerable blood* (see

> **The importance and interrelationship of psychosocial factors in heart disease.**
> - Psychosocial factors are linked to cardiovascular risk factors
> - They are significant factors by themselves
> - They may trigger a heart attack sooner
> - They commonly masquerade as cardiovascular symptoms, such as palpitation
> - They are very common among cardiac patients
> - They form a barrier to medical interventions and treatment

Source: Rozanski, A. Ref. 3.60.

Chapter I, Section 1). Although people readily admit to feeling stressed, they often deny their hostility perhaps because it has a more negative connotation. Nevertheless, the telltale signs of hostility include losing one's temper easily, uncontrollable shaking anger, or feelings of hatred expressed through rage. Interventions aimed at anger management and stress reduction, along with risk factor modification, may be helpful to hostile patients.

Low socioeconomic status

Heart disease was once considered a disease of the rich. Our understanding of it is more precise today: Heart disease is more accurately a disease of the poor in rich countries, and conversely of the rich in poor countries. (The rich in rich countries, who tend to read a lot and to be highly educated, have on the whole taken many measures to lessen their risk factors.) For all practical purposes, low socio-economic status is now considered a nonmodifiable risk factor in terms of cardiac risk assessment. Low education level is correlated with several important risk factors including smoking, hypertension, obesity, low physical activity, high carbohydrate intake, and diabetes. The two- to three-fold higher rate of lower extremity amputation in blacks and Hispanics in the US is largely attributable to poverty and low socioeconomic status. Another reason why low socioeconomic status is a risk factor is that many developing-world hospitals—most hospitals in India, for example—will not provide medical care unless the patients or their families deposit adequate funds in advance. This applies even to the care of heart attack patients, as well as those who require emergency blood transfusion or surgery.

Obstructive Sleep Apnea (OSA)

OSA is a common medical condition characterized by recurrent episodes of breathing cessation during sleep, associated with the temporary collapse of the upper airway. Such episodes of apnea may be associated with oxygen desaturation and are often terminated by brief arousal from sleep. People who have OSA typically snore. Because it deprives the sufferer of a restful sleep, OSA also results in high rates of automobile accidents related to excessive day-time sleepiness. It is strongly associated with known cardiovascular risk factors such as obesity, metabolic syndrome, hypertension, dyslipidemia, as well as heart disease and stroke. Weight loss can reduce the severity of OSA. CPAP (continuous positive airway pressure), the current standard treatment, eliminates apnea. Despite the availability of effective therapy, OSA remains an underdiagnosed and undertreated condition.

Air pollution

Epidemiological studies have demonstrated a consistent increase in cardiac risk in relation to both short- and long-term exposure to air pollution. This may be particularly important in large cities in India where air pollution remains very high.

Tooth loss and infection

Periodontal disease, a strong determinant of tooth loss, is associated with heightened inflammation of the gums and high levels of C-reactive protein (see Chapter III, Section 2). This condition is common among Indians, although tooth loss has not been linked to heart disease among this population. Several infectious agents have been implicated in atherosclerosis but many studies completed in the last five years have shown that antibiotics have no role in preventing and treating atherosclerosis or heart disease.

Emerging risk markers

A risk marker helps to identify people at high risk of heart disease without actually causing it. In some cases a risk marker may even be a consequence of heart disease. For example, erectile dysfunction is not a risk factor but a risk marker of endothelial dysfunction or silent heart disease. There is an ongoing debate as to whether C- reactive protein (CRP) is an emerging risk marker or risk factor.

Erectile dysfunction

Endothelial dysfunction of penile and coronary arteries often coexists. A request for a prescription for erectile dysfunction may be a red flag for silent heart disease, since 80% of this condition is caused by atherosclerotic disease. A recent European study showed a 57% 10-year risk of heart disease among those with erectile dysfunction, compared to 33% in the control group. Erectile dysfunction is eight times more common in patients with silent heart disease (ischemia) than in those without it (40% versus 5%).

Preeclampsia and recurrent miscarriages

Preeclampsia, a complication of pregnancy with severe hypertension has now been linked to the development of metabolic syndrome and premature heart disease. Women of childbearing age are usually protected from heart disease, even if they have never been pregnant and have had no children. However, certain risk factors such as *antiphospholipid syndrome, elevated levels of lipoprotein(a), and homocysteine*, are associated with an increased tendency for the blood to clot in these women. Many of these risk factors are also implicated in heart attack during or following pregnancy. These factors not only produce miscarriages in susceptible individuals, but also produce heart attack at a younger age – in the thirties and forties. A two- to three-fold higher rate of heart attack has been reported in women with recurrent miscarriages.

Peripheral vascular disease (PVD)

Peripheral vascular disease or PVD is condition characterized by progressive narrowing of peripheral arteries, The classical sign of PVD is intermittent claudication, which refers to severe cramping pain in the calf muscles produced with walking and relieved immediately with rest. If left undiagnosed and untreated, it eventually leads to the loss of a limb. It is unusually common among diabetics, who have a risk of amputation 400 times higher than non-diabetics. PVD can be diagnosed noninvasively with an ankle-brachial index (see Chapter VII, Section 3). PVD affects 12 million Americans, compared to 13 million with heart disease and the two conditions often coexist together. PVD is associated with severe generalized atherosclerosis. Individuals with PVD have a *three-fold higher* risk of coronary events, regardless of other factors. Although Indians have an excess burden of heart disease and diabetes, PVD is somewhat uncommon among Indians.

> **The signs and symptoms of peripheral vascular disease**
>
> - Cool temperature of the leg or foot.
> - Dry and scaly skin of the leg
> - Decreased hair on the leg and toenail growth.
> - A sore on the foot that does not heal.
> - Reddish-blue color of the leg when sitting.
> - Pallor (paleness) when the leg is elevated.
> - Little or no pulse in leg or foot.

Carotid bruit or femoral bruit

(Bruit pronounced BROO-ee) is a medical term for abnormal sounds that can be heard at certain arterial sites. Bruit is the result of the significant narrowing of the arteries from severe plaque build-up that restricts blood flow. A bruit can be heard years before the person develops any symptoms. It is readily heard at the femoral (main artery to the leg) or carotid (main artery in the neck that supplies the brain). A bruit indicates advanced atherosclerosis of the affected arteries. Since atherosclerosis is a systemic disease affecting all arteries, a bruit in the carotid or femoral arteries also indicates advanced atherosclerosis in all other arteries of the body, especially the coronary arteries.

Aneurysm

An aneurysm is a bulging or ballooning-out of the wall of an artery. Often the arterial wall is weakened by disease, injury or an abnormality present at birth. Aneurysms are often made worse by high blood pressure. Aneurysms usually occur in the abdomen (abdominal aortic aneurysm), but may occur in the chest cavity (thoracic aortic aneurysm). Rupture of most aneurysms is frequently fatal. (See glossary). The causes of aneurysms are usually the same as heart disease and the two often co-exist.

Aortic sclerosis and aortic calcification

Aortic sclerosis is a common condition affecting senior citizens. Recent studies suggest that the same risk factors that produce atherosclerosis of the coronary arteries also produce sclerosis of the aortic valve. This is particularly true in the presence of elevated levels *of lipoprotein(a),* and LDL and a low level of HDL. Calcifications of the aorta seen on x-ray are strong indicators of subclinical (asymptomatic) vascular disease and heightened risk from cardiovascular disease.

Baldness

Men with male-pattern baldness have a 36% greater risk of heart attack compared to men with full heads of hair or with receding hairlines. The risk is more pronounced in the presence of other risk factors, particularly hypertension or high cholesterol.

Low birth weight

Low birth weight usually signifies poor prenatal nutrition which is associated with permanent changes in the programming of the functioning of several organs. Long term follow up of more than 100,000 babies for up to 50 years has shown a significantly higher rate of metabolic syndrome, diabetes, and heart disease as young adults. The risk is further increased if the low birth weight is followed by overweight and obesity in childhood and as adults.

Short height

In general, short men and women have a higher risk of heart disease than their taller colleagues. Similar to baldness, this is mostly genetic and not modifiable. Men in the tallest (above 73 inches) compared with the shortest (below 67 inches) height category have a *35% lower risk* of heart attack. For every inch of added height, there is an approximate 2% to 3% decline in risk of heart attack.

Elevated white cell count

Inflammation is a key feature of atherosclerosis and its clinical manifestations. The leukocyte count is a marker of inflammation that is widely available in clinical practice. Numerous studies have shown elevated white cell count to be an independent predictor of future cardiovascular events, both in healthy individuals free of heart disease and in patients with stable angina, unstable angina, or a history of heart attack

Other risk factors

Abdominal obesity, high levels of lipoprotein(a), homocysteine, and C reactive protein are emerging risk factors of great importance in the Indian population. A section is devoted to each of these risk factors in this book. As mentioned earlier, more than 300 risk factors have been identified for heart disease. However, the search for all these numerous and unusual risk factors would be very time-consuming and unrewarding. They would pose only a minor threat to heart disease risk and strategies for dealing with them have not been developed.

Protective factors

Although physicians and researcher pay more attention to risk factors that increase the risk of heart disease, there is a growing evidence regarding various protective factors. These protective factors include large HDL particles, a diet rich in fruits and vegetables, regular physical activity, and judicious use of alcohol. These are discussed in subsequent sections.

KEY · POINTS · IN · A · NUTSHELL

♥ Abdominal obesity, sedentary lifestyle, lipoprotein(a) and homocysteine are emerging risk factors of outstanding importance among Indians (see following sections).

♥ Erectile dysfunction and peripheral vascular disease are strong indicators of heart disease.

♥ Preeclampsia, recurrent miscarriage and antiphospholipid syndrome are predictive of premature heart disease in women.

♥ A wide pulse pressure (above 40 mm Hg) indicates stiffness of the arteries and confers a high risk of stroke, heart attack, and heart failure, even when the blood pressure levels are within the normal range.

♥ Short men and women have higher risk of heart attack than their taller counterparts

♥ The risk of a heart attack is double among those with microalbuminuria, and triple among those with macroalbuminuria (large amounts of protein in urine).

♥ Most people with chronic kidney disease die of cardiovascular disease before they ever need dialysis treatment .

♥ Risk markers do not increase the risk of heart disease, but help identify the probable presence of the disease.

♥ Protective factors include regular physical activity, increased consumption of fruits and vegetables and consumption of small amounts of alcohol.

3.2 ▶ L-P-Little-a: The Deadliest Cholesterol of All

IN MAY 1990, DR. SUDARSHAN SADHASIVAM, dean of one of India's most prestigious medical schools, in Tamil Nadu State, visited the US to see his newborn granddaughter. That visit marked a turning point in my research on heart disease among Indians. Dr. Sadhasivam kept an almost perfectly healthy lifestyle. A strict vegetarian, he ate cautiously, exercised *14 hours* a week, and took an aspirin everyday. Yet somehow heart disease had caught up to him—and in a dramatic way. During his short visit, he developed persistent chest pain, severe enough that he could not eat or even talk. In my office, his electrocardiogram showed not one *but two* simultaneous heart attacks in progress. The following day, he developed crushing chest pain and went into shock while undergoing a coronary angiogram, a procedure that takes x-rays of the heart's major arteries (*see* Chapter VII, Section 3).

Despite his emphasis on health, Dr. Sadhasivam had one of the most extensive cases of heart disease I had ever seen. His coronary angiogram (*See* **Color Plates 3.2. and 3.3.**) showed that plaque had completely blocked one of his largest arteries, the right coronary artery, and almost completely blocked two other large arteries—the left main and the left anterior descending arteries. He was immediately scheduled for surgery. Fortunately, his three-vessel coronary artery bypass went well.

Puzzled by this unusual case of severe atherosclerosis in an otherwise healthy, and health-oriented, middle-aged man, I started searching for clues in the form of overlooked cardiac risk factors. More than that, Dr. Sadhasivam's case brought into sharp focus many other clinical cases of relatively young Indians with heart disease that I had seen over the years, but among which I had not consciously discerned any overarching pattern. Could a full diagnosis of his coronary artery disease more broadly account for what was turning out to be a distinctive, almost unique pattern of premature, severe heart disease among Indians, even those who lead healthy lifestyles? It turned out that Dr. Sadhasivam had a altogether normal lipid profile, except

So Then, Why Bother At All? Having under gone emergency bypass surgery, Dr Sadhavisam has resumed his active, productive life. One might wonder if his strongly health-oriented lifestyle before his heart attacks had all been a waste then. Given his genetic predisposition to heart disease from a high level of Lp(a), his-emphasis on health certainly had not been a waste. Like Dr. James Fixx, author of The Complete *Book of Running*, who died right after seting a master's record in a 3000-meter run (see Chapter I, Section1) Dr. Sadhasivam's superb diet and exercise regimen may have postponed his heart attack by several decades—by slowing atherosclearosis and miximizing the blood-carrying capacity of his coronary arteries.

for a somewhat low level of (good) HDL cholesterol—32mg/dL—and a high level of something called *lipoprotein(a)*, which measured at 42mg/dL. Normal levels are in the 20-30 range. I took a closer look, and instinctively realized that I was on to something. Herein, I said to myself, lay the key to this patient's paradoxical health profile: *L-P-Little-a.*

Always referred as "L-P-Little-a", whether in its abbreviated or full form, Lp(a) is one of the most widespread and important emerging risk factors for premature heart disease. High levels of Lp(a) are found in more than 40% of Indians, compared to less than 20% of whites. Indeed, for people from the Indian subcontinent, Lp(a) may be as important as the traditional heart disease risk factors. And in many Indians with premature heart disease and/or stroke, an excess of "L-P-Little-a" may be the *only* risk factor they have—as was the case with Dr. Sadhasivam. Two striking features of heart disease among Indians are its extreme prematurity and extreme severity. These are also the most salient features of heart disease in patients with Lp(a) excess. In this section, we will discuss what Lp(a) is, how you get it, and why it has had such a devastating effect on the Indian population.

Just what is lipoprotein(a)

To understand what a lipoprotein is, let's first briefly talk about the lipids in your blood. HDL (or good) cholesterol, LDL (or bad) cholesterol, VLDL cholesterol, and triglycerides are all lipids—meaning fats—that your body uses for a variety of important functions. But as every cook and budding lab scientist knows, oil and water don't mix. Your blood is essentially water, while your lipids are essentially oil. That means that to get around your body, cholesterol and triglycerides need to hire a taxicab, as it were. They need to climb inside some sort of a vehicle that *can* travel through water. To put it another, it's as if cholesterol and triglycerides don't have an entry visa, and they need some sort of outer jacket with a badge that gives them free passage through your bloodstream. That outer jacket, or vehicle, is **lipoprotein**, a structure consisting of an outer coat of protein and an inner core of lipid: hence, *lipo + protein.*

Once lipids like cholesterol or triglyceride take on the form of a lipoprotein, they can finally travel around your body's highway system—your arteries and veins—without restriction. Your body no longer sees them as oil trying to mix into water. (option to move to Chapter II section 3 cholesterol subheading lipoproteins to avoid duplication

Now here is the problem: That outer coat of protein that transforms a lipid into a lipoprotein also makes the lipid either very good or very bad for you, depending on the characteristics of the outer coat. Low-density lipoprotein (or LDL) cholesterol is simply cholesterol that is wearing a particular kind of outer coat that makes the cholesterol dangerous to you. High-density lipoprotein (or HDL) cholesterol is cholesterol that's wearing an outer jacket that makes cholesterol beneficial to you.

Lipoprotein(a)'s outer coat is like that of LDL cholesterol, except even worse. A genetic variant of LDL cholesterol, Lp(a) has an abnormal protein called apo(a) attached to it. Like a tiny snake fang, this small attachment transforms "L-P-Little-a" into the most dangerous lipoprotein

High Lp(a) magnifies the risk from other risk factors Even if you have no other risk factors, a high level of Lp(a) (above 20-30 points) increases your risk of heart disease two to four times. Your risk rises eight-fold if you also have *low HDL*, 12-fold if you have *high Lp(a)* plus *high LDL*, and 25-fold if you have all three. In people with several more risk factors, Lp(a) excess can raise the risk of heart disease as much as 100 times, compared to someone with normal Lp(a) and no other risk factors.

of all. Because of its biochemical characteristics, Lp(a) *has the effect of promoting the two things most responsible for heart attacks:* plaque buildup (atherosclerosis), and abnormal blood clotting (thrombosis).

Is L-P-Little-a really worse than LDL cholesterol?

The evidence thus far suggests that, all things considered, L-P-Little-a *is* worse than LDL cholesterol, but there is good news and bad news. (For the good news, turn to Chapter VI, Section 5, *Managing High Levels of Lipoprotein(a)*.) First, the bad news: Your Lp(a) level is largely genetically deter-

Lp(a) is one of the strongest, most readily measurable biological markers for premature heart disease.

mined, meaning that you are born with it. You have to have the gene that causes excessively high levels of Lp(a). Excess Lp(a) is therefore 5 to 10 times more common in individuals with a strong family history of premature heart disease. Given Lp(a)'s genetic basis, it is not surprising that Indians living in India, the UK, the US, Australia, and Singapore all have similar levels of Lp(a), and that studies have found that Indian siblings living in the UK and India, or in the US and India, have **identical levels.**

However, not every sibling or child in a family that has high levels of Lp(a) and a history of premature heart disease inherits the gene for it. Those who do not inherit the gene will have a normal Lp(a) level and perhaps a normal lifespan, all things being equal. Those who do inherit the "Lp(a) excess" gene, however, usually have an Lp(a) level identical to one of their parents, grandparents, or great grandparents, rather than the *average* of their parents or grand parents. Screening a person's closest blood relatives is therefore highly informative because Lp(a) is passed on as a dominant gene, meaning that *at least half* of the children of someone who has it will inherit the gene.

Second, maximum levels are reached as early as 24 months of age and are maintained throughout life. The level of "L-P-Little-a" in your blood never falls with positive lifestyle changes such as weight loss or vigorous exercise, but it can go up if you consume large amounts of trans fats. Trans fats are found in fried foods and the partially hydrogenated oils used in making crispy foods, non-dairy coffee creamers, commercially baked products such as donuts, and many other bakery or grocery store processed foods. Because of their **love of fried foods,** Indians consume particularly high amounts of trans fats, raising their Lp(a) level even higher. The frying process itself creates tons of trans fats, especially when the frying oil is reused (*see* Chapter V, Section 4).

More bad news: Excess Lp(a) is perhaps the only risk factor that promotes *both* plaque formation *and* blood clot formation. It also inhibits the normal breakup of blood clots. (Recall from Chapter I that the cause of most heart attacks is not just the formation of a plaque but the rupture of a soft plaque that then results in a blood clot.) High levels of Lp(a) can stimulate early and massive plaque buildup, leading to a heart attack and/or a stroke at a very young age. In the lab, it has been observed that animals that have the gene for Lp(a) develop spontaneous atherosclerosis even on a normal diet. On a high cholesterol, high saturated fat (that is, atherogenic) diet, these lab animal develop very severe plaque buildup. Unfortunately, the same thing happens in humans as well.

Table 3.4. Strong links: How Lp(a) predicts cardiovascular disease

- High levels of Lp(a) strongly predict early, advanced heart disease and stroke.
- In fact, depending on the presence of other risk factors, high Lp(a) can raise one's risk of heart disease anywhere from three-fold to 100-fold.
- Lp(a) levels exceeding 20 to 30mg/dL increase your risk of heart disease three to four times, even if you have no other risk factors.
- High levels are common among people with a family history of early heart disease.
- In both diabetics and non-diabetics, level of Lp(a) strongly predicts how severe their heart disease will be.
- In people who have undergone balloon angioplasty and/or bypass surgery, high Lp(a) strongly predicts re-narrowing of their coronary arteries and recurrent cardiac events.
- Excess levels are present in almost one out of every two Indians.

Lp(a)'s magnifying effect on other cardiac risks

What all of this means is that "L-P-Little-a" is one of the strongest, most readily measurable biological markers for premature heart disease, as shown in Table 3.4. Even if you have no other heart disease risk factors, a high level of Lp(a)—higher than 20 or 30 points—raises your risk of heart disease 2-4 times. Your risk rises eight-fold if in addition to high Lp(a) you also have low HDL; 12-fold if you have high LDL *and* high Lp(a); and 25-fold if *you have all three.* When people have several additional risk factors besides low HDL and high LDL, a high level of Lp(a) can raise their heart disease risk anywhere from five-fold to as much as 100 times, compared to people with normal Lp(a) and no other risk factors. Similarly, excess Lp(a) multiplies a smoker's cardiac risk two-fold, a diabetic's risk three-fold, and the risk of someone with high cholesterol or high blood pressure by a factor of four, over and beyond the risk conferred by these factors by themselves (*see* Figure 3.4). In

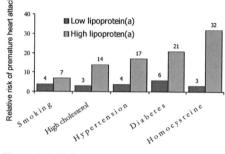

Figure 3.4. **Relative risk of premature heart attack as a function of lipoprotein(a) excess and other risk factors.** Note that lipoprotein(a) magnifies the risk three to 10-fold among those with traditional risk factors. The median Lp(a) was 40 mg/dl, which was used as the cut point for high and low levels. Source: Hopkins, PN. Ref. 3.32.

Interpreting the Statistics
Unlike other lipoproteins such as HDL and LDL cholesterol, the distribution of Lp(a) in a population is highly skewed and uneven. As a result, median levels are more accurate than mean levels, because the unevenness affects the median much less than it affects the mean.

the landmark Physicians Health Study (*see* Appendix B), high levels of Lp(a) were associated with a three- to four-fold higher risk of severe heart disease. The relative risk further rose to 12-fold when the person's LDL cholesterol was also high (*see* Figure 3.5). Lowering LDL with a statin may cut one's relative risk from 12-fold to four-fold, but that is still very high. Reducing it further requires lowering Lp(a) itself, with niacin. In short, high Lp(a) has a magnifying effect on many traditional risk factors. Through this synergistic action, elevated levels of Lp(a) stimulate abnormal clot formation and accelerate plaque buildup, laying the ground for heart attacks, strokes, and other major cardiovascular events. L-P-Little-a's influence on atherosclerosis and thrombosis produces several effects in the body—particularly premature, severe cardiovascular disease marked by restenosis (the rapid re-narrowing of an artery after it has been widened through balloon angioplasty and/or a stent). Let's look at these.

The effects of Lp(a) in the human body

Elevated Lp(a) has several serious effects, especially these:

► **Prematurity:** The higher the level of Lp(a), the lower the age of a first heart attack or stroke. Lp(a)'s role, however, diminishes with increasing age. The excess risk is highest before age 45, decreases after age 55, and disappears after age 65.

► **Severity:** Lp(a) is one of the few risk factors—along with low HDL and diabetes—that are directly associated with extensive plaque buildup and severe heart disease, as evidenced in studies such as the Physician's Health Study. The higher your Lp(a), the greater the number of narrowed coronary arteries you are likely to have, and the more severe the narrowing is likely to be. As a result, high Lp(a) can cause massive heart attacks that are more likely to be fatal.

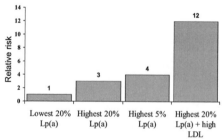

Figure 3.5. **Relative risk of severe heart disease requiring angioplasty or bypass surgery in the landmark Physicians Health Study.** This graph shows that, compared to the risk faced by people in the lowest 20% of lipoprotein(a) levels, people in the highest 20% have a three-fold risk of severe heart disease. Those in the highest 5% of lipoprotein(a) levels have a four-fold risk of heart disease compared to those in the lowest quintile. As the fourth box shows, however, when both high lipoprotein(a) and high LDL (above 160 mg/dL) are present, the risk of developing severe heart disease is 12 times higher than the risk faced by those in the lowest quintile. Source: Rifai, N. Ref. 6.49.

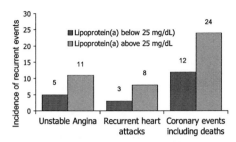

Figure 3.6 How the presence or absence of lipoprotein(a) excess influences the relative risk of recurrent heart attack and major acute coronary events (Cardiac death, heart attack, or unstable angina requiring hospitalization) among patients who have had coronary stents placed following a heart attack or acute coronary syndrome. Note that in three years there is a significant increase in such events in persons with lipoprotein(a) above 25mg/dL. Source: Zairis, N. Ref. 3.73.

▶ **Coronary artery re-narrowing:** Elevated Lp(a) is one of the few risk factors associated with high rates of coronary artery re-narrowing (restenosis) after balloon angioplasty or bypass surgery, especially when the person also has low HDL (*see also* Chapter II, Section 4). Lp(a), therefore, powerfully predicts the need for repeat angioplasty or surgery. The good news is that, in studies, reducing high Lp(a) levels with medications such as niacin reduced the rate of re-narrowing by up to 50% (*see* Chapter VIII, Section 2). People who have undergone bypass surgery or angioplasty at a young age ought to be tested for Lp(a) excess.

▶ **Recurrent heart attacks:** As shown in Figure 3.6, elevated Lp(a) strongly predicts recurrent heart attacks that may require hospitalization, even in patients with acute coronary syndrome who were successfully treated

with a coronary stent and were on all the best cardiac medications, including statins (*see* Chapter I, Section 1).

Lp(a) levels among Asian Indians

Lp(a) levels vary markedly by ethnicity, as might be expected of a trait with genetic origins. The level among Indians is second only to that of blacks, and five times higher than that of native Americans (*see* Figure 3.7). Lp(a) levels above 20 to 30 points are found in 40-45% of Indians globally, compared to less than 20% of whites and less than 1% of Native Americans. As shown in Figure 3.8, a study of 542 male and 468 female Indian and Chinese newborns which measured differences in their Lp(a) levels using

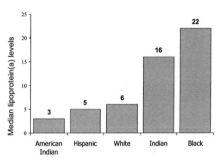

Figure 3.7. Median lipoprotein(a) levels (mg/dL) among Americans of different ethnicities. Source: Enas, EA. Ref. 3.21. *Reproduced with permission© British Journal of Diabetes and Vascular Disease.*

umbilical cord blood, large ethnic differences in Lp(a) levels—as much as three-fold—are present at birth. The Lp(a) levels were independent of the infant's birth weight and gender, but were significantly influenced by ethnicity. The difference in Lp(a) levels among these Singaporean babies parallels the marked difference in adult heart disease mortality rates between Indians and Chinese observed over the past 40 years in

Singapore, underscoring the idea not only that Lp(a) is inherited genetically but that its levels persist through life.

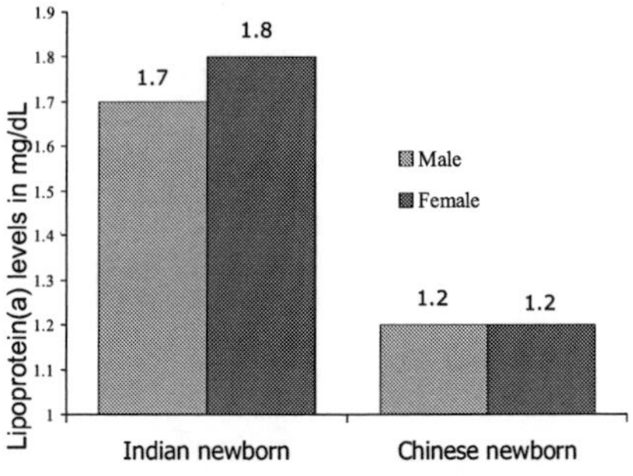

Because of the synergies mentioned above in the sub-section on Lp(a)'s magnifying effect, heart disease is even more severe when elevated Lp(a) is accompanied by diabetes, high homocysteine, and/or low HDL, high LDL, high triglycerides—in other words, metabolic syndrome. Diabetes, high homocysteine, and metabolic syndrome are, of all the heart disease risk factors, among the most prevalent in Indians. Lp(a) is particularly lethal in Indians because of a near-universal presence of low HDL, high triglycerides, and other emerging risk factors among them. Although African Americans and other blacks have the highest levels of Lp(a), the adverse effect of Lp(a) is almost neutralized by their high HDL and low triglyceride levels. blacks also have a different *and less dangerous* form (more properly called an isoform of Lp(a)—large-particle lipoprotein(a). There are actually 34 different

Figure 3.8. Differences in lipoprotein(a) in umbilical cord blood samples between Chinese and Indian newborns in Singapore. Note that the differences are consistently present in both boys and girls. The lipoprotein(a) levels are presented on the y axis on a logarithmic scale, so the differences are actually more dramatic than they even appear. Source: Low, PS et al. Ref. 3.44. *Reproduced with permission©Lippincott, Williams & Wilkins.*

isoforms or "versions" of Lp(a) that differ primarily by size, with the smaller ones posing the greater risk. Among Indians, however, both small and large isoforms are associated with heart disease, the small most likely being worse.

Taken together, these six risk factors—diabetes, high triglycerides, low HDL(particularly the most cardio protective large HD), high LDL, and high Lp(a) along with high homocysteine, provide the fullest, most persuasive explanation of the prematurity and severity of diffuse, multi-site, multi-vessel coronary artery disease among Indians worldwide. When one synthesizes together all these facts, it does not come as a surprise that more than 15 studies in India have confirmed that elevated Lp(a) is a powerful risk factor for heart attack, especially in Indians younger than 45.

> Taken together, the synergistic effects of six risk factors—diabetes, high tritlyceries, low HDL, high LDL, high Lp(a), and high homocysteine, provide the fullest, most persuasive explanation of the prematurity and severity of diffuse, multi-site, multi-vessel coronary artery disease among Indians worldwide.

Lp(a) and stroke: High Lp(a) is an equally strong predictor of premature stroke, including strokes in children. In several Japanese, Chinese as well as Indian studies of stroke occurring in people under 40 or 45 years old, elevated Lp(a) was the sole risk factor.

Measuring and treating high Lp(a)

It is worth highlighting that your Lp(a) levels need to be measured accurately, consistent with the recent guidelines issued by the National Heart Lung & Blood Institute, and the World Health Organization (*see* Chapter VII, Section 2). The first three reports from the Physicians Health study showed no relationship between Lp(a) excess and cardiovascular disease, but a more recent fourth report by the same investigators showed a very strong association with the onset and the severity of heart disease. The absence of correlations in the first three reports was attributed to the use of inaccurate commercial tests to measure Lp(a) levels.

Although Lp(a) levels above 30 are widely considered the cut-point for high risk, more recent studies suggest that the risk increases sharply after 20 mg/dL, not 30. In the National Asian Indian Heart Disease Project, *44% of Indians* without heart disease had Lp(a) levels above 20 compared with 25% of whites without heart disease. A cut-point of 20 may therefore be a more appropriate measure of high risk from Lp(a) excess, particularly among Indians.

Treatment: Treating Lp(a) is more difficult than other lipoproteins such as LDL and HDL cholesterol. The good news is that niacin, a relatively inexpensive drug, has been shown to lower Lp(a) effectively. (*See* Chapter VIII, Section 2 for a detailed discussion of niacin.) Niacin is also the most effective agent for raising HDL. At a daily dose 2 grams, niacin can decrease Lp(a) by 25% and increase HDL by 40%.

Chapter VI, Section 5 addresses the management and treatment of high Lp(a) levels. The Section 3 of this Chapter, will address homocysteine, another important emerging risk factor which is common among Indians and markedly increases the risk of premature heart disease when a person has high levels of both Lp(a) and homocysteine.

Table 3.5. How Lp(a) levels affect the prevalence of atherosclerosis

Lp(a) levels	CIMT	Carotid artery plaques
Low	16%	2%
Medium	20%	5%
High	30%	12%

Note: Carotid intimal medial thickness (CIMT) and carotid plaques are both measures of atherosclerosis. Source: Velmurugan, K. Ref.3.68.

KEY · POINTS · IN · A · NUTSHELL

♥ Always referred to as L-P-Little-a, lipoprotein(a) is a genetic variant of LDL cholesterol with an abnormal protein called apo(a) attached to it, that turns Lp(a) into a more dangerous risk factor than LDL cholesterol.

♥ One of the strongest biological markers for premature heart disease, Lp(a) may be the only risk factor that promotes both plaque buildup and abnormal blood clotting, the two features of heart disease most responsible for heart attacks.

♥ Lp(a) is therefore strongly associated with premature, severe cardiovascular disease that often leads to massive heart attacks and strokes at very young age.

♥ Lp(a) is strongly associated with rapid restenosis (arterial re-narrowing of the artery) following coronary angioplasty, with or without stent placement and bypass surgery. The risk is particularly high in people who also have low HDL as most Indians do.

♥ Elevated Lp(a) has a magnifying effect on many traditional risk factors. It raises heart disease risk two- to four-fold even in the absence of other risk factors, but raises it eight-fold if you also have low HDL, 12-fold if you have high Lp(a) and high LDL, 25-fold if you have all three, and up to 100-fold if you have these risk factors plus others.

♥ Largely genetically determined, Lp(a) levels are high in people with a family history of early heart disease.

♥ Your long-term adult Lp(a) level is reached by age two, persists throughout life, and does not fall with exercise, but rises if you eat a lot of trans fats, as most Indians do.

♥ Elevated Lp(a) levels are found in 40-45% of Indians worldwide, a level second only to that of blacks. Strikingly, Lp(a) is particularly dangerous among Indians due to common occurrence of low HDL , high triglycerides and high LDL levels.

♥ Unlike Indians, blacks are somewhat protected against the dangers of Lp(a) by having a less dangerous form of it and by their high levels of HDL, which Indians typically lack.

♥ The combination of high Lp(a), excess homocysteine, diabetes, and metabolic syndrome (i.e., high triglycerides, high LDL, and low HDL)—and the synergistic interaction among these risk factors—best explains the high prevalence of premature, severe, diffuse, multi-vessel coronary artery disease among Indians globally.

♥ Lp(a) above 30 is widely considered the cut-point for high risk, but a level of 20 may be a more appropriate cut-point, particularly for Indians.

♥ Cholesterol-lowering statins do not lower Lp(a) directly, but they help insofar as Lp(a) is more harmful when working in concert with high LDL cholesterol.

♥ Prescription niacin, a relatively inexpensive medication lowers Lp(a) safely and effectively. Two grams a day reduces it by about 25%, and 4 grams by almost 40%.

♥ Recent studies show that fenofibrate (Tricor) increases Lp(a).

3.3 ▶ Homocysteine - The Quasi-cholesterol

At the tender age of 39, Dr. Peter Chacko had his first heart attack. A young, busy, Indian physician, Chacko had no cardiac risk factors, except that his father had died young from a heart attack. When asked, he attributed his own heart attack to what he called "the stress" of his busy medical practice—a common misconception among many Indians. It was not his stress. So what was it? His total cholesterol was 208 mg/dL, just above the desired level of 200 mg/dL. Three months after the heart attack, he had had a near-normal coronary angiogram that revealed no obvious blockage or narrowing of coronary arteries that might require bypass surgery. However, yet within five years, *and without suffering a heart attack*, his atherosclerosis progressed so rapidly to and resulted in total blockage of all three of his major coronary arteries. His condition was dire. Two surgeons refused to operate on him, but a third agreed to perform a quintuple bypass surgery to find alternate routes around Chacko's five blocked coronary arteries. His heart disease, however, was so far advanced that he was permanently disabled. At the prime of his career, Peter Chacko was forced to quit a successful medical practice.

Advanced blood tests for emerging risk factors showed that Dr. Chacko had high levels of homocysteine and lipoprotein(a), along with a low level of HDL. This combination is a terrible triad that is all too common among Indians but not in any other populations. As a result of aggressive medical treatment directed at both traditional and emerging risk factors, Dr. Chacko has been able to regain a reasonably normal life. Although he had not spent a single day as a patient in the hospital in the last 15 years, he was never able to return to his practice. His story illustrates the importance of testing for and treating emerging risk factors among Indians. Had Dr. Chacko's abnormalities been detected and treated in his twenties, his heart attack, bypass surgery, disability, and premature retirement could have been avoided. His second angiogram is shown first deliberately, followed by the first angiogram (Color plate 3.4. and 3.5) to dispel the pervasive myth that Indians have small coronary arteries. A cursory examination of the first angiogram would reinforce this myth. His first angiogram five years earlier shows large coronary arteries which were completely occluded by the time the second angiogram was done. This section discusses the importance of testing for and managing homocysteine.

What exactly is **homocysteine**? Homocysteine is an amino acid produced by the body from the breakdown of another amino acid, methionine. It is found in the blood. A high level of homocysteine is associated with a heightened risk of heart attack and death. The risk is particularly magnified in the presence of high lipoprotein(a) levels, which we discussed in the preceding section, and smoking. Although an elevated homocysteine level in blood is an easily modifiable independent risk factor for cardiovascular disease, similar in importance to traditional risk factors, nearly half of people with very high homocysteine levels (above 100 micromol/L) develop heart attack or stroke or lose a limb—often a leg— before age 30 if they are not treated. Amputation attests to the extraordinary damage homocysteine can do to one's arteries.

Table 3.2. Relative risk of heart attack with high homocystene and other risk factors	
	Relative risk
High homocysteine alone	2-fold
High homocysteine plus smoking	12-fold
High homocysteine plus two standard risk factors	12-fold
High homocysteine plus High lipoprotein (a)	32-fold

Source: O'Callaghan, Ref. 3.53; Hopkins, RN. Ref. 3.32.

Indians have higher levels of homocysteine than other populations, and this contributes to their excess burden of heart disease. Nutritional factors appear to be more important than genetic factors among in raising the homocysteine level among Indians. Homocysteine levels can be lowered safely and effectively with prescription medications containing adequate doses of folic acid, B_{12}, and B_6.

Although homocysteine is not cholesterol, it functions as what I would call "quasi-cholesterol" because it increases the risk you face from high cholesterol and other risk factors. As a *predisposing risk factor*, homocysteine powerfully increases the magnitude of risk factors such as diabetes, smoking, and hypertension in many different populations. A normal level of homocysteine is below 10 micromol/liter in adults and below 5 micromol/liter in children. People with homocysteine levels above 12 have double the risk of heart attack. Homocysteine levels are often high in children with a family history of premature heart disease. High homocysteine levels often coexists with lipoprotein(a) excess and may partly explain the excess risk of heart disease in those with family history of premature heart disease. For example, in Dr. Chacko's case (above) his son, who was 15 at the time, had nearly identical levels of homocysteine and lipoprotein(a). This underscores the importance of these two factors in children with a family history of heart disease.

Persons with very high levels of homocysteine develop serious complications at a young age. In 1969 Kilmer McCully, pioneer of the homocysteine theory, observed the high risk of extremely premature heart disease in children with very high levels of homocysteine (above 100 micromol/L). Remember that normal is below five. Postmortem studies of children as young as eight with very high levels of homocysteine showed advanced atherosclerosis (plaque build-up) of the coronary arteries, similar to that observed among 80-year-olds. Subsequent studies extended these findings to adults as well.

Table 3.3. Relative risk of death from high homocysteine, regardless of other factors

Homocysteine level (micromol/L)	Relative risk of death
9 to 14.9	2
15 to 19.9	3
Above 20	5

Source: Nygard O. Ref. 3.52.

Whereas earlier studies focused on patients with very high levels, more recent studies have shown that even mild elevations of homocysteine are associated with a high risk of a heart attack. Each five micromol/L increase in homocysteine level confers the same increase in risk for cardiovascular disease as a 20mg/dL increase in total cholesterol level: namely, a 50% increase in cardiac risk. High blood levels of homocysteine are also related to a high risk of restenosis following coronary angioplasty. More than 100 studies comprising more than 15,000 patients have shown that elevated homocysteine level in blood is an independent predictor of death in people with and without the presence of other risk factors.

The cardiac risk is increased two-fold with mild, three-fold with moderate, and four-fold with severe elevation of homocysteine levels. Smoking increases a person's homocysteine levels and also increases the risk of a heart attack 12 times. The highest risk is among those with elevations of both homocysteine and lipoprotein(a), which confers a 32-fold increase in risk.

In patients with heart disease, homocysteine is a significant predictor of death, independent of traditional risk factors, number of severely diseased coronary arteries, and heart muscle function. Compared to patients with homocysteine levels below 9 micromol/L, the death rates were increased five-fold for those with levels above 20 micromol/L. (See Table 3.3).

A recent study from the Cleveland Clinic found that those with homocysteine levels above 14 micromol/L had a three-fold higher rate of death during a three-year follow-up period. The risk from elevated homocysteine level is not limited to heart disease; it also aggravates non-cardiovascular diseases (Table 3.4.). All these complications are magnified several fold in the presence of lipoprotein(a) excess. Homocysteine damages blood vessels in several ways:

Table 3.4. Complications related to elevated homocysteine levels

Cardiovascular diseases	Non-cardiovascular diseases
• Premature heart disease • Premature stroke, especially in children • Premature peripheral vascular disease • High risk of amputation • Restenosis following coronary angioplasty • Sudden and non-sudden death	• Chronic kidney failure • Dementia • Bone health and bone fracture • Deep-vein thrombosis • Proclivity for blood clots • Birth defects

- It injures and burns the endothelium (the layer of cells lining the inside of arteries). It appears that the effect is similar to the burns produced by powerful sulfuric acid.
- It can disrupt normal blood-clotting mechanisms, increasing the risk of clots that can bring on a heart attack or stroke.
- It also stimulates the growth of smooth-muscle cells, an integral component of plaque formation and growth.

Homocysteine levels among Indians and other populations

Among Americans, an elevated homocysteine level is present in less than 10% of patients without heart disease, 15% with heart disease, 35% of patients with stroke, and 47% of patients with peripheral vascular disease. Indians have higher levels of homocysteine than whites and Chinese all over the world, including the US, Canada, Singapore, and the UK. In one study in India, more than 70% of both vegetarians and non-vegetarians had high levels of homocysteine.

Homocysteine levels have declined in the US, following the 1998 FDA rule that flour and other specified grains must be fortified with folic acid at levels ranging from 0.43 mg to 1.4 mg per pound of product. However, homocysteine levels among Indians in the US are substantially higher than in whites. It is unclear whether flour bought from Indian grocery stores contains the required amount of folic acid.

> Dietary factors such as not eating enough foods that are rich in folic acid (like deep-green leafy vegetables), and the leaching or destruction of so much of their nutrient content through overcooking, are likely to be the primary factors that account for the destructively high levels of homocysteine in Indians.

Causes of homocysteine elevation

Homocysteine levels are controlled by genetic and nutritional factors, notably folate, vitamin B_{12} and vitamin B_6 intakes., insufficient dietary intake of the these vitamins can be caused by losses of these nutrients during processing of foods. Heavy alcohol intake, heavy coffee intake, and smoking all raise homocysteine levels. Intake of one to two drinks a day of any type of alcohol is usually associated with cardiac protection. However, an intake of one drink per day of hard liquor (rather than wine or beer) can elevate homocysteine. Low levels of B vitamins explain the high levels of homocysteine in smokers and alcoholics.

Vegetarians have lower levels of vitamin B_{12} than nonvegetarians. Nonvegetarians obtain most of their vitamin B_{12} through meat, whereas vegetarians obtain it from milk, dairy products, and eggs. Many commonly-used medications increase homocysteine levels, including metformin, niacin, fenofibrate (Tricor), cholestyramine (Questran), thiazide diuretics, and Dilantin. Increase in the homocysteine with these medications can be easily managed with multivitamins containing adequate amounts of B vitamins, as discussed below.

Unlike in other populations, high homocysteine levels among Indians are related more to depressed levels of *vitamins B_{12} and B_6,* than to low levels of folic acid. Dietary factors, such as not eating enough foods that are high in folic acid (like green leafy vegetables), and the destruction of so much of their nutrient content through prolonged cooking, appear to be the major factors among Indians. Mutations in the gene that result in elevated levels of homocysteine are less common among Indians than whites and other populations. Homocysteine levels are elevated even with mild kidney disease. It is markedly elevated in patients undergoing maintenance dialysis and contributes to the five to 10-fold increases in the risk of a heart attack or a stroke among these patients. People with kidney failure are somewhat resistant to the homocysteine-lowering effect of B vitamins. Therefore, very high doses of B vitamins are required to lower homocysteine levels in patients with kidney dialysis and kidney transplant recipients.

Table 3.5. Amount of folic acid and vitamin B in some common medications and supplements. Note that most supplements do not contain sufficient amounts of B vitamins to lower homocysteine

Brand	Folic acid	B12	B6	Betaine
Metanx	2.8 mg	2 mg	26	
Foltx	2.5mg	1000 mcg	25 mg	-
Folgard Rx	2.2 mg	500 mcg	25 mg	-
Folgard	800 mcg	115 mcg	10 mg	-
Cardio B	5 mg	1000 mcg	50mg	500 mg
Vitaplex plus	800 mcg	50 mcg	25 mg	-
Centrum silver	400 mcg	30 mcg	6 mg	-

Treatment of high homocysteine

Foods high in folate, such as spinach, asparagus, beans, peanuts, orange juice, and enriched grain products can prevent homocysteine elevation, as well as lower it slightly. In fact, following the Folic Acid Fortification Program, which began in 1998, high homocysteine levels among Indians have declined by 50%.

Folic acid lowers homocysteine by 25%. However, folic acid alone is not sufficient in most Indians as well as other populations. Homocysteine levels can be lowered to normal levels by safe, simple, and inexpensive treatment with a combination of vitamins B_6, B_{12}, and folic acid. In some resistant cases, riboflavin and biotin may be required. Recent studies indicate that daily administration of 2 mg of B_{12} orally per day has the same efficacy as 1 mg given as an intramuscular injection every four weeks. Preliminary studies indicate that the n-3 polyunsaturated fatty acids containing fish oils can lower homocysteine levels by 50%.

There are several on-going trials to determine if reduction of homocysteine blood levels with folate, B_6 and B_{12} translate into a reduction in cardiovascular events in high-risk patients. Results are expected by 2006.

KEY · POINTS · IN · A · NUTSHELL

♥ A high level of homocysteine is associated with a heightened risk of heart attack and stroke.

♥ The risk is highest in association with elevated lipoprotein(a) and smoking.

♥ Nearly half of the people with very high homocysteine levels develop a heart attack or a stroke, or undergo a leg amputation before age 30, if not treated.

♥ Indians have higher homocysteine levels than all other populations.

♥ Nutritional factors appear to be more important than genetic factors, especially among Indians for elevated homocysteine levels.

♥ Many medications for the treatment of diabetes and dyslipidemia can raise homocysteine levels.

♥ Homocysteine levels can be lowered safely and effectively with prescription medications containing adequate doses of folic acid, vitamin B12, and vitamin B6 (Metanx, Foltx, Folgard, etc.).

3.4. ▶ C-Reactive Protein- A Sign of Silent Inflammation

Mrs. Thresiamma Joseph, a diabetic for 20 years, had three-vessel bypass surgery following a heart attack which was the first clue of her heart disease. Within seven months, two of the three bypasses failed with recurrence of severe chest pain and inability to walk more than half a block. A repeat coronary angiogram showed diffuse disease (narrowing of key arteries at several locations) rendering them unsuitable for angioplasty, stent, and repeat bypass surgery. She was told that *nothing could be done* to improve her chances of survival and quality of life. She was told to come to the emergency room upon severe worsening of symptoms so the doctor could relieve them. The patient was given no hope and began preparing for imminent death.

I had the opportunity to evaluate this desperate woman. The underlying problem was identified as a combination of high C-reactive protein and low HDL, high lipoprotein(a), in addition to long-standing diabetes. She was treated aggressively with multiple medications so that she can now walk two hours at a stretch without symptoms. More importantly, she has had a repeat stress test which showed no evidence of vulnerable heart muscle and a repeat angiogram three years later showing improvement in her plaque build up.

Of all of the emerging risk factors, an elevated level of C-reactive protein (CRP) has received the most scientific attention in the past decade. C-reactive protein is a specific protein that indicates inflammation. An elevated CRP level predicts and precedes the development of diabetes, heart attack, and stroke, decades before such a catastrophe. Among people with heart disease, a high CRP is a *strong determinant of complications* following a heart attack, angioplasty, and stent. The formation of a blood clot that triggers a heart attack is almost always due to a rupture of a lipid-rich unstable plaque. Such plaques are often inflamed. CRP is a readily measurable marker of inflammation, which makes these plaques vulnerable and prone to rupture. Thus CRP serves as a surrogate marker for a vulnerable plaque. Indians have higher levels of CRP than other populations - roughly twice the levels of CRP whites do. Among Indians, it is related to a sedentary lifestyle and *abdominal obesity* but not general obesity. Physical activity with or without weight loss can significantly reduce CRP. This section highlights the importance and implications of elevated CRP among Indians.

Atherosclerosis is now considered a chronic inflammatory disease (though not necessarily an infectious disease that can be treated with antibiotics). The degree of elevation in CRP level is correlates highly with the extent of inflammation, as well as the presence and severity of unstable vulnerable plaques.

In general, people with high CRP alone have twice the cardiac risk of people with normal CRP levels (Table 3.6). This risk increases to four-fold when high CRP is present with low HDL (or high total cholesterol to HDL ratio), and five-fold with high LDL levels. The risk due to elevated CRP levels is higher in women than in men. In the Women's Health Study (see Appendix B), the risk of a first heart attack was 50% higher in those with a CRP level of more than 4 mg/L as compared to those with normal CRP and high LDL (above 154 mg/dL). Among those with high levels of both CRP and LDL, the risk was 50% higher [than the control group]. The risk of a heart attack from elevated CRP is markedly increased in the presence of an elevated white blood cell count and or metabolic syndrome. Efforts are underway to incorporate CRP levels in the Framingham Risk Score (see Chapter II, Section 7)

Table 3.6. Cardiac risk according to CRP levels

CRP level	Risk category
Below 1mg/L	Low
1 to 3mg/L	Average
3 to 10mg/L	High
above 10mg/L	Very high

CRP, metabolic syndrome, and diabetes

A high CRP level correlates strongly with the presence of metabolic syndrome, as well as its severity. (Metabolic syndrome is discussed in Section 7.) The CRP level increases as the number of the components of metabolic syndrome rises; those with all five components have the highest CRP levels. High CRP is also a powerful predictor of diabetes. The risk of developing diabetes increases three-fold independent of other risk factors and as high as 25-fold when accompanied by metabolic syndrome. Many experts believe that the time has come for a careful consideration of adding CRP as the sixth clinical criterion for metabolic syndrome.

Indians and CRP

CRP level correlates highly with increased fat mass CRP levels are generally two-fold higher among overweight people and four-fold higher among obese people. Yet, even though Indians have much less total bodily obesity than other populations, CRP levels are the highest among Indians—nearly double the levels in whites in the UK and Chinese in Canada. This paradox is primarily due to the high prevalence of *abdominal obesity* in Indians. Several studies have shown CRP levels correlate strongly with abdominal obesity, measured as waist circumference, than total obesity measured as weight or body mass index.

Causes of elevated CRP

The causes of elevated CRP include obesity, particularly abdominal obesity, smoking, diabetes, metabolic syndrome, hypertension, excess coffee consumption, and estrogen treatment in women. Obesity, particularly abdominal obesity, markedly increases CRP levels.

CRP levels are elevated in all inflammatory conditions, including all infections. Certain types of arthritidies are associated with some of the highest levels of CRP. Extensive periodontal disease, an inflammatory condition associated with inflammation of the gums and tooth loss and common among Indians, is associated with increased CRP levels as discussed earlier. Thus, CRP may not be a true marker of vulnerable plaques, but an indicator of inflammation from a variety of causes.

Testing for CRP

The standard CRP test (used for detecting chronic inflammatory conditions, such as arthritis) does not detect low levels of CRP associated with cardiac risk. A high-sensitivity CRP (hs-CRP) test has been developed to overcome this problem. It is available in most hospitals and laboratories in the US. Some, but not all, insurance companies and managed care plans pay for an hs-CRP test. In people, who have any kind of infection or inflammatory condition, the test can be markedly abnormal and needs to be repeated after the acute condition has subsided to accurately determine the stable CRP level.

Treatment for high CRP

Increased physical activity and weight loss are the most effective strategies for lowering high CRP levels. Weight loss can reduce its levels by half. Exercise lowers CRP by one-third even when the body weight is not lost. Regular physical activity and weight loss together have the greatest effect on lowering CRP. Marathon runners have half, and lean marathon runners have one-fourth the level of CRP of an average adult.

One aspirin (325 mg) a day may lower CRP; the benefit of aspirin in cardiac protection is greatest among those with high CRP levels. All cholesterol lowering statin medications lower CRP by 25% in two weeks. Since people with high CRP constitute a group with heightened risk, such individuals should be treated more aggressively with statins and other medications. A recent study has demonstrated the benefit of aggressive lowering of both LDL and CRP levels. A high dose of potent statins was compared to an average dose of a moderately potent statin (Lipitor 80 mg versus Pravachol 40 mg). Patients, who achieved a dual goal of LDL less than 70 mg/dL and CRP less than 2 mg/dL, had the best clinical outcome. Those, who achieved either the CRP or LDL goal but not both, had a 40% higher risk, and those, who achieved neither, had a 90% higher risk (Table 3.7).

Other studies have shown that reductions in both LDL and CRP levels are associated with greater regression of coronary plaques (see Chapter VII, Section 7). The totality of the data suggests the potential role of high-dose statins in reducing the risk in patients who have both LDL and CRP.

Table 3.7. Relative risk of recurrent MACE (major acute coronary events) according to CRP and LDL levels

Subgroups		MACE categories		
LDL (mg/dL)	CRP (mg/L)	MACE %	MACE/100 person-yr	Risk ratio
Below 70	Below 2	5%	2.4	1.0
Below 70	2 or more	7%	3.1	1.3
70 or above	Below 2	7%	3.2	1.4
70 or above	2 or more	10%	4.6	1.9

Notice that the lowest risk occurs in persons with LDL below 70mg/dL and CRP below 2mg/dL. Note that the risk increases 50% with an elevation of any one of these two factors and it doubles when both are elevated. Source: Ridker, PN. Ref. 3.56.

KEY · POINTS · IN · A · NUTSHELL

♥ Atherosclerosis is now regarded as a chronic inflammatory disease.

♥ A high level of C-reactive protein (CRP) is a strong marker of inflammation.

♥ High CRP is a predictor of future risk of heart attack and diabetes in healthy individuals.

♥ High levels of CRP confer a heightened risk of recurrent heart attacks and complications among people with heart disease.

♥ Both general and abdominal obesity are common causes of elevated CRP.

♥ Other causes of elevated CRP include smoking, metabolic syndrome, hypertension, excess coffee consumption, and estrogen treatment in women.

♥ High CRP levels are twice as common among Indians as non-Indians, and are probably related to abdominal obesity and physical inactivity.

♥ Physical activity with or without weight loss can reduce CRP by more than 50%; lean marathon runners have the lowest levels of CRP

♥ Statin and aspirin therapies are more beneficial among people with high CRP levels.

3.5 ► Obesity - The Price of Sedentary Lifestyle

An epidemic of obesity is sweeping the developed countries of the west, with the US leading all nations. At least one in three Americans is obese and two in three are overweight. If the current trends are not reversed, it is projected that almost all Americans will be overweight by 2050 and obese by the end of the century. Obesity is primarily due to a lack of physical activity and overeating, but the relative contribution varies among individuals. A weight gain of 10 pounds a year requires only a mere extra 100 calories a day. Most Indians are not obese by the standard criteria, but nearly half have obesity by the *Asia-Pacific Criteria of Obesity* issued by the World Health Organization (WHO). Obesity is correlates highly with dyslipidemia, metabolic syndrome, and diabetes. This section discusses the effects of obesity and highlights the difference in criteria for obesity between Asians and other populations.

It only takes eating an extra 100 alories a day to see a weight gain of 10 pounds at the end of the year.

Over the past 40 years, the average American woman gained one inch in height (went from 5'3" to 5'4") and the average American man 1.5 inches (5'8" to 5'9.5"). However, both men and women gained an average of 25 pounds during that time. In 1998, the American Heart Association upgraded overweight/obesity to its list of major cardiac risk factors. The WHO has recently coined the term "globesity" to describe a global epidemic of obesity affecting at least 300 million people—a three-fold increase since 1980s in many parts of the world.

Obesity is a predisposing risk factor that markedly increases the risk posed to you by all other cardiac risk factors, except smoking. These include dyslipidemia, metabolic syndrome, diabetes, and hypertension. Obesity accounts for one-fourth of the disease burden of diabetes, hypertension, and heart disease. People with obesity have double the risk of heart disease and stroke and more than triple the risk of diabetes, compared to those who are of normal weight. The prevalence of degenerative arthritis, kidney stones, gastroesophageal reflux disease (GERD), erectile dysfunction, gout, reduced amount of sleep, and obstructive sleep apnea (snoring and periodic stopping of breathing during sleep) increases in proportion to the degree of excess weight. Other complications (particularly among women), include poor self-esteem, poor social life, anxiety, depression, and stress. In addition, childhood obesity has recently been linked to cancer. In short, obesity reduces the quality of life in almost everyone it affects.

Immigrants and weight gain

Although severe obesity often has a genetic basis, the major factor driving obesity is *excess food intake* in comparison to one's physical activity level. In other words, it is usually very much a question of lifestyle. The 2000 report of the National Health Interview Survey involving 32,374 respondents, 14% of whom were immigrants, found that the prevalence of obesity among immigrants increased steadily and approached that of US-born adults within 15 years of immigration. Their lifestyle, in short, had changed. The average weight gain was nine pounds for a typical immigrant woman measuring 5'4", and 11 pounds for a typical immigrant man 5'9" tall. Trends in obesity among immigrants may, therefore, reflect **acculturation.** Acculturation, in the context of immigrants, refers to the way they assimilate to and adopt the lifestyle of the country of immigration. Like other immigrants, most Indians also show similar or even greater weight gain after immigrating to the US. More importantly, however, the adverse effect of this weight gain is two to three times greater among Indians than it is in other populations. Why is that? We will approach this shortly.

Fast foods and fast weight gain

A 15-year study has found that young adults, who frequently eat fast food, are more likely to gain weight and develop diabetes than those who do not. Young adults, who consumed fast food more than twice a week, gained 10 additional pounds and had twice the risk of developing diabetes than those, who ate fast food less than once a week. In response, many fast-food chains are beginning to offer healthy alternatives. For example, McDonald's now buys more apples than any other restaurant chain in the US, and it began selling 99 cent Apple Dippers last year as an alternative to fries, ice cream, and pies. Unfortunately, many people eat the Apple Dippers *on top of* the fat-rich fast food, defeating the entire purpose.

The price of obesity

The impact and cost of obesity is substantial. It accounts for 20% of the $1.7 trillion spent on healthcare in the US. Obese persons spend nearly four times as much on prescription medications as normal-weight persons. This translates into a difference of $700 per year per person. By the time they are 50 years of age, those who choose to eat whatever they want and do not bother to exercise regularly, usually end up taking, on average, four different medications to control blood pressure, three medications to control diabetes, and two to control dyslipidemia. Physiologically, with just 15 pounds of extra fat added on, your blood pressure, cholesterol, and triglycerides levels all begin to go up and your HDL level comes down. By the time most people have added an extra 30 pounds, they have begun developing hypertension, diabetes or dyslipidemia.

Standard criteria for obesity

How fat is fat? For an average man (150 pounds), adding an extra 15 pounds of body fat is medically regarded as being overweight, and 30 pounds as obese. Obesity is defined as a body fat content of more than 25% in men and more than 33% in women. Since the accurate measurement of body fat is very laborious and expensive, body mass index or BMI is used as a surrogate yardstick for obesity in clinical practice. BMI is the ratio of body weight in kilograms divided by height in meters squared. The corresponding formula for body weight in pounds and height in inches is given below:

$$BMI = 704 \ \frac{Weight\ (lbs)}{Height\ (in)\ X\ Height\ (in)}$$

BMI can also be obtained from published tables. Free charts for BMI are downloadable from the internet: for example, at www.nhlbi.nih.gov. In non-Asian adults (whites, blacks and Hispanics), a normal healthy weight is currently defined as a BMI of below 25, overweight as 25 to 30, and obese as above 30. Morbid obesity is defined as a BMI above 40, or above 35 if you have other metabolic abnormalities such as diabetes, high blood pressure, or metabolic syndrome. About 5% of the US population is morbidly obese; many of them may be candidates for gastric bypass surgery (see below).

The cut point that defines obesity is likely to be lowered because new data shows a high risk of hypertension, diabetes, and metabolic syndrome among many people with "normal BMI." For example, women 18 years of age with a BMI of 24 developed hypertension twice as often and diabetes five times as often as women with a BMI below 21.

Metabolic syndrome and obesity

Metabolic syndrome refers to a constellation of several abnormalities including high triglycerides and large waist size. It is intimately associated with high risk of heart disease and diabetes (see Section 7). Although obesity and high BMI are not considered among the criteria for metabolic syndrome, the risk is markedly elevated with increasing BMI, even in the range considered normal (BMI below 25). The NHANES III study found a high prevalence of metabolic syndrome among people with a BMI below 25, which is considered normal by current standards. Men and women with BMI of 21-23 had a **four-fold higher** rate of metabolic syndrome than those with a BMI below 21. Similarly, women

In both men and women, a simple rule of thumb for calculating your optimum weight is: 107 pounds for the first five feet, and four pounds for each additional inch thereafter. Example: If you are 5 ft 6 inches, your optimal weight is 107 + 24 = 131 punds or lower.

with BMI 25-27 had 17-fold higher rate and men had a nine-fold higher rate than those below 21. Screening in individuals with normal or slightly elevated BMI is, therefore, important to prevent diabetes and cardiovascular disease.

WHO's Asia Pacific Criteria for Obesity

As discussed earlier, obesity is defined as an excess of body fat. A desirable fat content is 12% to 20% for men, and 20% to 30% for women. For a given BMI, women have more fat than men. A similar situation exists for Asians as compared to whites and blacks. At a given BMI, Asians have *3% to 5% higher* body fat than other populations. Also, for a given amount of body fat, the **BMI is 2 to 3 units lower in Asians** than in whites. This phenomenon is attributed to the smaller body frame of Asians. Therefore, the standard cut-points of obesity may not be appropriate for Asians in general and Indians in particular. Singapore has adopted new cut-points for obesity. Under Singapore's new system, people with a BMI more than 27.5 are considered at high risk of metabolic disease, while 23 to 27.4 signals moderate risk and 18.5 to 22.9 is healthy. The WHO recommends different cut-points for obesity in Asians (Asian Pacific criteria). **A BMI more than 23 is considered overweight for Asians,** as opposed to more than 25 in other populations. A BMI **more than 25 is considered obese for Asians and Indians** in contrast to 30 for other populations.

Conversely, blacks have less body fat and metabolic abnormalities at a given BMI. The optimum BMI appears to be below 23 for Asians, 23 to 25 for whites and 23 to 30 for blacks. A simple rule of thumb for optimum weight in both men and women is 105 pounds for the first five feet and five pounds for each additional inch. The BMI cut-point for overweight and obesity in Indians are given in Table 3.8.

Compared with whites, blacks, and Hispanics, Indians have a substantially lower rate of obesity, particularly among those who live in the rural areas. However, the metabolic abnormalities and the risk of diabetes and heart disease is not fully reflected in obesity measured as BMI. Current evidence indicates that the distribution of fat is more important than total amount of fat in a given individual. The next section addresses the importance of fat distribution and abdominal obesity with special attention to Indians.

Table 3.8. Cut-points for BMI for overweight and obesity for Indians and whites at selected heights.

Maximum weight in pounds					
Indians	Normal	Overweight	Obesity	Severe Obesity	Morbid Obesity
Height in inches	BMI below 21	BMI above 23	BMI above 25	BMI above 30	BMI above 35
60 (5 ft)	107	118	128	153	179
61	111	122	132	158	185
62	115	126	136	164	191
63	118	130	141	169	197
64	122	134	145	174	204
65	126	138	150	180	210
66 (5 ft 6")	130	142	155	186	216
67	134	146	159	191	223
68	138	151	164	197	230
69	142	155	169	203	236
70	146	160	174	209	243
71	150	165	179	215	250
72 (6 ft)	154	170	184	221	258
whites	Normal	Normal	Overweight	Obesity	Severe Obesity

Note. the differences in cut-points for obesity between Indians and whites. This table may not be appropriate for individuals who have significant muscle mass due to resistance training or high level of fitness.

KEY · POINTS · IN · A · NUTSHELL

- ♥ Two in three Americans are overweight, and one in three is obese.
- ♥ Obesity is primarily due to overeating in relation to physical activity.
- ♥ Asians have a greater amount of fat than whites, for the same weight and BMI.
- ♥ The optimum BMI is lower among Indians and other Asians than whites.
- ♥ A BMI above 23 is considered overweight and BMI above 25 obese among Asians, compared to 25 and 30 for whites, respectively.
- ♥ A 5'6" Indian, who weighs more than 155 lbs, is considered obese, compared to 185 lbs, for whites.
- ♥ Obesity correlates highly with dyslipidemia, metabolic syndrome, and diabetes.
- ♥ Obese persons spend nearly four times more on medications than people of normal weight.

3.6 ► Abdominal Obesity - The Shape of Cardiac Risk

Extensive research over the past decade has identified abdominal obesity—defined simply as having a large waist—as a strongly predictive risk factor for diabetes, heart disease and sudden death. In particular, abdominal obesity is a substantially better predictor of diabetes and heart disease than general obesity. So compelling is waist measurement as a predictor of heart disease that the lower risk of heart disease in women has been found to correlate with their smaller waist size. Indeed, gender is not the primary issue: men and women of equal waist size have a similar risk of heart disease and diabetes. Abdominal obesity is two to three times more common in Indians than is general obesity, measured as Body Mass Index (BMI). For any given waist size, Indians have double the risk of dyslipidemia and diabetes of other populations. This section discusses the dangers of abdominal obesity, with a focus on the Indian population.

> Body Types: Fat distribution is almost everything when it comes to fat and heart disease, better to be pearshaped—like a woman with fat hips—than apple-shaped—like a man with a fat belly

General obesity versus abdominal obesity

The risk from a large waist—measured at the largest circumference between your belly button and the top of your hip bone, wherever that circumference occurs—exceeds that from high BMI). In the landmark INTERHEART Study, abdominal obesity was the third most important risk factor after abnormal lipids and smoking, accounting for 20% of the risk of a first heart attack (rising to 24% among women and younger individuals). (Abnormal lipids refer to the ratio of your good to bad cholesterol.) Other studies have also shown that the importance of obesity in heart disease actually declines and disappears once abdominal obesity has been factored in.

Abdominal obesity assumes greater importance in people whose BMI puts them in the normal weight or mildly overweight categories. The risk of biochemical abnormalities, including metabolic syndrome, are observed in children, adults, and the elderly with abdominal obesity. In one study, abdominal obesity without generalized obesity increased the risk of diabetes two-fold in men and three-fold in women. In contrast with generalized obesity, abdominal obesity clearly has a lot to do with how fat is distributed on your body, as we are about to see.

Pears are better than apples!

It is well-known that women have more fat than men at any given weight and height, but this excess fat does not necessarily translate into high cardiac risk. Distribution of body fat rather than the absolute amount of fat is what determines heart disease. Fat around the abdomen or waist is the most dangerous form of fat for cardiovascular and diabetic risk, compared to fat in the thighs and buttocks. Recent studies (2005) indicate that large hips (both fat and muscle) may indeed be protective against diabetes and heart disease. In other words, when it comes to fat, it is better to be pear-shaped (like a woman with a fat hip) than apple-shaped—(like a man with a fat belly).

The two commonly identified patterns of obesity are apple-type obesity (also called central obesity, abdominal obesity, android obesity, or upper body obesity) and pear-type obesity (also called lower body obesity, peripheral obesity, gynoid obesity, or gluteo-femoral obesity). Abdominal obesity accumulates in three places: It includes (i) subcutaneous fat (fat located in the front of the abdomen and under skin), (ii) retro-peritoneal fat (fat around the kidney region) and (iii) visceral fat

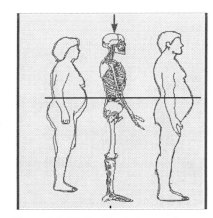

Figure 3.9. Distinct body types of persons suffering from metabolic syndrome. Most of these people have large bellies but may not be overweight by conventional standards. This combination of unhealthy abdominal girth despite "desirable weight" as determined by a body mass index of less than 25 is unusually common among Indians.

(fat deep inside the abdomen itself and surrounding your vital organs, such as liver and intestines). The main problem is the third—visceral fat—and most men put on fat in their belly early on.

The problem with a big belly is that visceral fat serves as an active chemical factory. It produces

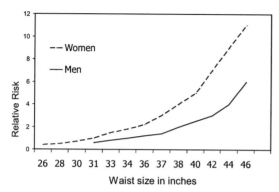

numerous biologically active molecules and hormones that lead to the development of metabolic syndrome, diabetes, and heart disease. The more visceral fat you have, the worse off you are. Visceral fat can be reduced with exercise and caloric restriction, but is not accessible by liposuction, which removes the less dangerous subcutaneous (surface) fat.

The only accurate way to measure visceral obesity is with expensive imaging procedures such as Computerized Tomography (CT) or Magnetic Resonance Imaging (MRI) scans. However, abdominal girth is considered a fairly accurate surrogate for these more expensive procedures.

When women first become obese, they show a pattern of lower body obesity—fat in their buttocks and thighs—which is intended primarily by Mother Nature for use during lactation (breast feeding), and even in times of starva-

Figure 3.10 . The relative risk of obesity-associated risk factors (metabolic syndrome diabetes and/or hypertension) at different levels of waist size for men and women. Women tend to have a higher risk as compared to men at any given waist size. Source: Zhu, SK. Ref. 3.74. *Adapted with permission. © American Journal of Clinical Nutrition.*

tion. This fat is not metabolically active and does not produce any harmful effects. It is, in a sense, "storage" fat—warehoused and inactive. It is only as obesity increases in women that, as in men, excess fat begins to accumulate also in the abdomen. After menopause, women catch up with and often overtake men in putting on belly fat. Occasionally, women have upper body (apple-type) obesity without lower body obesity before menopause, but this is not common. It must be stressed that such women have very high risk of diabetes and heart disease, as high as or higher than for men.

Waist girth: a powerful predictor of diabetes and heart disease

Rising waist girth is usually accompanied by decreasing cardiovascular fitness, as well as increased risk of osteoarthritis of the knees. Waist girth is strongly related to hypertension and diabetes in men and

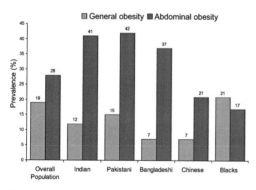

women in diverse populations. In an analysis of the records of 27,270 men in Health Professionals Follow-up Study (See appendix B) those in the highest quintile of waist had a 12-fold risk of diabetes compared to the lowest quintile. But, the risk of diabetes was only eight-fold n the highest versus the lowest quintile of body mass index. Thus waist size is stronger red flag than body weight.

Usually waist girth is five inches smaller in women than men, **irrespective of height.** Accordingly, cut-points for abdominal obesity are different in men and women. An abdominal girth above 40 inches (102cm) in men and above 35 inches (88 cm) in women puts whites, blacks, and Hispanics at a very high risk of diabetes and heart disease, even when their weight and BMI are normal. At a given abdominal girth, the risk of diabetes and heart disease is identical in men and women. Thus, body fat distribution may help to explain the gender differences in heart disease. Figure 3.10 shows the relative risk of obesity-associated risk factors (metabolic syndrome diabetes

Figure 3.11. Diffrences of the prevalence of general obesity and abdominal obesity in men by ethnicity in the UK. Most Indians and other south Asians have less obesity by BMI standards but markedly increased rates of abdominal obesity. In this study, a waist-to-hip ratio greater than 0.95 for men was used for defining abdominal obesity. Note the that the prevalence of abdominal obesity is four-fold higher than general obesity among Indians and other south Asians. Abdominal obesity among women showed similar pattern. Source: Heartstat.org. Ref. 3.29.

and/or hypertension) at different levels of waist circumference. Notice how rapidly the risk rises after reaching a waist size of about 36 inches.

Abdominal obesity among Indians

As stated, abdominal obesity is two to three times more common among Indians than total or general obesity. This is in sharp contrast to whites, who have only a slightly higher rate of abdominal than general obesity, and blacks who have actually a lower rate of abdominal obesity than total obesity (see Figure 3.11.). Earlier studies focused on waist-to-hip ratio (WHR), whereas newer studies have found waist girth to be as good as WHR as a predictor. The prevalence of abdominal obesity using waist circumference is higher than that with WHR.

Result of the studies published in the last two years indicate that waist to hip ratio may indeed may be better predictor of cardiovascular risk and heart attack, since this ratio integrates the heightened risk of abdominal girth and protective effects of hip girth. This is particularly true among Indians but not among the Chinese or blacks.

For any given abdominal girth, abdominal obesity in Indians is associated with greater cardiovascular risk and metabolic abnormalities not only in adults but also in children. For example, Indian children with a waist size of just 32 inches (80 cm) had a higher level of insulin (a strong predictor of metabolic syndrome and future risk of diabetes) than White children with a waist girth of 36 inches (90cm) (see Table 3.9).

Table 3.9. The influence of waist girth on fasting insulin levels among Indian and White children aged 8 to 11 in the UK

	Log Insulin levels			
Waist size (in inches)	20	24	32	36
Indians	2.7	3.8	5.2	6.2
whites	2.5	3.1	3.9	4.4

Note that Indian children with a waist of 32" have higher insulin levels than White children with a waist of 36". Waist size affects the insulin levels of Indian children more than it does White children. Source: Whincup, PH. Ref. 3.70.

Asia Pacific criteria for abdominal obesity

The World health Organization (WHO) Asia Pacific criteria for abdominal obesity is different than the usual criteria used for non-Asian populations such as whites and blacks. Among Asians, a waist girth above 32 inches (80 cm) for women and above 36 inches (90 cm) in men qualifies for abdominal obesity, compared to 35 inches and 40 inches respectively among non-Asian populations.

Although BMI is the yardstick to assess obesity, it does reflect body fat percentage. As stated earlier, Asians have 3 to 6% higher body fat than whites, at any given BMI. Among Asians who have the same BMI, Chinese have the lowest percentage of body fat, while Indians have the highest. This is the rationale behind the more restrictive definition of abdominal obesity for Asians than the standard definitions for non-Asian populations, such as Americans and Europeans. At a given waist size, Asians have greater body fat and metabolic abnormalities.

A recent Japanese study found optimum waist size to be 32 inches for women and 36 inches cm for men in this population – nearly identical to the WHO Asia Pacific Criteria. A recent study, in Singapore, has clearly demonstrated the importance and implications of the Asia Pacific criteria on the rates of abdominal obesity in Indians. Despite very high rates of heart disease and diabetes, the prevalence of abdominal obesity as defined by the standard criteria was only 9% among Indian men and 26% among Indian women in Singapore, a rate substantially lower than expected. When the Asia-Pacific criteria were applied, the prevalence of abdominal obesity increased nearly five-fold to 41% in men and two-fold to 54% in Indian women. The Chinese who have low rates of heart disease have a rate of abdominal obesity that is less than half that of Indians at every age group. Abdominal obesity is particularly

Did you know...
The World Health Organization (WHO) Asia Pacific criteria for abdominal obesity are different than the usual criteria used for non-Asian populations such as whites and blacks. Among Asians, a waist girth above 32 inches (80 cm) for women and above 36 inches (90 cm) in men qualifies for abdominal obesity, compared to 35 inches and 40 inches respectively among non-Asian populations.

When the Asia-Pacific criteria were applied, the prevalence of abdominal obesity increased nearly five-fold to 41% in Indian men and two-fold to 54% in Indian women in Singapore.

predictive of high-risk status among Indians whose BMI falls *between 20 and 30*. Many Indians may appear relatively "skinny" but their enlarged waist size may put them at high risk for diabetes and heart disease. This difference in the criteria for abdominal obesity has a significant impact on the prevalence of metabolic syndrome, which will be discussed in the next section.

KEY · POINTS · IN · A · NUTSHELL

♥ Abdominal obesity is a much better predictor of dyslipidemia, diabetes, and heart disease than general obesity.

♥ Cut-points for abdominal obesity vary by gender and ethnicity.

♥ The usual cut-point for abdominal obesity is 36 inches in women and 40 inches in men but are 4 inches lower among Asians 32 inches in women and 36 inches in men

♥ Abdominal obesity is two to three times more common than general obesity among Indians.

♥ At a given waist size, Indians and other Asians have greater dyslipidemia, diabetes, and heart disease than it does on Americans and Europeans.

♥ The lower risk of heart disease in women is primarily due to their smaller waist size, not their gender per se.

♥ Men and women of equal waist size have similar risk of heart disease and diabetes.

♥ Increasing waist size is accompanied by increasing insulin levels, even among children; this increase in insulin levels is greater in Indian children as compared to white children.

♥ Indian children with a waist size of 32 inches have higher insulin levels (a strong predictor future risk of diabities) than white children with a waist size of 36 inches.

♥ An unhealthy abdominal girth is unusually common even among Indians with "normal" weight and body mass index.

3.7 ▶ Metabolic Syndrome—The Ticking Time Bomb

If you have never heard of metabolic syndrome, you are not alone. Although 55 million Americans and nearly 50% of Indians over the age of 60 have it, few people know anything about it. Yet metabolic syndrome predicts a very high risk of heart attack and stroke, almost as high as diabetes. The term "metabolic syndrome" refers to a cluster of metabolic abnormalities that include abdominal obesity (large waist size), high triglyceride levels, low HDL (good cholesterol), prehypertension, and prediabetes. It is considered a *prediabetic state,* with most of the affected individuals developing diabetes within a decade or two. In 1988, Dr. Gerald M. Reaven, an endocrinologist at Stanford, was the first to describe a cluster of low-level risk factors that increase heart disease risk and called it *syndrome X.* The term metabolic syndrome came into wide use only after the National Cholesterol Education Program (NCEP) renamed it and proposed criteria for recognizing it in 2002.

The metabolic syndrome predicts your lifetime risk of heart attack, whereas the Framingham Risk Score calculates the 10- year risk of heart attack from traditional risk factors.

In the US, metabolic syndrome is present in 24% adults and 42% of those above 70 years of age. It is most common among Hispanics (32%), followed by whites (24%), and least among blacks (22%). The overall prevalence of metabolic syndrome in adult Europeans is 15% versus 24% in the US. Indians have a high prevalence of it, especially when the Asia Pacific criteria are used (See

Table 3.10 in Section 7).The original cut-point for abnormal blood sugar in the definition of metabolic syndrome was 110mg/dL, but this has subsequently been lowered to 100. At this new cut-point, 64 million Americans have metabolic syndrome.

Metabolic syndrome is not limited to adults. It affects one in eight children compared to one in four adults. It is found in a third of obese children, and in half of severely obese children and adolescents. Its presence increases with worsening obesity. As in adults, it is associated with a clustering of risk factors that markedly increase the risk of heart disease and diabetes. People with metabolic syndrome have a low rate of survival following angioplasty and bypass surgery. This section highlights the importance of metabolic syndrome with particular emphasis on the Indian population.

Metabolic syndrome is really a group of lifestyle and emerging risk factors. The emerging epidemic of metabolic syndrome is attributed to increasing obesity and a sedentary lifestyle. The main factors that precipitate it are, therefore, weight gain and a lack of regular physical activity. Below are its five major components (See box). Note that you need to have only three of these five to be diagnosed with metabolic syndrome. For example, many of us have a large belly with high triglyceride and low HDL levels. That is a recipe for metabolic syndrome, putting us at heightened risk of heart disease and diabetes.

The five key features of metabolic syndrome	
1.	Abdominal obesity • Waist size exceeding 36 inches (90 cm) for men • Waist size exceeding 32 inches (80cm) for women
2.	Triglycerides above 150mg/dL
3.	Low HDL level • below 40mg/dL for men • below 50mg/dL for women
4.	Blood pressure above 130/85mm Hg
5.	Prediabetes or impaired fasting glucose (100 to 125mg/dL)

Note that the criteria for abdominal obesity is different among Indians and other Asians

Thrifty gene and food abundance

The thrifty genotype hypothesis offers one explanation for the late twentieth century epidemic of obesity, metabolic syndrome, and diabetes. In 1962, Jerald Neal, a British scientist proposed that obesity in populations like the Pima Indians might be the expression of a "thrifty gene" that served well in our prehistoric past, conserving bodily resources in times of famine and scarcity, but which became detrimental with a steady and abundant supply of food. Longitudinal studies over the past two decades have confirmed that we may in fact have a thrifty gene that can lead to a "thrifty" metabolic rate that can play a role in the development of obesity. The hypothesis is that, as hunter-gatherers, our ancestors adapted to alternating cycles of feast and famine. When food became much more plentiful with better technology, the same thrifty genes that once promoted temporary obesity to preserve caloric energy began to contribute to insulin resistance and, ultimately, metabolic syndrome.

A recent study investigated the time line for the development of metabolic syndrome from adolescence (age 13) to young adulthood (age 36) among 364 people enrolled in the Amsterdam Growth and Health Longitudinal Study. At age 36, there was a 10% prevalence of metabolic syndrome, as defined using modified NCEP criteria. Compared with those who never developed the syndrome over the studied time period, those, who developed metabolic syndrome by the age of 36, had the following:
(1) A greater increase in total body fat
(2) A substantial decrease in cardiopulmonary fitness level
(3) A greater decrease in hard physical activities
(4) A trend toward a higher intake of food throughout the years

This study shows that body fat and fat distribution, cardiopulmonary fitness, and lifestyle are the major determinants of metabolic syndrome among young adults, and that these represent separate potential targets for its prevention. This study further suggests that intervening early in life may be a particularly effective strategy for prevention of metabolic syndrome.

Abdominal obesity

Metabolic syndrome is caused by the body's inability to use insulin efficiently. The hallmark of the condition is excessive abdominal fat. The criteria for abdominal obesity is different in men and women as shown above. The criteria are also different between Asian and non-Asian populations (see section 6).

Metabolic syndrome among Indians

In Canada, the prevalence of metabolic syndrome using the NCEP criteria, is higher in Indians (26%) than whites (22%) and double that of Chinese (11%). The prevalence of metabolic syndrome among Indians in the US is yet to be reported, but is likely to be one in three compared to one in four for the general US population, when *WHO Asian-Pacific criteria* are used (waist size above 36 inches in men and above 32 inches in women; see section 6).

These narrower Asia Pacific criteria for abdominal obesity result in a 50% increase in the prevalence of metabolic syndrome from 22% to 32% in Indian men and from 20% to 29% in Indian women in Singapore **(Table 3.10)**. At every age group, Indians have at least double the rates of metabolic syndrome as compared to the Chinese. This parallels their contrasting rates of heart disease (Figures 1.13 and 4.8). Approximately 50% of Indians over the age of 60 have metabolic syndrome. It is likely that this may be the case for Indians worldwide if the Asia-Pacific criteria are used. This book strongly recommends that you should not wait until you meet the more generous NCEP criteria before you increase your physical activity and decrease your caloric intake.

Table 3.10. Differences in the prevalence of abdominal obesity and metabolic syndrome by NCEP and Asia-Pacific criteria among Indians in Singapore.

	Abdominal obesity		Metabolic syndrome	
	NCEP Criteria*	Asia-Pacific criteria**	NCEP criteria	Asia-Pacific criteria
Indian men	9%	41%	22%	32%
Indian women	26%	54%	20%	29%
Chinese men	4%	26%	11%	18%
Chinese women	7%	21%	9%	15%

*waist more than 40 inches for men and 35 inches for women
** waist more than 36 inches for Asian men and 32 inches for Asian women. Note a 500% increase in the prevalence of abdominal obesity and 50% increase in metabolic syndrome using the correct criteria among Indian men. Source: Tan, CE. Ref. 3.60.

High triglycerides

Triglycerides are fats consisting of three molecules of fatty acid combined with a molecule of the alcohol glycerol. Calories not immediately needed by the body are converted into triglycerides and then transported to fat cells for storage. These triglycerides are released to satisfy your body's energy needs between meals. Triglycerides not used can lead to excess fat buildup in the body. Most triglycerides are transported through the blood stream as very low density lipoproteins (VLDL), a carrier of both cholesterol and triglycerides. LDL is formed when triglycerides are shed from VLDL.

Why fast before a testing for triglycerides?

Unlike cholesterol and HDL, levels of triglycerides are markedly affected by the timing of blood testing: for example, non-fasting triglyceride levels are two to three times higher than fasting triglyceride levels. For this reason, fasting (no calories) for eight to 12 hours before drawing blood is recommended for this test.

Women have lower levels of triglycerides as compared to men, but a higher overall risk at any given level of triglycerides. High levels of triglycerides increase the risk of a heart attack, when accompanied by at least some elevation of total cholesterol (above 130mg/dL). (See Chapter VI Section 2 and 4).

Although levels of triglycerides below 150mg/dL are considered normal, about 50% of Americans have levels below 100mg/dL. Recent studies indicate that the risk of premature heart attack and diabetes increases when levels of triglycerides exceed 100 mg/dL. In a recent case-control study, the researchers analyzed blood samples from 653 individuals who had suffered a heart attack or had undergone angioplasty or bypass surgery. Each of these patients also had a close family member with heart disease. The blood test results were compared with those from 1,029 control subjects who were enrolled in two community health studies. The risk of heart disease with an elevated triglyceride level rose progressively until 800 mg/dL with an 11-

fold risk of heart attack compared with those whose triglycerides were below 100mg/dL People with high triglyceride levels should make appropriate lifestyle changes. They can be lowered through weight loss, a lower carbohydrate diet, and exercise (see Chapter VI section 4).

Hypertriglyceridemic waist

Hypertriglyceridemic waist refers to the condition in which a large waist size is accompanied by a high level of triglycerides. It is a forerunner to metabolic syndrome. The risk of heart attack appears to be greater with a hyper-triglyceridemic waist than prediabetes (elevated blood sugars between 100 and 125mg/dL). The risk of a heart attack is increased two-fold with prediabetes, five-fold with hypertriglyceridemic waist, and nine-fold when both conditions coexist. (See Table 3.11). The principal cause of hypertriglyceridemic waist among Indians is the urban lifestyle, marked by low physical activity and consumption of unhealthy foods (high in calories, saturated fats, and refined carbohy-drates) although genetic predisposition may also play a small role.

Table 3.11. Relative risk for heart attack as a function of blood sugar, triglycerides and waist size in men.

	Normal blood sugar	High blood sugar
Waist less than 36 inches and normal triglycerides	1	2
Waist more than 36 inches and high triglycerides	5	9

Note that even among whites, a waist size of more than 36" is more strongly associated with a high risk of heart disease than is elevated blood sugar Source: St-pierre, J. Ref. 3.65.

HDL and metabolic syndrome

The cut point for low HDL in metabolic syndrome is below 40mg/dL in men and below 50mg/dL in women. Compared to whites, low HDL is twice as common among Indian men, and three times more com-mon among Indian women. Women in general have 10mg/dL higher HDL than men. However, the differ-ence is narrower or non-existent among Indian women. Low HDL partly explains the excess burden of heart disease among Indian women (see Chapters II section 4 and Chapter IV section 3).

Elevated blood pressure

The optimum blood pressure is now defined as below 120/80 mmHg. More than 140/90 mmHg is consid-ered high blood pressure. Levels of 130 to 139 systolic or 80 to 89 diastolic are defined as prehypertension. The criterion for abnormal blood pressure for metabolic syndrome is more than 130/85 mmHg.

Elevated fasting blood sugar

Although elevated fasting blood sugar is one of the five components of metabolic syndrome, this is the least common of the five diagnostic criteria. For example, among Americans with metabolic syndrome, abdominal obesity is present in 36% to 46% of them, compared to 10% to 16% who have elevated fasting blood sugar. Moreover, high levels of triglycerides and low levels of HDL are twice as common as an elevated fasting blood sugar. **Impaired fasting glucose**, has recently been renamed **"prediabetes"** because so many of these individu-als become diabetic in 10 to 15 years.

C-reactive protein

People with the metabolic syndrome also tend to have high levels of a protein, known as C-reactive protein, or CRP, which is released during inflammation and has recently been linked to heart disease see section 4). Many experts believe that CRP is an important part, cause or consequence of the metabolic syndrome. People with metabolic syndrome and high CRP are particularly at high risk for heart disease and diabetes. CRP is currently not one of the five criteria for the diagnosis of the syndrome, but is likely to be included with the next revision of these criteria.

Blood sugar level between 100 and 125mg/dL, once called impaired fasting glucose, has recently been renamed "predia-betes" because so many of these individuals become diabetic in 10 to 15 years.

Crucial link between metabolic syndrome and diabetes

Metabolic syndrome often heralds diabetes. It is a prediabetic state, even if one's blood sugar level is absolutely normal. Diabetes is diagnosed when the fasting blood sugar is above

125mg/dL. Blood sugar level between 100 and 125mg/dL, once called

It appears that metabolic syndrome identifies a group of very high risk individuals 20 years before they become diabetic, and 10 years before a diagnosis of prediabetes. Currently, metabolic syndrome is present in 10% of people with normal blood sugar levels, 50% with prediabetes, and 80% with diabetes (Table 3.10). In short, if you have metabolic syndrome, there is a good chance that you will get diabetes. In a large British study, over a short span of just five years, the risk of diabetes increased seven-fold among those with metabolic syndrome and 25-fold when C-reactive protein was also elevated (See section 2).

Table 3.12 Prevalence of metabolic syndrome according presence of diabetes and prediabetes

	Men	Women
Normal blood sugar	15%	10%
Prediabetes	64%	42%
Diabetes	84%	78%

Source: Isomaa, B. Ref. 3.33.

Metabolic syndrome and heart disease

Approximately one in 10 cardiovascular deaths is directly attributable to metabolic syndrome. It is particularly common among people with premature heart disease. It is associated with a two- to three-fold risk of developing and dying from heart attack. The most recent NHANES (2004) study suggests that the risk of heart disease in people with metabolic syndrome is higher than patients with diabetes. The prevalence of heart disease was 14% in persons with metabolic syndrome as compared to 8% in persons with diabetes alone. Another study found evidence of early atherosclerosis in 71% of people with metabolic syndrome only, compared to 59% of patients with diabetes only, and 88% of patients with both.

About 20% of diabetics do not have metabolic syndrome and have a substantially lower risk of heart disease. Conversely, people with metabolic syndrome have a markedly increased risk of heart disease even in the absence of diabetes (see Figure 3.12.). In Pakistan, metabolic syndrome and lipoprotein(a) levels were stronger predictors of the presence and severity of heart disease, than LDL level. Metabolic syndrome not only increases the risk of a heart attack, but also death following coronary bypass surgery. Those with metabolic syndrome were four times more likely to have died within eight years of their surgery than those without it.

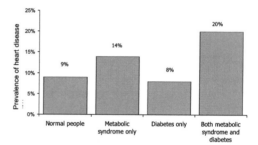

Figure 3.12 . Prevalence of heart disease as a function of diabetes and metabolic syndrome. You can see that a combination of diabetes and metabolic syndrome carries a greater risk of heart disease than diabetes alone. Source: Alexander, CM et al. Ref. 3.01.

Did You Know... Metabolic syndrome not only increases the risk of a heart attack, but also death following coronary bypass surgery. Those with metabolic syndrome were four times more likely to have died within eight years of their surgery than those without it.

Among people with metabolic syndrome, those who also have calcified plaque in the coronary arteries identify a group at particularly high risk of heart attack. Coronary calcium indicates the presence of plaque build-up in the arteries supplying the heart. The amount of coronary calcium is measured using computed tomography (CT) and is called a calcium score. Calcium scores of zero are the best; scores from one to 100 are mild; scores of 100 to 400 are moderate; and scores over 400 indicate extensive coronary calcium. People with high calcium scores are at high risk of heart attack. Those with mild calcium scores are considered at low risk for any cardiac event over the following five years, while those with moderate scores are at intermediate risk for cardiac events. However, people with *low calcium score and metabolic syndrome* have a three-fold higher rate of abnormal stress test indicative of ischemia, than people without metabolic syndrome and thus help identify those at the highest risk for a heart attack.

Impact of metabolic syndrome on coronary angioplasty and bypass surgery

Metabolic syndrome has been shown to increase the risk of death after angioplasty. In a study of 2,300 patients, who had undergone angioplasty at Cleveland Clinic, those with metabolic syndrome, had double the rate of recurrent heart attack, including death. The presence of metabolic syndrome also has a negative impact on those, who have undergone heart bypass surgery. In a study of 6,428 patients, who had bypass surgery, those with metabolic syndrome were four times more likely to have died within eight years of their surgery than those without. About 10% of men and 20% of women had four components of metabolic syndrome. Women with four components of the syndrome were 10 times more likely to have died than those with none. A high prevalence of metabolic syndrome offers another explanation for the higher rate of complications found among Indians following coronary angioplasty and bypass surgery.

Severity of metabolic syndrome

Although a combination of three components results in a diagnosis of metabolic syndrome, those with four or more components face substantially higher risk. Increasing the number of components of metabolic syndrome confers an increase in the severity of heart disease. In one study, the risk of a heart attack increased four-fold with four or more components of metabolic syndrome compared to those with none; the risk of diabetes increased 24-fold (see Table.3.13.) Metabolic syndrome is also a predictor of death from heart disease. Compared to the general population, those with metabolic syndrome have a two-fold greater risk of cardiac death, which increases to four-fold when four components are present compared to those with none.

Table 3.13. Relative risk of developing heart attack or diabetes according to the presence and severity of metabolic syndrome

Metabolic syndrome status	Relative risk Heart attack	Diabetes
No metabolic syndrome (fewer than 3 components)	1	1
Metabolic syndrome (three components)	3	7
Metabolic syndrome (four or more components)	4	24

Note that even among whites, a waist size of more than 36" is more strongly associated with a high risk of heart disease than is elevated blood sugar Source: St-pierre, J. Ref. 3.65.

Controlling metabolic syndrome

People with metabolic syndrome needs to reduce his or her caloric intake and increase physical activity to prevent the development of diabetes and early heart attack. This topic is discussed in Chapter VI section 6.

KEY · POINTS · IN · A · NUTSHELL

- ♥ Metabolic syndrome identifies individuals at a very high risk of developing heart disease.
- ♥ The risk of heart disease in people with metabolic syndrome is almost as high as those with diabetes.
- ♥ Abdominal obesity, high triglycerides, low HDL, prehypertension, and prediabetes are the five key components of metabolic syndrome.
- ♥ The presence of any three of these components means you have metabolic syndrome; four or more greatly increases the risk of heart disease and diabetes.
- ♥ Metabolic syndrome is found in one-third of obese children and one-half of severely obese children.
- ♥ Metabolic syndrome is present in one-third of Indians and nearly one-half of Indians older than 60 years of age.
- ♥ The prevalence of metabolic syndrome may be underestimated by one-third if the Asia pacific Criteria for abdominal obesity are not used.
- ♥ People with metabolic syndrome have a higher rate of complications including low rates of long-term survival following angioplasty and bypass surgery.

Chapter IV

Heart Disease in Particular Populations

hapter I introduced the Indian Paradox—the observation that Indians worldwide have high levels of premature, severe, multi-vessel heart disease, despite having low-to-average levels of the traditional risk factors. Chapters II and III, which discussed the traditional and the emerging risk factors, respectively, presented the pieces we might use to explain the puzzle. **Cracking the Indian Paradox**, the opening section of Chapter IV, turns to the task of trying to resolve the paradox. Examining key evidence from different countries, immigrant cultures, and ethnic groups, Section 1 argues that the most compelling explanation for the paradox is the elevated levels of various emerging risk factors among Indians all over the world, and the particularly harmful way in which these emerging factors interact with traditional risk factors. Because of the synergy between the traditional risk factors and emerging factors (such as LP(a), C-reactive protein, and homocysteine), Indians typically face a higher cardiac risk from a 10-pound weight gain or 10 more cigarettes a day than members of other groups who do not have elevated emerging risk factors.

Section 1 also discusses whether nature or nurture is more to blame for Indians' excess burden of emerging factors, the role that rapid urbanization has played in the epidemic, and how physical inactivity, abdominal obesity, and an unhealthy diet have contributed to the precursors of heart disease—such as dyslipidemia, insulin resistance, and metabolic syndrome. ◆

The Indian Paradox illustrates a striking truth: Cardiovascular disease risk factors affect different ethnic groups differently. *Section 2*, **Ethnicity and Heart Disease**, examines several populations around the world that have lower-than-expected levels of cardiovascular disease to try to explain the paradoxical relationship between their relatively low disease rates and their sometimes high risk factor levels. Several lessons surface: First, HDL's protective effect, and Lp(a)'s harmful effect, are both more important than we may have acknowledged. Second, emerging risk factors, as a whole, play a vital role in producing stark ethnic differences in atherosclerosis and, ultimately, in heart disease rates. ◆

Third, there appear to be tipping points in the risk level profile of an ethnic group before which the group was protected from high rates of heart disease, but beyond which the addition of just one more elevated risk factor—perhaps through immigration, urbanization, or a change in lifestyle—can suddenly tip the scale and start to compromise the protective shield an ethnic group had enjoyed until then, triggering the acceleration of cardiovascular disease. Before the tipping point is reached, nature protects against the adverse effects of nurture and lifestyle. After the tipping point is passed, nature seems to amplify the adverse effects of nurture and lifestyle, heightening vulnerability and hastening disease. In short, the complex interplay of lifestyle and genetic factors that can be protective or harmful. We can do little about our genetic inheritance, but there is a lot we can do to control our other risks. ◆

Like Section 2—ethnicity—the last two sections of Chapter IV each considers heart disease in a particular population. *Section 3*, **Women and Heart Disease**, makes one thing abundantly clear: men and women differ considerably in their vulnerability to cardiovascular risk factors, in the typical symptoms they exhibit, in the developmental timeline of disease, and even in how healthcare providers perceive the urgency of their disease. This has implications for both diagnosis and treatment because, even in high-information societies such as the US, the myth that heart disease is a man's disease has been a slow-dying myth. As the section explains, more women die from heart disease than men, and a woman is eight times more likely to die from this cause than from breast cancer. Women have a better risk factor profile than men at younger ages, but much worse after menopause when their LDL cholesterol and triglyceride levels rise and their HDL starts to fall. Examining specific risk factors—from height, obesity, abdominal obesity, and hypertension to smoking, diabetes, metabolic syndrome, and Lp(a)—Section 3 shows how, in many instances, elevated levels of the risk factor are more harmful to a woman than to a man. It also highlights which factors are particularly prevalent among Indian women. The sections ends by discussing the prevention and management of heart disease in women. ◆

A Word about Terminology

Throughout this book, the term Indian refers to people who trace their origin to the Indian subcontinent—meaning Bangladesh, India, Pakistan, and Sri Lanka—including those who now live abroad but originate from one of these four countries. "Indian" in this context is ethnically interchangeable with "South Asian," "Indo-Asian," or "Asian Indian." The term thus excludes native Americans but includes more than people from the nation of India.

Measurement Units: As is conventional, blood glucose levels, triglyceride levels, and cholesterol levels are stated throughout this book in milligrams per deciliter (mg/dL). Blood pressure is stated in millimeters of mercury (mmHg).

Citing key studies, including postmortem studies done of young military servicemen and angiograms of hearts donated for transplant, *Section 4*, **The Pediatric Foundations of Heart Disease**, makes the case that the foundations of heart disease are laid very early on indeed, perhaps even as early as in the womb. Yet children and adolescents are not miniature versions of adults; they are biologically different. As you will learn, certain risk factors such as dyslipidemia are thus even more harmful to younger adults than to older people. Exposure to them can set up young people for a lifetime of struggle against cardiovascular disease. Building on a foundation of early exposure to risk factors, atherosclerosis tends to progress rapidly especially from one's mid-teens to mid-30s. Despite this, an epidemic of childhood obesity, inactivity, and diets laden with fats and sugar has resulted in a high prevalence of metabolic syndrome and diabetes, which in turn work in concert with other factors such as hypertension to lead to heart disease. The section ends by showing parents what they can do to help their children reduce their risk of heart disease and its precursors, thereby giving them a positive start in life. ◆

4.1 ► Cracking the Indian Paradox

O NE WOULD EXPECT INDIANS to have low rather than high rates of heart disease. Many are long-term vegetarians, are physically active throughout the day, are not particularly plagued by high blood pressure, and are not obese by traditional standards. As we saw in the CADI Study of Indian doctors living in the United States (Chapter I, sections 2 and 4), the prevalence of obesity and of smoking among them was very low—each less than 5%. Yet despite low levels of the traditional risk factors, an alarming number of Indians the world over develop severe, premature and malignant heart disease. What accounts for this excess burden of heart disease among Indians everywhere? In 1998, I coined the term **"the Indian Paradox"** to describe this phenomenon of malignant heart disease in the absence of high rates of traditional risk factors.

Some research suggests that there is perhaps no Indian Paradox at all. After all, Indians do have high rates of diabetes, a powerful heart disease risk factor, and many Indian men do smoke. Other explanations based on lifestyle have been suggested: For example, the Indian diet is particularly high in saturated fats and cholesterol, such as from *ghee* and coconut oil, and perhaps urban Indians tend to be particularly sedentary. These proposed explanations all have some merit, but ultimately they are dissatisfying because they do not adequately account for the high rates and malignant nature of heart disease among Indians.

This does not mean lifestyle factors do not matter. They do. Studies done on immigrants show that, within two or three generations, the difference between the heart disease rate of new immigrants and that of the dominant culture virtually disappears as the immigrant group adopts the diet, daily patterns, and other lifestyle choices of the main culture. Surely, this attests to the powerful influence of environmental, "nurture" factors on the genesis of disease. Change a population's cultural environment, and their disease rates often change as well.

All true—except for Indians. Indians abroad have been the single exception to this general rule. Their death rates from heart disease, instead of converging toward non-Indian rates as expected, have persistently remained 50% to 300% higher than existing rates in the countries to which they emigrated—be it Europe, North America, or other Asian countries. This is especially so among younger Indians. Equally telling is that when the lifestyle of the entire culture begins to undergo transformation toward increased sedentariness, urban stress, and richer food—as has happened in rapidly modernizing countries such as Singapore—the cardiovascular health of that country's Indians is affected more by the harmful changes than that of the non-Indian groups. This phenomenon is discussed further below (*see* also Chapter I, Section 2).

These observations tell us that genes may play a stronger role in Indian heart disease than among other groups. This genetic component partly explains the persistence of high rates of heart disease among Indian adults of all socioeconomic classes and all ages, both men and women, over large geographical distances, and through time. Yet genes do not tell the full story. Without a more sophisticated understanding of risk factors and how they interact, the Indian Paradox will remain an enigma.

This first section of Chapter IV looks beyond the standard explanations of heart disease to examine the most plausible candidate for the paradox: the high prevalence among Indians of several emerging risk factors which not only are harmful on their own, but also interact synergistically with the conventional risk factors in a particularly damaging way when both kinds are present in an individual.

In particular, Indians worldwide appear to be predisposed toward having an

What is Lipoprotein(a)?
Lipoprotein(a)—or Lp(a) for short, pronounced *L-P-little a*—chemically resembles LDL cholesterol. People with elevated Lp(a), such as millions of Indians, are at substantial risk for developing heart disease because the presence of high levels of Lp(a) in the blood makes other heart disease factors like LDL cholesterol more active in causing atherosclerosis. In a way, Lp(a) is like a catalyst — magnifying the effects of other risk factors. Diet and exercise have no influence on Lp(a), unlike on your cholesterol and triglyceride levels. People with high Lp(a) thus need to initiate a comprehensive risk factor modification program to minimize the factors that Lp(a) intensifies.

excess of several non-traditional risk factors—namely, C-reactive protein (CRP), homocysteine, lipoprotein(a), and metabolic syndrome. Some of these may be partly the result of lifestyle and partly genetically inherited.

> The persistence of high rates of heart disease among Indian adults of all socioeconomic classes and all ages, both men and women, over large geographical distances, and through time, points partly to a genetic foundation.

High levels of Lp(a) clearly point to a genetic component to Indian heart disease, but it is not clear, besides Lp(a), what else may be genetic. What we do know is that not only do these factors, by themselves, heighten Indians' risk, they also intensify the harmful effects of the standard factors when both are present, thereby countering the cardioprotective benefits Indians might normally have enjoyed from having low levels of the standard risk factors.

It is this synergy between the emerging and standard risk factors that may be most responsible for the Indian Paradox. For example, a high level of either Lp(a), homocysteine, or CRP, by itself, can **double** a person's risk of heart disease, even if he or she does not have high levels of the traditional risk factors. Their risk, however, rises **four to eight** times when several emerging risk factors are present together with traditional factors.

Nature versus nurture: The role of genes and environment

To grasp why this is, we must understand that most chronic diseases—including heart disease—involve nature-nurture, or gene-environment, interactions. They persist and progress because factors in your lifestyle or environment—such as smoking, unhealthy diet, lack of exercise, obesity, or stress—conspire with factors in your biology to keep the disease going. As medical scientists like to say: "*Genetics loads the gun, but environment pulls the trigger.*"

> The susceptibility of Indians to a number of emerging risk factors, some of which may be partly genetic, markedly magnifies the harmful effects of the standard risk factors such as physical inactivity, low HDL, and diabetes.

Indians appear to be in double jeopardy from the nature-nurture duo. First, nature appears to have endowed them regrettably with high levels of Lp(a), small-particle HDL, which is dysfunctional and less protective than large-particle HDL, and a body type characterized by abdominal obesity (*see* the Risk Factors box, *below*). High levels of CRP, homocysteine, and metabolic syndrome may also have a partially genetic basis. Nurture, presented with this loaded magazine, then "pulls the trigger" through unhealthy lifestyle choices such as living a sedentary life or eating a diet overly rich in saturated fats, trans fats, and cholesterol—changes associated with rising affluence, urbanization, and mechanization.

Let's look more closely at this idea that there may be a genetic foundation underlying the heart disease data we are seeing among Indians everywhere. To do that, let's briefly examine two other cases—Japanese immigrants in the United States, and Irish immigrants. The impact of immigration on heart disease rates has been studied in several populations because it enables us to separate the influence of lifestyle and environment (nurture) from the influence of genes, and see which one, if any, is making the greater contribution.

Case Number One: The Japanese, who are among the longest-lived people in the world, traditionally have very low rates of heart disease. This seems to be due to a combination of both genes and culture, particularly diet. However, when many Japanese emigrated to the United States in the middle of the 20th century and adopted a more or less western lifestyle—including western food, with its

Table 4.1. Important Risk Factors for Indians

Traditional factors with prevalence comparable to or lower than that of other groups	Traditional factors with high prevalence	Emerging risk factors with high prevalence
High total cholesterol High blood pressure Smoking Overall obesity	Diabetes Physical inactivity Low HDL level	High level of Lp(a) Abdominal obesity High triglyceride level Small, dysfunctional HDL Metabolic syndrome High level of homo cysteine High level of CRP High level of fibrinogen

high fat and low fish content—their heart disease rates ratcheted up two to three times in very little time, compared to the rates of Japanese who did not emigrate. The heart disease rates among the Japanese emigrants, however, remained lower than those of non-Japanese Americans (*see* section 2). What accounts for this? Although nurture had deteriorated for the Japanese upon changing their lifestyle, nature—their genes—was still partially protecting them from the full impact of their new, less healthy western lifestyle. *Good nature countered bad nurture.*

Did You Know ...
Diabetics with the lowest 20% of cholesterol levels face a higher risk of heart attack than the non-diabetics with the highest 20% of cholesterol levels!

Case Number Two: When large numbers of the Irish, who traditionally have very high rates of heart disease, emigrated to the US, their heart disease rates continued to remain high and *did not change much.* Why not? In this case, they emigrated from one relatively unhealthy dietary environment (Ireland) to another (the US), and nature neither worsened nor protected against nurture.

Case Number Three: After emigrating to the US or other countries, heart disease rates among Indians, as noted in the opening paragraphs, have risen sharply—up to three times higher than the average rates in their new country. This suggests gene-environment interactions, as does the fact that the high rates persist through *several generations* even when lifestyle factors and social habits in that country have undergone large-scale change. The result: Indians around the globe have the highest heart disease rates—even though nearly half of them are lifelong vegetarians, and even though they have about the same or fewer traditional risk factors than people of other ethnic origins, particularly whites.

Nature and nurture lessons from Singapore

Indians living in Singapore (an example presented in Chapter I, Section 2) illustrate the issue well, because the nation's population is manageable enough for its well-organized public health department to have collected good data for several decades.

Even as far back as the late 1950s, **three to four times** as many Indian Singaporeans had heart disease and heart attacks as Chinese Singaporeans. In the past three decades, as Singapore has become more developed and urbanized, adverse changes in lifestyle—such as greater rates of obesity, inactivity, saturated fat intake, and smoking—have increased the risk factor levels of *both* Chinese and Indian Singaporeans to a similar degree. Yet unexpectedly, this similar increase in risk factor levels across the board has had a *greater* adverse effect on Indian Singaporeans than on Chinese Singaporeans! It has caused proportionately more heart disease among the Indians than among the Chinese, as measured in the incidence of heart attacks and deaths from heart disease.

The result is that the 300-400% difference that existed in heart disease rates between the two groups has remained. Heart disease rates for both groups (indeed, for the entire national population) have doubled in the last three decades.

Multiple Risk Factors Driving Towards Danger—A Vehicle Analogy
When several risk factors are simultaneously present, the smart thing to do is to reduce the ones you can control. Few people would quarrel with the idea that driving an old unreliable car (*risk factor 1*) down the highway at 75mph (*risk factor 2*), on very little sleep (*risk factor 3*), in icy conditions (*risk factor* 4), in foggy weather (*risk factor 5*), while you have major issues on your mind (*risk factor 6*) is to court disaster.

By itself, each of these risk factors does not pose a great risk of an accident. But the same action that might be reasonably safe in one circumstance—driving at 75 on the highway—is suddenly no longer safe when you add a new risk factor: an old unreliable car. To maintain the same margin of safety, you now need to reduce speed to perhaps 50. Add a third factor-sleep deprivation-and you may have to cut your speed down to 40. Include icy conditions, and you may not be safe over 30 mph. Toss in the factor of foggy weather, and you are down to no more than 20 mph. And so on.

Heart disease risk factors work much the same way. Whether genetic or lifestyle-based, when several are present, they gang up to raise your risk. But researchers are discovering that there may be a further dimension: Unlike the standard risk factors—smoking, hypertension, diabetes, high LDL, and low HDL—the emerging risk factors don't just *add cumulatively* to your risk. They seem to *multiply* your preexisting risks *synergistically.*

A Pernicious Pact between Two Powerful Adversaries

Analysis of data from numerous studies over several years makes it increasingly compelling that, for Indians, some of the key **emerging risk factors** of heart disease are as dangerous as the **conventional** factors. Not only that, but the simultaneous presence of the two kinds of factors magnify their harmful effects, dramatically heightening risk. In essence, they team up against the person. It is this synergistic, mutually reinforcing effect of emerging and standard risk factors on one another that may best explain the Indian Paradox.

This very telling, and simple quantitative illustration will help us see why. Suppose that in the 1970s, before the urbanization-driven increase in risk factor levels, one Chinese Singaporean died every year from heart disease for every three Indian Singaporeans. And assume that, after the similar increase in risk factor levels for both Chinese and Indians, one additional Chinese Singaporean now dies every year, making two a year. If this rise in the level of harmful risk factors *affects Indians the same way as it affects Chinese Singaporeans*, as we would assume, then one additional Indian a year would similarly die, making 3 + 1 = 4.

Right? Wrong. What the data show instead is that, for every two Chinese dying from heart disease after the rise in risk factor levels since the 1970s, *six* Indians are dying! Amazingly, the 3-to-1 ratio that existed several decades ago has stayed virtually the same! The Chinese went from one to two a year; but instead of the Indians also going from three to four year, *they* went from three to six.

These and other data suggest that, with many risk factors, a higher level of the same one factor causes an increase in cardiac risk that is

three times greater in Indians than in Chinese. The same increase in the level of a risk factor typically creates a higher risk among Indians than among Chinese and other racial groups. To offer an example: The cardiac risk faced by Indians from a 10-pound weight gain or smoking 10 cigarettes a day, is three times greater than that faced by Chinese from the same

Table 4.2. Risk factor levels needed to produce the same amount of heart disease risk in Indians as in other groups

	Indians	Other groups
Weight gain	10 pounds	30 pounds
Increase in waist size	10 cm	30 cm
Rise in blood pressure	10 mm Hg	30 mmHg
Rise in blood sugar	10 mg/dL	30 mg/dL
Rise in total cholesterol	30 mg/dL	90 mg/dL
Increase in smoking	10 a day	30 a day

Note. Indians face greater risk from the same risk factor levels. For example, the risk conferred on Indians by gaining 10 pounds is similar to that of a non-Indian person gaining 30 pounds.

An At-Risk Population

Often, higher levels of the same risk factor increase cardiac risk **three times** as much in Indians as in Chinese. The amplified effect that even a modest rise in risk factor levels has on Indian heart disease rates, compared to non-Indians, helps to explain why the rates of heart attacks and heart disease have risen two to three times on the Indian subcontinent in the past three decades. The lethal combination of phisical inactivity and an overly rich diet encouraged by urbanization first leads to insulin resistance, then to the metabolic syndrome, followed by diabetes and heart disease. The profound contribution of urbanization to heart disease among Indians has not received the kind of urgent attention a true crisis such as this properly deserves.

weight gain or number of cigarettes. In loose terms, the risk an Indian faces from gaining 10 pounds in body weight or increasing cholesterol by 30 mg/dL is similar to the risk a Chinese faces from gaining 30 pounds or increasing *cholesterol by 90 mg*(*see* Table 4.2).

The amplified effect that even a modest rise in risk factor levels has on Indian heart disease rates, helps to explain why these rates have, over the past three decades, risen threefold in urban areas of the Indian subcontinent, and twofold in rural areas. Let's examine one of the most overlooked of these risks: urbanization, and the ill effects it triggers.

Urbanization—the underappreciated risk factor

Like other developing regions, the Indian subcontinent has been undergoing rapid urbanization and modernization. This is often depicted in the media as a positive sign of development. What receives less attention is the fact that, along with heightened stress and environmental pollution, this transformation has been accompanied by reduced physical activity and unhealthy changes in diet—particularly the over-consumption of higher-calorie foods; refined, high glycemic load carbohydrates, and saturated fats, and the under-consumption of "low status" whole-grain products, fruits and vegetables that are associated with a lowly farming existence. This lethal combination of inactivity and an overly rich diet first leads to insulin resistance, then to the metabolic syndrome,

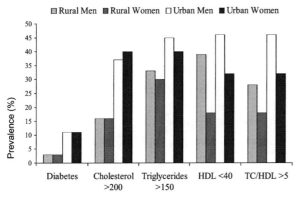

Figure 4.1. Differences in selected risk factors between urban and rural men and women. The risk factor profile in urban India, much worse than in rural India, explains the higher heart disease rates in urban areas. TC /HDL = Total cholesterol/HDL ratio. Source: Reddy, KS. Ref. 4.46.

followed by diabetes and heart disease.

Among Indians living abroad, high rates of heart disease can similarly be traced to the ill effects of inactivity, unhealthy diet, and urbanization—especially metabolic abnormalities. Studies show significantly higher levels of cholesterol,

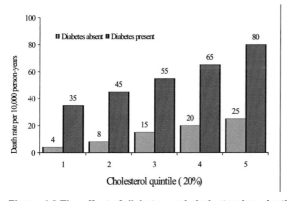

Figure 4.2. The effect of diabetes and cholesterol on death rates from heart disease, per 10,000 person-years. Diabetics with the lowest cholesterol have a higher risk than non-diabetics with the highest cholesterol. Source: Bierman EL Ref. 4.5.

triglycerides, blood sugar, and blood pressure among Indians abroad than among those living in rural India. These data are clearest and most irrefutable in comparisons between siblings. In turn, the adverse effects of these metabolic abnormalities

Lessons from: Japanese, Irish and Indian immigrants
Let's summarize in a slightly oversimplified way what we can learn from the three immigrational cases we have discussed, because it is vital to grasp the underlying nature-nurture dynamic that is at work here.

i. The **Japanese** went from good (cardioprotective) nature and average nurture in Japan to good nature and worse nurture in the US, with the result that their heart disease rates went up. These rates, however, remained lower than those of non-Japanese Americans, suggesting that their genes continued partly to protect them despite high rates of cardiac risk factors. (This is further explained in Section 2.)

ii. The **Irish** went from average nature and bad nurture in Ireland to (once again) average nature and bad nurture in the US, with the result that nothing much happened to their rates. The rates remained high as before. Unlike the genes of Japanese-Americans, Irish genes did little to protect them from their unhealthy lifestyle choices.

iii. Finally, **Indians** emigrating to the US and other countries have typically bad nature and moderately good nurture (particularly if they did not live in large cities) to bad nature and worse nurture (a more westernized lifestyle, for example). The result is a substantial increase in heart disease rates. Not only have Indian genes not protected them from their new unhealthy environment as Japanese genes did, but even unlike those of the Irish, their genes (or some mix of genes and emerging risk factors) have uniquely conspired with their new unhealthy lifestyle choices to send their heart disease rates sky-rocketing. Nature merely failed to protect the Irish from poor habits. In the case of Indians, by contrast, emerging risk factors, along with a genetic makeup that includes factors such as lipoprotein(a), team up with unhealthful lifestyle choices to raise heart disease rates to unprecedented levels. One might say that, among the Japanese, nature **counters and protects against** the adverse effects of nurture. Among Indians, nature seems to **worsen** the adverse effects of nurture.

Compared to whites and other populations, even though Indians have similar or lower levels of conventional risk factors such as high cholesterol, high blood pressure, and tobacco abuse, an excess of emerging risk factors magnifies the adverse effects of the conventional factors (see also Chapter I, Section 4). The result is the epidemic of heart disease we are now seeing among Indians worldwide.

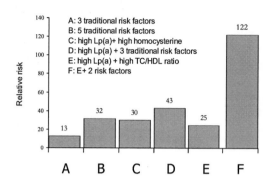

Figure 4.3 Relative risk of developing premature heart disease from traditional and emerging risk factors. Lp(a) = lipoprotein(a). TC = total cholesterol. TC/HDL = total cholesterol to HDL ratio. Note that risk having homocysteine and lipoprotein(a) excess is similar to those who have all five traditional factors. Source: Hopkins PN et al, Ref 4.26.

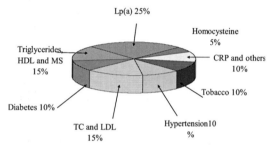

Figure 4.4. The relative contributions of different cardiac risk factors to premature heart disease in Indians. Figure 4.4. estimates the relative contributions of various risk factors to premature heart disease among Indians. Approximately 25% of premature heart disease among Indians is due to Lp(a) excess, and another 25% comes from a combination of metabolic syndrome and diabetes.

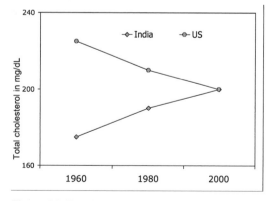

Figure 4.5. Trends in cholesterol levels in India and the US. Between 1960 and 2000, cholesterol levels decreased by an average of 30 points in the US, but increased 30 points in India—equivalent in cardiac risk to a 90-point increase in cholesterol elsewhere. This may explain 50% or more of the excess burden of heart disease in India.

are markedly magnified by Indians' underlying genetic predisposition toward both metabolic syndrome and heart disease.

Urbanization's contribution to the epidemic of heart disease among Indians has not received the level of attention a true crisis such as this rightly deserves. The effects of urbanization have led to an average weight gain of 25 to 30 pounds and an extra 6 inches in waistline—a change associated with a marked increase in metabolic abnormalities.

Not surprisingly, although rural-based Indians smoke more than urban Indians, they have lower heart disease rates. Why? The prevalence of diabetes and high cholesterol in urban areas is 2-3 times higher than in rural areas, and high triglycerides and low HDL are nearly 50% higher. Having diabetes raises the cardiac risk from traditional risk factors two to threefold. In fact, the risk of a heart attack among the 20% of diabetics with the lowest cholesterol levels exceeds the risk among the 20% of nondiabetics with the highest cholesterol (*see* Figure 4.2).

A similar phenomenon of risk magnification occurs with elevated levels of emerging factors such as homocysteine, Lp(a), and CRP. The relative risk of developing heart disease rises two to threefold when *either* lipoprotein(a) *or* homocysteine is elevated (compared to someone who has normal levels of them); but this risk rises **30-fold** when both are elevated. Furthermore, the risk of heart disease rises only 13-fold when any three of the traditional risk factors are present in a person, but this increases 43-fold when elevated Lp(a) is combined with just three of the traditional risk factors. A person's heart disease risk becomes particularly extreme, 122 times higher, when the person has elevated Lp(a), a high total cholesterol to HDL (TC/HDL), and two other risk factors.

Because of the amplifying effect that emerging risk factors such as homocysteine and Lp(a) have on the traditional risk factors, the cardiac risk faced by Indians from the traditional factors may be as high as, or higher than, in other populations, even though Indians have a lower prevalence of the traditional risk factors. Why? Because of the prevalence of high levels of emerging risk factors. Even if one conserva-

> **Did you know...**
> In the past three decades, cholesterol levels in India have risen by about 30 points, but fallen by the same amount in the US. The figure is even worse than it sounds. Why? Because other risk factors highly prevalent among Indians - such as Lp(a), homocysteine, CRP, and metabolic syndrome - worsen the harmful effects of bad cholesterol, it is likely that this 30-point increase in cholesterol has had the same impact on cardiac risk as a 90-point increase would have among non-Indians.

A Dangerous Synergy

Heart disease risk rises 2-3 times when either LP(a) or homocysteine is elevated; but it rises 30-fold when both factors are elevated!

tively estimated that the presence of high levels of either CRP, homocysteine, or Lp(a) doubles the relative risk of heart disease in each case, the *combination* of any two of these results in a risk four times higher than created by whatever level of traditional risk factors the person has at the time. The presence of all three can raise the risk eightfold. As we discussed above, the synergistic effects of emerging and standard risk factors best explains **the Indian Paradox**.

Traditional risk factors are doubly important

Although the traditional risk factors do not fully explain the high levels of heart disease among Indians, these factors, for reasons that have been discussed, are *especially important* in Indians and remain the principal targets for prevention and treatment. This is particularly true of cholesterol, which is on the rise. Over the past 30 years, cholesterol levels have fallen by about 30 points in the US—and *risen* by the same amount in India. Recall from previous paragraphs that the rise in cardiac risk from a 30-point increase among Indians is similar to that from a 90-point increase in other populations. The evidence of risk magnification from extensive data, such as those yielded by population group comparisons in Singapore (*see above*), underscores the need for both physicians and patients to *address conventional risk factors among Indians well before they reach the levels currently thought to be dangerous.*

Did You Know...

Excess weight and physical inactivity are the main contributors to the onset of metabolic syndrome, which accelerates atherosclerosis and other harmful changes in the body, leading to coronary artery disease.

Similar cholesterol, yet differing risk levels

The Seven Countries Study, involving almost 13,000 American, European, and Japanese men (*see* Appendix B), is one of the first major longitudinal studies that clearly showed that members of different ethnic groups who have the same number and severity of traditional risk factors can have different degrees of coronary heart disease, as evidenced by the rates of major coronary event among them. In particular, for any given level of risk factors,

Urbanization and Metabolic Syndrome

Metabolic syndrome is a cluster of disorders that strongly predict heart disease, stroke and diabetes. You are said to have the syndrome if you have three or more of the following disorders:

- insulin resistance, evidenced by a high blood sugar level (more than 100mg/dL)
- high blood pressure
- abdominal obesity (a waistline exceeding 36 inches in Indian men and 32 inches in Indian women)
- unhealthy HDL cholesterol levels—less than 50 in women and less than 40 in men
- high triglyceride levels

Having one of these disorders makes it more likely that you have, or will develop, others. In effect, they form a **chain reaction**, one leading to another. Furthermore, each has a **multiplying**, not just **additive**, effect on the others. The result is that having three or more dramatically increases your cardiovascular risk. As if that is not bad enough, high levels of lipoprotein(a) in the blood of Indians appears to give them a genetically-based predisposition toward heart disease that further magnifies the harmful effects of metabolic syndrome.

One reason urbanization has increased the prevalence of metabolic syndrome on the Indian subcontinent is that genes adapt to change slowly —over centuries—but urbanization has altered the lifestyle and environment of Indians in a matter of years. Thus, in many ways, the heart disease epidemic among Indians is the body's reaction to environmental overload upon a background of genetic vulnerability! It reflects the inability of the human body to adapt at the tissue level to excessively rapid and radical change. Our **genes** are telling us that we still live in an agrarian society characterized by physical work, fresh air, and *just enough* calories to get us through long tough days—mainly fruits, vegetables and grains, with the occasional catch of wild game. The **lifestyle** of many urban dwellers, on the other hand, is telling them to park themselves in front of the TV and reach for another beer. It is only a question of time before the body sends out a red alert. And on the Indian subcontinent, it has.

The cardiac risk from traditional factors such as smoking, high blood pressure, and high cholesterol is two to three-fold higher among diabetics than nondiabetics. A similar phenomenon of risk magnification occurs with elevated levels of homocysteine and/or lipoprotein(a). All three—diabetes, homocysteine, and LP(a)—are particularly common among Indians and contribute substantially to their heightened risk or heart disease.

such as cholesterol, the Japanese and Southern Europeans had a lower risk of developing heart disease than the Americans and Northern Europeans.

Table 4.3 compares the cardiac risks faced by Northern and Southern European male smokers, all of whom had hypertension (with a systolic, or upper number, of 180). Despite identical levels of the three major traditional risk factors—namely smoking, high blood pressure and high cholesterol—the risk of getting a heart attack or dying from one was *twice* as high among the Northern Europeans as among the Southern Europeans.

As one can see, for any given age, the incidence of coronary heart disease in Southern Europeans with cholesterol of 240 is *lower* than that for Northern Europeans with cholesterol of only 160. Note secondly, that the cardiac risk faced by a 40-year-old with cholesterol of 320 is roughly similar to that faced by a 60-year-old from the same ethnic group who has cholesterol of 160.

The first of these facts tells us that genes matter. The second tells us that, despite this, your cholesterol level also matters. A person's genes can **protect** them against certain risk factors—as observed among Southern Europeans and Japanese in the Seven Countries Study, and Chinese in the longitudinal medical data from Singapore. But genes can also **worsen** the harmful effects of a risk factor such as cholesterol, even if the person has only a moderately high level. Having a high degree of the risk factor only makes matters worse.

This appears to be the case with Indians. As Table 4.4 shows, the cardiac risk from a cholesterol level of 160 among Indians is similar to that faced by Americans with cholesterol of 260. Data from the European and Singapore studies indicates that recommended cholesterol levels should be at least 20% lower for Indians than the level recommended for Americans and Europeans.

Table 4.3. Differences in coronary event rates among Northern and Southern European male smokers with hypertension

Total cholesterol (mg/dL)		Coronary events per 1000 over 10 years	
		Southern Europe	Northern Europe
At age 40	160	29	51
	240	48	84
	320	77	135
At age 60	160	87	193
	240	137	288
	320	288	407

Source: Menotti A. et al. Ref. 4.35 Note that, at every age, the risk of heart disease in Northern Europeans with cholesterol of 240 is actually higher than that of Southern Europeans with the cholesterol of 320. Note also that the risk faced by a 40-year-old with cholesterol of 320 is similar to that of a 60-year-old person with cholesterol of 160.

The difficulty of measuring risk across ethnicities

Because heart disease risk factors affect different ethnic groups differently, a risk measurement tool developed for one population may not be accurate for other groups. Indeed, two British studies released in 2005 both concluded that the Framingham Risk Score, one of the most widely cited risk prediction models in the western world, does not accurately predict cardiac risk among Indians. Although it is accurate for white and black Americans, the Framingham model underestimates the cardiac risk for Indians, and overestimates it for Japanese-Americans, Hispanic-Americans, Native Americans, and Chinese-Americans—in the case of Chinese, by as much as 300% or more.

Table 4.4. Cholesterol levels among Indians to produce the same amount of heart disease risk among Americans

Total cholesterol level, Indians	Comparable cholesterol levels in Americans
120 mg/ dL	220 mg/ dL
160 mg/ dL	260 mg/ dL
200 mg/ dL	300 mg/ dL
240 mg/ dL	340 mg/ dL
320 mg/ dL	429 mg/ dL

Source: Adapted from Aarabi, M. Ref. 4.1.

To be used for Indians, the studies found, the Framingham formula should be adjusted upward—by adding 10 years in age, 50 points of systolic blood pressure, and 100 points of total cholesterol. The model, once recalibrated, has also been shown to be accurate for predicting risk in Chinese, British, and Spanish men.

Until new data become available, Dr. Michael Davidson, a co-investigator in the CADI Study (*see* Appendix B), recommends multiplying the Framingham Risk Score by 1.5 for Indians. I recommend multiplying it by 2. Millions of high-risk Indians who would benefit from aggressive lipids treatment may be missed if such a modification is not made to correct for the underestimation.

> Small people have small arteries; large people have large arteries. Indians are no exception. Smaller arteries **will not** make it more likely that you will get heart disease. If you do, though, it may be harder to thread a catheter down the artery because it is small—similar to finding a vein to draw blood on a newborn.

Improving on Framingham

Studies done in the UK have found that nondiabetic Indians have an **80% higher** risk of getting a heart attack than the Framingham model predicts. As mentioned earlier, the Framingham model overestimates cardiac risk for Southern Europeans and underestimates it for Northern Europeans. In response to its poor predictive value for the European population, a new model called SCORE—it stands for the Systematic Coronary Risk Evaluation—was developed.

SCORE improves on Framingham in one area, but not in another. On the plus side, SCORE uses different formulas for high-risk and low-risk European countries to enhance its accuracy. The Framingham model, on the other hand, uses different formulas for predicting risk among men and women. On the minus side, SCORE predicts only the 10-year risk of actually dying, whereas the Framingham model predicts heart attacks *as well as* deaths from cardiac disease. Since SCORE excludes non-fatal heart attacks, it substantially underestimates a European's overall cardiac risk, since many people have heart attacks they do not die from.

SCORE's use of different formulas for high- and low-risk countries is an important advance because, as discussed in the next section, heart disease rates vary markedly among Europeans. The United Kingdom, for example, has rates four times higher than France. Other low-risk countries besides France include Belgium, Greece, Italy, Luxembourg, Portugal, Spain, and Switzerland.

Framingham did not do well when applied to South Asians; has the SCORE prediction model fared any better? A British study published in 2005 convincingly demonstrates that SCORE substantially underestimates cardiovascular risk among all South Asians. In short, the major existing prediction models all underestimate the risk of heart disease among Indians, by as much as 50%.

Common myths and misconceptions about heart disease among Indians

- **Myth** *Indians suffer from heart disease because they have smaller coronary arteries.*

- **Fact** Artery size is correlated to body size, not to ethnicity. Smaller individuals of any ethnic group have smaller arteries; larger individuals have larger arteries. Indians are no exception. (*See* **Color Plate 3.4**, *Indians Have Small Coronary Arteries . . . The Myth*, and **Color Plate 3.5**, *Indians Have Small Coronary Arteries . . . The Facts*.) British-based cardiologist and researcher Dr. Jatinder Dhawan confirmed this in a study of male Indian patients undergoing coronary angiography. On average, they had smaller-diameter coronary arteries than whites, but this difference disappeared when the results were adjusted for the differences in body size and fatness. At the same body mass index (BMI) and weight, Indians have similarly-sized arteries as whites, blacks, and other Asians. Similar observations have been made in Pakistani heart disease patients.

The risk of heart disease in Indians with a cholesterol level of 160 appears to be similar to that of Americans with cholesterol of 260.

Not only do Indians not have small arteries for their build, but small arteries do not raise your risk of developing heart disease (although shortness in height, it should be noted, has been identified as a heart disease risk factor). Women, for example, have smaller coronary arteries yet develop heart disease 10 to 20 years later than men. Similarly, Chinese and Japanese typically have smaller arteries than, for example, white Americans, yet have less heart disease. Small-sized arteries, however, do matter in one way: They are associated with significantly higher rates of complications during coronary angioplasty, stenting, and bypass surgeries because it is harder to thread a catheter down a small artery.

■ **Myth** Indians abroad have high rates of heart disease because of the stress of immigration and adjusting to a new culture.

■ **Fact** Cultural adjustment following emigration is stressful to all groups because it is often accompanied by low social support, loss of self-esteem, and isolation. However, countries such as the US attract immigrants from all over— Africa, Europe, Latin America, the Middle East and other Asian countries. Yet, unlike Indians, many of them have heart disease rates similar to, and often half that of, the overall US population. If anything, English-speaking immigrants from Commonwealth countries, including Indians, should have an advantage because they do not have to learn a new language.

Undoubtedly, chronic stress and other psychosocial factors do contribute to heart disease and heart attacks, especially when they take the form of hostility, an angry personality, or bottled-up rage. This makes stress and anger management an important cardioprotective skill to learn. But stress should not be overrated as a contributor to heart disease. Scandinavian countries are, in some ways, among the lowest-stress societies in the world, yet they tend to have high rates of heart disease. More likely, immigration sometimes correlates with greater heart disease because new immigrants exchange their physically active life in their home country for a much less active lifestyle. In that sense, immigration has a similar effect to urbanization.

■ **Myth** *Indian vegetarians don't have to worry about heart disease. They are protected.*

■ **Fact** Vegetarians worldwide have extremely favorable lipid profiles and low rates of heart disease, except Indians. For example, nearly half of the participants in the CADI study were lifelong vegetarians, yet, they had heart disease rates similar to those of non-vegetarians (*see* Chapter I, Section 2). The rates of diabetes were actually higher among the vegetarians, possibly because of a higher glycemic load from a higher intake of refined carbohydrates. Moreover, Indian non-vegetarians, who have high heart disease rates, tend not to eat a lot of meat (2-4 ounces once or twice a week), so the differences between them and Indian vegetarians are not that great.

Vegetarians worldwide have extremely low rates of heart disease, with the exception of Indians. Although nearly half of the participants in the CADI study were lifelong vegetarians, they had heart disease rates similar to those of non-vegetarians.

The Indian vegetarian diet needs "adjustment" for it to be healthy (*see* Chapter V, Sections 1-7). Besides high glycemic index carbs, Indian vegetarians typically consume generous amounts of full-fat dairy products, butter, and *ghee* (clarified butter), all of which is laden with saturated fat. In addition, because they fry foods so frequently, and frequently reuse the oil, their intake of trans fat is often as high as, or higher than, that of non-vegetarians. Finally, most Indian vegetarians *avoid fish*—one of the most cardioprotective foods on the planet, especially oily fish high in omega-3 fatty acids. This phenomenon, which I have termed *contaminated vegetarianism*, is paradoxical because a central goal in becoming vegetarian is usually to achieve greater health.

In contrast, many western vegetarians do eat cardioprotective amounts of fish that is high in omega-3 acids, and they avoid dairy products, substituting them with soy-based and nut-based products. Not surprisingly, the lipid profile of western vegetarians is strongly anti-atherogenic, with high HDL and low LDL. The vegetarian diet is very healthy—*if* it is done right. Indians, both vegetarians and non-vegetarians, should model their nutrition after the most healthy western (or Mediterranean) vegetarian diets—meaning lots of fruit, raw or lightly cooked vegetables, whole grains, legumes, nuts, and healthy oils—adding moderate amounts of fish and lean meats if they are non-vegetarian. Chapter V outlines such a nutritional plan.

KEY · POINTS · IN · A · NUTSHELL

♥ Heart disease risk factors often affect different ethnic groups differently. For any given level of risk factors, some groups—e.g., Chinese, Japanese, Southern Europeans—have a surprisingly low risk of developing heart disease, while others (e.g., Indians) have a particularly elevated risk.

♥ Compared to other groups, even a modest rise in any risk factor levels appears to have an amplified effect on heart disease among Indians.

♥ Rapid urbanization on the Indian subcontinent, accompanied by physical inactivity and unhealthy diet, has led to a high prevalence of lipid abnormalities, insulin resistance, metabolic syndrome, and increasing rates of diabetes and heart disease.

♥ The same phenomenon was first observed among Indian immigrants abroad.

♥ High rates of diabetes and metabolic syndrome, however, only partially explain the excess of heart disease among young Indians.

♥ The most compelling explanation for the epidemic among Indians worldwide is their excess burden of several emerging risk factors, and the synergistic interaction of these with traditional risk factors.

♥ Lp(a), for example, makes Indians susceptible to heart disease at a young age by magnifying the effect of high LDL and low HDL cholesterol, hastening atherosclerosis.

♥ Because of these synergies, heart disease risk rises four- to eightfold when multiple emerging risk factors are present.

♥ A high level of either Lp(a), homocysteine or CRP, for example, can by itself double the risk of heart disease, with or without the presence of any traditional risk factors.

♥ There is an important genetic component to Indian heart disease. Elevated levels of Lp(a) are among the factors genetically inherited, but it is not clear what other risk factors are part of the Indian genetic makeup.

♥ Some of the other emerging factors in Indians may be partly genetic and partly lifestyle-related.

♥ This high prevalence of emerging risk factors among Indians neutralizes the advantage they might have enjoyed from their somewhat lower prevalence of traditional risk factors.

♥ In addition, all the current major heart disease risk prediction models underestimate the risk faced by Indians by up to 50%. This can lead to under-diagnosis and under-treatment of at-risk Indians.

♥ High homocysteine levels are associated with improper diet and cooking practices, while high levels of CRP are associated with abdominal obesity and physical inactivity.

♥ A vegetarian diet can be strongly cardioprotective, if done right, but the Indian vegetarian diet typically has large amounts of saturated and trans fats, along with high-glycemic carbohydrates and little fish.

♥ Contrary to popular opinion, Indians have normal-sized arteries for their build, because artery size depends on body size, not ethnicity. Smaller arteries, in any case, do not raise one's heart disease risk. They do, however, contribute to more complications following coronary angioplasty or bypass surgery.

4.2 ► Ethnicity and Heart Disease: Resolving the Paradoxes

ALL HUMANS SHARE a set of genes that can be traced back to a single evolutionary line that emerged in the Olduvai Gorge, on the highlands of tropical East Africa. Despite this shared origin, the risk of a person developing heart disease varies more than tenfold from one ethnic group to another, and threefold just within the United States. How can our genes be so similar, yet lead to such different outcomes? Blacks, for example, have the highest rate of hypertension, kidney disease, and stroke, yet low rates of heart disease. Indians, on the other hand, have low rates of hypertension and are often vegetarian, yet have high rates of heart disease. For any given degree of atherosclerosis, people from the Indian subcontinent have higher rates of coronary disease than other groups.

> Race and ethnicity are not risk factors—like cholesterol. They are risk markers (that is, outward signs) that help us to predict, based on a person's ethnicity, what risk factors they are likely to face, and how harmful those risk factors are likely to be.

These differences in disease rates and risk levels offer us a unique opportunity to understand the complex genetic-environmental interactions that underlie heart disease. After emigrating to the US, for example, the rates of stroke in Asians fall, yet their heart disease rates rise—a reflection of new changes in lifestyle and environment. As a melting pot of immigrants and Native Americans, the US is a natural laboratory to study the relative roles of nature and nurture in the development of coronary disease. A greater understanding of why heart disease rates differ among ethnic groups, and why some groups seem more protected than others, will help us understand heart disease itself. It will also help us to identify those risks we should be more aggressive about reducing through prevention and treatment strategies.

This section discusses ethnic differences in heart disease, the risk factors that underlie and drive these differences, why some groups appear to be enjoy greater protection than others, and what Indians and other ethnic groups can learn from these data.

Diseases vary primarily by ethnicity, not race

The terms "racial" and "ethnic" are often used interchangeably in the medical literature, but they are not the same. Indeed, many experts today believe that the entire concept of race is illegitimate when applied to humans, because a race is, biologically, a different sub-species—eagles versus sparrows, for example, or poodles versus Great Danes. Humans are much more similar to one another than that. Genetically, we are

> Although Indians are, strictly speaking, Asians, this book follows common linguistic practice in using the term "Asian American" to refer to non-Indian American Asians, such as Southeast Asians and Japanese and Chinese Americans.

much more closely related than the superficial differences that many people regard as so meaningful when they draw distinctions between racial groups—differences like skin color, hair texture, body shape, and eye color. For historical reasons, many of these distinctions have acquired inflated social meaning, yet most of these features do not reflect genetically significant differences among groups—either in susceptibility to disease or anything else. Human "races," in short, are far more *visually* distinct than *genetically* distinct.

That is not to say that all genetic differences are merely superficial, only that the ones we often use to distinguish racial groups from one another are not the important ones. They are often just that: skin deep. There could well be deep genetic differences between the races waiting to be discovered by future researchers; we do not know. What we do know is that there are differences in how *ethnic* groups respond to diseases and risk factors, and that some of these differences may be genetic, or part-genetic and part-environment.

So what is the difference between a racial and an ethnic group? Largely one of degree. Both have an environmental as well as a genetic component, but a **racial group** is the more purely biological classification, while an **ethnic group** is more of a societal entity that shares common cultural traditions, values, lifestyle preferences such as dietary practices, and other personal behaviors. Because environmental and behavioral factors have heavily influenced how our genes interact with disease, this makes ethnicity a more accurate predictor of the diseases to which particular ethnic groups are vulnerable and the way they will respond both to disease and to treatment. Diseases, in other words, vary more by ethnicity than by race because ethnicity better captures how different environments and lifestyles have altered the way a people's genes respond to disease.

For classification and data management purposes, humans nevertheless continue to be divided into three racial groups—Mongoloid, Negroid, and Caucasian. By contrast, there are *hundreds* of ethnic groups, each of whom may be a mix of one or more of the three races—in other words, multiracial. Racial classifications are, therefore, less useful than ethnicity in understanding the impact of disease on populations, simply because race is too broad. It overgeneralizes. blacks, for example, constitute a "race" as the term is used; yet heart disease, stroke, and other disease rates *vary markedly* among blacks from Africa, Europe, the Caribbean, Australia, and the US. This variation reflects ethnic (and thus environmental) diversity, even though they are all from the same so-called "race." Asian Indians, similarly, are not a single race but a collection of related ethnic groups that loosely share a cluster of genetic commonalities, along with various sociocultural practices—including a nearly incorrigible love for fried foods and high-fat vegetarian foods.

Despite the inaccuracies introduced by over-generalization about "races," many different ethnic groups continue to be lumped together in medical databases (including even *death certificates*, which often wrongly record the ethnicity of a deceased person simply because "he looks close enough"). Asian Americans, for example, are often lumped with Pacific Islanders as a broad category labeled Asian American/Pacific Islanders, or AAPI. Ethnically, AAPI is actually a highly heterogeneous collection of more than 40 ethnic groups, and any disease statistics imputed to the entire group are likely to be gross overgeneralizations. For example, heart disease rates are the lower among AAPI than whites, blacks, or Hispanics, but within the group itself, there is great heterogeneity. Indians, for instance, have heart disease rates three to six times higher than the Chinese. Publishing "average" heart disease rates for large, multiracial, multiethnic groups such as AAPI is, therefore, a bit like stating that the "average" height of American basketball players and pygmies from Papua New Guinea is five feet. It may be statistically true. Diagnostically, it is unhelpful.

Why Ethnicity is Superior to Race as a Diagnostic Category
Compared to race, ethnicity is a superior indicator of the diseases to which a group is particularly vulnerable, and how they respond to illness and treatment, because ethnicity better reflects the nature-nurture interaction. The world's ethnic groups are not susceptible to the same diseases, and even the same diseases take slightly different forms in different groups because of differences in lifestyle and environment as well as in genetic inheritance.

The wide variations in the prevalence and incidence rates of diseases from one ethnic group to another reflect a complex set of gene-environment interactions that go well beyond race. Racial categories are, therefore, too broad a stroke to capture the distinctions we need to draw to be able to assess risk levels, explain why disease rates differ from ethnic group to group, and create prevention and treatment strategies targeted to specific ethnic groups.

Did you know...
In some populations, high rates of risk factors are accompanied by low rates of heart disease. In others, it is just the opposite: low risk factors rates are accompanied by high heart disease rates.

Publishing average heart disease rates for a large, multi-ethnic group such as Asian American/Pacific Islanders, is somewhat like stating that the "average" height of pygmies and American basketball players is five feet. It may be statistically true, but it is diagnostically unhelpful.

Heart disease and stroke rates: Western versus Asian populations

Differences in the incidence of heart disease and stroke in the East and the West give us a glimpse into the impact of ethnicity on disease risk. Recall that heart disease and stroke are both cardiovascular diseases typically caused by atherosclerosis and blockages that cut off blood supply and oxygen to the heart or the brain. Yet people in the west die from heart disease *three to four times* more often than from stroke—while the exact reverse is the case for Asians; they die three to four times more often from stroke. Genes, environment, and behavior all play a role. Among Americans and Europeans, elevated cholesterol levels from a high consumption of saturated fats probably constitutes the single most important cause of their high rates of heart disease. By contrast, the high incidence of stroke among Asians can largely be attributed to unmanaged hypertension caused primarily by excessive salt in their diet, although some genetic factors are also involved.

> Americans of European descent die three to four times more often from heart disease than from stroke. In contrast, Asian death rates from stroke are three to four times higher than from heart disease. Such variations suggest not only that the same risk factors have a different impact on heart disease than on stroke, but also that ethnic groups respond to these risk factors in different ways, even after you take into account differences in diet.

Another difference: Stroke among Asians is frequently fatal because it tends to take the form of hemorrhagic stroke—in contrast to thrombotic stroke, common in the West, which leads more often to paralysis and disability than death.

The huge variations in heart disease and stroke rates around the world suggest that, in different ethnic groups, the same risk factors— such as cholesterol and hypertension—have a different impact on heart disease than on stroke, because different groups respond to these risk factors in different ways, even after you take into account differences in diet. For example, the risk of developing and dying from a stroke varies fivefold by ethnicity and tenfold from country to country, and the rates of heart disease exhibit a similarly wide variation. Regional variation is similarly large: Unlike heart attack, two-thirds of stroke deaths occur in developing countries. Mortality is particularly high in Eastern Europe, South America, and Asia.

Tid bits

Upon emigrating to the US, Asians typically increase their intake of saturated fats. This results in high levels of blood cholesterol and rising rates of heart disease.

Trends in heart disease among immigrants

As might be expected from the discussion of the influence of cultural and geographical environment, data on immigrants show that, despite sharing a common genetic background, ethnically related people acquire different cardiovascular disease rates when they live in different geographic and cultural environments. Thus, heart disease rates among recent immigrants—people who have left one country, but have not quite yet integrated into their adopted country—are generally intermediate between the rates found in the two countries. The implications of this will be further discussed in the later paragraphs on trends in heart disease among Japanese Americans.

Upon immigration to the US, Asians typically increase their consumption of saturated fats, resulting in elevated levels of cholesterol and raised rates of heart disease. Nevertheless, heart disease rates among Japanese Americans, Chinese Americans, Korean Americans, and most other Asian Americans are about half that of whites. Immigrants from the Indian subcontinent are an exception: their heart disease rates are three to four times higher than whites, and six times higher than the Chinese (*see* section 1).

> Acculturation is the modification of an immigrant culture's lifestyle through contact with their adopted country's dominant culture. The degree and speed of acculturation, along with the cardiovascular disease rates prevailing in the country of origin and the country of adoption, determine the new rates of CVD among an immigrant group.

Ethnic differences in cardiac risk factors

Of course, changes in diet or other cultural and behavioral practices do not by themselves elevate or lower heart disease rates. These influences are mediated through risk factors. It is because the prevalence of risk factors such as elevated cholesterol, blood pressure, smoking and diabetes varies markedly by ethnicity that cardiovascular disease rates differ from one ethnic group to another. For example, hypertension is more common among blacks, whereas diabetes is more common among Native Americans and other minority populations. Asian Americans have similar rates of diabetes as whites, despite lower rates of obesity (5% versus 22%) and being overweight (33% versus 39%). Once you adjust for the lower rates of obesity, the rates of diabetes in Asian Americans are actually 60% higher than in whites.

The *traditional* risk factors of cholesterol, blood pressure, smoking and diabetes, however, fail to explain the marked differences in heart disease rates among people of different ethnicities (Table 4.5). It appears that the strength of the connection between these risk factors and cardiovascular disease varies from group to group. For example, hypertension is more dangerous and more resistant to treatment among blacks than in members of other populations, who have similar levels of blood pressure, cholesterol, body weight, smoking, and diabetes.

In short, not only do some groups have higher levels of risk factors, but also similar levels of risk factors seem to have more detrimental effects in some groups than in others. In some groups, certain risk factors seem to have surprisingly little effect. Examining the relationship between risk factors to heart disease in various ethnic groups, therefore, reveals several paradoxes. In some populations, high rates of risk factors are accompanied by low rates of heart disease. In others, low rates of risk factors are accompanied by high rates of heart disease.

> Approximately 15% of US residents are foreign-born. The proportion of whites is expected to decline from the current level of 67% to 50% by about 2050. Hispanics, the largest and fastest-growing minority, now represent 14% to 15% of the population. blacks account for 12%, and Asians make up 4%.

Table 4.5. Age-adjusted mortality rates from heart disease for Americans of different ethnicities, during 1998

Ethnicity	Mortality per 100,000
African Americans	187
whites Americans	183
Hispanic Americans	124
Native Americans	124
Asian Americans	100

Source: CDC and AHA

Table 4.6 below summarizes examples of this paradoxical relationship between risk factors and heart disease among people of different ethnicities. **One key lesson** that emerges from these comparisons is that the powerfully protective effects of HDL against heart disease, and the damaging effects of Lp(a), are both much more important than we have perhaps recognized.

A second lesson is that we need to undertake more research not just on how the total *amount* or level of particular risk factors in the blood promote disease, but also on the *qualitative* differences that exist within these risk factors and how these protect or heighten a person's vulnerability. For example, the relative proportions of large HDL versus small HDL, or large LDL versus small LDL, or large Lp(a) versus small Lp(a), make a huge impact on overall risk. Most blacks, for instance, not only have relatively more of the cardioprotective large HDL, as well as more of the benign large LDL rather than the dangerous small LDL, but *also* appear to have relatively less of the dangerous small Lp(a). Indians, on the other hand, may have higher proportions of the small dangerous Lp(a), in addition to their known elevated levels of small dangerous LDL and low levels of large beneficial HDL. In short, qualitative differences matter. And when they are not in your favor, you need to double your efforts in other areas to reduce your overall risk.

Ultimately, the comparative data summarized in Table 4.6 reinforce a fundamental thesis of this book: that several emerging risk factors—many of them not yet very well studied—interact synergistically with more standard risk factors (and possibly with one another) to dramatically raise a person's overall cardiovascular risk if he or she has several of these risk factors and few protective factors.

The Notion of a Tipping Point: Whether you will develop cardiovascular disease, and how quickly, is, therefore, often a question of balance. Like the straw that broke the camel's back, there appear to be **tipping points** in a person's risk factor profile. Before the tipping point was reached, the "camel's back" seemed to be doing just fine. However, the

> **Within Six Inches of Your Life**
> Like the straw that broke the camel's back, there appear to be "tipping points" in an individual's cardiovascular disease risk factor profile. If you jump off a cliff at the end of a bungee cord and come within just six inches of the ground, you are *technically* still safe and healthy! But it would not take much—just a few more inches—to cross the gap between "still safe" and catastrophic outcome. The introduction of just one more elevated risk factor, however, can cross that gap and accelerate cardiovascular disease.

addition of one just more risk factor, or an increase in the level of an existing risk factor—perhaps through a change of cultural environment from rural to urban, or migration from East to West, or a promotion to a more sedentary desk job—can suddenly **tip the scale** and trigger an acceleration in the progression of cardiovascular disease.

Each of the high risk factor/low heart disease paradoxes displayed in Table 4.6 depict an ethnic group that, on average, has not reached its tipping point (although, of course, there are people in each group who do get cardiovascular disease). If you jump off a cliff at the end of a bungee cord and come within just six inches of the ground, you are technically-speaking still "safe" and healthy. But it would not take much—just a few more inches—to cross the gap between "still safe" and catastrophic outcome.

The paradoxes discussed below suggest that many ethnic groups are, in a sense, bungee-jumping to within a few feet of catastrophe. That is, they still have low heart disease rates despite the dangers coursing through their blood in the form of risks from various dietary choices, behavioral practices, and genetic factors, but it may not take much to tip the scale. To employ another metaphor: they are skating on thin ice—but often, that thin ice has been surprisingly stable and it has protected them for decades and even centuries.

With the rapid pace of modernization and globalization, however, ethnic groups are modifying or discarding centuries-old practices very quickly, thereby altering the risk factor balance that had once protected them. Even Chinese in Beijing today can be seen wolfing down greasy fast-food hamburgers and fried chicken like the heartiest of Americans—unheard of just 30 years ago. In short, what medical researchers are observing is that many ethnic groups—Indians, for example—are beginning to introduce just enough new harmful changes to tip their risk factor balance—and extend the bungee cord that extra six inches that results in disease rather than mere risk.

Taking Charge - It's Possible
It is not set in stone that societies must remain high stroke cultures or high coronary disease cultures. Over the past three decades, for example, the US and Japan have dramatically reduced their death rates from heart disease and from stroke, respectively. This has been achieved through better testing, wider use of medications, and changes in diet, salt intake, smoking, and physical activity levels. Japan's stroke mortality rate, for example, is now comparable to that of the general US population—almost unimaginable two decades ago. Although both nations still have a long way to go, they have essentially taken charge of their cardiovascular health at the individual, public health, and societal levels. The challenge is for South Asians to do the same.

The bright side of these observations is that, by actively reducing your controllable risks all around, you can give yourself the kind of robust margin that is likely to protect you from cardiovascular disease well into your golden years.

▶ The Japanese Paradox

For the past 50 years, despite high rates of smoking and hypertension, the Japanese have had some of the lowest rates of heart disease mortality among all industrialized countries. Their heart disease rates are less than one-fourth that of Europeans. Yet 63% of Japanese men and 13% of Japanese women smoke, compared with 24% and 22% of American men and women, respectively. The Japanese also have high rates of diabetes (13%) and prediabetes (20%).

Explanation: So why do they have low heart disease rates? Somewhat greater physical activity, lower obesity, and a healthier diet—particularly lower consumption of saturated fats, less dietary cholesterol, more fish, and more grains and fiber—combine with genetics to give the Japanese lower triglyceride levels, total cholesterol levels that are about 10% lower than Americans, and HDL levels that are 20% higher, to protect them against higher rates of heart disease.

Lessons: The effects of immigration have been studied extensively among Japanese Americans, particularly in states such as Hawaii and California. These studies typically all point to classic interactions between genes and environment. The relative immunity of the Japanese to heart disease is progressively lost upon emigration to the US as they become acculturated and adopt western food practices such as high dietary cholesterol. Yet, although heart disease rates *triple* among Japanese American

Table 4.6. Paradoxical Relationships between Risk Factors & Heart Disease In different Ethnic Groups

The Group	The Paradox	Factors that help explain the paradox
The Japanese	Low heart disease despite high rates of smoking, hypertension, and diabetes	Strongly antiatherogenic lipid profile made up of high HDL, low LDL, and low TG, plus fish consumption and low obesity
The Chinese	Low heart disease despite high rates of smoking, salt intake, and hypertension	Strongly antiatherogenic lipid profile made up of high HDL, low LDL, low TC, and low TG. Low Lp(a) and low obesity (though beginning to change)
The French	Low heart disease despite high-fat diet, including saturated fats	Regular consumption of cardioprotective monounsaturated fats and folate-rich fresh fruits and vegetables; moderate red wine consumption; low homocysteine; low obesity through portion control; moderately high daily physical activity. Genetically low Lp(a)
African Americans	Low heart disease despite high rates of obesity, smoking, and diabetes; a high-salt, high-fat diet; low socioeconomic status; the highest hypertension and stroke rates in the US, and the highest levels of Lp(a)	Strongly antiatherogenic lipid profile made up of high HDL, low LDL, and low TG. Low rates of abdominal obesity and metabolic syndrome (men). Moderately high daily physical activity
Hispanic Americans	Low heart disease despite high rates of obesity, diabetes, low socioeconomic status; and lower HDL, higher triglycerides, and higher prevalence of metabolic syndrome than whites	Lower levels of Lp(a) than whites
Native Americans	Low heart disease despite high rates of obesity, abdominal obesity and diabetes, high rates of physical inactivity and unhealthy diet, and low socioeconomic status and access to treatment	Low levels of LDL and Lp(a)
Filipinos	Low heart disease despite high rates of obesity, diabetes, and hypertension	More study needed
Asian Indians	Highest heart disease rates despite high rates of vegetarianism and low rates of risk factors other than diabetes	Atherogenic lipid profile (low HDL, high TG). Small dense LDL, small dysfunctional HDL; high levels of Lp(a), CRP, fibrinogen, PAL-1, homocysteine, and Apo B. High prevalence of abdominal obesity, physical inactivity, insulin resistance, and metabolic syndrome

Key: Apo B = apolipoprotein B; CR = C-reactive protein; Lp(a) = lipoprotein(a); PAL-1 = plasminogen-activator inhibitor type 1; TC = total cholesterol; TG = triglycerides.

immigrants after leaving Japan, their rates continue to remain less than half that of white Americans because they have not lost all their immunity.

Reflecting the west's relatively low rates of stroke, however, Japanese American men in Hawaii have higher rates of *heart disease,* but lower rates of *stroke* than men living in Japan. Because of improved detection and treatment of *high blood pressure* and reduced smoking, stroke rates among some Japanese American have fallen by more than half compared to those in Japan, and are now comparable to stroke rates among whites. Data from two very carefully designed prospective studies, the Ni-Hon-San Study and subsequently the Honolulu Heart Program, have shown that, between 1966 and 1984, the overall mortality rate from cardiovascular disease (meaning heart attack plus stroke) among Japanese Americans fell *by 40%* compared to native Japanese. Reason: The dramatic decrease in number of deaths from stroke far exceeded the increase in deaths from heart disease.

Essentially, they moved from a high-stroke, low-coronary disease culture to a low-stroke, high-coronary disease culture. As recent immigrants, not only are Japanese Americans somewhere in between the two poles—Japan and US—but also differences within their cardiovascular disease rates reflect in an almost linear way just where they are on that immigrational gradient. Acculturation studies show that Japanese-Americans who maintain a more traditional Japanese lifestyle (and are therefore closer to the Japanese end of the spectrum) have lower heart disease risk factor values and, not surprisingly, lower heart disease rates than those who have adopted a more American lifestyle and diet. In short, changes in risk factor levels following immigration reflect the gradient of westernization the immigrants and their descendants experience—a powerful testament to the influence of lifestyle choices on a person's risk factor profile and thus vulnerability to disease.

Greater westernization in middle-aged Japanese Americans, for example, is associated with more severe atherosclerosis—equivalent to as much as a **20 year increase in age,** meaning that atherosclerosis among 50-year-old Japanese Americans is on average comparable to that of 70-year-olds living in Japan.

Acculturation studies have also shown that the Japanese Americans engage in significantly less physical activity than Japanese in Japan. In addition, there were telling dietary changes: Japanese Americans consumed 60% more animal fat, *60% more saturated fat,* 40% more cholesterol, and 60% more refined, non-complex carbohydrates than those living in Japan. They ate more fat, and they ate more bad fat. These changes all result in a threefold higher rate of diabetes and a twofold higher rate of dyslipidemia.

It is not fixed in stone that Asia must inevitably remain a high-stroke culture while the West is condemned to remain a high coronary disease culture. Change is clearly possible. Heart disease death rates, for example, have fallen substantially in the US over the past three decades through both prevention and treatment. Yet another set of data that show the powerful effects of lifestyle modification are Japan's cardiovascular disease trends. For many decades, two to three times more Japanese died from stroke than from heart disease. Over the past 30 years, however, deaths from stroke have fallen by two-thirds because of a concerted effort by Japanese to reduce their salt intake, together with improvements in the detection and control of high blood pressure. During the past 30 years, there has been a sevenfold increase in the use of high blood pressure medications. Heart disease deaths in Japan have also declined by one-third from advances in the detection and control of cholesterol. The most recent data, from 2003, show that the stroke mortality rate in Japan is now comparable to that of the general population in the US and in the UK.

▶ The Chinese Paradox

Heart disease: As with the Japanese, smoking and hypertension are major risk factors among the Chinese, and smoking rates continue to increase. In contrast, Chinese Americans have the lowest rates of smoking—12%—compared to 22% among Americans overall. In the Minhang District of China, for example, 67% of men smoke on average about 17 cigarettes a day, spending as much as 60% of their total personal income on cigarettes. Despite this, heart disease rates are *three to five times* lower than those observed among Europeans and Americans. Fewer than 1 in 10 deaths in rural China are attributed to heart disease, as compared to one in three in the US. The overall rates, however, are two to three times higher among urban Chinese than rural Chinese.

What accounts for the low heart disease rates? Like the Japanese, the Chinese have an *anti-atherogenic lipid profile* that tends to retard atherosclerosis: low total cholesterol, low LDL, low triglycerides, low lipoprotein(a), and high HDL levels. Total cholesterol levels in some rural regions are in

What is Epidemiologic Transition?
Epidemiologic transition refers to the transition from a rural sustenance economy to an urban economy. It is characterized by decreased physical activity and increased consumption of highly refined and energy-dense foods. This results in a decrease in deaths among children due to infections, and an increase in cardiovascular and other chronic diseases.

the 80-112 range, which is very low indeed. In one study, 2% of Chinese had a total cholesterol level below 100 and only 6% of males and 8% of females had cholesterol above 200—again very impressive. Total cholesterol-to-HDL ratio, an even stronger predictor of heart disease than low total cholesterol or low LDL alone, is below 4 in both urban and rural Chinese, compared to 5 or more among the general American population (*see* Table 4.7). This favorable lipid profile protects against their high levels of smoking and hypertension.

Recent studies indicate, however, that with China's rapid modernization, cholesterol levels among urban Chinese in many regions of the country are fast approaching—and in some cases even surpassing—western levels. On average, cholesterol levels have risen by 40 points, BMI has increased by one unit (equivalent to five to six pounds per person), and diabetes has tripled (3% to 9%). As a result, death rates from heart disease have risen since the 1980s. Treatment following a heart attack is also less than optimal.

The rise in risk factors most likely results from lifestyle changes brought on by modernization, dietary changes accompanying the adoption of "western" habits, and inadequate preventive strategies. Called *"epidemiologic transition,"* this phenomenon is occurring in many developing countries undergoing economic transition. In China, there has been a fivefold increase in the consumption of red meat and eggs, along with a significant decrease in the consumption of fruits and vegetables. On the plus side, the Chinese still have a low prevalence of abdominal obesity (25%) and metabolic syndrome (15%).

Stroke: The Chinese have *five* times as many strokes as heart attacks, and *three* times as many Chinese die from stroke as from heart attack—a very high rate of stroke mortality. The main reason is that they tend to have **hemorrhagic strokes** (a blood vessel bursting in the brain), which are far more lethal than **ischemic strokes** (a clogged blood vessel starving brain cells of oxygen). Their rates of hemorrhagic stroke are two to three times higher (25% to 35%) than those of white Americans (6% to 12%).

Table 4.7. Urban and Rural Differences in the Prevalence of Selected Risk Factors in 50-year-old Men and Women in China

	Men			Women		
	Average	Urban	Rural	Average	Urban	Rural
Age	50	50	50	50	50	50
BMI	23	24	23	24	24	23
Waist girth (inches)	32	33	31	30	31	30
Waist to hip ratio	0.86	0.88	0.86	0.83	0.83	0.83
Total cholesterol	184	193	182	188	196	186
LDL	108	117	106	111	118	109
HDL	51	47	52	55	55	55
Triglycerides	129	155	122	128	133	126
Total cholesterol to HDL ratio	3.6	4.1	3.5	3.4	3.6	3.4
Triglyceride to HDL ratio	2.5	3.3	2.3	2.3	2.4	2.3

Source: Gu, D. Ref 4.24.

▶ The French Paradox

The French enjoy a reputation around the world—tinged perhaps with some envy—for having Europe's lowest rates of obesity and heart disease, despite their high intake of butter, cream, cheese, and other saturated fats (above 16% of their daily caloric intake). Their heart attack rates are one-fourth that of England, one-sixth that of the former Russian states, and one half that of the US.

The Wine Factor: The French Paradox is often attributed to their daily consumption of alcohol (20 to 30g per day), particularly wine, but the evidence of this is not strongly convincing. Wine consumption appears to explain only a small part of it. Red wine has become associated with a lowering of heart disease rates partly because it is considered to be rich in antioxidants that may play a role in inhibiting the oxidation of LDL cholesterol, which is what makes LDL cholesterol dangerous. The evidence for this anti-oxidation effect on LDL, however, is not yet that strong and is still being gathered.

Second, one of the reasons why it may be wrong to associate wine with cardiac health is that, in the US and many European countries, it is consumed primarily by people with higher incomes, and this socioeconomic bracket tends to have other good health habits—like regular exercise, low rates of smoking, and healthful diets—that may be the protective factors rather than the wine. In France, by contrast, almost everyone drinks wine daily irrespective of their socio-economic status, but little can be inferred from this.

Third, alcohol in general is believed to protect against heart disease by increasing HDL, but HDL levels among the French are no higher than among other Europeans and Americans, so this does not seem to be the factor that accounts for their low heart disease rate. Moreover, alcohol tends to increase the *non*-cardioprotective fraction of HDL (small-particle HDL). Finally, there are many countries (such as Germany) with high alcohol consumption rates but without low heart disease rates; so alcohol consumption cannot possibly be a *strong* beneficial factor, although it is beneficial in moderate amounts.

Did You Know...
The French tend to drink wine daily regardless of socioeconomic status. In the US and in other European countries, wine is consumed mainly by those with a higher socioeconomic status, many of whom have other good habits (such as exercise, low smoking rates, and health-conscious eating) that may be the factors protecting their cardiac health, rather than the wine they drink.

Explanation: So what underlies the French cardiac story? Wine consumption is only one factor. The French also have a lower prevalence of many conventional risk factors. Obesity is one example. They eat smaller portions and invest more time and energy in the quality and presentation of the food than the quantity. By comparison, American restaurant portions are 25% to 75% larger than those in French restaurants; and if you visit an American fast-food franchise you are most likely to be asked at the counter whether you want your order "super-sized." Many say "yes".

Although the average age of a first heart attack in the US is 49 for African Americans compared to 54 for Hispanics and 63 for whites, once you adjust for the risk factors levels of the three groups, African Americans have far *less heart disease than expected.* High levels of **large-particle HDL** protects them. For any given level of risk factors, African Americans have lower-than-expected heart disease, but in absolute terms they have fairly substantial rates of heart attack because their risk factor levels are often higher than other groups.

For example, blacks are often less attentive about managing hypertension, avoiding unhealthy foods, or managing body weight. This explains why they have the lowest average age of a first heart attack in the US. Given their high levels of Lp(a), their heart attack rates might have been even higher were it not for the genetic protection they get from high HDL.

Although blacks have lower-than-expected heart disease rates, however, when they do get heart disease their mortality rates—particularly out-of-hospital mortality—are high. The reasons: Lower average socioeconomic status, less timely recognition of the symptoms, poorer access to good-quality treatment, and less adequate insurance coverage.

The French are also more physically active and consume more *monounsaturated* fat than other Europeans. Among Europeans, they have the highest levels of folate and lowest levels of homocysteine, which parallel their highest-in-Europe intake of fruits and vegetables, rich sources of folate. Finally, their low levels of lipoprotein(a) may render them genetically less susceptible to heart disease.

▶ The African American Paradox

African Americans have a high prevalence of several cardiovascular disease risk factors—including hypertension, diabetes, smoking, obesity, left ventricular hypertrophy, and in some cases a fast food-oriented diet that is high in trans and saturated fats. Their low socioeconomic status also means that they have inadequate insurance coverage and less access to preventive services such as anti-hypertensive and cholesterol-lowering medications. Following a heart attack, African Americans are also likely to receive less medical care that might arrest the progress of their heart disease. One would, therefore, expect them to have high rates of heart disease, yet despite all this, they have lower-than-expected rates. In the 1960s, heart disease rates among African Americans were *four times lower* than among whites in rural southern Georgia.

A reversal: Reaching the tipping point Underscoring the idea that there is a *tipping point* in the balance of risk factors and heart disease, however, by the 1990s African Americans had almost completely lost their *protective advantage* over other groups against heart disease because of a rapid adoption of unhealthy lifestyles since the 1960s, and slower adoption of heart-healthy behaviors since the 1970s. Thus currently, death rates from heart disease are 35% *higher* among African American women than among white women—a historic reversal. For stroke, the figure is 71%.

Compared to African American women, African American men are doing a bit better and appear to have retained somewhat more of the protective advantage they once had. For example, while the incidence of heart disease is now higher in African-American women aged 25 to 54 years than in similarly aged white women, it is lower in African American men aged 25 to 74 years than in similarly aged white men. The age-adjusted incidence of heart disease is 22% lower among African American men than among whites Partly reflecting poorer treatment, however, deaths from heart disease are 15% higher in African American men than in white men. African Americans also have higher rates of cardiac arrest than whites, particularly at younger ages—for example, twice as high as whites, in the 32- to 36-year-old group.

In contrast, blacks in Africa, the Caribbean, and the UK continue to have extremely low rates of heart disease—a finding that, along with others, gives some credence to the notion that some genetically-based protections against heart disease go beyond the ethnic group level and penetrate down to the level of race. For example, in South Africa, the heart attack death rate among black men is *30 times lower* than among South African Indians, and 20 times lower than among South African whites. In the UK, the heart disease death rate among black men is approximately half that found in the general population; among black women, it is two-thirds the general population rate. All around the world, even blacks with diabetes have low rates of heart disease because their diabetes typically is not accompanied by metabolic syndrome—except for African Americans.

Atherosclerosis: Despite a higher prevalence of diabetes, African Americans have less severe and less extensive coronary atherosclerosis. In a study of patients undergoing coronary angiogram for chest pain, almost three times more African Americans (48% versus 17%) had a normal angiogram than whites. Discuss explanation over the phone blacks also have a lower prevalence of left main artery disease (6% versus 11%) and three-vessel disease (32% versus 45%) and, consequently, a lower rate of bypass surgery (*see box*). Despite these lower rates, in-hospital mortality is similar between blacks and whites after a heart attack. This may be due to higher pre-hospital mortality (sicker blacks dying before reaching the hospital).

Stroke: Given their high rates of obesity, diabetes, cigarette smoking, low socioeconomic status, but especially hypertension—including untreated hypertension—it is not a complete surprise that African Americans, particularly men, have the highest rates of stroke and stroke deaths in the US. The so-called "Stroke Belt" is a cluster of 11 southeastern states, including South and North Carolina and Georgia, that all have a high concentration of blacks. Since the 1930s, stroke mortality rates in the Stroke Belt have exceeded the national average by 10% or more. Today, their mortality rates run 33% higher.

In general, the risk of having a stroke, or dying from one, is twice as high for African Americans as for whites. Most strokes in white Americans occur in the elderly. Elderly blacks **certainly** also suffer from strokes, but the *excess* stroke mortality in blacks beyond the rate one would expect as a predictable occurrence in the elderly occurs mainly at younger ages, between 45 and 55. The risk is greater for blacks younger than 60 compared to blacks older than 60.

As with Asians, blacks have a higher burden of hemorrhagic stroke than ischemic or thrombotic stroke. Compared to whites, high blood pressure in African Americans—the chief underlying cause of stroke—is characterized by higher incidence, earlier onset, longer duration, higher prevalence, lower treatment rates, and higher rates of mortality and morbidity.

> African Americans develop high blood pressure earlier than other groups in the US, and their hypertension is more severe. It is also more prevalent, with an overall age-adjusted prevalence of 40%, and 70% among African Americans over 60. Compared to whites, hypertension in blacks is a stronger predictor of heart disease; diabetes is a weaker predictor. In whites, it is the opposite.

Explanation: What accounts for the lower rates of heart disease among African Americans? First, it appears that the *antiatherogenic lipid profile*—low LDL, low triglycerides, and high HDL—shared by blacks around the world offsets the adverse effects of African Americans' high levels of lipoprotein(a), hypertension, diabetes, smoking, and frequently unhealthy, high-fat, high-salt diet. While African Americans have a higher rate of generalized obesity, this is offset by the fact that blacks in general have a lower prevalence of *abdominal* obesity (24% in blacks versus 35% in whites). The average waist size of African American men is two inches less than that of white American men, but African American women have not kept weight off so successfully. Their average waist size is two inches greater than that of white women. In addition,

Why Do blacks Have Fewer Bypasses?

Do African Americans have fewer bypass surgeries than whites because they have less medical coverage and access to healthcare, or because they have less severe heart disease?

Studies done at Veterans Administration hospitals, where patients have equal access to healthcare, have shown that, compared to whites, African Americans have just half the prevalence of severe coronary disease such as left main artery disease, and just two-thirds the prevalence of three-vessel disease. Their lower coronary bypass surgery rates point to less severe heart disease rather than inadequate insurance coverage.

Other studies, in which cardiologists evaluated angiograms blindly (that is, without knowing the patient's ethnicity) and categorized them by severity of heart disease have produced the same results: angiograms of African Americans show less severe heart disease. This points especially to the powerful protective effect of their high levels of HDL cholesterol.

African American men have the country's lowest rates of metabolic syndrome, 16%; this low level is not shared by African American women (26%).

Excess burden does not just mean "too much," as in "excessive." It is a comparative term used in epidemiology (the study of how disease spreads in populations) that means a level *over and above* something else. It refers to the level of a disease or a risk factor over and above what is observed in other populations. The term captures the idea that there is often a certain amount of a disease or risk factor in virtually all ethnic groups, but one or more groups may have a particularly elevated level (or *excess* burden) of it—beyond the average.

For example, the hypertension rate in African Americans is 40%, compared to 25% in the white population and less in other ethnic groups. This results in an **excess burden** of hypertension among blacks that is nearly double. In short, excess burden roughly means elevated level.

These gender differences in abdominal obesity and metabolic syndrome help to explain why African-American women 25 to 54 years old now have a higher incidence of heart disease than similarly aged white women, while African American men of the same age range have a lower incidence than white men. In short, more African American women than men have reached the **tipping point** where their risk factors begin to neutralize and overwhelm the **protective advantage** that their antiatherogenic lipid profile and naturally low abdominal obesity once conferred upon them.

▶ The Hispanic American Paradox

Hispanic Americans, at 37 million the largest and fastest-growing minority group in the US, have a higher prevalence of obesity and diabetes than whites. They also have lower socioeconomic status, lower health insurance coverage, and lower utilization of preventive services than whites. Regarding their lipid profile, Hispanics have lower HDL, higher triglyceride levels, and a higher prevalence of metabolic syndrome than whites. The prevalence of hypertension in Hispanics is similar to that of whites.

The paradox: On the basis of their risk factor profile, Hispanic Americans would be expected to have a greater incidence of heart disease than whites. Yet statistics show that, compared to white Americans, they have significantly less atherosclerosis as measured by calcified plaques in their coronary arteries (*see* Chapter VII, Section 3) as well as 20%-30% fewer deaths from heart disease. Twice as many whites as Hispanics have a calcified plaque score above 400, which typically signifies severe narrowing of coronary arteries. Their lower heart disease mortality rate is all the more significant because, like African Americans and other low-income minorities, Hispanics are significantly less likely to receive treatments such as angioplasty following a heart attack.

What accounts for the lower rates of cardiovascular disease even among Hispanic diabetics? The clues have not been studied well, but one strongly compelling factor is the fact that Hispanics have lower levels of Lp(a) than whites.

▶ The Native American Paradox

Native Americans have low rates of heart disease despite a high prevalence of several risk factors. Fundamental changes in lifestyle in the past 100 years—especially the adoption of a higher-fat, lower-fiber diet and a less active lifestyle—have resulted in a much higher increased prevalence of diabetes and obesity and an excess of other risk factors. Indeed, Native Americans today (population: approximately 2 million) have the world's highest rates of diabetes and obesity, with diabetes rates (mainly type 2 adult-onset diabetes) running three to five times higher than in the general US population. The overall prevalence is more than 30%, much of it undiagnosed. This tragedy is particularly poignant because the great Native American horse cultures of the past were among the most active people's in the world. The rates vary from tribe to tribe, with Pima Indians in Arizona having the highest prevalence of both obesity and diabetes. About 50% of Pima Indians aged 30 to 64 are diabetic. Diabetes was virtually non-existent among them during the early part of the 20th century.

Paradoxically, Native Americans today have the highest rates of diabetes and obesity in the world, yet low rates of heart disease.

According to the NIH and CDC, American Indians and Alaska Natives are two times as likely to develop diabetes as similarly aged non-Hispanic whites, and four times more likely to die than non-Hispanic white if they do develop diabetes (often from heart disease or other diabetes-related complications). Many of them feel discouraged by the high rates of diabetes among them, and by the inaccurate perception that developing diabetes is an almost inevitable fate.

As you might already have surmised, obesity is a powerful predictor of diabetes among Native Americans, as is true of all other populations. The prevalence of diabetes among Native Americans rises from 20% in those with a body mass index (BMI) below 20 to 60% in those with a BMI above 40. Despite their high rates of diabetes and obesity, hypertension is no more prevalent in Native Americans than in whites. Obesity, for some reason, does not affect their blood pressure as much.

Ethnicity is an even stronger predictor of diabetes than obesity among Native Americans, although it should be noted that ethnicity can mark both genetic and lifestyle factors (*see box on right*). Most Native Americans are not full-blooded and are partly Hispanic, black, or white. The prevalence of diabetes is low (below 10%) in those with less than 25% Native American ancestry even if they are obese, and increases with the degree of Native American ancestry. For example, for any given degree of obesity diabetes is four times higher in full-blooded Native American than those who are less than a quarter ancestry.

The Paradox: Despite their high risk factor levels, heart disease rates among Native Americans remain low. The most recent data show a 38% lower heart disease and 36% lower stroke mortality in Native Americans than whites, although recent incidence data show that mortality rates are on the rise.

Explanation: The Native American Paradox can be best explained by their low levels of LDL, non-HDL cholesterol, and Lp(a). Their LDL levels are 20 to 30 points lower than in whites. Only 3% of Native American men and 6% of women have LDL above 160 versus 20% of the general US population. However, Native American are more likely to develop heart disease at much lower non-HDL cholesterol levels (below 80). Bad cholesterol, in other words, seems to affect them more than it affects others, but the good thing is that they generally have low levels of bad cholesterol. Most importantly, they have the lowest levels of Lp(a); fewer than 1% of Native Americans have high Lp(a).

▶ The Filipino Paradox

Filipinos have higher rates of obesity, diabetes, metabolic syndrome, and hypertension than whites, yet lower heart disease rates. The reasons for this phenomenon have not been studied extensively.

▶ Other Paradoxes

Almost everyone "knows," or believes, that fat is bad. Yet people in many Mediterranean countries such as Spain, Greece, and Israel have some of the highest intake of fat—as high as 45% of daily calories—but low rates of heart disease. Their secret? Unlike Indians, who typically consume a lot of trans fats and saturated fats (both highly dangerous to cardiac health),

Genes or Lifestyle?
Obesity is strongly linked to diabetes. Among Native Americans, however, ethnicity is an even stronger predictor of diabetes than obesity. **Normal weight** people who have more than 50% Native American ancestry have twice the diabetes rate as **obese** individuals with less than 50% Native American ancestry.

This does not point entirely to a **genetic** basis for their diabetes, since people who have more than 50% Native American blood are also more likely to have a culture and lifestyle more typical of Native Americans than others with less Native American ancestry. It is believed that Native American diabetes is both genetic and related to unhealthy diet, obesity, and physical inactivity.

There are, nevertheless, several genetic pointers: *One* is the fact that Pima Indians have low rates of metabolism, which predisposes them to obesity. *Second*, excess fat tends to be centrally located, meaning they have high rates of abdominal obesity. *Third*, among tribes such as the Pima Indians, diabetes rates are highest in children whose parents became diabetic at an early age.

It is interesting to note that Pima Indians are also the fullest-blood Native Americans in the United States.

much of the fat Mediterranean people consume is olive oil, which is rich in heart-healthy monounsaturated fat and antioxidants. The Mediterranean diet also emphasizes foods of plant origin, which means they consume low amounts of saturated fat and high levels of foods rich in vitamins and other micronutrients.

Likewise, despite a high fat intake, in part because of the cold weather, and long winter months that force them into physical inactivity, many Scandinavian countries have relatively low heart disease rates, and their life expectancy rates are among the highest in the world, just below Japan's. **Some** reasons: First, their diet emphasizes fish, particularly cod and herring, both of which are high in omega-3 fats. Very cold weather also means that they do not have to use herbicides and insecticides on virtually any produce, and they believe that this contributes to their health. Third, high socioeconomic levels mean that Scandinavians are generally aware of the need to make lifestyle modifications such as getting exercise and managing weight. Along with Japan and South Korea, the Scandinavian countries (Norway, Denmark, Sweden, and Finland) together with Holland and Switzerland, have the lowest rates of obesity in the world.

Some Final Reflections

These paradoxes, considered together, underscore the role that emerging risk factors—such as Lp(a) and homocysteine—play in producing wide variations in the incidence, prevalence, and mortality rates for heart disease in different ethnic groups. In each case, however, it is also clear that the low heart disease rates of that group are not a random accident. When we look closely, we find that they

Better Drugs, Better Prevention: The Promise of Personalized Medicine
The Science Behind It

Your cells each have a nucleus, or core. Inside the nucleus are 46 chromosomes that look like strands of hair. Inside each chromosome are thousands of genes. Inside each gene are DNA molecules made up of thousands of "letters" called base pairs. These groups of letters—you have probably seen them; they are always A, T, G and C—essentially constitute "words" that, like the software that runs your computer, carry all the instructions that tell your body how to run itself: whether you should become a boy or a girl, white, black or Indian, when a particular protein should be made, whether your body should identify a foreign substance as a disease and attack it or leave it alone.

All those letters in all those DNA strands in all of those genes in all those chromosomes, together, make up your genome. Your entire genome is about three billion letters long. It is the software application suite that makes you who you are, and determines which diseases you will be susceptible to or protected from. It carries the instructions that determine how your body will respond biologically to the outside world.

That genome has now been cracked—meaning that scientists have succeeded in "reading" the entire three-billion-long sequence of letters that make up the DNA code of someone's genome, and put it on a computer. As Dr. Francis Collins, director of the National Human Genome Research Institute, wrote in *The Boston Globe*

("Personalized Medicine and Designer Drugs," July 17, 2005): By 2020, it is projected that people will be able to have their genomes read (meaning sequenced) for about $1,000 or less. That information could then become part of their file at their doctor's office.

Other than sounding like interesting science fiction, why does this matter to you? Here is the thing: Currently, we know that genes make some people more susceptible than others to disorders such as heart disease and diabetes. We know that, like cancer and sickle cell, heart disease is partly inheritable and that it runs in families and ethnic groups. We also know that genes determine why people respond differently to the same medication: For some people, it works like a charm. Others get side effects and can even die from it.

What we did not know, genetically, is why. The human genome project is changing that. Instead of just being able to say that ethnic groups and families vary in their susceptibility to disease, doctors will be able to use your genome information to tell if you are susceptible to heart disease, what kind of risk factors are most dangerous to you, and what medications will work best for you. In short, the day of personalized medicine is within sight.

The Implications

Personalized medicine carries many implications for healthcare delivery, but three aspects in particular are worth summarizing: Prevention, medications, and dosage.

I. Preventive strategies: Currently, physicians do not understand genes well enough to create risk-reduction strategies tailored to patients based on their susceptibilities. Genome information will almost certainly change that. By 2010, it is likely that genetic tests will become available for many common disorders, allowing patients to work with their doctors to develop a lifelong plan of prevention personalized and fine-tuned for their particular genetic makeup. Doctors will be able to tell what disorders patients are at highest risk of developing, and what lifestyle choices will magnify or minimize that risk. We already know that if you are African American, for example, you are more likely to develop high blood pressure than if you were, let's say, white. With your genome sequenced, your doctor will be able to offer not just a general speculation based on ethnicity, but a specific prediction based on your genes.

Gene analysis may help us better understand why some people have a strongly antiatherogenic lipid profile—low triglycerides, high levels of large-particle HDL, low levels of small, dense LDL—while others have the opposite. It may also help us better understand what exactly emerging risk factors such as Lp(a), C-reactive protein, and homocysteine do that predisposes some to coronary artery disease. Indeed, with a better understanding of the genetic basis of cardiovascular disease, there will be no such thing as "emerging" risk factors, only standard ones.

II. Medications: Today, doctors typically give patients a different drug to see if that one will work better if the first one did not work well. In an era of personalized medicine, much of this trial-and-error will be eliminated as custom-tailored "designer drugs" are developed for cardiovascular diseases and diabetes. Just as we now know that cholesterol comes not in one but in several forms, as HDL, LDL or VLDL, each with many subclasses within it, so scientists may also discover in the next decade or so that there are eight or ten different sub-classes of hypertension—some that are particularly sensitive to salt intake, or to stress, or to weight gain, or to inactivity. These sub-classes will lead to newer, more targeted medications.

Like your DNA fingerprint, every individual's genome is unique, but the genomes of the world's six billion people do fall into some broad types. There are not six billion types of genome. The Human Genome Research Institute has recently created a map of the common patterns of human genetic variation—called the HapMap—the first phase of which was completed in February 2005. The HapMap is likely to become the genetic basis for doctors to predict what particular kind of hypertension or diabetes you are at risk of developing, or whether you are genetically more likely to develop hard stable plaques or soft vulnerable plaques. The HapMap will also become the basis for pharmaceutical companies to develop medications that, like birth control pills, are targeted to specific kinds of patients—but this time, patients with a particular type of genome, or "haplotype" (similar to phenotype).

According to a 2005 study published in *The New England Journal of Medicine*, scientists have recently identified a gene that helps to determine whether it is safe or dangerous for you to take Warfarin, a blood thinner often prescribed for heart patients and people with blood-clotting abnormalities. Their work is likely to become the basis for developing a genetic test that could help physicians adjust the dose of warfarin, and help companies create more targeted types of blood thinner based on common patterns of genetic variation.

III. Drug dosage: People's bodies process and eliminate drugs at very different rates, some more quickly or slowly than others (see Chapter VIII, Section 1). Tiny variations in the letter sequences in their genes appear to be responsible for this. With your genome on file, your doctor could tell if you have the kind of gene that makes you process, for example, cholesterol-lowering statins or codeine quickly or slowly, then use this to adjust the dose. Japanese and Indians, for instance, tend to metabolize statins such as Zocor and Crestor more slowly than others, and therefore need less because the statin stays in their blood longer. On the other hand, about 7-10% of whites have a variation of a gene—the CYP2D6 gene, a type of P450 gene, for those who want to know—that cannot process certain medications very effectively, including some heart disease drugs and some antidepressants. Gene analysis could put this information at doctors' fingertips, helping them to select not only the right medicines but the right doses. In fact, the US Food & Drug Administration recently approved a genetic test to help doctors prescribe medications and doses. Called the AmpliChip, the test analyzes two genes that carry the instructions for making the enzymes that the liver uses in processing about a quarter of all current prescription drugs.

Clearly, every new technology carries a potential for abuse, and the medical, scientific, insurance, and legislative communities will have to work together to reduce that likelihood. If, however, humanity proves itself capable of handling genetic information responsibly and ethically, the age of personalized medicine promises far more in terms of quality of life than any of its potential costs.

either are doing something right, or have protective genes, or both. Several compelling examples emerge: A strongly antiatherogenic overall lipid profile, consumption of cardioprotective monounsaturated fats, high fish consumption, daily physical activity, low obesity, a body type that produces low abdominal obesity, moderate red wine consumption, high HDL levels or large HDL particles, naturally low levels of Lp(a), and so on.

Taken together, these factors explain a great deal of the paradoxes we have considered. Global data nevertheless indicate that, as members of different ethnic groups increasingly migrate to other cultures, or change their diet and physical activity patterns in response to rapid urbanization, many of them are losing the essential balance of factors that had once protected them from high rates of heart disease. They are, in other words, reaching the tipping point.

> As members of different ethnic groups migrate to other cultures, or change their diet and activity patterns in response to urbanization, many are losing the essential balance of factors that once protected them from heart disease. They are, in other words, reaching the tipping point.

Among the paradoxes (*see Table 4.6 again*), the Indian Paradox is the only one that actually presents worse than expected heart disease rates—signifying a population that has already reached its cri-tical tipping point, and in some ways is already well past it. Nevertheless, the counter-story presented here is that concerted, focused lifestyle modifications can and will reverse this dire trend. The message is one of hope, because the human body is in fact a finely-tuned machine that responds magnificently to the right inputs—*if* you make them. Section 1 of this Chapter discussed the Indian Paradox in greater detail. The next section, Section 3, will address gender differences in heart disease, and what women in particular need to know about this killer dissease.

KEY · POINTS · IN · A · NUTSHELL

♥ Ethnicity is a better indicator than race of the cardiovascular diseases to which a population is vulnerable because ethnicity better captures how environment and lifestyle change the way a group's genes respond to disease.

♥ The same cardiovascular risk factors often have a different impact on heart disease than on stroke depending on the ethnicity.

♥ Europeans are three to four times more likely to die from heart disease than Asians, while Asians are three to four times more likely to die from stroke than Americans and Europeans.

♥ After Asians emigrate to the US, their stroke rates fall but their heart disease rates rise, attesting to the influence of their new cultural environment.

♥ The interaction of ethnicity and heart disease points to numerous paradoxes, and to a complex interplay of lifestyle choices and protective or harmful genetic factors.

♥ Blacks, for example, have high rates of hypertension, kidney disease, obesity, and stroke yet lower-than-expected rates of heart disease, partly because of the protective effect of high HDL.

♥ Similarly, despite the world's highest rate of diabetes, obesity and kidney disease, Native Americans have low rates of heart disease, partly because of their low levels of LDL and Lp(a).

♥ Being full-blooded Native American, however, puts you at a much higher risk for developing diabetes even if you are normal weight than being obese but having less than 50% Native American ancestry. This indicates how strongly ethnicity can correlate with cardiac risk factors.

♥ Hispanics, on the other hand, have high rates of obesity and diabetes, yet, low rates of hypertension, stroke, and heart disease.

♥ Japanese and Chinese Americans have lower rates of heart disease than European Americans but higher than Japanese/Chinese living in Japan and China.

♥ Because of the paradoxical interplay of genetics, ethnicity, and lifestyle, heart disease rates vary more than 10-fold among people of different ethnic origins.

♥ In all, the evidence indicates that the protective effect that genes confer on some ethnic groups appears to be both strong and yet fragile.

♥ There appear to be tipping points beyond which the addition of just one more elevated risk factor begins to break down the protective shield and neutralize the advantage that an ethnic group enjoyed until then. Cardiovascular disease may then begin to accelerate rapidly.

♥ This has occurred, for example, among African Americans since the 1960s, particularly women, among Native Americans over the past decade, and among Japanese and Chinese immigrants to the US.

♥ While many ethnic groups have largely protective risk factor profiles, Asian Indians possess the opposite: a combination of lifestyle factors and genetic inheritance that is highly atherogenic.

♥ Overall, the paradoxes explored in this section point to the key role that emerging risk factors play in generating wide ethnic differences in coronary heart disease rates around the world.

♥ Finally, several risk emerging factors appear to interact synergistically with standard risk factors, working in concert to dramatically raise a person's overall cardiovascular risk, if he or she has several risk factors and few protective factors.

4.3 ▶ Women and Heart Disease

WOMEN STILL FEAR BREAST CANCER as their greatest health risk and are much less likely to worry about heart disease. Yet a woman's lifetime risk of dying from heart disease is more than *eight times higher* than from breast cancer. In 2002 as many as 42,000 American women died from breast cancer, compared to 356,000 from heart disease. This is over 80,000 more deaths than the total combined number of women who died from breast cancer, lung cancer, stroke, and pulmonary disease in 2002. Researchers estimate that only about 10 percent of Americans are at low risk for heart disease.

Heart disease is an "equal opportunity" disease that rarely discriminates between the sexes. Although health-threatening heart disease develops 10 to 15 years later in women than in men, and women overall have fewer heart attacks than men, they are more likely to die when they do have one. In addition, their risk rises steeply after menopause. In fact, since 1984 more American women than men have died from heart disease (*see* Figure 4.6). Similarly, the excess of heart disease appears to be greater in Indian women than in Indian men.

Despite these numbers, many people, both male and female, including physicians, seem unaware of the grave threat heart disease poses to women. Because high rates among women are a relatively recent discovery, women are less likely than men to obtain preventive recommendations from doctors, who tend to perceive their heart disease risk as lower. Following menopause, women's LDL and triglycerides levels increase and their HDL

The Knowledge Gap
Heart disease is now the leading killer of women in most countries. Polls show that, as recently as 2004, fewer than **one in five** physicians, and just 8% of primary care doctors, were aware that more women than men die each year of heart disease. In fact, the lifetime—risk of a woman dying from heart disease is *eight times higher* than from breast cancer.

levels decrease significantly, heightening their risk. Add to that, the fact that most women having a heart attack do not experience the "typical" symptoms of chest pain. In all, this is not the time for complacency.

Gender versus sex: different, but both matter

The terms sex and gender are often used interchangeably, but they are not quite the same. Men and women differ not only physically and reproductively but also in the way they think, feel, and act. The biological differences are called **sex**, and are determined by genes and chromosomes. The psychological and behavioral differences constitute **gender**. Cultural and social factors, pressures, and expectations play a prominent part in determining our gender roles and what their boundaries are. These roles, like one's sex, often influence cardiovascular health.

*Your **sex**, male or female, was assigned to you by biology. Your **gender**—your masculinity or femininity—is determined by the roles and expectations that your culture defines for your sex. Both affect your cardiovascular health*

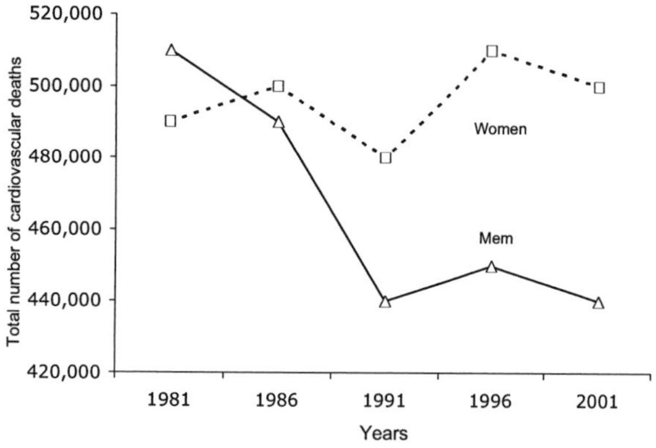

Figure 4.6. Cardiovascular mortality trends for males and females 1981=1991. Source: Center for Disease Control and National Center for Health Statistics

For example, while the female hormone estrogen—a *biologically*-based difference—has a cardioprotective benefit on a woman's health, some *gender expectations*—such as the expectation in some cultures that women should not been seen jogging and exercising outside—can be a hindrance to their cardiovascular health. On the other hand, other expectations such as that women should not smoke can be helpful. In short, both our biological sex and our sociocultural gender role influence our cardiovascular health. In some cases, it is not clear whether differences in male and female heart disease characteristics are caused more by genes and hormones, or more by gender differences, or both.

Some differences, however, are fairly clear. For example, a recent British study found that, between ages 18 and 70, men lose up to a quarter of their heart's pumping power but women seem to lose less. This may help explain why women on average outlive men by up to five years. It is projected that, in many developed countries, women's life expectancy will rise to 90 years by 2025. This, however, would give many women an even longer time to develop heart disease at an advanced age.

Women are often perceived as lower risk

Women's physicians, as well as women themselves, tend to underestimate the risk of heart disease in women. In a 2004 national online survey of 100 cardiologists, 100 obstetricians-gynecologists, and 300 primary care physicians, researchers gave each doctor profiles of patients who have the same heart disease risk level, and asked the doctors to make recommendations. The study found that the doctors were much more likely to classify a female patient as lower risk once they knew she was female, even though she had the same risk level profile as male patients on the list. However, once a physician placed a particular woman patient in her appropriate risk category, she was then likely to be recommended for the same treatment as a man. The bias, in other words, was not against giving women care; it was against recognizing that they need care in the first place.

In a national study, doctors reviewing patient profiles were more likely to classify a woman's heart disease risk as lower than that of a man with the same risk level. This reflects a widespread societal bias against recognizing that women are as much at risk for heart disease and heart attack as men.

Gynecologists Many women regard their gynecologists more or less as their primary care doctor. Yet in the study, gynecologists were especially likely not to score themselves well on providing adequate care that would prevent cardiovascular disease and help women manage their risk factors. Gynecologists were often much less aware of national guidelines for cholesterol and blood pressure levels than primary care physicians. Yet gynecologists also reported that they provided primary care to two-thirds of their patients, indicating their important role in the battle against heart disease.

The Centers for Disease Control reports that the average life expectancy for Americans reached 77.6 years in 2005. Women are now expected to live on average 80.1 years, compared to 74.8 for men.

Heart attack characteristics: Differences between men and women

On average, women get a heart attack 10 to 15 years later than men, but women are more likely to die when do have one. A high proportion of heart attack deaths among women—more than half—occur outside a hospital, possibly because women have less familiar heart attack symptoms or are more often misdiagnosed, and thus are not hospitalized in time. A 2005 study found that women under 55 who came to the emergency room with chest pain that suggested a heart attack were seven times more likely than men to be sent home from the Emerganci room (RM) without proper treatment. The study also found that non-hospitalized patients who have heart attacks were twice as likely to die as those who were hospitalized. In addition, women do not do as well as men after a heart attack. Of the women who survived a heart attack, 42% died within a year compared with 24% of the men. Women were almost twice as likely to suffer a second heart attack after the first one. Additionally, more women than men tend to become partially disabled after a heart attack. Compared to men of the same age, women also have double the mortality following bypass surgery.

The Red Dress Symbol Around 1997, a shift in awareness of heart disease as the leading killer of women began to emerge. In 2003, 46% of women, themselves, identified heart disease as the leading cause of death in women, up from only 20% in 1997. You may have seen the "Red Dress" symbol used by the US National Heart, Lung, and Blood Institute (NHLBI) as part of **The Heart Truth**, a national campaign to raise awareness about the facts of heart disease in women.

Thus, besides having heart attacks later in life than men, women's heart attack data are not very favorable to them on most other dimensions—including timely symptom recognition, likelihood of receiving the appropriate level of care, mortality rates, post-attack morbidity, likelihood of a second attack, and medical community perceptions and attitudes. Women, therefore, often miss out on lifesaving diagnoses and treatments for heart disease, even though it kills them more often than any other illness, and kills more of them than men.

The onset of heart disease in women is 10 to 15 years later than in men and usually 10 years after menopause. This advantage is lost if they have had premature menopause or diabetes, or if they smoke.

The data also appear suggestive that somewhat more women than men are prone to developing soft, fragile, lipid-rich, vulnerable plaques that are more likely to rupture or erode and cause a heart attack, while men are more prone to developing large, hard, stable, fibrous plaques that do not rupture but can narrow a coronary artery and cause chest pain. For example, studies show that women who suffer an acute heart attack are more likely than men to have coronary arteries that look "normal" on an angiogram—meaning arteries with either no visible plaque, plaque with less than 50% narrowing of the artery, or non-obstructive disease. A 2005 study found such "normal" coronary arteries in 10-25% of women who had had an acute heart attack, compared to only 6-10% of men.

Heart attack data are not very favorable toward women regarding mortality rates, post-attack morbidity, likelihood of a second attack, and physician attitudes. Women's symptoms are also less often recognized, and they are less likely to receive timely care. Women tend to have a better risk factor profile than men at younger ages, but worse at older ages.

Chest pain and other predictors of coronary events in women

Chest pain (angina) is a poorer predictor of heart attack in women than men. More women than men get cardiac-related chest pain that does not lead to a heart attack, partly because estrogen protects them from heart attacks. Women are more likely than men to come to the hospital complaining of chest pain that turns out to be their first symptom of heart disease.

Men, by contrast, are much more likely to come to the hospital with an actual heart attack, perhaps because men are more likely to brush off chest pain in an act of *machismo*. Smoking and diabetes are stronger predictors of heart attack in women than in men.

Chest pain, however, seems to be a poorer predictor of heart attack in women than in men. In the Framingham Heart Study, only 17% of women with typical angina went on to develop a heart attack, compared with 44% of men. In the Coronary Artery Surgery Study (CASS), only 50% of women with typical angina had significant coronary blockage, compared with 83% of men. Whether this discrepancy is due to over-reporting of chest pain by women or under-reporting by men is unclear. There are currently no studies that specifically address these issues for Indian women.

Heart attack symptoms and sudden death: How women differ

Because women's heart attack symptoms are substantially different from men's, this tends to lead to delayed diagnosis and treatment. As stated earlier, women suffering a heart attack often reach the hospital significantly later than men because women tend **not experience** the so-called "classic" symptoms of chest pain that radiates into the shoulders, neck, or arms. Some experience mid-back pain as their only symptom. They also sweat less while having a heart attack. Other women report extreme fatigue about a month before the attack, but no chest pain (*see* Table 4.8). Delayed arrival at the hospital often undermines the benefit of clot-busting therapy that might help **abort a heart attack** and minimize its damage. Caregivers need to become more familiar with female heart attack symptoms to save the lives of women victims.

Sudden death: More than half of sudden deaths in both women and men occur within six hours of the onset of symptoms. (Sudden death means death within 24 hours of the symptoms or the underlying causal coronary event.) Early diagnosis of heart disease is particularly important in women because two-thirds of women, who die suddenly, had no previous symptoms of heart disease, compared to about half of men.

The risk factors and mechanisms of sudden coronary death differ for younger and older women. Younger women who die of heart disease are often smokers with minimal coronary narrowing. Older women who suddenly die of heart disease often have dyslipidemia, with severe coronary narrowing and plaque ruptures. In contrast, **young Indian women** who die suddenly of heart disease tend to be nonsmokers with advanced and extensive atherosclerosis resembling the disease found in older non-Indian women.

Menopause and heart attack

Because of estrogen's cardioprotective effect, women typically do not start developing life-threatening heart disease until about 10 years after

Table 4.8. Most Commonly Reported Symptoms of Heart Attack in Women

Before the heart attack
- Unusual fatigue - 71%
- Sleep disturbance - 48%
- Shortness of breath - 42%
- Indigestion - 39%
- Anxiety - 35%

During the heart attack
- Shortness of breath - 58%
- Weakness - 55%
- Unusual fatigue - 43%
- Cold sweat - 39%
- Dizziness - 39%

Other symptoms
- Nausea and vomiting
- Jaw pain
- Fainting spells
- Abdominal pain
- Heart palpitation
- Loss of appetite

Women's symptoms are more diverse and less predictable than the so-called "classic" symptoms typically found in men—cevere acute chest pressure or pain that may radiate to shoulders, neck, arms or jaw, and making the person clutch his chest. In a recent NIH study of 515 women, 43% reported having no chest pain during the attack, and fewer than 30% reported having chest pain before. Almost all the women (95%), however, reported having early warning signs in the form of new or unusual physical symptoms a month or longer before the heart attack. Note, however, that many women do get chest pain, and both men and women can experience atypical symptoms.

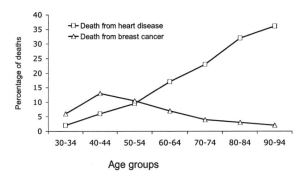

Figure 4.7. Percentage of deaths due to breast cancer and heart disease in the U.S by age groups in 2002.
Source: National Center for Health Statistics

menopause—10 to 15 years later than men. This advantage is lost if they are diabetic or smoke and, of course, premature menopause shortens the timeline. For example, 2-3 times as many post-menopausal women have heart disease as pre-menopausal women of the same age. Between ages 45 and 80, women's death rate from heart disease rises 40-fold. At 80, the rates become identical in men and women. The substantial and steady rise in deaths from heart disease with advancing age contrasts sharply to breast cancer deaths, which peak between ages 40 to 50 years and declines steadily thereafter. (*See* **Figure 4.7**). Although the incidence of heart attack in women younger than 50 is about 10 times lower than in men of the same age, women under 50 face a substantially higher risk of complications following a heart attack than older women. For this reason, they need to be evaluated for emerging risk factors such as lipoprotein(a) and homocysteine levels. After menopause, the increase in heart disease risk is related more to a higher incidence of *standard* risk factors such as hypertension, diabetes, obesity and dyslipidemia.

Menopause and dyslipidemia

Although most women have an exceptionally good lipid profile until age 40, menopause is associated with a marked deterioration in their lipid profile. Unlike in men, whose LDL levels plateau around age 50, women's LDL levels continue rising steadily—on average about 2 mg/dL every year from age 40 to 60. A woman's LDL level may, therefore, rise a total of about 40 points over that 20-year period. A woman's total cholesterol is about 10 points lower than a man's before age 45, but 20 points higher than a man's after 65.

Besides higher LDL, menopause is also associated with a 40-point increase in triglycerides and a 10-point decrease in HDL, possibly related to weight gain that results in an increase in abdominal fat. Having HDL below 40 increases a woman's cardiac risk five times, compared to have HDL above

> **Did you know...**
> Women typically have an excellent lipid profile before menopause. From ages 40 to 60, however, most women begin to develop dyslipidemia. Their LDL and triglycerides both rise by about 40 points, and their HDL (good cholesterol) falls by about 10 points, sharply raising their cardiac risk. High triglycerides are more harmful to women than men, and more harmful to Asians than non-Asians—thus putting Indian women at particularly high risk.

80. Rising triglycerides and falling HDL further stimulate a woman's body to produce larger numbers of the most dangerous type of LDL—small-particle, dense LDL. All of these lipid-level changes together contribute to the higher incidence of heart disease in postmenopausal women.

High triglycerides levels more strongly predict heart disease in women than men. In general, a 90-point increase in triglyceride level raises cardiac risk by 75% in women, versus 30% in men. Among Asians, the risk is double for both men and women with high triglycerides compare to those with low triglycerides. In a 20-year follow-up study of Swedish women, a high triglyceride level was also significantly associated with death from cardiac and other causes.

In its recent guidelines, the American Heart Association (AHA) has changed the cut-point for what constitutes low

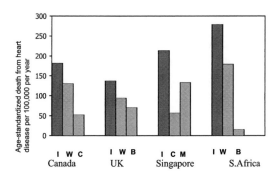

Figure 4.8. Age-standardized death rates from heart disease among Indian women per 100,000 per year compared to other ethnic groups in Canada, UK, Singapore and South Africa. Note that in each of these four countries, Indians have the highest mortality rates. (I= Indians, B=blacks, W=whites, C=Chinese, M= Malays) Source: Enas, EA. Ref. 4.21.

HDL in women from "less than 40" to "**less than 50**." Women, in other words, should aim at making lifestyle changes that bring their HDL level above 50. In the CADI Study of Indians living in the US (*see* Chapter I, Section 2), 70% of Indian women had HDL below 50. Indian women in general have an HDL level about 10 points lower than whites (45 versus 55) and 20 points lower than blacks, Chinese, and Japanese women (65 mg/dL). This low level of HDL in Indian women parallels their high rates of heart disease.

> A high **SMR** tells us that proportionately more Indian women die from heart disease than non-Indian women who die from it. A high **PMR** tells us that proportionately more Indian women die from heart disease than the number who die from other things

Heart disease among Indian women in and outside India

The elevated rate of deaths from heart disease among Indians compared to other groups is as great in Indian women as in the men, and possibly worse. Consider Figure 4.8. In all the four featured countries, Indian women have substantially higher death rates from heart disease than any other group, particularly when the rates are age-adjusted. This is especially significant because smoking—which is strongly linked to heart disease—is rare among Indian women and common among Indian men, both in India and abroad. This suggests that other perhaps non-standard risk factors are putting Indian women at high risk. Before looking at particular groups of Indians abroad and at home, however, let's look at two measurements or concepts that give us an overall picture of the seriousness of heart disease among Indian women: the *Standardized Mortality Ratio*, and the *Proportional Mortality Ratio*.

► Standardized Mortality Ratio (SMR)

A **mortality ratio**, as the name suggests, compares two mortality rates. It compares the death rate in a given population to the death rate in the general population. This gives us an idea how well the population under study is doing compared to everyone else. A concrete example always helps: Let's take heart disease among Indians in the UK in 1997. Mathematically, the **mortality ratio** for Indians in the UK for heart disease that year is the number of Indians who died from heart disease out of every 100,000, divided by the total number of people who died from heart disease out of every 100,000 people living in the UK. The ratio is then multiplied by 100 simply to turn it into a percentage instead of a fraction.

Mortality ratio for Indians = (death rate among Indians) / (death rate in general population) x 100

A mortality ratio of 150, for example, means that 50% more people died per 100,000 from a particular disease in the population being studied than the number who died per 100,000 in the general population.

A *standardized* **mortality ratio**, or SMR, similarly compares two death rates, but adds an adjustment: It compares *age-standardized* (*age-adjusted*) death rates. Why is this significant? Because age-standardizing the death rates makes comparisons between different populations more realistic by minimizing the effect of any possible differences *in the age composition* of different populations. For example, a population that has a long life expectancy—such as Japanese or whites—is likely to have a higher incidence of heart disease and thus higher death rate from it simply because it has so many more older people in it. By contrast, a population with a very high birth rate and, therefore, many youngsters and teenagers will have an "artificially" low death rate from heart disease or cancer or stroke, because relatively few young people die from these.

> *An age-adjusted rate tells you how many people in a particular population would have died had they had the exact same age composition (neither younger nor older) as the general population.*

> The technicalities of calculating SMR and PMR should not obscure the larger point that emerges from all these data: Regardless of which country you study, which age range you choose, or which other ethnic groups to whom you compare them, Indians, both men and women, have strikingly high mortality rates from cardiovascular disease.

Age standardization adjusts the death rates so that the differences are not simply due to a population having many more older or younger people in it. To put it another way: An age-adjusted rate tells you how many people in a particular population *would* have died *had they had* the exact same age composition as the general population—called the "standard" population in research because it usu-ally serves as the reference group. Figure 4.8, for example, tells us that, during the years studied, the age-adjusted death rate among Indian women in the UK was 151 per 100,000. That means 151 Indian women could have been expected to die from heart disease out of every 100,000, if Indian women in the UK had the same age distribution as the general population. Indian women in the UK also had an age-adjusted mortality rate from stroke of 141 per 100,000 standard popu-lation. Again, this means that their death rate can be expected to have been 41% higher than that of the general population had the two populations had the same age composition.

> Like age-adjusted death rates, you can also have *gender-adjusted* death rates. Not surpris-ingly, they are adjusted for possible variations in disease incidence or mortality rates that are introduced by differ-ences in the gender dis-tribution of the popula-tions being studied.

Standardized mortality ratio = (*age-adjusted* death rate among Indians) / (*age-adjusted* death rate in the general population) x 100

It should be clear, however, that the age-adjusted death rate for the general population is just the death rate in the general population! Why? Because the age distribution in the general population itself is what is being used as the standard. *Other* population's age compositions are standardized against *it*. This is the same as saying that the general population is always assigned an SMR of 100, (because age-adjusted death rate of the general population, divided by age-adjusted death rate of the general population, times 100, is a 100). In short, because it is age-standardized, an SMR gives us a better idea of how well the popu-lation under study is doing compared to everyone else than just a straightforward mortality ratio.

Table 4.9. It tells us that, between 1990 and 2000, Indian women living in California had an SMR for heart disease of 164. If this were a straightforward mortality ratio, it would mean that 64% more Indian women died per 100,000 than the number of women who died

Table 4.9. Standardized Mortality Ratio and Proportional Mortality Ratio for Heart Disease among Women in California, 1990-2000

	Percentage change in death rates, 1990 to 2000	Standardized mor-tality ratio (SMR)	Proportional mortali-ty ratio (PMR)
Total	-14%	100	100
White	-10%	98	109
Black	-11%	103	99
Hispanic	-9%	106	94
Japanese	-18%	78	80
Chinese	-10%	84	81
Indian	+5%	164	144

Source: Palaniappan et al. L Ref. 4.42
Note that Indian women have a substantially higher SMR and PMR than other eth-nic groups, and they are the only group whose death rates from heart disease rose during the 1990s.

per 100,000 in the general population. In contrast, a *standardized* mortality ratio of 164 tells us that, *if the Indian population had had* the same age composition as the general population, then compared to the rate for all women in the general population, 64% more Indian women would have died from heart disease out of every 100,000 of them.

> From 1990 to 2000, the death rate from heart disease among Indian women in California rose by 5% compared a 10-15% decrease among all other women.

▶ Proportional mortality ratio (PMR)

Like the SMR, the Proportional Mortality Ratio for a particular disease tells us the proportion of deaths from that disease in a given population, compared to deaths from all causes (*see* Table 4.9, as well as Appendix A for more on this). In effect, it tells us how dangerous that disease is in that population, as compared to all the other things that kill them. Thus, for heart disease, for example, a PMR gives us a sense of how large a contribution heart disease is making to the overall death rate, and, therefore, how much people in a given ethnic group should worry about heart disease. It tells us how high heart disease ranks among fatal diseases and other causes of death.

Data such as those in Table 4.9 tell us that, compared to other groups, Indian women in California—and by extension, elsewhere—have a substantially higher Proportional Mortality Ratio, as well as a substantially higher Standardized Mortality Ratio, for heart disease. High SMR tells us that proportionally more Indian women die from heart disease compared to non-Indian women who die from it. High PMR tells us that proportionally more Indian women die from heart disease compared to the number who die from other things. Together, these data indicate that Indian women have a higher burden of heart disease than other populations, and that heart disease has become a particularly serious cause of death among Indian women, compared to other causes. This excess burden of heart disease appears to be caused by elevated levels of abdominal obesity, metabolic syndrome and diabetes, and high levels of lipoprotein(a) and homocysteine.

■ **India:** Currently, about 10% of Indian women in India have heart disease—a rate identical to that of Indian men. Multivessel disease—involving two or three coronary arteries—is common among Indian women: it is found in more than 50% of clinical cases. Heart disease in young premenopausal Indian women is also common, despite their low smoking rates.

■ **United States:** In the 1980s, Indian women in California had the highest death rate from heart disease among women in that state—30% higher than whites and 325% higher than Chinese Americans. A more recent study showed that the death rate from heart disease among Indian women actually increased by 5% between 1990 and 2000, while decreasing 10-15% for women from all other ethnic groups in California (*see* Table 4.9).

■ **United Kingdom**: As in the US, Indian women in Britain have a higher death rate from heart disease than all other women. A 1991 study of heart disease deaths across the UK during the preceding 12 years found that British immigrants from India had a heart disease death rate three times higher than immigrants from the US (an age-adjusted death rate of 151 versus 56). Indian women in the study were the only group whose death rate actually went up over the years studied (13%); it declined for all other women, by up to 36%.

IMPORTANT RISK FACTORS IN WOMEN

All the traditional and emerging risk factors currently identified in men are equally important in women. Women tend to have a better risk factor profile than men at younger ages, but worse at older ages. Certain risk factors—including *diabetes, low HDL, high triglycerides, high blood pressure, high uric acid,* and *smoking*—are more harmful to women than men.

Of these particularly harmful factors for women, Indian women have a higher prevalence of three of them—*diabetes, low HDL,* and *high triglycerides*—than white women, but a lower prevalence of *high blood pressure* and *smoking* than white women.

Additionally, compared to white women, Indian women have a higher prevalence of *abdominal (centralized) obesity* but a lower prevalence of *general obesity* and *high total cholesterol*. With the exception of tobacco use, the prevalence of most risk factors is lower in rural India than in urban.

I. Height, general obesity, and abdominal obesity

A number of bodily characteristics affect a woman's risk for heart disease:

■ **Height:** As in men, shortness is associated with heart disease in women: the taller you are, the lower your risk. In a large study involving about 2,000 women, women shorter than 59 inches had a risk of heart disease *three times* higher than women taller than 69 inches. The difference persisted even after statistical adjustments were made for age, weight, educational status, religion, and other factors.

Waist Size: Smaller is Healthier
For Indian women, optimum waist size is no more than 32 inches, compared to no more than 35 inches for non-Asian women.

■ **Obesity:** As stated in Chapter III, Section 5, the optimum body mass index (BMI) for Asians is below 23; 23-25 is considered overweight, and above 25 is considered obese. In the Nurses' Health Study (*see* Appendix B), death rates due to heart disease were *four times* higher in obese women with a BMI above 32 than in slim women with a BMI below 21. A weight gain of even 15 to 24 pounds after age 18 was associated with a doubling of risk for diabetes and heart disease in women. Conversely, middle-aged women who lose about 10 pounds of weight significantly reduce their risk for diabetes.

■ **Abdominal obesity:** Several studies in the past two decades show that waist size may be an even better predictor of heart disease than body weight. For Indian women, the optimum waist size is below 32 inches, compared to 35 inches for non-Asian women. This recommendation holds true regardless of the person's height.

II. Smoking

Smoking is an even stronger risk factor for women than men: It quadruples the risk of a heart attack in young premenopausal women. In one study, women under 45, who smoked 35 or more cigarettes a day, increased their risk of heart attack and other coronary events by a factor of seven. More than 50% of heart attacks in middle-aged women in most populations (but not Indian women, few of whom smoke) is attributable to cigarette smoking. Smokers, who quit, lowered their cardiovascular risk to that of a non-smoker within three to five years. Women, however, apparently have a harder time quitting than men; their rates of successful quitting have been less than half those of men.

Although the overall smoking rate is still low among women in India, recent studies show an 18% increase in the past decade, much of which can be attributed to aggressive marketing campaigns directed toward women by tobacco companies. Furthermore, although only 8% of women in Asian countries smoke, more than 60% of the men do, exposing vast numbers of women and children to the harmful effects of secondhand smoke.

> **What Family History tells about a Woman's Heart Disease Risk**
> A piece of research that strongly suggests that heart disease risk factors affect women quite differently than men is that a history of heart disease, heart attack, or sudden death before 55 **in a sister** is more strongly predictive of a heart attack in a woman than the same history in her **brother or parent**. For example, a family history of premature heart disease in a sister is associated with a **12-fold higher** risk, versus sixfold for a brother and threefold for a parent.
> In practical terms, this means women with a family history of premature heart disease—especially in a sister—need to have their risk levels evaluated, particularly for emerging factors such as lipoprotein(a) and homocysteine.

III. High blood pressure (hypertension)

Having hypertension raises a woman's risk of heart disease fourfold, and her risk of dying from a coronary event sevenfold. Hypertension affects a woman's cardiovascular health more severely than a man's, although the reasons for this are not entirely clear. It also tends to be more common in women than men after age 45: the prevalence among white American women over 45 is 60%, and 79% for African American women.

> **Did you know...**
> *A diabetic woman's risk of getting a heart attack is nearly as high as that of a diabetic man, and as high as 16 times that of a non-diabetic woman.*

What promotes high blood pressure in women? Besides the usual factors—salt intake, inactivity, age, and genetics—hypertension in women is particularly closely correlated with obesity. It is six times higher in women with a BMI over 30 than in those with a BMI under 20. Blood pressure continues to increase in women until the age of 75, when its prevalence exceeds 80%. Also, control of hypertension remains poor in women in general and in elderly women in particular, among whom only 30% have their high blood pressure under management.

IV. Diabetes

More than 9 million women in the US have diabetes, a condition that greatly increases their risk of developing heart disease and/or dying from a heart attack. Other studies show that women with diabetes have a greater risk of dying from heart disease than women who had a prior heart attack. In a 13-year follow-up study of 1,296 nondiabetics and 835 diabetics aged 45 to 64 who had no cardiovascular disease, the researchers found that the coronary event rate per 1,000 person-years was 12 and 2 in nondiabetic men and women, respectively, versus 36 and 32 in diabetic men and women, respectively (*see* Figure 4.9). Some of this excess risk may be explained by the lower rates of heart disease for nondiabetic women in contrast to nondiabetic men. For example, in this study, compared to nondiabetic subjects, the risk of coronary events rose 16-fold in diabetic women but only three-fold in diabetic men.

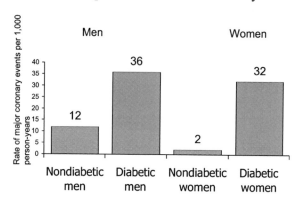

Figure 4.9. Differences in the incidence of major coronary events such as heart attacks in men and women according to the presence and absence of diabetes. Note that the incidence of heart attacks is only one-sixth among nondiabetic women compared to non-diabetic men. However the incidence rates of coronary events among diabetic women is almost as high as diabetic men. Source: Juutilainen, A. Ref 4.30.

V. Metabolic syndrome

Metabolic syndrome is the most common cardiac risk factor among women with premature heart disease. About 73% of American women have it, compared to 31% of American men. Even among normal-weight women, metabolic syndrome confers a threefold risk of premature heart attack. Like smoking, hypertension, diabetes, low HDL, and high triglycerides levels, metabolic syndrome is a stronger predictor of heart disease in women than men. Women in harmonious, happy marriages are less likely to develop this syndrome than dissatisfied, widowed or divorced women, suggesting that stress and its behavioral effects may play a role.

> **Metabolic syndrome** is a cluster of five or six elevated risk factors, such as high blood pressure and abnormal lipids, that are all caused by physical inactivity, unhealthy diet, and inherited genes. These risk factors first lead to insulin resistance, and then to the syndrome. Metabolic syndrome dramatically raises a woman's chances of developing either diabetes, stroke or heart disease, or several of these.
>
> Like smoking, diabetes, hypertension, high triglycerides, and low HDL, metabolic syndrome predicts heart disease more strongly in women than men. In other words, it is worse for a woman to have any of these other risks, than for a man to have them.

VI. Lipoprotein(a)

Diabetes is widely considered among the foremost predictors of heart disease, yet in younger women, lipoprotein(a) appears to be, if anything, an even more powerful predictor for heart disease than diabetes. Among premenopausal women who have heart disease, an elevated level of Lp(a) is three to four times more common than diabetes. Secondly, women who have a combination of high Lp(a), low HDL, and a high total cholesterol-to-HDL ratio face a 100-fold greater risk of having a premature heart attack.

Although a person's Lp(a) level is largely genetically determined, it does not necessarily remain constant throughout life: It increases by about 10% in postmenopausal women. Lp(a) can also be lowered. In both men and women, niacin has been shown to be a safe and effective medication for lowering Lp(a) levels. Niacin is also highly effective in raising HDL, particularly the most cardioprotective large-particle HDL. Niacin, therefore, seems ideally suited for use in combination therapy with statins for Indian men and women (*see* Chapter VI, Section 5 and Chapter VIII, Section 2).

VII. Other factors

Depression, extreme hostility, and low social support are also associated with higher levels of heart disease. Because women are more prone to depression than men, this may complicate their heart health. Among women, depression is associated with a post-heart attack, death rate 50% higher than that of non-depressed women. Low socioeconomic status and/or low literacy rates are also associated with a 30% to 50% higher prevalence of heart disease risk factors and rates.

Married women, whose husbands have suffered a heart attack have more risk factors, and have them more often, compared to married women in the general population. This suggests that a shared family lifestyle can put both adults at a higher risk of heart disease.

Women, who have had recurrent miscarriages, also have a higher risk of premature heart disease. This excess risk is attributed to high levels of certain emerging risk factors such as antiphospholipid antibodies, homocysteine and Lp(a).

DIAGNOSING HEART DISEASE AMONG WOMEN

i. Treadmill stress testing

The crucial link between detection of heart disease and its optimal management is accurate, safe diagnosis. Yet many at-risk women who would benefit from heart disease-screening tests are simply not getting them, partly because they are not referred for the right tests as often as at-risk men are. In addition, ordinary exercise treadmill tests are of less diagnostic value to women than to men, because women yield more "false positives"—in other words, the test suggests they have heart disease when in fact they do not. An ordinary treadmill test, nevertheless, can be useful as a screening device for women with a normal ECG and who can exercise vigorously enough: In this case, a negative result can effectively exclude severe heart disease.

Women, who have an abnormal ECG, however, need something more than a garden-variety treadmill test. A stress test with nuclear or echocardiography imaging is more accurate in their case. Even there, however, such a test can result in a false negative because, compared to men, women more often have non-obstructive disease (with only mild narrowing) and one-vessel disease.

Exercise capacity is the major yardstick for how fit one's heart is and for measuring one's long-term risk of death from heart disease and other causes. One problem is that women generally have a lower exercise capacity than men, implying inaccurately that they automatically also have less cardiovascular fitness. A typical 50-year-old woman, for example, has an exercise capacity of about 7 METS, compared to 8 for a similarly aged man. A MET measures the intensity of physical activity (*see* Chapter V, Section 8). For this reason, a new exercise nomogram—a chart for calculating or interpreting a person's cardiovascular fitness in terms of his or her exercise capacity—has been developed specially for women.

> Angiograms tend to be more useful in detecting coronary heart disease in men than in women, because atherosclerosis in women tends to be more **diffuse** than in men. Second, women have **smaller** coronary arteries. Both factors — diffuse atherosclerosis and smaller coronary arteries—make it harder to perform an angioplasty or bypass surgery on women. Thus, in both **detection** and **treatment**, there is currently a male-female gap to be bridged.

ii. Heart scans

A heart scan—more formally known as an Electron-Beam Computed Tomographic test, or EBCT—can detect calcified plaques in the coronary arteries of people, who have no known heart disease. The test gives you an overall "calcium score" on a scale of 0 to 4000. A score above 3000 suggests you need bypass surgery, or even that you have advanced inoperable disease. A score above 1000 usually indicates the need for an angiogram. On the other hand, if your calcium score shows that you have no calcified coronary plaques, it is very unlikely that you have any severely blocked coronary arteries. For practical purposes, a low-risk woman with a total calcium score below 100 can in most cases avoid having to undergo a coronary angiogram, even if she came in with atypical chest pain and indications of borderline abnormalities from an exercise stress test.

iii. Coronary angiograms

The Gender Gap
Examined in its entirety, women's heart disease risk profile means that prevention must receive even greater emphasis. Yet according to a major 2005 study, only one-third of women at high risk of heart disease are getting the medications they need to reduce their risk of heart disease, including statins and niacin. Women, in short, are lagging behind in screening, detection, treatment, and preventive strategies including the achievement of basic lipid level goals.

Coronary angiograms are most effective in detecting large, hard plaques that bulge into the inner channel of the artery. They are much less effective in spotting soft plaques buried deep inside the wall of the artery itself. This poses a problem for screening at-risk women, because atherosclerosis in women tends to be more diffuse—occurring at multiple sites along the full length of the artery. It tends to be less obstructive at any one particular point and, therefore, less likely to show significant narrowing at a specific site when an angiogram is done.

When a coronary angiogram is done on women with chest pain and cardiac risk factors, only about 35% of them show any significant narrowing, compared to 80 to 90% of men. Since a coronary angiogram on average ranges between $15,000 and $20,000, these findings underscore the need for better use of noninvasive tests such as a stress test with imaging to identify women who would truly benefit from getting a full-fledged angiogram.

Diffuse plaque buildup in women may also help to account for the lower rates of coronary angioplasty and bypass surgery among women, both of which are best performed on patients who have severe but more localized narrowing and a good post-procedure prognosis. In addition to diffuse atherosclerosis, women often have coronary arteries that are too small for angioplasty or bypass surgery. A woman with the same body mass index (BMI) as a man will tend to have smaller coronary arteries than he does.

TREATING AND PREVENTING HEART DISEASE IN WOMEN

The undertreatment of women

As the preceding paragraphs have shown, heart disease is worse in women than in men along several dimensions, and many heart disease risk factors have a more harmful effect on women than on men. It is also often harder to detect advanced plaque buildup in women on an angiogram, because their coronary artery disease tends to be more diffuse. Additionally, conventional exercise treadmill tests are less helpful to at-risk women because they yield more "false positives" than do men. Furthermore, gender perceptions often make it less likely that a women at serious risk of cardiac disease will receive the level of urgent care she needs, or that people around her will even recognize her symptoms if she begins to have a heart attack.

All of this means that even greater weight needs to be placed on *prevention* in both sexes, but perhaps particularly even more so in women. Yet according to a 2005 study of more than a million members of a major managed-care organization (*see* the Kaiser Study, Chapter I, Section 2), only a third of women at high risk of heart disease are actually getting statins or other cholesterol-lowering medications that help patients cut their risk of developing life-threatening atherosclerosis. Even fewer women, the study showed, received niacin to boost their HDL (good) cholesterol levels, or fibrate therapy to lower their triglyceride levels.

Following a heart attack, women are only half as likely as men to receive aspirin, beta blockers, or thrombolytic (clot-dissolving) therapy. In 2004, about 50% of US women above 55 had lipid and blood pressure levels and other clinical indicators that qualified them for drug treatment, yet only 12% of women were meeting their NCPE-defined (see Appendix B) guidelines for LDL cholesterol level, compared to 31% of men. This underscores the need for a more aggressive, more comprehensive approach to the treatment of dyslipidemia in women.

Coronary angioplasty and stent: Differences between women and men

Before 1990, women were referred for coronary angiograms, angioplasty or bypass surgery only half as frequently as men. That began to change. Studies undertaken between 1990 and 2000 indicated that women were now nearly as likely to undergo coronary angioplasty or stent as men, but still less likely to undergo coronary artery bypass surgery. It is not clear whether this difference in bypass surgery rates represented *only* under-treatment of women, or over-treatment of men *as well*. Evidence since 2000 suggests, however, that the gender bias against aggressive intervention and treatment of heart disease in women is disappearing in the US, but not necessarily in other countries, including India.

Although men and women have similar success rates after angioplasty and stent, in the *short-term* the rates of morbidity and mortality associated with these procedures are three times as high in women as they are in men. This may point to the severity of women's underlying disease, as well as to their smaller-sized coronary arteries. The likelihood of an embolism forming—meaning blockage of an artery, for example, by a detached blood clot—during an angioplasty or stent procedure is about five times greater in women because women tend to form larger blood clots than men. In the *long-term*, however, women tend to have an excellent prognosis after successful angioplasty and stent, as good as that observed in men—once they are over the short-term risks.

Preventing and managing heart disease in women

• **Screening:** Because many of the risk factors of heart disease have a genetic basis, screening the blood relatives of someone, who has premature heart disease is an important part of an effective prevention strategy. Such screening, however, should include the wives of men who have had a heart attack or have heart disease because studies show that such women have a higher prevalence of risk factors, possibly because they share many features of their husband's environment and lifestyle, including diet, not to mention secondary smoke.

• **Physical Activity and Weight Management:** As with men, proper nutrition and regular vigorous physical activity are crucial in at-risk women for losing excess weight, maintaining proper weight, improving lipid profile, and slowing down the process of atherosclerosis. Prolonged sitting—at a desk job or factory job or at home—significantly increases cardiac risk. It has been found that women with higher physical fitness scores have fewer cardiac risk factors and a 50% lower risk for heart attack than sedentary women. Exercise helps to prevent not only heart disease but diabetes and metabolic syndrome.

To achieve weight loss, many women prefer diet to exercising. But note that even though physical activity promote weight loss/weight management, the two are each *independently* important factors. Achieving both doubles your cardiovascular benefits. To really reduce your heart risk, you need to pursue both exercise and weight management, not just one or the other (*see* Chapter V, Section 8 for tips on how to structure physical activity into your daily life). Losing just a few pounds can make a huge difference to your health, and exercising vigorously or even walking briskly for at least two and half hours per week (30 minutes a day times five) can reduce your risk of having a major coronary event by about one-third. Additional benefits of regular exercise in women include a reduction in the risk of breast cancer by as much as 72%.

• **Aspirin:** The benefits of taking an aspirin a day in reducing cardiac risk appear to be less in women than men. Aspirin can promote internal bleeding because it *damages the lining of the stomach*. In the Women's Health Study, nearly 40,000 healthy women were treated with 100 mg of aspirin on alternate days or dummy pills for 10 years. On the plus side, there was a 17% reduction in the risk of stroke in the aspirin group. The results indicated, however, that except in those older than 65, there were no reductions in heart attacks. More ominously, despite the very small dose of the aspirin used—a normal aspirin tablet is 325mg— for every three cardiac events prevented there was one case of major bleeding that required a blood transfusion.

• **Hormone Replacement Therapy:** As a heart disease prevention strategy, Hormone Replacement Therapy, or HRT, was until recently considered a good alternative to cholesterol-lowering therapy in post-menopausal women. Although HRT increases a woman's good (HDL) cholesterol, however, it also increases the levels of two risk factors: C-reactive protein and triglycerides. Several large studies completed in the last 10 years have demonstrated that the harm from HRT outweighs its benefits. All the major recommending and regulatory agencies have now advised against its use for heart disease prevention and treatment. It is now limited to women with severe menopausal symptoms.

The only group of women at risk for heart disease for whom the benefits of HRT may outweigh the risks are women with high Lp(a), such as Indian women. HRT reduces Lp(a) levels by an average of 20%, and up to 50% in women with high levels of it. More studies are needed to ascertain the potential role of HRT in the management of Lp(a) among Indian women.

• **The pill** Unlike the first (pre-2000) generation of birth-control pills, the newest generation of oral contraceptives is not associated with a high risk of heart attack or stroke, except among smokers and those with genetic abnormalities that predispose them to excessive blood clotting. Some oral contraceptives do raise blood pressure, but this rise disappears upon withdrawal.

KEY · POINTS · IN · A · NUTSHELL

♥ A woman's lifetime risk of dying from heart disease is eight times greater than from breast cancer.

♥ Although heart disease develops 10 to 15 years later in women than in men, more women die from heart disease each year than men.

♥ A woman's risk of a heart attack increases steeply after menopause, when her LDL and triglyceride levels begin to increase and her good cholesterol (HDL) level begins to fall.

♥ Most women having a heart attack do not experience typical chest pain symptoms.

♥ Following a heart attack, women have a higher rate of complications, including death and disability, than men.

♥ Women, who have had recurrent miscarriages, have a higher risk of having a heart attack at a young age than those who have not.

♥ Metabolic syndrome is a very strong predictor of premature heart disease in women, and is a stronger predictor in women than in men. Happily married women are less likely than dissatisfied, widowed or divorced women to develop it.

♥ Women with a high level of Lp(a) and a high total cholesterol-to-HDL ratio are at very high risk of developing heart disease (a 100 times more likely than those who do not).

♥ The optimum waist size for Indian women is no more than 32 inches, versus no more than 35 inches for non-Asian women.

♥ Diabetic women face a risk of heart attack up to 16 times greater than non-diabetic women. The increase in risk for diabetic men is only threefold.

♥ Particularly for high-risk women such as post-menopausal Indian women with a family history of heart disease, proper nutrition and regular physical activity are crucial priorities in promoting weight loss, maintaining proper weight, improving their lipid profile, and slowing down atherosclerosis.

♥ The gender bias against aggressive intervention and treatment of heart disease in women is disappearing in the US, but not necessarily in other countries, including India.

4.4 ▶ The Pediatric Foundations of Heart Disease

SEVERAL STUDIES CONVINCINGLY DEMONSTRATE that heart disease begins in childhood and that the presence of risk factors in a child often triggers the onset of heart disease—sometimes advanced disease—as a young adult. Obesity, which is increasing more quickly in children than in adults, has resulted in a dramatic rise in metabolic syndrome and diabetes, both of which are precursors to heart disease. Some studies have even detected fatty streaks, the earliest sign of atherosclerosis (or plaque buildup), in the coronary arteries of preschool children. And significant heart disease has been found in hearts donated for transplant from young children. There are some indications that heart disease may even begin before birth. It has been found, for example, that a high level of blood cholesterol in a woman during her pregnancy is associated with atherosclerosis in her unborn child. This Chapter summarizes the most important things you need to know and do to identify and minimize heart disease risk factors in your own or others' preteen or teenage children.

The PDAY Study showed that the prevalence and extent of plaque buildup both rise rapidly between the ages of 14 to 35.

Early plaque buildup: Evidence from postmortem studies

Heart disease starts much earlier than has traditionally been thought. A study of 200 young American servicemen, who died during the Korean War, for example, found atherosclerosis in 77% of them, despite their average age of just 22. About 12% of them had substantial atherosclerosis, with one or more coronary arteries showing more than 50% narrowing. Another 3% had at least one artery that was completely blocked with plaques. Similarly, about half of all servicemen who died during the Vietnam War and were autopsied showed evidence of atherosclerosis. Their heart disease did not develop overnight, suggesting that it started much, much earlier—during childhood.

Several studies undertaken in the past decade indicate that the overall prevalence of coronary atherosclerosis in young people is similar to that observed in young servicemen 50 years ago. The Pathobiological Determinants of Atherosclerosis in Youth Study (or PDAY, *see* Appendix B), which examined nearly 3000 persons ages 15 to 34 who had died in accidents, found a dramatic increase in the extent of plaque buildup with increasing age. Significant plaques were present in 20% of 15- to 19-year-olds, increasing to 40% for 30- to 34-year-olds.

This all but confirms the pediatric origins of atherosclerosis. Consistent with our knowledge that women lag men by 10 years in developing heart disease, young girls possessed fewer plaques than young boys.

Early plaque buildup: Evidence from heart transplant donors

A fascinating coronary ultrasound study from The Cleveland Clinic, one of the world's foremost cardiac centers, showed evidence of atherosclerosis in the coronary arteries of 17% of otherwise healthy heart donors younger than 20. This proportion rose to 85% among donors 50 and older (*see* **Figure 4.10**, *Heart Transplant Donors with Substantial Coronary Plaque Buildup*). None of these donors had been diagnosed with heart disease before they died, and only 8% of them had given any evidence of atherosclerosis on their coronary angiograms. In fact, the angiograms of all the donors younger than 30 were completely normal, yet ultrasound

Measuring plaque buildup in children

As several studies have demonstrated, two additional markers of plaque buildup in children as well as adults are **(i)** the calcification of plaques inside your coronary arteries, and **(ii)** the thickening of the walls of your two carotid arteries—two major arteries that run up into your neck and head.

Plaque calcification is measured by a test called electron beam computed tomography, or EBCT for short. Carotid artery thickness—more properly called common carotid artery intimal-medial thickness, or CIMT—is measured by ultrasound. Both EBCT and ultrasound are very sensitive tests that can be done repeatedly to monitor the development and progression of a person's atherosclerosis. Both are also noninvasive, meaning that the doctor or lab tech will not be sticking anything into you (see Chapter VII, Section 3 for more on these procedures).

showed that 28% of them had atherosclerosis. This attests both to the extent of early atherosclerosis and to the fact that a "normal" coronary angiogram does not necessarily mean you are off the hook. The best offense against heart disease is still prevention, not detection followed by treatment.

Risk factors during childhood: strongly predict later heart disease

Studies such as the Bogalusa Heart Study (*see* Appendix B) have shown having cardiovascular risk factors in childhood, particularly high LDL levels and high Body Mass Index (BMI), strongly predict atherosclerosis in adult life. Similar conclusions were reached in a Finnish study of 2,229 white adults aged 33 to 39 who had first been examined at ages 12 to 18. It was found that risk factors measured in adolescence predicted the development of atherosclerosis better than those measured in their adult life.

Risk factors in childhood predict later heart disease
Studies show that risk factors measured during childhood and adolescence predict heart disease during adulthood better than those measured during adult life.

Risk Factors among Medical students
The impressive cardiac risk profile of 3,800 medical students in a major study attests to the powerful effect of **a)** being aware of the danger posed by cardiovascular risk factors, and **b)** the benefit of becoming part of a sub-culture that maintains strong negative perceptions unhealthy habits such as over-consumption of saturated fat, and positive perceptions of healthy ones, such as exercising regularly.

In a third study that measured cardiac risk factors during childhood (15 years or younger) and twice again during young adult life (on average, at 27 and at 33), it was found that calcified coronary plaques had developed in 31% of the men and 10% of the women. It was also found that the plaque buildup during adulthood correlated with increased BMI (weight gain), high blood pressure, and decreased HDL during childhood and adolescence. These risk factors were observed among those who had developed plaques when first measured at 15 years old or younger. The study reinforced the findings of other studies—that risk factors measured in childhood and adolescence predict the development of atherosclerosis better than those measured in their adult life.

Taken together, these studies advance the view that the presence of elevated levels of traditional cardiac risk factors during childhood and adolescence correlates strongly with the severity and extent of atherosclerosis, both during youth and later in life. As the number and/or level of risk factors increase, so does the pace and severity of plaque buildup. In addition, the presence of some risk factors—such as obesity—in childhood tends to predict their ongoing presence during adulthood.

This emphasizes the need for aggressively reducing risk factors in children, beginning at a young age. Not only does beginning early lay a foundation of later benefits, but also it predicts a higher rate of success because the mind of a child is more trainable and pliable than that of an adult set in his or her ways.

Intervention can be done through conscious modification of lifestyle choices. A 1990 study of more than 3,800 American medical students, for example, showed that young people can go against the trends that are overtaking their generation and initiate prudent changes in diet and exercise levels that produce a highly favorable risk factor profile. Total cholesterol levels among the medical students ranged from 173 to 180 points, well below the national average. Triglycerides levels ranged from 56 to 101, and HDL levels ranged from 51 to 57 in males and 62 to 70 in females. LDL levels were also low, ranging from 92 to 112. Smoking was extremely low—just 2% in men and 3% in women. Half of them

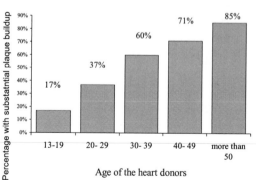

Figure 4.10. Percentage of heart transplant donors who have substantial coronary plaque buildup, by age range. Note the steady progression from early adolescence onward, suggesting that the process begins in childhood, well before age 13. Source: Tuzcu, EM. Ref 4.52. *Reproduced with permission* © Lippincott Williams & Wilkins

exercised more than three times a week. Hypertension was observed in 6% of the men and 3% of the women—moderately low, but perhaps reflecting the fact that hypertension can be inherited—but diabetes was present in less than 1%.

The excellent cardiovascular risk profile of these medical students paralleled the very low rates of heart disease observed among American physicians (with the exception of Indian physicians in the US; *see* section 1 of this Chapter). Their superior profile attests to two things—first, the powerful effect of awareness: being medical students, they had read about the ill effects of cardiovascular risk factors and internalized the message, resulting in a powerful motivation to change. Second, it appears that these students had become part of an entire subcultural, high-achievement, college environment that maintained negative perceptions of smoking and other unhealthy habits, and reinforced positive perceptions of the benefits of selecting low-fat foods and "working out."

In short, learning about and really understanding the way risk factors function matters greatly. In addition, your cultural environment—which includes your family, workplace, school, neighborhood, and even place of worship, not just your country or state—also matters: your daily network of friends, family, and workplace colleagues constitute a cultural "microenvironment" that can make it easier, or alternately more challenging, for you to break bad habits and substitute healthful ones.

Let's look at a few specific risk factors that can affect children and their future cardiovascular health.

I. High blood pressure

> **Choose Your Friends Wisely ...**
> Your daily network of friends, family, and colleagues form a "microenvironment" that can make it easier, or harder, for you to break bad habits and substitute health-promoting ones. The same holds true for your kids. It is not always possible for them to choose their associations, but it helps to encourage them to put some thought into whom they surround themselves with. As the 1990 medical student study and numerous immigration studies have shown, your environment profoundly affects how you act and what you see as important. Ditto your children.

Children's blood pressure values are normally lower than those of adults, but they are not entirely immune to high blood pressure. About 1-3% of preadolescents and 5-6% of adolescents have hypertension, although a study of 10,215 children ages 5 to 14 in New Delhi found that 12% of the boys and 11% of the girls had hypertension. Diabetes is a serious but underappreciated sequel to high blood pressure. A 38-year follow-up study of 1,152 medical students has shown that developing high blood pressure precedes the onset of type 2 diabetes in middle age by 20 to 25 years. Higher blood pressure in the prediabetic state may contribute to the presence of vascular disease at the time of diagnosis of type 2 diabetes.

A serious but underappreciated sequel to hypertension is diabetes.

What leads to hypertension in children? One factor positively associated with it is the body mass index (BMI) of a child's parents as well as his or her own. Smoking by mothers during pregnancy is also associated with increased blood pressure in children, while breastfeeding for at least six months is associated with a lowering of blood pressure. Although hypertension does not begin to accelerate atherosclerosis until around age 30, childhood hypertension does track into adulthood. It is, therefore, important to initiate interventions aimed at reducing a child's early-life risk factors: these include breast-feeding, quitting smoking during pregnancy, and helping all family members to keep their weight under strict management. Reducing the widespread prevalence of high blood pressure would go a long way toward helping cut the risk of cardiovascular disease.

II. Tobacco use

As in adults, tobacco use among children accelerates plaque buildup and the onset of coronary events by at least 10 years. This is a particular problem on the Indian sub-continent, where a recent survey revealed that more than 50% of Indian school children, both boys and girls, regularly or sometimes use tobacco, particularly in the form of chewing tobacco (*gutka*). The survey found that even some eight-year-olds use tobacco. Contrary to common opinion, smokeless tobacco is just as harmful to the user's cardiovascular health as smoking is.

III. Dyslipidemia

Research indicates that dyslipidemia—meaning having lipid levels that are seriously out of balance—is even more harmful to younger person's cardiac health than to that of an older adult. Carefully designed studies such as the Johns Hopkins Precursors Study (*see* Appendix B) have shown that every 1% elevation in total cholesterol raises a **young adult's** risk of heart disease by 4% to 5%, compared to a 1% rise in the risk of an older adult. In the Johns Hopkins study, 1,017 young men (average age 22 years) were followed for 27 to 42 years after having their cholesterol levels measured. The study found that their cholesterol levels at age 22 were strongly associated not only with the onset of heart disease later on in life but with the likelihood of dying from it. A 36-point increment in total cholesterol—perhaps a 15% to 25% rise—was associated with a 100% increase in cardiovascular risk.

Table 4.10. Markers in at-risk children and adolescents who require
• Has parents or grandparents who had a premature* heart attack or stroke • Has a family history of unexplained sudden premature* death • Has parents or grandparents who have undergone angioplasty or bypass surgery at a premature age* • Has at least one parent with high cholesterol • Has a cigarette smoking habit • Has hypertension • Is obese or overweight • Has metabolic syndrome • Has diabetes

* Below 55 in men, and below 65 in women

Runs in the family: Dyslipidemia in children not only identifies the child's own risk of future heart disease, but often also that of his or her family members. The Muscatine Study, which examined 2,874 American school-age children, found that a relationship existed between children's cholesterol levels and heart attack deaths among their adult relatives. Twice as many young male relatives (ages 30 to 59) of children who had high cholesterol died from heart attack compare to young male relatives of children who had lower cholesterol levels. Among female relatives of high-cholesterol children, heart attack death rates ran 10 times as high as those of female relatives of low-cholesterol children.

The relationship, of course, does not specify a causal direction one way or the other. Most likely, the pathway is a combination of genetics and lifestyle: High-cholesterol children may partly inherit their dyslipidemia from their relatives. On the other hand, children may have high cholesterol also because they eat the same kinds of high saturated fat, high cholesterol, high calorie diet their family members eat at home. The relationship between the child's cholesterol level and the relative's cardiovascular health may be stronger among the *female* relatives perhaps because there is a stronger caretaking bond between them and the child, and thus the likelihood that they both eat the same things is stronger. Regardless of the precise causes, the discovery that a child has high cholesterol should lead to the testing of his or her immediate relatives, and vice versa.

Screening for high cholesterol: Children or teenagers with any of the personal or family traits outlined in Table 4.10.

IV. Maternal cholesterol promotes fetal atherosclerosis

Like the harm caused by smoking or excessive alcohol consumption during pregnancy, a high level of maternal cholesterol during pregnancy is associated with fatty streaks in the arteries of the unborn child, the earliest stage of atherosclerosis. In one study, fatty streaks were present in the aortas of 50% of the fetuses of mothers, who had abnormally high cholesterol (maternal hypercholesterolemia) during pregnancy. This condition induces changes in the fetus that make the newborn child more susceptible to accelerated atherosclerosis both during childhood and in later years.

Studies suggest that every 1% jump in a young adult's total cholesterol raises his or her risk of heart disease by 4% to 5%, compared to only a 1% increase in an older adult.

The documented finding that toxins and other chemicals in the fetal environment can affect the child's future morbidity and mortality well into adulthood underscores the importance of screening and treating women even before they become pregnant. It takes time to reverse dyslipidemia and bring down elevated levels of various bodily substances. Although statins and most other cholesterol-lowering medications **should not be** used during pregnancy, there are many cholesterol-lowering interventions that women with high cholesterol can initiate during pregnancy to decrease atherogenesis in their baby.

V. Obesity, metabolic syndrome and diabetes in children

> **Did You Know?**
> Childhood obesity tends to predict obesity during adulthood. About 1 in 10 children and teens are obese and have metabolic syndrome. Because such children tend to become obese as adults, interventions need to begin early in life.

Childhood obesity has literally become a sprawling national problem that now threatens children's health and, ultimately, their life expectancies. The average American child is bombarded by more than 20,000 food advertisements a year, each carrying a message to eat more, often more of the wrong thing. Childhood obesity is now even more common among rural than urban children: (20% versus 16%. In rural North Carolina, for example, it is as high as 50% of all children.

Denial is only worsening the overweight problem: Fully one-third of the mothers of overweight children do not consider their child overweight. Denial, however, does little to disguise the harm: Obesity accelerates the severity and extent of plaque buildup, and recent studies have linked childhood obesity to another powerful cardiovascular risk factor—the development of left ventricular hypertrophy in adulthood—as well as to some cancers.

The obesity-diabetes connection: Excess weight is the force driving the twin epidemics of childhood metabolic syndrome and childhood diabetes, both of them dangerous cardiovascular risk factors. Diabetes diagnosed before age 40, for example, is associated with a *12-year decrease* in a person's lifespan and quality of life. Currently, approximately one in 10 children and adolescents (from 2 to 19 years old) are obese and have metabolic syndrome, and one in 50 is prediabetic. Few pieces of data more strongly stress the importance of early, aggressive risk prevention strategies. Low consumption of fruits and vegetables and over-consumption of high-sugar drinks are both associated with the alarming prevalence of metabolic syndrome in children.

Type 2 diabetes: The incidence of type 2 (adult onset) diabetes—hitherto uncommon in children—has increased tenfold in the past decade in children and adolescents in the US, and now accounts for 33% to 46% of all diabetes among 10- to 19-year-olds. Girls are twice as likely as boys to develop type 2 diabetes.

The role of genes: As we saw in Chapter IV, Section 2, diabetes has a strong genetic foundation, and it tends to get passed on from parent to child. Since genes change very slowly, however, the current pediatric epidemic of diabetes cannot be caused by a large increase in genetic predisposition. It instead reflects a population that had a certain amount of relatively unexpressed predisposition toward diabetes but is now reaching its *tipping point* as a result of unhealthy lifestyle changes among its children—especially in the area of diet and physical inactivity.

In the UK the risk of developing type 2 diabetes is 14 times greater among South Asian children than white children, despite a lower rate of obesity among them.

Its genetic basis, nevertheless, is unquestionable: Siblings of diabetic children, for example, have a 175- to 250-fold increased risk of developing diabetes compared to siblings of nondiabetic children. In the UK, the risk of developing type 2 diabetes is *14 times* greater among South Asian children than white children, despite a lower rate of obesity among the South Asians. Bolstering the notion of parent-child generational transmission, a study conducted among native Canadian Indians showed that one out of every three children of a mother, who had diabetes herself as a child, develops diabetes as early as by **age seven**. The evidence for its genetic basis means that individuals, doctors, and public health agencies need to engage in much more diligent early screening to identify the most vulnerable cases and nip the disease in the bud. Early intervention will be a key to a successful national strategy.

What you can do: On the individual level, there are several simple but extremely effective things you can do to forestall type 2 diabetes in your child, and they center on nutrition and exercise.

First, tackle the tendency toward inactivity by limiting to less than two hours a day the amount of time your child spends watching TV or playing video games.

Second, add a carrot to the stick: Help your children to find interesting things to do that will encourage vigorous daily physical activity.

Third, if they are overweight or obese and increased activity by itself does not solve the problem, help them reduce their weight. Note that weight management confers a separate independent benefit from physical activity. Physical activity without weight loss is great. Weight management without physical activity is great. But the two together are far better than just one. Here are some effective weight reduction strategies:

▶ *Increase* the range and times spent engaged in physical activity that induces sweat.

▶ *Encourage them* to drink lots of fluids, especially water. This should come naturally with increased activity.

▶ *Help them* to avoid the "Super-Size" mindset: serve smaller portions of food that are not laden with sugar and fat.

▶ *Pay attention* to your children's "lifestyle." If their closest friends spend much of their leisure time at the mall eating fast food, candy, and pastries, chances are your kids will do the same. No one wants to feel like the odd man out. In short, your children's social and psychological environment matters.

▶ *Read* Chapter V for a more extensive discussion of health-smart nutritional choices and physical activity plans.

VI. Prematurity, low birth weight, and "catch-up growth"

Low birth weight is associated with a heightened risk of diabetes and heart disease in middle age. For example, in a study of 16,000 persons, the death rate from heart disease was significantly higher among people whose birth weight was less than 5.5lb (2,500g) than in those who were 9.5lb (4,310g) or heavier. Scientists have known about this link. The question is why. Evidence is mounting in support of a theory, called the *Fetal Origins Hypothesis,* that says that under-nutrition of the unborn child during mid to late gestation not only results in low birth weight, but makes different organs of the child grow at disproportionately different rates, programming the child for future diabetes and heart disease. The foundations for heart disease, in other words, may sometimes be laid during fetal life.

Low birth weight, a risk factor that may reflect fetal under-nutrition, often leads into a second risk factor, *forced catch-up growth*, as the child's parents and physicians try to "help" the little tyke along by overfeeding him or her. Overfeeding is as harmful to a child's development as mild under-nutrition—indeed, possibly more.

If low birth weight is a risk factor, it often soon leads to another one—*Catch-up growth*. Like the 4 foot 7 boy in sixth grade who shoots up to become a 6 foot 7 senior, catch-up growth refers to an accelerated growth that occurs naturally in babies born with low birth weight. The problem arises when physicians and parents often try to "help" the low birth weight child along by *overfeeding* him or her. In one study, "forced" catch-up growth between one to five years of age was associated with hypertension, diabetes, and heart disease later in adult life. (The risk tends to be small during the child's first year) Overfeeding during this period—when babies need a lot of fat and calories anyway—was not associated with a subsequent heightened risk of high blood pressure in the study. What is important is not to try to push a physically small child along by continuing to overfeed him or her. The adverse effect of "forced" catch-up growth is worst among children, who continue to gain excess weight and who become obese by age 15.

Prevention: Giving your child a positive start in life

This section, if nothing, should have made it clear that any effective approach to prevention and intervention must target multiple risk factors and must begin in early life. Why? The reason is simple: Obesity, unhealthy dietary habits, a sedentary lifestyle, dyslipidemia, metabolic syndrome, hypertension, accelerated atherosclerosis, insulin resistance, and prediabetes all form an interrelated nucleus of risk factors that worsen the effects of one another, feeding back into each other like a flow chart with multiple loops. The good news is that they are also all highly modifiable.

*Excess weight, unhealthy diet, physical inactivity, out-of-balance lipids, metabolic syndrome, high blood pressure, premature atherosclerosis, insulin resistance, and prediabetes all form an **interrelated nucleus of risk factors** that intensify one another's harmful effects, feeding back into each other like a flow chart with multiple loops. The good news is that these risk factors are all highly modifiable.*

It is not enough for your child simply to be not obese, or even to be normal weight and eat healthily. Every child should be normal weight, *and* eat a low saturated fat, low-sugar diet centered on low-glycemic, carbohydrates, *and* exercise daily. Since the foundations of the conditions that later turn into full-blown diabetes or heart disease begin to be laid almost from the day you are born—some studies indicate even in the womb—prevention and intervention *must* start early in life—2 years of age.

The irony is that many parents pour their lives into their children, spending substantial amounts of resources on tennis and piano lessons, summer camp, tutoring, and nice-looking clothes—only to introduce the child to a series of lifestyle choices that sets them up for a lifetime of struggle with weight and health problems.

The findings of carefully structured investigations such as the landmark Bogalusa Heart Study reinforce the medical community's conviction that your lifestyle choices in early life have a profound impact on your cardiovascular risk in adulthood. Starting your child on a heart-healthy diet and program of activity *by age two* is the best way to prevent not only obesity but atherosclerosis, while keeping cholesterol and blood pressure at normal levels. It is also the best way to delay or avert serious coronary events later in life. Ideally, some preventive strategies—such as lowering your own cholesterol levels as a mother, and avoiding toxins that can cross the placental barrier, such as nicotine—should begin during pregnancy, not just after.

Children as young as age 2 can and should, get a jump start on eating behavior that's healthy for the heart, according to 2005 dietary recommendations released by the American Heart Association (AHA) and endorsed by the American Academy of Pediatrics

Optimum levels of lipids, blood sugar, blood pressure, waist size, and body mass index during childhood are associated with markedly reduced risks of metabolic syndrome and cardiovascular disease in adulthood. This alone should be enough to encourage parents to give their children the best chance they can have to develop into healthy, long-lived adults.

KEY · POINTS · IN · A · NUTSHELL

♥ Heart disease begins in childhood, possibly even before birth, and progresses silently for decades before manifesting as a heart attack.

♥ A mother's high blood cholesterol during pregnancy is associated with early atherosclerosis in the arteries of the unborn child. Similarly, smoking during pregnancy and not breast-feeding increase a newborn's risk of developing hypertension later.

♥ Having risk factors as a child often leads into heart disease in early adult life, and coronary disease has been found in more than a third of hearts donated for transplant from children.

♥ The prevalence and extent of plaque buildup both rise rapidly especially between the ages of 14 to 35, particularly in males, but the foundations for it are laid much earlier than that.

♥ An epidemic of childhood obesity (often denied by the parents) has resulted in a dramatic rise in metabolic syndrome and diabetes, both precursors to heart disease. Approximately one-third of obese children have metabolic syndrome and are likely to become diabetic before 30.

♥ Dyslipidemia is even more harmful to younger adults than to older. Every 1% rise in total cholesterol boosts a young adult's heart disease risk by 4-5%, but only by 1% in older adults.

♥ Obesity, inactivity, hypertension, dyslipidemia, metabolic syndrome, prediabetes, and diets laden with saturated fats and refined sugar all form an interrelated cluster of risk factors that worsen one another's effects, feeding back into each other like a flow chart with multiple loops.

♥ On the other hand, low levels of risk factors during childhood markedly reduce a person's risk of cardiovascular disease as an adult.

♥ Prevention and intervention need to target multiple risk factors and begin in early life. The best offense against heart disease is aggressive prevention, not expensive treatment.

♥ Over 50% of school children in India, both boys and girls, regularly or sometimes use tobacco, putting their cardiovascular health at serious risk.

♥ Children, spouses and close relatives often share a similar gene-environment profile (diet, activity levels, other lifestyle choices). Discovering that a child has high cholesterol should therefore lead to the testing of his or her immediate relatives, and vice versa.

♥ Ultrasound (which can used to measure carotid artery thickness) and EBCT (used to measure plaque calcification) are both sensitive, noninvasive, repeatable tests that can be done to monitor atherosclerosis progression in a child or young adult.

Part Two

Taking Action

Chapter V

Practical Steps for Preventing Heart Disease

Section 1, **Developing a Broad Strategy**, presents a broad outline of half a dozen important preventive strategies for reducing your risk of heart disease, and why an approach that combines and pursues several strategies simultaneously is particularly effective and synergistic. The section also discusses why it is often important for you to go beyond population-based recommendations and cut-points—which may reflect the practical realities of a resource-constrained healthcare system—and take charge of your health decisions by actively discussing with your doctor what these numbers mean for you. ◆

Drawing on scientifically tested principles of motivation that are based on the identification and visualization of the benefits of change, Section 2, **Finding the Motivation to Change**, discusses how to motivate yourself to design, initiate, and sustain a balanced, realistic lifestyle modification program. Short practical assignments are included that will assist you to recognize the strengths you have used on previous occasions to achieve success in other areas of your life, and transfer them to nutrition and exercise. ◆

The third section, **Introducing the Prudent Nutrition Program**, sets out the main components of this Program, the dietary guidelines that underpin it, and what makes this nutritional program different from and superior to the dozens of fly-by-night diets that come and go. The only kind of weight-reduction diet that is both healthy and sustainable is a high-fiber, low-calorie, carbohydrate-balanced, cardioprotective diet composed of great-tasting, nutrient-rich, low glycemic ingredients that you can readily find and with which you are already familiar. ◆

Sections 4, 5 and 6 address fats, proteins, and carbohydrates, respectively. Fats range from very healthy and cardioprotective to very unhealthy and harmful to your health. Section 4, **Fats! The Good, the Bad, and the Deadly**, explains the huge difference between good and fats, and why the Prudent Diet is a *balance* between fats, carbs and proteins. Using tables and figures, the section concisely summarizes the features of various meats and fish, different cooking oils, the new generation of cholesterol-lowering margarines, and the factors that make some favorite components of the Indian diet, like coconut oil and palm oil, unhealthy. Section 4 tells you why monounsaturated fats are so much better for you than saturated and trans fats, why it is dangerous to reuse cooking oil, why omega-3 fats, found in oily fish, is such an effective weapon against atherosclerosis. ◆

Section 5, **The Right Carbs**, presents a centrally important discussion: What do glycemic index and glycemic load mean, and why are these concepts critical to creating a balanced nutritional program that can help you keep your blood sugar level stable? It outlines the two fundamental criteria for choosing any carbohydrate, and how to apply these two principles to selecting fruits, vegetables, legumes, and whole grains that are rich in vitamins, antioxidants, and phytosterols. The section explains why eating the wrong carbs can not only doom you to low HDL cholesterol levels, high triglycerides, and excess body weight that you cannot lose, but also predispose you to developing diabetes and, ultimately, heart disease. ◆

Like Sections 4 and 5, **Healthy Protein Choices**, the sixth section, guides the reader through the maze of conflicting opinions and unscientific "advice" out there and distils the essential principles for making superb protein selections. Proteins are the building blocks of life itself. The section addresses questions such as "How much protein do I need?" "Are there any low-fat, high-protein sources?" and "How can the best sources of protein lower my cholesterol?" ◆

Building on Sections 4, 5 and 6, the next section, **Designing a Prudent Nutritional Program**, brings together the building blocks of the preceding sections—carbs, fats, and proteins—to help you design a personalized nutrition program that will dovetail perfectly with your tastes, needs, budget, and lifestyle. Section 7 shows you what to avoid, what to maximize on, and what to watch out for; offers you a step-by-step analysis of what the different numbers on a typical food label mean; and discusses how to troubleshoot the nutritional program you are developing. ◆

The last section, **Physical Activity: The Other Half of the Equation**, addresses the second great component of the diet-and-exercise duo: how to burn calories. It covers virtually everything you need to know to design a physical activity program that you can enjoy and sustain over a lifetime—one that fits into your lifestyle, produces results without overstressing your body, and helps you improve on all the three dimensions of training: flexibility, strength, and aerobic capacity. One of the hardest things to get right is knowing how hard to exercise: Too casual, and you don't see results. Too hard, and you risk quitting, injury, and even immune system suppression. This section will show you how to subjectively measure intensity, using a number of up-to-date, effective, easy-to-use scientific tools. You will be introduced to different types of enjoyable activity and shown how to achieve a balance between frequency, intensity and duration. Finally, the section outlines both the non-cardiovascular and cardiovascular benefits of exercise, and offers you a full range of practical do's and don'ts. ◆

5.1 ▶ Developing a Broad Strategy

DR. TIMOTHY GILL, the Asia-Pacific regional coordinator for the International Obesity Task Force, on a visit to India, recalls that a driver he had hired to take him around told him that his plan for staying healthy was to save enough money now so that when he had his inevitable heart attack at some point in the future, he would be able to pay for the very best bypass surgeon available. His focus was entirely on treatment, not prevention. "I don't think it ever struck him that he could do something about it or change what could happen," Gill reflected. "Of all Asians, South Asians have by far the worst [heart disease] problems."

As Benjamin Franklin once remarked, "An ounce of prevention is worth a pound of cure." The truth is that it is far more expensive, and more risky, to **treat** heart disease once you have it than to **prevent** it from developing in the first place. One obstacle to more widespread prevention, however, is that too many patients and even physicians are treatment-focused rather than prevention-oriented. For millions of people, the urgency of heart disease—and the crisis it poses not only to an individual but often to an entire family—does not become evident until the disease is at their very doorstep

The lifetime risk of developing heart disease is 49% for men and 32% for women in the US. About 335,000 Americans die of heart disease every year before reaching a hospital.

and is in an advanced stage. Consider this: The US healthcare system, all told, devotes about 99% of its budget to treatment, and just 1% to prevention. From salaries to departmental budgets, prevention is massively underfunded at all levels. Most healthcare plans are similarly more willing to spend far more on covering expensive invasive procedures needed by a very sick person with heart disease than on covering less costly preventive measures that would have helped to keep the person from becoming sick, such as advanced lipid tests, a smoking cessation program, or health club membership. It has been said that healthcare in many countries, including western countries, focuses more on "disease care" than on the proactive promotion of healthful living through aggressive preventive strategies.

Although the tools of high technology can be lifesaving, and bypas surgery can be dramatic and heroic, consistent, daily, aggressive management of cardiac risk factors is in the long run the most effective and sensible strategy.

In the industrialized nations of the west, great strides have been taken to reduce the death rate from heart disease. In the US, for example, the incidence and mortality rates of heart disease have declined nearly 60% in the past three decades despite a doubling of the rates of diabetes and obesity. Similarly, over the course of the 20th century the lifespan of Americans rose from 50 to 75 years. It needs to be pointed out, however, that much of this progress has come from advances in *treatment* that require a great deal of money as well as a relatively high level of technology—neither of which is readily available throughout much of the developing world.

In 2000, for example, according to the Centers for Medicare and Medicaid Services (CMS), healthcare spending in the United States amounted to 13.2% of US economic output (gross domestic product) and may climb to 17% of GDP by 2011—an astonishing amount of money. If the populations and governments of the Indian sub-continent are to make real headway against heart disease, they will need to lay more emphasis on prevention than the west has done. South Asia cannot afford the number of bypass surgeries and angioplasties performed in the US, however effective these interventions often are in bringing heart disease symptoms under control.

A Word about Terminology
Throughout this book, the term Indian refers to people, who trace their origin to the Indian subcontinent—meaning Bangladesh, India, Pakistan, and Sri Lanka—including those who now live abroad but originate from one of these four countries. "Indian" in this context is ethnically interchangeable with "South Asian," "Indo-Asian," or "Asian Indian." The term thus excludes native Americans but includes more than people from the nation of India.

Measurement Units: As is conventional, blood glucose levels, triglyceride levels, and cholesterol levels are stated throughout this book in milligrams per deciliter (mg/dL). Blood pressure is stated in millimeters of mercury (mmHg).

Heart disease is highly predictable, preventable, and controllable—but it is not *curable* once you have developed it, and there is no single "magic bullet" that can eliminate your risk of dying from a heart attack. Your goal should be to improve your cardiovascular health and quality of life through prevention, detection, and management of risk factors. Although the tools of high technology can be lifesaving, and although bypas surgery can be dramatic and heroic, consistent, daily, aggressive management of cardiac risk factors is in the long run the most effective and sensible strategy. This section provides a broad outline of the most important preventive measures for reducing your risk of heart disease.

Prevention strategies: Populations versus individuals

Physicians, governments, and public health specialists use two fundamental approaches to reduce the incidence of serious diseases such as heart disease. One is to try to identify the highest-risk *individuals* and treat them. The second is to adopt an across-the-board, population-based strategy, without looking at who is or is not at risk, and try to change the behavior, values, and risk factors of the entire population through broad-based policies such as public awareness programs, dissemination of information in the media, changes in school lunches and the regulations that govern what food companies can make and sell. The population-based approach obviously takes much longer, because it involves changing how the cultures views itself, its future, and its values, but when successful it can have a profound effect on an entire nation and its economy. In the US, a 50% reduction in smoking rates and a 30-point decrease in cholesterol levels over the past half century are prime examples of the monumental triumph of a population-based strategy. These two single changes account for 50% of the decline in heart disease in the US in the past three decades. Cary Grant or Sean Connery casually lighting up a cigarette in a hotel lobby simply looks out-of-place, dirty, and old-fashioned to most American teenagers today. Thirty years ago, those same teenagers would have thought it looked "cool." In many parts of America today, a smoker has the image of someone who is shady, not clean-shaven, out of touch with modernity, and slightly out of control. Smoking is no longer the "in-thing."

This is the kind of large-scale, wholesale, across-the-board, cultural change that needs to take place in regions such as South Asia if the tide of heart disease is to be reversed. At the moment, that tide is going in the wrong direction—as Asians become more urbanized, more sedentary, and more fat, and begin to adopt unhealthy practices that western countries are discarding or have discarded.

Tid Bits

It is estimated that just a 2 mm Hg reduction in blood pressure in the entire US population, achievable through salt restriction, would reduce the incidence of heart attack by 6%, stroke by 15% and the prevalence of hypertension by 17%.

This will take time. In the mean time, there is *you*—the individual. My focus is to introduce to you a personal strategy to reduce your risk of heart disease to a far greater degree than you might have thought possible. Take a look at the table below for a summary of these strategies.

Implementing lifestyle changes

The following sections of Chapter V are written in a workshop format. There are several assignments to help you apply the knowledge provided in this book, and detailed research substantiates the value of these ideas. It would be very beneficial to start a journal and track your activities.

If you are the **creative, intuitive** type and require just a few key ideas to get going, then focus on any one part—either the nutrition or the exercise program—and work through some of the ideas. You will get an immediate payoff. Select the suggestions that work for you, and defer those that do not appeal to you right away. If you are open-minded, try each of the ideas presented in this section and see if they work well for you. On the other hand, if you are the **analytical, systematic** type, working through each of these Chapters with a pencil your first time through may be helpful. Spend 30-45 minutes per day, a mini-

Slow Death, by Choice

What exactly is wrong with eating food that is too rich? Not to put too fine a point on it, but basically, you are slowly dying. Imagine falling off the edge of a tall cliff in slow motion: Just because you currently feel fine because you have not yet hit the ground does not mean all is well.

Many people look at heart disease in much the same way that they look at lung cancer: "There's a chance I will get lung cancer if I smoke," they say, "but then again, there's a chance I won't. No one can say beforehand. It happens suddenly." It is a mistake to think of heart disease in such maybe, maybe not terms. Saturated fats, trans fats, and cholesterol cause atherosclerosis slowly, gradually, and systematically, with every single dab of *ghee* you spread on bread. You do not stay disease-free and suddenly develop heart disease one day.

Others have an attitude of fatalism: "I'm young, I'm sure my arteries can stand a little bit of hardening and narrowing. After all, atherosclerosis is just like developing gray hair. It's just natural. It's like slowing down as you grow old." Wrong. Atherosclerosis is *not* "just like gray hair." There are 90-year-olds in rural China and rural Africa who have no plaque at all in their arteries! Hardened, narrow arteries are not inevitable. Aging is; plaque is not.

Fatalistic resignation is precisely what promotes disorders such as coronary artery disease that you could avoid, retard or reverse if you aggressively took hold of the major risk factors in your life-especially having fat around your middle, lack of exercise, smoking, diabetes, having unbalanced levels of cholesterol, triglycerides, homocysteine, and lipoprotein(a), and eating food that is too rich. Dying from heart disease is *not karma*. It is really a slow death by choice.

mum of four times a week on different assignments. Work on improving your mental habits, eating healthy foods suited to your taste, and enhancing your life with appropriate physical activity.

What on Earth is Primordial Prevention?
"Primordial" used in this context does not mean prehistoric, like a primordial forest. It means basic or fundamental first-line prevention. It is a technical term used in the public health literature by organizations such as the World Health Organization.   The goal of Primordial Prevention is to help you avoid developing high-risk factors from the get go. Primordial Prevention is what *everybody* should do, whether you are 14 or 74, at risk or fit as a fiddle.

EIGHT PREVENTIVE STRATEGIES

The following sub-section summarizes eight strategies to successful, sustainable prevention.

1. Quit smoking

Smoking is one of the most important risk factors of heart disease and lung cancer. Only an estimated 9% of Americans aged 65 and older are smokers, yet this group accounts for two-thirds (300,000 of the 440,000) of Americans who die every year from smoking-related diseases. If you smoke, it is important that you make the most concerted effort you can to stop right now! No single step you take can improve your cardiovascular outlook more than quitting smoking. With that one change, you can reduce your risk of heart attack by more than 50% within one year. Passive or "second-hand" smoking can be almost as bad for you. Fortunately, in the US, most workplaces are smoke-free, and increasingly, other public spaces such as movie theaters, restaurants, airports, museums, and subway and train stations have joined this trend. In many developing countries, however, this is not always true, and even children are exposed to secondary smoking.

The American Heart Association currently has an initiative to reduce smoking rates throughout the US by 50% and deaths from stroke and heart attack by 25%, by 2010. Many conveniently administered, nicotine-replacement medications and programs are available to help you minimize the physical discomfort caused by nicotine withdrawal when you stop smoking, but the most important first step is for you to make the decision to quit. Most users find that this psychological challenge is the biggest hurdle in quitting. The physical symptoms themselves, while annoying, are not life-threatening. Several methods that slowly wean you off nicotine to minimize withdrawal cravings are available—including gums, lozenges, nasal sprays, inhalers, patches, and the drug bupropion (Zyban). The following websites are among the many that offer helpful information about quitting smoking: www.cancer.org, www.quitnet.com, www.quitsmokingsupport.com, and www.whyquit.com. In addition, Medicare's 2005 prescription drug benefit will cover smoking cessation treatments that are prescribed by a physi

Table 5.1. Categories of Prevention	
Primordial Prevention For healthy people without risk factors or heart disease and normal waist and weight (to avoid having high risk factors)	Regular physical activity (4 to 5 hours/week) Prudent Nutrition Program Prevention of weight gain in childhood and adult life Maintenance of ideal body weight and waist line Lifetime avoidance of smoking Maintenance of low-risk status
Primary Prevention For people who have substantial cardiac risk factors such as smoking, diabetes, dyslipi demia and/or hypertension (to ward off heart disease)	Basic prevention as listed above, plus Physical activity (6 to 7 hours/week) Weight loss and its maintenance Smoking cessation Control of blood pressure Control of dyslipidemia Control of blood sugar
Secondary Prevention For people who have survived a heart-attack, undergone angioplasty or bypass surgery or have been diagnosed with heart disease	Primary prevention as listed above, plus Aspirin (81-325mg daily) ACE inhibitors Beta-blockers Tighter control of dyslipidemia Cardiac rehabilitation
Tertiary Prevention For immediate control of severe symptoms of heart disease	Balloon angioplasty Bare-metal stent or drug-releasing stent Coronary bypass surgery

2. Consider aspirin therapy, but also its potential risks

In a recent study of high-risk men, aspirin reduced the risk of a heart attack by 32% and stroke by 13%. However, many people take aspirin daily to prevent a heart attack without realizing its risks and potential side effects. Your physician may recommend that you take daily low-dose aspirin (81mg) if you are in the medium- or high-risk category. However, because of potential gastrointestinal problems such as stomach upsets, perforation, and bleeding, daily aspirin is not recommended to healthy individuals who do not have at least two traditional cardiac risk factors. In such low-risk people, aspirin's risks may outweigh the benefits because, unlike statins, it is associated with significant side effects. This is discussed in greater detail in Chapter VIII, Section 3.

3. Load up on fruits and vegetables

In 2000, 81% of men and 73% of women stated that they ate fewer than five servings of fruits and vegetables a day, according to data from the Centers for Disease Control. Greater intake of fruits and vegetables is associated with up to a one-third lower risk of cardiovascular disease, cancer, and several other diseases. This finding supports the general health recommendation to consume 10-12 servings (5-6 cups) a day of fruits and vegetables. Sections 3 to 7 discuss nutrition in much greater detail.

4. Eat nuts

Nuts are nutritious snacks that fit well into a busy schedule. In the past, many people have avoided nuts because of their high fat content. However, most of the fat in nuts is unsaturated and thus healthy (see Chapter V, Section 4). Several studies have shown that the modest consumption of nuts is associated with a 30-50% reduction in heart disease. It is not completely understood why, but possible mechanisms include a reduction in LDL, the antioxidant action of vitamin E, which is abundant in many nuts, and improved platelet function that decreases the tendency for unwarranted blood clotting.

Microwaving nuts for a few seconds enhances their taste and texture. It is important to stick with the unsalted variety to control your intake of sodium. Roasted nuts purchased from the grocery stores may contain a significant amount of unhealthy oils and salt. Check the label. Caramelized nut products are not recommended because of their high sugar content. Eating nuts daily will not promote weight gain if you do not eat too much of them, and if you make room for them by cutting down on other calories.

Table 5.2. Fat composition in selected foods

Nuts	Calories (per 100g)	Total fat (g)	Monounsaturated fat (g)	Polyunsaturated fat (g)	Saturated fat (g)
Pecan	710	74	44	21	6
Almond	597	53	34	13	4
Cashew	574	46	27	8	9
Flax seed	492	34	7	22	3
Coconut meat	684	69	3	1	61
Avocado	177	17	11	2	3

Source: Enas EA. Ref 5.9. Note that most nuts are high in heart-healthy monounsaturated fats. Note by comparison how little unsaturated fat and how much saturated fat coconut contains.

5. Use alcohol judiciously

Moderate alcohol consumption appears to reduce the risk of heart attack and stroke. No more than two servings of alcohol for men and one for women per day is cardioprotective. These recommendations should not be exceeded. Some studies suggest that even one or two drinks per week is sufficient. Alcohol, though, is not without dangers. Binge drinking (defined as three or more drinks in one sitting) is harmful to the heart, liver, and brain. It may increase blood pressure, homocysteine and triglyceride levels, and can precipitate a heart attack or stroke. Those who do not like drinking are not encouraged to start drinking for cardiac protection. This topic is discussed in Section 3.

6. Take personal initiative

"*Buyer beware*," as the commercial law saying goes. The public is constantly bombarded with confusing, often conflicting advice on how to prevent and treat heart disease, and the press often reports on new medical findings that will have "a dramatic impact" on your life. Stories of medical miracles and breakthroughs crowd front pages of newspapers and magazines. "According to the latest studies…" has become a mantra in the media.

It is important to keep these new findings in perspective and read them in context. Often, the whole story is not fully evident. A large, single, multi-year study of 28,000 people conducted across 52 countries, such as the INTERHEART study, is likely to have much greater scientific merit than 30 small studies each done on just 100 people in one country or at one institution. Before you accept the quick interpretations of the media, you should read the original scientific publication for yourself. If you find it convincing, the next step is to check with your physician before you act on the publication's conclusions.

This book provides guidelines on important risk factors, such as cholesterol level and hypertension, that are collated from a large number of major studies and are current as of June 2005. Bear in mind also that, as new scientific knowledge emerges, scientific bodies such as the CDC or WHO may raise or lower the cut-points for various risk factors. What was considered acceptable just 50 years ago—for example, a systolic blood pressure of 250 mm Hg—may today seem outrageously high, even irresponsible. Currently, a blood pressure of 115/75 mm Hg is considered optimum; this is down from the 120/80 standard that had held for many years. Similarly, the current optimum LDL is 40mg/dL, which corresponds to a total cholesterol level of just 115. Again, when I was in training to become a cardiologist at Cook County Hospital in Chicago, *cholesterol of 330* was considered normal. Ask your physician about the latest guidelines for your particular problems and insist that he or she finds out what they are. Your physician will review your current status of health and often recommend an appropriate prevention strategy.

> The existing threshold for when to initiate treatment for a specific risk factor may not reflect how dangerous it is to you, but rather a judgment about whether the health system has the means to treat you. This is why you must actively engage your doctor in probing discussions about what these numbers all mean—for you

Depending on what the current cut-points are, the thresholds for initiating drug treatment of blood pressure, cholesterol, and overall cardiovascular risk require careful case-by-case consideration. Since the benefit you will gain from obtaining treatment increases as the cut-point for a particular risk factor is lowered, any across-the-board advice in a book would be somewhat arbitrary. A small reduction in the threshold can substantially increase the number of people who need treatment, as well as the urgency with which they need it. The question of what thresholds should be issued is thus partly a matter of practical resource constraints and social values. Countries of different economic status may recommend different thresholds, and often, the thresholds are simply not aggressive enough.

What this means is that the threshold that exists in your particular country, or state, for initiating treatment for a particular risk factor may not reflect how harmful that risk factor is to you, but rather whether your community's public health system has the resources to treat you. Risk factors, however, are real, not just policy numbers. They represent real organic conditions in your body that could be hastening your progress toward the crisis point of a major coronary event. This is why it is important that you not let yourself become a passive healthcare consumer. You need to stay on top of health issues and actively engage your physician in probing down-to-earth conversations about what these numbers all mean, for you.

7. Know your numbers

Checking and remembering the results of your blood pressure, blood sugar, total cholesterol, and HDL levels are more important than you realize. Asking for these tests and being able to recall these numbers are more important to the quality of your life, certainly your health, than remembering even the dates of birthdays and wedding anniversaries! A 2004 survey found that, in the preceding 12 months, 58% of Americans had had their blood pressure checked and 83% had had their cholesterol checked. Those numbers are good, but the percentage of people who actually remember their blood pressure and cholesterol numbers is far less encouraging. Approximately one-third of the general population never bother to find out at all. Another third do, but then do not remember which number is which. Only a third find out and remember these values as well as what they mean.

8. Adopt a multi-pronged approach: Take aim at several risk factors

Advances in medicine over the last 50 years have identified several lifestyle factors as well as medications that, acting together, are capable of reducing the risk of a first heart attack by **more than 95%** (see Table 5.2). Quitting a smoking habit, for example, can cut your risk of a first heart attack by up to 70%, compared to those who continue to smoke. Bringing your LDL cholesterol level to less than 100 can lower your risk by up to 65%, compared to if you did not. Clearly, quitting smoking *and* lowering your LDL to below 100 will not result in reducing your heart attack risk by up to 70% plus 65%! Your risk reduction cannot go down by more than 100%, because 100% represents zero risk. You cannot add them up that way. In addition, some of the factors are not necessarily independent variables. Exercising (#4), for example, contributes to and overlaps with maintaining ideal body weight (#5). Rather, the way to read this chart is that the more risk-reduction strategies you follow, the closer your risk of a first heart attack will approach zero.

Note, too, that many of these risk-reduction strategies are synergistic, interactive, and mutually reinforcing. They strengthen the effect of one another. A corollary to this is that the risk factors themselves are also synergistic. One risk factor tends to make the effect of another risk factor worse, and they work together to accelerate atherosclerosis and hasten heart disease. This synergistic interaction of both health factors and risk factors is why you are strongly encouraged to reduce your risks by following *multiple* strategies rather than just limiting your efforts to just one or two.

The reason is that the combined effect of cardiac risk factors on your health are not just additive but exponential. For example, a diabetic smoker who also has hypertension increases his or her risk of a first heart attack by **16-fold,** compared to someone who has none these three risk factors, even though each of the risk factors, individually, conveys only a two-fold to three-fold risk. The addition of elevated LDL cholesterol and low HDL cholesterol to the existing three factors increases the risk further to **32-fold.** Adding obesity to the existing four risks increases the person's risk to **64-fold.** Cardiovascular risk factors, in other words, act in concert, intensifying each other's effect in a multiplicative way. As a result, a comprehensive strategy aimed at all these six risk factors yields far better benefits than focusing on just one or two of these.

Table 5.3. How much specific lifestyle changes reduce your risk of a first heart attack, compared to those who do not make that change

	Change in Lifestyle	Risk Reduction
1	Smoking cessation	50-70%
2	Lowering your LDL level to below 100mg/dL	35-65%
3	Controlling blood pressure to no more than 120/80	30%
4	Physical activities that burns more than 2000 calories per week	45%
5	Maintaining an ideal body weight and waistline	35%
6	Increasing HDL to 60mg/dL	50%
7	Eating five servings of fruits and five servings of vegetables daily	30%
8	Eating 30-50g of nuts a day	30%
9	Alcohol consumption in small quantities (fewer than 2 drinks per day for men, 1 for women)	25 to 45%
10	Taking low-dose aspirin (81mg a day in moderate and high-risk individuals)	25 to 33%
	Benefit of all changes combined	more than 95%

KEY · POINTS · IN · A · NUTSHELL

♥ Heart disease has become the most predictable, preventable, and treatable of all chronic diseases.

♥ The four major categories of prevention are primordial, primary, secondary and tertiary prevention.

♥ The most effective and least expensive prevention strategy is to stop smoking. An important point, however, is that non-smokers should not become complacent, particularly Indians, because emergent risk factors can still put them at high risk.

♥ The risk of a heart attack can be reduced by more than 95% by controlling the key modifiable risk factors. These include diabetes, high LDL cholesterol, low HDL cholesterol, high lipoprotein(a), high blood pressure, excess body weight, and large waist size.

♥ Smoking, having hypertension, and having diabetes increases your risk of a first heart attack by 16-fold, compared to someone who has none of these risk factors—even though each factor individually conveys only a two-fold to three-fold higher risk.

♥ The addition of elevated LDL and low HDL increases the risk to 32-fold. The addition of obesity to all these increases the risk to 64-fold.

♥ Eating generous amounts of fruits and vegetables everyday, along with a small amount of nuts, is highly effective in preventing heart disease.

♥ Moderate use of alcohol has a protective effect, but excess consumption and binge drinking raise your triglyceride and blood preasure levels are counter-productive.

♥ As new scientific knowledge emerges, the cut-points for various risk factors may be lowered even further. The long-term trend over the past several decades indicates that the medical community has systematically underestimated how dangerous various risk factors are.

♥ The best action plan is for you to be as aggressive in lowering your cardiac risk factors as you can.

5.2 ▶ Finding the Motivation to Change

The complex software of the mind

If our brains worked like the electronic chip in a robot or a computer, every overweight person at risk of developing heart disease could simply drive themselves to a nearby Service Center, have a technician plug them into the latest Learning Module, press a few keys, and reprogram their brain with a concise set of instructions: "Exercise more. Eat less. Avoid harmful fats." And that would be that. Unfortunately, or fortunately, our minds do not work that way. We are complex beings with complex motivational structures.

Everyone knows the benefits of a healthful lifestyle; but look around and you will see that few follow it regularly. Most of us can easily list the times—weeks, months, sometimes years—that we have failed to exercise or eat healthfully. Yet these embarrassing memories of personal failure rarely motivate us to do better. Everyone has successes, yet rarely do we focus on our successes and use them as launching pads to attain a more optimal level of health.

In this section, I will show you powerful ways to motivate yourself by identifying your strengths and driving forces of success toward a healthy lifestyle. Given our busy schedules and multiple commitments, healthy eating and regular exercise are undoubtedly challenging tasks. And I cannot offer you a $49.95 Software Learning Module that you can instantly plug into your brain to reprogram it, the way Neo and the rest of the crew do it in the movie *The Matrix*. I believe, however, that with the right desire and motivation, you will be able to find the appropriate balance of satisfaction, enjoyment, goal achievement, and discipline to create and maintain a healthful lifestyle. Knowledge, in its own way, does rewire the mind. And that is what this book offers you.

This section examines the importance of motivation in pursuing a realistic yet effective risk-reduction program based on balanced, real-world nutritional changes. Even more important, it discusses how to find that motivation. A few assignments have been provided to help you identify your inner strengths and the possible barriers that have in the past thwarted your attempts to pursue such goals.

Benefits of healthy eating and regular exercise

A healthy lifestyle provides many physiological, biochemical and metabolic benefits:

- You will feel energized within one to two weeks of implementing a regular exercise and a nutrition program.

- Your mood will improve as a result of endorphins released in your brain.

- Your blood pressure will come within a desirable range, and if you take blood pressure medications, you may be able to reduce their number or dosage.

- If you have dyslipidemia, you will improve your lipid profile. With regular exercise, high triglycerides will come down by 30% within two to three months; HDL will increase 10% in about 10 months.

- If you have diabetes, you will have better control of your blood sugar because your insulin resistance will fall as your muscles begin to use insulin better in response to exercise; if you are taking medications, you may be able to lower your medication dosage and sometimes eliminate them altogether.

- Your immune system will be strengthened; you will be less susceptible to flu, the common cold, and repeat infections. If you do get a cold, you will recover faster.

- In the long run, you will reduce your risks for heart disease, cancer, and other ailments.

What are the challenges to a healthy lifestyle?

Many of us cheat ourselves out of the benefits of a healthy life. How many times have you heard these excuses?

1. "I'm always on the move. My schedule doesn't permit me to exercise regularly or eat healthy."
Response: With regular exercise and appropriate nutrition, you become more productive and enjoy your increased energy level. Presidents George Bush Sr. and Bill Clinton **found time** in their busy schedules to exercise 45 to 60 minutes a day, as does the current president George W. Bush. If *they* can find the time, so can you.

2. "I have tried it before and failed."
Response: Focusing on the past cannot provide solutions to the future. Perhaps you tried too hard, or approached it the wrong way. There are many dysfunctional approaches to nutrition and exercise. Have faith in yourself and try it once more—my way. Every time you eat healthy or exercise, you are providing significant benefits to your body and mind even if you are not aware of it. Focus on these benefits, and you will be motivated to continue your health improvement program.

3. "What's the point? A friend of mine exercised regularly but still suffered a heart attack."
Response: Your friend may very well have died from a heart attack 10 to 20 years earlier had he *not* exercised. Statistics indicate that regular exercise and proper nutrition can add 10 to 20 productive and disability-free years to your life. Regular exercise has a significant protective effect against sudden death; and exercise strengthens your heart's ability to survive a heart attack because, among other things, it increases both your heart's ability to pump blood and your blood's capacity to carry oxygen. There is no way to completely eliminate the risk of heart disease, but you can definitely reduce the risk substantially.

4. "Something just tells me that a heart attack will never happen to me."
Response: Really? Statistics say otherwise! If you are over 20, chances are that a biopsy or angiogram

of your arteries would show that atherosclerotic plaques have *almost certainly* started to develop! You just can't see them. In addition, there is no correlation between symptoms and severity of heart disease. You can feel perfectly fine yet still be seriously sick—until something suddenly strikes. Half of all patients who die suddenly have no prior symptoms of heart disease. Among people with heart disease, sudden death is the first symptom of heart disease that about one-third ever experience, and heart attack is the first symptom that another third experience. One-third of people stricken with a heart attack die within three months. And heart attacks do not wait for you to be conveniently near a hospital before they occur: Two-thirds of all deaths from heart attacks occur before the person ever reached the hospital.

5. "I'll definitely make the changes—after my 60th birthday or retirement."
Response: This excuse is more of an expression of chronic procrastination than a real plan. It is the mind's way of fooling itself into thinking that you are serious about making the changes. The sooner you make these changes, the sooner will you get the benefits. Besides, like childbirth, it is much harder to start exercising or to make other fundamental changes at 60 than at 30.

Assignment 1

What are *your* top three excuses? Don't just verbalize them. Write them down here and consider what you can do to transform them from a mountain to a mole hill:

My favorite excuse	What can I do about it?
1.	
2.	
3.	

Mental training and motivation

It is important to realize that lifestyle changes occur only when your mind sees an emotional benefit to the change (not necessarily a logical benefit). You have probably heard or read about people quitting smoking, heroin, or alcohol-drinking cold turkey. To offer you a bit of personal detail: I quit smoking cold turkey after two years of smoking. The cold turkey method works for some but, not for all. Be prepared for a possible relapse, especially if you are will-power challenged. As Michael Dell of Dell Computers has said, there is a distinction between a dreamer and a visionary. Both have dreams, but the visionary has the will, the focus, the persistence, and the means to achieve that dream. *Are you a dreamer or a visionary?*

Knowing what you really want is half the battle. The other half, however, is making the right changes in your life. Your mind is a powerful machine. You can use its power to help you reach your goals.

The need to change

Next, consider the implications of good versus poor health in your life. Some people are motivated by the negative implications of their unhealthy lifestyle or habits and will work to prevent potential health incidents. Others are motivated by the pictures of good health and well-being. Ask yourself the following questions:

- If I get a heart attack at this moment, what impact will it have on me, my family, my friends, and loved ones?

- What would life look like if I were extremely healthy, with abundant energy and enthusiasm? How would I feel?

- What images or thoughts come to your mind? Which of these strongly affects you on an emotional or cognitive level? We all want to be free of pain and discomfort—the big question is whether you feel the positive benefits of a health-oriented program outweigh the pain of pursuing it, or is keeping the same unhealthy lifestyle easier? What is the price of not pursuing a proactive pathway to better health? If you ask yourself these questions on a daily basis, you will find the motivation to change! Remember, an unfit and unhealthy body may not allow you to enjoy the fruits of your labor in retirement or spend quality time with your grandchildren.

Drawing on your past successes: What drives you?

How do you achieve success? What personal methods do you use? You can use the answers to these questions to make the necessary nutritional and physical activity changes in your lifestyle. The same emotions and personality traits that enabled you to achieve success in other areas of your life are the ones that will assist you in the area of health-oriented lifestyle changes. Examine some of your personal successes over the past three to five years. What are your strengths and skills?

For example, you may be persistent, methodical, and detail-oriented at work, and you like to take one thing at a time. Or perhaps you are someone who is driven by the Big Picture, by blue-sky inspiration, the way a sail catches the wind. Perhaps you are someone who needs a support group of nurturing friends who offer gentle encouragement. Or just the opposite: you need a locker-room buddy who challenges you to achieve difficult goals and says, "I'll bet you $30 you can't do this." What drives you?

It is important that you identify what emotions, ideas, and values drive you to make productive changes in your professional life or in your relationships. You can use those same emotions and aptitudes to launch a powerful nutrition and physical activity program. In turn, your success in staying on your nutrition and activity program may feed back into other areas of your personal and professional life, revealing to you hidden strengths and reserves that you did not know you had.

Strengths and traits that drive people to success
Flexibility
Competitiveness
Analytical skills
Discipline
Planning & Execution
Focus
Creativity
Perseverance
Other skills

Assignment 2

Write down three specific successes or achievements in your recent past. They could be related to your professional or personal life. Picture the events that led to that achievement as if they were a movie. What did people say when you achieved your goals? Were there any emotions that were associated with that time period that helped motivate you to work to those goals? Was it fear/anxiety, anger, passion, enthusiasm, a cause, or perhaps hope? Was it just being tired of mediocrity, a desire to make a positive difference in other people's lives, a sense of self-worth, a desire for vindication, or possibly a drive to be recognized as capable, self-willed, and disciplined? Are you driven more by internal or by external cues, and what kind?

Assignment 3

Success or achievement	Key emotions associated with working toward or achieving this goal
1.	
2.	
3.	

For each of these three successes, write down the skills and talents you used or had to learn in order to achieve that goal. Pick out the top two to three characteristics in you. It is essential to keep these strengths in mind when you create a successful lifestyle change program.

The importance of rewards

Regardless of what our particular personality type is, we are all driven, either consciously or subconsciously, by the idea of achieving some kind of benefit when we successfully make a change. The benefit may be self-esteem: for example, losing weight and appearing attractive to someone in our life. Or achieving a greater measure of existential security: for example, avoiding serious illness or premature death. It could be religious: for example, honoring and respecting your body as a temple of God's Spirit, and having the feeling of receiving God's approval for doing so. Each of these benefits is a type of reward.

I suggest that, in your path toward the ultimate goal of excellent health and very low risk factors, if that is your goal, you pick out a number of intermediate, along-the-way goals, and figure out how to reward yourself for reaching each of these smaller, midway goals. For example, if you plan to lose 30 pounds in one year, set an intermediate goal of losing 10 pounds in three months. The reward may be almost anything you like: a party, a trip to Las Vegas, or a shopping spree for new clothes, or something less ambitious. Here is another idea: Promise yourself a trip to the movies or to a play with your spouse or significant other if you succeed in sticking to eating at least one bowl of salad as part of your meal everyday for two weeks.

Rewards, even small ones, reinforce habits, as the behavioral psychologist Ivan Pavlov demonstrated through his experiments with dogs a century ago. Rewards have a powerful conditioning effect on the mind. (That, in fact, is the basis of addiction.) According to Thorndike's Law of Effect, if you perform an activity and are **rewarded** for it, you are more likely to do it again and again, because a response to a given situation that produces satisfaction becomes associated in the mind with that situation. It is amazing that once you reward yourself, the reward becomes psychologically associated at a deep level with the behavior, and you will be motivated to continue making progress.

Another form of reward is to focus on the short-term benefits of regular physical activity and eating healthy. You will find that the consistent combination of these two will provide you with a powerful natural healing power and method of regeneration.

What happens when you slip up? As you make these changes, you may find that you are not 100% compliant with your nutrition or exercise program. Don't worry about minor setbacks and temporary failures. In fact, do not strive to be a perfectionist! Just focus on picking up from where you left off and being *consistent over time*. You are human, not a machine. Gradually, you will be able to identify definite, specific changes in your psychology and physiology as you make steady progress.

KEY · POINTS · IN · A · NUTSHELL

- ♥ Lifestyle changes will remain a dream without proper motivation, planning, and action.
- ♥ Some people can motivate themselves by focusing on the negative consequences, others by the positive consequences or benefits.
- ♥ You can apply the skills and emotions that have helped you achieve your past successes in order to set goals and make appropriate lifestyle changes possible.
- ♥ Benefits of healthy lifestyle include more energy, improved immunity to diseases, and a sense of well being.
- ♥ An unfit and unhealthy body may not allow you to enjoy the fruits of your labor in retirement or spend quality time with your grandchildren.
- ♥ Other benefits include prevention and control of obesity, hypertension and diabetes.
- ♥ A consistently healthy lifestyle can lower your healthcare costs by 75% or more.
- ♥ Don't attempt to be a perfectionist; be a consistent pragmatist

5.3 ▶ Introducing the Prudent Nutrition Program

Numerous studies over the past fifty years have shown that a well-balanced, sensible diet can prevent heart disease and its complications to a degree similar to that observed with the most effective medications used to lower cholesterol, statins. The Prudent Diet presented in this section is rich in all the right things: fruits, vegetables, nuts, whole grains, legumes, low-fat dairy products, fish, and lean cuts of meat, while being low in saturated fats and high glycemic index food such as refined carbohydrates. Implementing the Prudent Diet is easier than you think. Because it is a balanced diet, you are much more likely to stay on it than on some of the more extreme diet that emphasize one food category at the expense of another. A diet that you cannot stay on for your entire life is a diet that will lead to failure, because eventually your body and your taste buds will rebel against it.

The purpose of this Chapter is to describe key aspects of a nutrition program that minimizes your risk of developing obesity, diabetes, and heart disease and controlling them if you are already suffering from these conditions. This Chapter describes the principles underlying a sensible, balanced, cardioprotective diet that emphasizes heart-healthy preventive nutrition, and how the Indian diet can be modified to embrace all of its nutritional requirements.

The Prudent Nutrition Program

Let's go over the key components of the Prudent Nutrition Program, outlined in the box below.

1. Hunger satisfaction

Do you get hungry again within a couple of hours after eating lunch or dinner? You are probably trying to lose weight on an excessively restrictive low-calorie diet. My Prudent Nutrition Program will leave you feeling satisfied even four to six hours after a meal, and one to two hours after a snack. I show you food choices that will keep you feeling full even though they are low in calories.

2. Great taste

Research shows that people stay on a nutrition program if they like the food they eat. So it is essential that you find foods that really appeal to you. The Prudent Nutrition Program encourages you to try out a wide range of fruits and vegetables that offer a variety many times higher than meat products.

3. Nutritionally sufficient

The Prudent program is geared to meeting your body's need for *macronutrients* (protein, carbohydrates, fat) as well as *micronutrients* (minerals, vitamins, antioxidants, phytonutrients, and other vital trace substances), both of which are essential for the healthy functioning of your body. There is no scientific basis for loading yourself with multivitamin supplements. You should be able to get all the micronutrients you need by eating 9-13 servings of fruits and vegetables as recommended by the 2005 Dietary Guidelines by US government. As discussed earlier, one ounce of nuts (a handful), the recommended daily amount, provides additional minerals, vitamins, and fiber. In special cases, fiber supplementation and omega-3 supplementation may be appropriate (see Chapter VI, Section 2). A meta-analysis of 136,000 people involving 19 studies has shown that taking no more than 200 IU of vitamin E a day is safe, but taking more than 400 IU a day can be dangerous. Most people get 15 units a day from their diet alone and another 30 to 60 IU if they take multivitamins. High doses of vitamin E may increase the tendency for blood clots and even death.

> **Key Components: The Prudent Nutrition Program**
> - Created to work synergistically with increased physical activity
> - Hunger satisfaction
> - Great taste
> - Nutritionally sufficient
> - Carbohydrate balanced
> - High in fiber
> - Moderate in healthy fats
> - Sensibly low in calories
> - Permits moderate use of alcohol

The 2005 Dietary Guidelines for Americans (DGA)

The Prudent Nutrition Program presented here is consistent with the 2005 Dietary Guidelines for Americans (DGA), recently issued by the US government. Here are the principal components of the DGA. In April 2005, the influential United States Department of Agriculture (USDA) unveiled its new food pyramid, which summarizes the DGA's recommendations. The food pyramid can be found at www.mypyramid.gov

- Get most of your nutrients by eating a variety of nutrient-dense foods which provide the highest vitamin and nutrient contents with the fewest calories
- Choose foods and beverages with little added sugar, or without caloric sweeteners
- Consume fewer sugary and starchy food to maintain good oral hygiene
- Prevent weight gain
- Get more exercise (60 minutes for normal weight people and 90 minutes for overweight persons most days of the week)
- Eat more vegetables and fruits (10-12 servings or 5-6 cups per day)
- Choose vegetables from five subgroups (dark green, orange, legumes, starchy vegetables, and other vegetables) several times a week
- Eat more whole grains
- Eat 3 cups of fat-free or low-fat dairy products per day
- Eat less saturated fat, cholesterol, and trans fat
- Choose healthy, low-glycemic carbohydrates, and avoid fat-laden, sugar-laden or refined carbohydrates
- Reduce salt consumption to 2300mg a day and increase potassium consumption
- Limit alcohol consumption to one drink per day for women and two for men
- Maintain good hygiene: Clean your hands, food contact surfaces, fruits and vegetables
- Avoid unpasteurized milk and juice, raw or undercooked eggs, and raw or undercooked meat and poultry

4. Carbohydrate balanced

In the wake of enthusiasm over the Atkins Diet, there has been a recent tendency to deride and misunderstand the role of "carbs" in the diet. This is terribly short-sighted. The Institute of Medicine of the Academy of Science recommends a minimum of 130 grams of carbohydrates per day for the proper functioning of the brain. As **Section 5** explains, however, all carbohydrates are not created equal. Some are much better for you than others.

5. High in fiber

The current recommendation is to eat between 25 and 35 grams of fiber a day. Fiber lowers the cholesterol and blood sugar, cleans out your digestive tract, and keeps you regular. High-fiber foods include fruits, vegetables, whole grains, and beans.

The only kind of weight-reduction diet that is both sustainable and healthy is a nutritionally sufficient, high-fiber, low-calorie, carbohydrate-balanced, cardioprotective diet composed around great-tasting, low glycemic index ingredients that you are already familiar with and can readily find.

6. Moderate in healthy fats such as nuts and fish

Nuts are a powerhouse of nutrients. They are perhaps the best natural source of vitamin E and are relatively concentrated repositories of dietary fiber, magnesium, potassium, and arginine, the dietary precursor of nitric oxide. The FDA has recently allowed a qualified health recommendation for the following nuts: almonds, peanuts, pecan, pistachio, hazel nuts and walnuts. Scientific evidence suggests that eating an ounce of any of these nuts a day, as part of a diet low in saturated fat and cholesterol, may help reduce the risk of heart disease. A healthy diet incorporating nuts has been shown to reduce the risk of heart disease by 25% to 35%. The Dietary Approaches to Stop Hypertension (DASH) Diet also recommends regular consumption of nuts along with seeds and dried beans (four to five servings per week) as part of a diet to control hypertension (see Chapter VI, Section 1). Some studies have found that substituting almonds and walnuts for other fats can reduce LDL by 8% to 12% and increase HDL 10% to 15%. Other studies show that macadamias and hazelnuts are beneficial. Almonds are high in protein and vitamin E, while walnuts are high in omega-3 fatty acids.

Until recently, peanuts were not considered as healthy as other nuts. We now know that the fat found in peanuts is actually good for us; for one thing, it does not clog arteries like saturated fat. Peanuts contain a respectable list of nutrients—vitamin E, niacin, thiamin, riboflavin, vitamin B_6, and essential minerals such as copper, phosphorous, potassium, zinc and magnesium. They also are a good source of fiber and protein and contain a small amount of resveratrol, the potent antioxidant in red wine.

As always, however, peanuts, like any other nuts, should be consumed in moderation: A single ounce of peanuts has 14 grams of fat, meaning that a handful can have up to 200 calories. One needs to be extremely careful to eat "peanut sized" portions of nuts to avoid overconsumption. If you can limit nuts to one ounce, however, it is a well-spent 200 calories.

Fish—a mouth-watering way to prevent sudden death

Have you noticed? Fish never die from heart attacks. Similarly, populations that eat large amounts of fish—Japanese and Eskimos, for example—have low rates of death from heart disease. Replacing high-fat meat with fatty fish can cut your risk of sudden death 40% to 60%. Eating 40 to 60 grams of fish a day (or two fish meals per week) is optimal. Eating 300 grams of fish per week also lowers inflammatory markers such as C-reactive protein by a third. A greater intake confers no additional benefit. Eating fish regularly also reduces the risk of diabetes. The beneficial effect of fatty fish is greater than that of lean fish or shellfish. In one study, consumption of fish one to three times per month was associated with a 40% reduction in diabetes, and a 64% reduction in diabetes was noted among those who consumed fish more than five times per month.

Fish also protects against stroke. In the Cardiovascular Health Study, eating tuna or other broiled or baked fish—but not fried fish, fish sandwiches, or fish burgers—one to four times a week was associated with a 27% lower risk of stroke, compared to people who ate fish less than once per month. In contrast, eating fried fish or fish sandwiches more than once a week was associated with a 44% higher risk of stroke compared with consumption of less than once per month. Another thing that may be even more dangerous is the repeated use of the *same oil for frying*, because it leads to the accumulation of dangerous trans fatty acids and oxidation products.

7. Sensibly low in calories

Calorie reduction is a central goal in any weight-reduction diet, and perhaps the most difficult one to achieve. Even a 10% reduction of your total calories (120 calories out of a 1200-calorie diet) can go a long way toward achieving and maintaining optimal weight. Agencies used to recommend 2000 calories per day for men and 1500 calories for women. America's obesity epidemic, however, has forced various national agencies to reevaluate the average person's caloric requirements. Table 5.4 gives the 2004 guidelines, recommended jointly by American Diabetes Association, the North American Association for the Study of Obesity, and the American Society for Clinical Nutrition. Note that since most Indians weigh less than 200 pounds, their average daily calorie requirement is only 1000 to 1200. These recommendations are not etched in stone and can be increased depending upon the individual's level of physical activity. It is also okay to indulge occasionally, but keep in mind that these are borrowed calories which you need to "pay back" before the end of the week.

Table 5.4. Calorie intake for healthy weight loss among adults: A joint recommendation by American Diabetes Association, the North American Association for the Study of Obesity, and the American Society for Clinical Nutrition.

Body weight (pounds)	150 to 199	200 to 249	250 to 300
Suggested daily calorie intake for healthy weight loss (1-2 pounds/week)	1000 to 1200	1200 to 1500	1500 to 1800

Source: Klein, S. Ref 5.27.

8. Judicious use of alcohol

Studies suggest that moderate alcohol intake helps to prevent heart attacks. The permissible limit is two drinks for men and one for women a day. Recently, it has been shown that just one drink per week provides the same amount of cardiac protection. More than two drinks per day do not provide any additional protection and may even be dangerous. Binge drinking is anything more than *five drinks per* occasion for men, or more than four for women.

Should you drink wine or beer? The greater protection wine appears to confer when compared to other types of alcohol may reflect healthier lifestyle habits among wine drinkers, who generally have a higher socioeconomic status. However, red wine's high antioxidant content may also be important. The antioxidant activities of one glass of red wine (150 ml) is equivalent to that of 12 glasses of white wine, four glasses of beer, two cups of tea, four apples, five portions of onion, six portions of eggplant, seven glasses of orange juice, or 20 glasses of commercial apple juice. The skins of red grapes are particularly rich in the antioxidant resveratrol, also found in white grapes but to a lesser degree, and in peanuts and raspberries.

Alcohol may have other additional harmful effects, particularly in men younger than 45 and women under 55. These include traffic accidents, alcohol dependence, liver disease, spousal abuse, high blood pressure, stroke, obesity, suicide, and breast and other cancers. Every year in the US, 75,000 preventable deaths are attributed to alcohol abuse. Although the death rate from alcohol was one-sixth that of smoking, most of the dead were teens and young adults, unlike smoking which kills middle-aged and older people. For these reasons, you should not start drinking alcohol if you do not already do so. And if you do, don't exceed the recommended limits.

9. An integrated program created to work synergistically with increased physical activity

I wish I could tell you differently, but you will achieve the full benefits of a nutrition program only if you combine it with regular physical activity. Lack of physical activity is the primary reason for the near-universal failure of virtually all commercial weight loss programs. If you are a normal weight adult or child, you should aim to achieve a daily minimum of 60 minutes of moderately vigorous physical activity, 90 minutes or more if you are overweight (see Chapter V, Section 8).

Tid Bits
*One American drink of alcohol is **45** ml of spirits, **120** ml of wine, or **350** ml of beer.*

If you need to lose weight, the recommended weight loss rate is one to two pounds a week. Healthy weight loss is a good indicator that your nutrition program is working for you. A combination of careful nutrition and physical activity can shave off 500 calories per day in food consumption (that is 3500 calories a week) and increase your caloric usage by 500 calories per day. Together, these changes would result in a net caloric deficit of 7,000 calories per week, meaning a weekly weight loss of two pounds.

How does this actually translate into practical terms? This could be achieved by replacing two cups of rice with one bowl of vegetable salad and walking five miles a day at moderate speed (90 to 120 minutes a day). Remember vigorous exercise, such as running or using "cardio" machines like elliptical cross-trainers, can cut the time by 50 to 75% (*see* Chapter V, Section 8).

KEY · POINTS · IN · A · NUTSHELL

♥ The only sustainable, healthy, weight-reduction diet is a nutritionally sufficient, high-fiber, low-calorie, carbohydrate-balanced, cardioprotective diet composed around great-tasting, low glycemic index ingredients that you are already familiar with and can readily find: the Prudent Nutrition Program.

♥ The Prudent Nutrition Program can reduce your risks of heart disease, obesity, and diabetes.

♥ Key aspects of this program include satiety, great taste, a wide range of food choices, and nutritionally balanced meals with adequate carbohydrates and fiber.

♥ To achieve and maintain optimum weight and waist size, caloric intake should be complemented with regular physical activity.

♥ The recommended intake of fruits and vegetables is nine to 13 servings per day.

♥ Consumption of 40 to 60 grams of fish a day, or two fish meals per week, reduces the risk of sudden death by 40 to 60%.

♥ An ounce of nuts per day has a variety of health benefits, including increasing your HDL level and supplying the necessary minerals and antioxidant vitamins .

♥ While regular consumption of small amounts of alcohol has cardioprotective effects, it should not be overindulged because of significant risks to health including alcoholism and automobile accidents.

5.4 ▶ Fats! The Good, the Bad, and the Deadly

I n the hysteria to counter the epidemic of obesity, fats have acquired a bad name. The record needs to be set straight: You would literally die if you had no fat in your body. Fat is a vital energy source and aids in several important and complex cell functions—including the production of steroids, the maintenance of the immune system, vision, blood clotting, the production of sex hormones, and various healing and anti-inflammation mechanisms. This section discusses the importance of choosing not only the right amount but the right *types* of fats in your diet. Yes, there *are* good fats. The real mystery is how, with so many health-promoting and even cardioprotective fats available, people find a way to eat so much of the bad kind of fat.

The terms "fats" and "fatty acids" are used interchangeably in this book. Fatty acids are organic acids made up of a carbon chain with hydrogen bonds. Triglycerides, which mean three fatty acids bound by glycerol, are the normal way we consume fat in our diet and the way our body circulates fat in the bloodstream.

Total fat consumption

In 2001, the National Cholesterol Educational Program (NCEP) raised the upper limit of total fat intake from 30% to 35% of your daily energy requirements. Since a gram of fat provides 9 calories of energy, this still translates to less than 40g of fat per day for an average Indian, who should consume about 1000 to 1200 calories per day. Consumption of excess fat (above 65g a day) has been shown to double the risk of heart attack and stroke. How much fat exactly do you need? Some experts recommend very low proportions—less than 10% in the Ornish Diet, for example. Others swear by very high protein—more than 40% in the Atkins Diet, for instance. But most animal proteins, such as meat, come mixed with fat. For example, virtually every kind of steak—even the leanest cuts—and every kind of cheese have more fat calories in them than protein calories. As a result, most high-protein diets designed around animal proteins are in reality *high-fat diets masquerading as high-protein diets*. And with animal fat calories comes high cholesterol.

Similarly, a very low-fat diet is essentially a very high-carbohydrate diet. There are several problems with this: First, it markedly increases the triglyceride levels in your blood, which is bad, and it drastically lowers your heart-protective (HDL) cholesterol. Both high triglycerides and low HDL are more common among Indians than other populations. Second, the ability of a meal to keep you from getting hungry again soon is often dictated by the fat and protein content of the meal. Very high carb diets can make you hungry, particularly if the carbs have a **high glycemic index** (see section 5), and cause your body to release more insulin than you need to break down the sugar in what you ate. And third, as indicated earlier, fat is essential for your body to work properly. Most experts, therefore, recommend a diet that is moderate in fat, like the one you will find here: the Prudent Diet.

Good fats and bad fats

First, let's talk about cholesterol. Early studies of the link between cholesterol and heart disease emphasized the importance of the total amount of cholesterol in your blood. Today, we know that there is good and bad cholesterol. Similarly, recent research has shown that the *type* of fat you eat is even more important than the *amount* of fat you eat. Not all fats are created equal. Some fats are healthy; others are downright dangerous. Some raise your bad cholesterol; others actually lower it.

There are essentially *four* kinds of fats (monounsaturated, polyunsaturat-

Americans Eating Somewhat Healthier Fats Today
The proportion of fat calories in the American diet that comes from beef, pork, dairy, and eggs fell to 33% in the 1994-96 period, from 50% in 1965. The proportion of fat calories from poultry rose to 7% from 4%. Calories from fruits and vegetables rose to 13%, from just 8%. According to USDA data, in 2001 the average American ate 194 pounds of red meat, poultry and fish —16 pounds more than in 1970. Of this, he or she ate 34 pounds more poultry and 3.4 pounds more fish than in 1970, but 21 pounds less red meat.

ed, saturated, and trans fats), with vastly different atherogenic (plaque-forming) and anti-atherogenic properties (*see* Table 5.5). Biochemically, why they differ depends on the nature of the hydrogen bonding between the atoms in these fat molecules. Why does something so seemingly insignificant as chemical bonding make such a difference? Look at it this way: There is a world of difference between a lightly roasted marshmallow and one that has been held in a fire for half an hour and has turned into a black crisp. The two are made of essentially the same thing: the only difference is that the *molecules* in the second have undergone a "slight" rearrangement that has suddenly made it virtually toxic to your system. Two molecules can look very similar under a microscope; but one could be a deadly poison simply because the chemical bonds that hold its atoms together are slightly different. Let's look at each of the four main kinds of fat.

I. MONOUNSATURATED FATS

Monounsaturated fats are very **healthy fats** that lower your LDL (or bad) cholesterol level and actually increase your HDL (good) cholesterol level. Because of the growing awareness of their beneficial effects, a liberal consumption (of up to 20% of your daily calories, or about 22 grams) is recommended. Since monounsaturated fats do not raise triglycerides, they may be particularly beneficial to Indians with high triglycerides. Olive oil, canola oil and avocados are great sources of monounsaturated fats, as are most nuts: macadamia nuts, hazelnuts, pecans, almonds, cashew nuts, pistachio nuts, peanuts. The major source of monounsaturated fats in the western diet is actually meat—particularly chicken, beef, pork, and lamb—but meat also has saturated fats, which are bad for you.

Type of fat	Comments	Sources
Monounsaturated fat (omega-9)	Very healthy	Olive oil, canola oil, avocados, nuts, meat
Omega-6 polyun saturated fat Omega-3 polyunsaturated fat (DHA, EPA, and ALA)	Moderately healthy Very healthy essential fatty acids	Vegetable oils and nuts DHA, EPA: Dark-meat oily fish. ALA: vegetable oils, particularly flaxseed and canola
Saturated fat	Unhealthy and dangerous	Animal fat such as in meat; high-fat dairy products; coconut and palm oils
Trans fat	The most dangerous	Fried foods, overused frying oil; partially hydrogenated oils such as in commercially baked cookies and donuts

II. POLYUNSATURATED FATS

A second type of unsaturated fats are the polyunsaturated fats. There are two kinds, omega-3 and omega-6, and they have both become buzz words in the field of nutrition. Let's look at omega-6 first and then omega-3, since we have gone over omega-9 (monounsaturated fats) above. The order will be 9-6-3.

Omega-6 fatty acids

Omega-6 lowers LDL cholesterol, but unfortunately it also lowers HDL cholesterol. Consumption of omega-6 has increased from next to nothing 50 years ago to 8% of people's daily calories in present-day America. The recommendation is to limit intake of omega-6 fats to no more than 10% of daily calories. Since the proportion of polyunsaturated fats in the Indian diet is unclear, it is difficult to make any kind of recommendation as to increase or decrease the intake of this fat in the Indian diet. Like the other unsaturated fats, omega-6 fats are liquid at room temperature. They are the major ingredient in most vegetable oils and some nuts.

Omega-3 fatty acids

Omega-3 is even better for you than omega-6, because unlike omega-6, omega-3 lowers LDL without lowering HDL. There are three kinds of omega-3: two are found in fish, DHA and EPA, and the third, ALA, is plant-based. We will look at ALA further down below. All three are essential fatty acids that regulate many cell functions in our body, reduce triglycerides levels, and decrease the

Tid Bits
DHA stands for docosahexaenoic acid. EPA stands for eicosapentaenoic acid. Both are found in fish oil. ALA stands for alpha linolenic acid, and it is found in plants.

risk of diabetes, but our bodies cannot make omega-3 fats, so we have to get them from food to maintain optimum health. (There is also evidence that, in cell membranes, EPA competes with and replaces the arachidonic acid, which is harmful.)

Fish in general is a good source of omega-3 fats, but the content varies markedly (see Table 5.6). The best sources are dark-meat, oily fish such as salmon and mackerel. These contain more than 0.4g of omega-3 fats per 100 grams of fish. Studies indicate that people who eat two to four servings of such fish per week have a 25 to 50% lower risk of sudden death (with or without a heart attack). However, the beneficial effects of fish are largely destroyed if it is fried. Omega-3 fatty acids are also available in fish oil capsules. Although it is catching on, the intake of omega-3 is still less than 1g per person per day in western countries compared to 2-3 grams in

Table 5.6. Total fat and omega-3 content per 100 grams of selected fish

	Fat (grams per 100g of fish)	Omega-3 polyunsaturated fat (grams)
Sardines	16	3.3
Mackerel	13.9	2.5
Lake trout	9.7	1.6
Salmon (Chinook)	10.4	1.4
Salmon (Atlantic)	5.4	1.2
Blue fish	6.5	1.2
Shrimp	1.1	0.3
Lobster	0.9	0.2

Source: Connor, S L. Ref. 5.7.

Japan, and 15 grams a day among Eskimos. The US recommended daily intake is 1 gram of DHA + EPA. A healthy diet have omega-6 and omega-3 fats in a roughly 2:1 to 4:1 ratio; the two substances work together in the body. In other words, for every 4g of omega-6, aim for at least 1 gram of DHA + EPA. Some experts feel that the typical US diet contains 10-30 times more omega-6 than omega-3. It is likely that Indians have a very low intake of omega-3, particularly vegetarians who avoid fish and fish oil.

ALA, the third omega-3 fatty acid

Even though DHA and EPA are far more potent omega-3 fats than ALA, most people get most of their omega-3 from ALA (or alpha-linolenic acid). ALA, however, is the "parent" fatty acid to DHA and EPA. That means you can make DHA and EPA from ALA because their chemical structures are similar. Your body can rapidly convert ALA into EPA, but only slowly into DHA. It needs roughly 11 grams of ALA to produce one gram of DHA or EPA. That is a lot. Additionally, eating trans fats (like the hydrogenated oils in biscuits, cakes, and cookies) can slow the conversion of ALA into EPA and DHA.

Oils high in ALA include flaxseed (50%), canola (10%), mustard (10%) and soybean oil (7%). Almonds, walnuts and peanuts are also good sources of ALA, as are tofu, soybeans, pinto beans, and flax seeds.

III. SATURATED FATTY ACIDS

Most of us know saturated fatty acids as "the bad fats." There is a high correlation between the amount of saturated fats consumed and the risk of heart disease. The contribution of saturated fats to blood cholesterol level is at least 10 times larger than that of dietary cholesterol. This is partly because we ingest so much more saturated fat than cholesterol, and partly because the body can make cholesterol from almost anything: fats, protein, carbohydrates, and dietary cholesterol itself. The intake of saturated fats in Japan is only 6% of Japanese total calories. Not surprisingly, Japan has one of the world's lowest rates of heart disease and blood cholesterol level.

Indian vegetarians and ALA

There are different kinds of vegetarians. Vegans are the pure vegetarians; they eat only plant foods. *Lacto*-vegetarians eat plant foods and dairy products. Ovo-vegetarians eat plant foods and eggs. *Peso*-vegetarians eat plant foods and fish. (Once you add red meat, however, you are no longer a vegetarian of any kind.) Most western vegetarians are lacto-, ovo-, or peso-vegetarians—or something in between, such as lacto-peso-vegetarian. Very few Indian vegetarians, however, are peso-vegetarians. Since they do not consume fish, Indian vegeterians have to derive all their omega-3s from ALA. This is one more reason why Indians must avoid trans fats, since trans fats hamper the ALA-to-DHA/EPA conversion in the body. Most Indians probably do not get enough omega-3.

Table 5.7. Major sources of saturated fat

Meat sources	Beef, lamb, pork, bacon, sausage, ribs, wings and skin of poultry
High-fat dairy products	Butter, ghee, cheese, ice cream, and full-fat milk.
Tropical oils	Coconut, palm, and cocoa butter
Commercial bakery products	Cakes, biscuits, cookies, donuts and rusk
Foods cooked in dalda or vansapathi	Most of Indians snacks, except those prepared with heart-healthy ingredients

In contrast, on average 15% of total daily calories in the UK comes from saturated fats, partly explaining their high rate of heart disease. In fact, the 10-fold difference that exists in heart attack death rates among different countries is *best explained by differences in the intake of saturated fats*, with only three exceptions: India (unexpectedly high rates of heart disease), Finland (unexpectedly high rates of heart disease), and France (unexpectedly low rates of heart disease).

In most countries and cultures, saturated fats come primarily from animal products such as meat and full-fat dairy products, especially butter and ghee. In India, however, tropical oils such as coconut and palm oil, both of which contain very high amounts of saturated fat, contribute heavily to saturated fat intake.

Meat's many faces: The good, the bad, and the neutral

Bear in mind that not all saturated fats raise cholesterol. For example, stearic acid, which comprises nearly half of the saturated fat in beef and lamb (mutton), is cholesterol-neutral. Meat is also a very good source of cholesterol-*lowering* monounsaturated fat (see Table 5.8). Moderate consumption of lean meat may therefore be beneficial. According to US Department of Agriculture, lean meat contains less than 9 grams of fat per 100 grams of meat. If you eat beef, consider loin or round cuts. They are the leanest. "Lean" and "select" cuts also tend to be low in cholesterol-raising saturated fat. Avoid portions that say "prime" or "rib"—these are the fattiest, with the highest marbling (fat that cannot be removed by trimming because it is distributed within the meat itself).

Table 5.8. Atherogenic, antiatherogenic, and neutral fatty acids in selected meats and butter

Type of fat	Saturated fat			Monounsaturated fat
	Total saturated fat	cholesterol-raising saturated fat	cholesterol-neutral saturated fat (stearic acid)	cholesterol-lowering (oleic acid)
		Bad for you	Neutral	Good for you
Lamb fat	54%	29%	25%	33%
Beef fat	51%	29%	22%	39%
Pork fat	39%	27%	12%	45%
Chicken fat	30%	24%	6%	42%
Butter	66%	53%	13%	28%
Ghee	Same as butter but with additional harmful cholesterol oxides			

Source: Enas, EA. Ref. 5.9.

Eat your dairy products—the smart way

Whole milk, cheese, and ice cream are high in saturated fat and cholesterol. However, they are also the richest source of calcium, a key nutrient for strong bones, especially in women and children . The solution is to consume low-fat dairy products: skim milk, 1% milk, low-fat cheese, low-fat buttermilk, and low-fat or non-fat yogurt. The 2005 USDA dietary guidelines recommend three servings of dairy products daily.

IV. TRANS FATS

The fourth and final kind of fat is the deadly **trans fat**. Pick up a packet of cookies, a bottle of salad dressing, or a carton of nondairy coffee creamer at the grocery store and read the food label. You will often see something like "partially hydrogenated soybean oil and/or cottonseed oil" among the ingredients. Most fats eventually become rancid and develop a disagreeable taste. Rancidity occurs mainly through the air oxidation of double bonds that form unpleasant-smelling aldehydes. Unsaturated fats, such as you might find in a nondairy coffee creamer, turn rancid much more quickly than do saturated fats. To make them stay fresh for longer, food companies use a commercial process called hydrogenation, which turns vegetable oil into solid or semisolid shortening. Hence, terms like "partially hydrogenated soybean oil."

The problem is that, during the partial hydrogenation of vegetable oil, trans fats are produced. Most people do not realize that trans fats are even worse than saturated fats in heightening the risk of heart attack, stroke, and diabetes. Both saturated fats and trans fats increase LDL. However, trans fats go further and *decrease* your HDL, whereas saturated fats at least increase your HDL level. In addition, trans fats are among the few non-genetic factors that can raise lipoprotein(a) to harmful levels (*see* Chapter III, Section 3).

Another process that transforms cooking oil into trans fats is deep frying. Ethnic groups that eat a lot of deep-fried foods and snacks, such as Indians, end up consuming large amounts of trans fats. Table 5.9 shows common sources of trans fats in diets. Indians urgently need to reduce their intake of trans fats and saturated

Table 5.9. Common sources of trans fats

Fried Indian snacks	Samosa, bajjis (fritters)
Commercial bakery products	Cakes, Danish pastry, donuts, crackers, rusk, croutons, biscuits, cookies, white bread
Fried foods	French fries and fried chicken
Other foods	Non-dairy creamer, tortillas, pizza and peanut butter Stick margarines, salad dressing

fats by avoiding ghee, fried foods, dalda (vanaspathi), and shortening. Like nondairy creamers, cookies, and salad dressing, many margarines contain partially hydrogenated oil. In recent years, the trans fats content of most US margarines has been substantially reduced through manufacturing advances. This, however, may not be the case in other countries and regions, including India.

The new margarines

If you use margarine or a cheese spread for your sandwiches, consider switching to one of the new sterol- or stanols-based margarines such as *Take Control or Benecol*. In addition to being a rich source of monounsaturated fats, these new-generation margarines contain plant substances that actually help to prevent the absorption of cholesterol in your body. These margarines lower cholesterol levels by as much as 5% when consumed at appropriate amounts. Smart Balance® Omega plus Buttery Spread is another great-tasting spread that is ideal for cooking, baking and table use. It contains no hydrogenated oils nor trans fats, and it provides a favorable omega-6 to omega-3 fat ratio of 4:1. One serving (1 table spoon or 14g) contains 550mg of omega-3 and 2200mg of omega-6. It is also available in a "lite" version that is lower in calories but can be used only for light frying, sautéing and table use, not for baking.

Choices, choices: Choosing a cooking oil

Monounsaturated fats are the major ingredients in two commonly used cooking oils: olive oil and canola oil. Extra virgin olive oil is the first round of oil that is pressed from the olives. In addition to tasting great, which makes it excellent as a salad dressing, it is rich in antioxidants. Regular olive oil is good for sautéing. Other sources of monounsaturated fats include mustard oil, peanut oil and sesamy seed oil. Coconut oil is a singular exception among vegetable oils having highest amount of saturated fat and the lowest of monounsaturated fat. Sunflower and safflower oils are usually high in polyunsaturated fats and low in monounsaturated fats. High-oleic

Table 5.10. Different types of fat in common cooking oils

	Monounsaturated fats	Polyunsaturated fats	Saturated Fats	Remarks
Olive oil	74%	8%	14%	Excellent. Use extra-virgin for salads and regular for cooking
Mustard oil	59%	21%	12%	Caution—very high in erucic acid, a cardiotoxic substance
Canola oil	59%	30%	7%	Recommended. High in omega-3 fats
Peanut oil	46%	32%	17%	OK to use
Sunflower oil	45%	40%	10%	See text; high-oleic versions are cholesterol-lowering
Safflower oil	13%	79%	8%	OK to use
Sesame oil	40%	42%	14%	OK to use
Palm oil	37%	9%	49%	Not recommended
Corn oil	24%	59%	13%	OK to use
Soybean oil	23%	58%	14%	OK to use, high in omega-3
Palm kernel oil	11%	2%	82%	Avoid at all cost
Coconut oil	6%	2%	92%	Avoid at all cost

Source: Enas, EA. Ref 5.9.

Effect of various cooking oils on cholesterol levels

Cooking oils have a huge impact on your cholesterol level. Data from several studies show that substituting a cholesterol-raising cooking oil for a cholesterol-lowering one can increase blood cholesterol anywhere from 14% to almost 80%, depending on the amount and kind of oil substituted. In one study, substituting 24% of daily calories from corn oil with coconut oil increased LDL cholesterol by 79 points over a period of six months. A Malaysian study that replaced two-thirds of dietary fat from palm oil (already bad for you but used extensively in that country) with coconut oil reported a 10% increase in LDL cholesterol over 5 weeks. Subsequent feeding of palm oil or corn oil significantly reduced the LDL cholesterol by, 20% and 42% respectively. And in Mauritius, banning the importation of palm oil and substituting it with soybean oil resulted in a 30-point decrease in total cholesterol (from 213 to 183) for the entire country over a five-year period, from 1987 to 1882. Finally, another study found that, in populations that consume a lot of coconut, reducing coconut intake from 18% to 9% of daily calories resulted in an 11% reduction in LDL cholestrol level

(cholesterol-lowering) safflower and sunflower oils are often available in health-food stores and directly from the manufacturers, but not from regular supermarkets or grocery stores.

Table 5.10 shows the proportion of monounsaturated fats, polyunsaturated fats and saturated fats in common cooking oils. On the basis of extensively analyzed data such as these, the best cooking oils are olive oil and canola oil. The worst are coconut oil, palm kernel oil, and palm oil—along with butter and ghee, which are not listed here because they are not from plants. Mustard oil (commonly used in states of Orissa and West Bengal), though a good source of monounsaturated fats, is very high in erucic acid, a cardiotoxic substance. Canola oil is a genetically modified form of mustard oil in which the erucic acid has been substituted with ALA. Figure 5.1 predicts how substituting various cooking oils in a particular diet (in this case, a typical Dutch diet) would affect HDL and LDL cholesterol levels, based on studies of how smaller amounts of these oils affect cholesterol levels. Replacing all fat in this diet with coconut oil would raise LDL cholesterol by 34 points in one year, while replacing all fat with safflower oil would decrease LDL by 30 points—a net difference of 66 points!

> ### Now That You Know...
> The **best** cooking oils are olive oil and canola oil, along with high-oleic safflower and sunflower oils, found in health food stores. The **worst** are coconut oil, palm kernel oil, and palm oil—along with butter and ghee.

Dietary cholesterol and blood cholesterol

Although the contribution that dietary cholesterol makes to blood cholesterol is much less than that of saturated fats, dietary cholesterol should not be ignored. You should keep your intake low. The current recommendation of cholesterol intake is less than 200mg per day. Dietary cholesterol is found only in the animal kingdom, particularly egg yolk, organ meats such as liver, brain, chicken skin, and shell fish (shrimp, crab, lobster). Two egg yolks have 560mg of cholesterol—almost three times your daily limit—and 100 grams of brain has 2000mg. Three ounces of beef, lamb, or pork contain 75mg. A cup of whole milk has 33mg. A partial list of foods that are major sources of dietary cholesterol is given in Table 5.11.

Most cholesterol in poultry is in the skin, although there is some in dark meat. As a result, chicken wings are worse than prime rib in cholesterol content. Shrimp and other seafood, although they have cholesterol, are generally healthy foods because they contain very little saturated fat

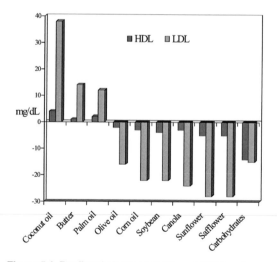

Figure 5.1. Predicted change in HDL and LDL levels when all the fat in a Dutch diet is replaced by a particular oil. Note the net difference of 66 mg /dl in cholesterol level from substituting safflower oil with coconut oil. Source: Katan, MB. Ref. 5.25 *Reproduced with permission © the American Journal of Clinical Nutrition* and American Society for Clinical Nutrition.

and a lot of very healthy omega-3 fats. Organ meats are a delicacy among Indians, but they are very high in cholesterol and saturated fat, and their consumption should be limited to a few times a year. Buffalo milk is very high in fat content, 8%, compared to 4% for cow milk and 0% for skim milk.

For a comprehensive website that offers concise yet complete nutritional analyses of virtually every common food available in the US, along with extensive advice and searching options, visit www.nutritiondata.com.

Table 5.11. Major sources of dietary cholesterol

- Egg yolks, but not egg whites
- Organ meats such as liver, kidney, heart, and brain
- Meat such as beef, pork, lamb, and goat
- Poultry, especially skins, but also dark meat such as thigh
- Shell fish such as shrimp, prawn and lobster
- All full-fat milk, but especially buffalo milk
- High-fat dairy products: butter, ghee, cream, ice cream, milk shakes, cheese, especially soft cheese, curd.

KEY · POINTS · IN · A · NUTSHELL

♥ The kind of fat you eat is far more important than the quantity. Some fats promote atherosclerosis, others slow it down, and yet others are neutral.

♥ Trans fats are the worst fats of all, followed by saturated fats.

♥ The 10-fold variation in heart attack death rates among different countries is best explained by differences in the intake of saturated fats.

♥ Saturated fats, which are found in particularly high concentrations in ghee, butter, full-fat dairy products, coconut, and fatty portions of meats, should make up less than 7% of your total calories (below 10 grams a day).

♥ Saturated fat intake, even more than dietary cholesterol, is the principal determinant of blood cholesterol level.

♥ Egg yolks, organ meats, and chicken skin are among foods especially high in cholesterol, but most foods that are high in saturated fats are also high in cholesterol.

♥ The best fats are polyunsaturated fats with high omega-3 (DHA and EPA) content, found in oily fish. Frying, however, destroys virtually all of the cardiac benefits of fish.

♥ The second-best fats are the monounsaturated cooking oils, especially olive oil, canola oil. They raise HDL and lower LDL.

♥ The worst cooking oils are coconut, palm kernel, and palm oil—second only to trans fats in the harm they can cause to cardiovascular health.

♥ Monounsaturated fats are also found in nuts, avocados, and lean meat, and should comprise up to 20% of your daily calories.

♥ Trans fats (produced during deep frying) increase cholesterol and decrease HDL.

♥ Avoiding fried or crispy foods is the best way to minimize the intake of trans fats.

♥ Replace full-fat dairy products with low-fat equivalents such as skim milk and fat-free yogurt.

♥ Avoid deep frying, especially with previously used oils.l

5.5 ▶ Identifying The Right Carbs

Carbohydrates, which include vegetables, fruits, bread, *dosai*, *rotis*, and rice, are the most common energy source worldwide, and they form a large part of the Indian diet. *Rotis* are a form of unleavened bread often cooked over a *tava* or griddle and often form the bulk of the calories in the north Indian diet. All forms of unleavened Indian bread – *paratha*, *kulchas*, and *naan* are included under the rotis category for the purposes of the book. On the other hand, rice constitutes the bulk of calories in the South Indian diet. This section discusses the principles that underlie the process of choosing the right types and amounts of carbohydrates in a balanced diet. You will learn why it is important to know what a carbohydrate's glycemic index is, why some carbohydrates manage to be low in calories yet leave you feeling full for several hours, how some carbohydrates promote cardiac health by lowering your bad cholesterol, and how to construct a nutritional program around high-fiber, high-nutrient, low glycemic index fruits, vegetables, and whole grains.

Did you know...
High glycemic index foods markedly raise your triglyceride and blood sugar levels, depress your HDL levels, and heighten your risk of diabetes and heart disease. This danger is under-appreciated by many Indians, including even physicians.

Glycemic Index: the all-important measure

Carbohydrate quality used to be described in terms of whether it was a simple or complex carbohydrate. It was a useful distinction, but today, nutritionists are more likely to talk about its Glycemic Index. Every food—but especially carbohydrates—raises your glucose sugar level as your body digests the food and sugar enters your blood stream. The Glycemic Index, or GI for short, is a published ranking of foods that refers to how quickly each food raises your blood sugar after you have eaten it. Pure glucose has the highest known GI. Many raw, uncooked vegetables are among the lowest-GI carbohydrates. Cooking raises GI by making the food more rapidly digestible. The Glycemic Index uses white bread as an arbitrary reference standard and assigns it a value of 100; every other food is then compared to it. Why does all this matter?

Many factors determine a food's Glycemic Index and load: fiber, protein and fat content. Processing raises GI, as does ripeness in fruits, and even storage methods. Prolonged cooking raises GI by disintegrating the cell wall and making the food more quickly digestible. Raw vegetables not only have low GI but also have more nutrients.

Let's cut to the chase: There are two fundamental goals in choosing any carbohydrate. It is these two criteria that distinguish truly superb carbohydrates from very bad ones. *The first goal* is nutritional value. Some carbs are packed with extremely powerful vitamins, minerals, antioxidants, and phytonutrients that act almost like "body armor" against disease, infection, atherosclerosis, and even aging. Other carbohydrates are nutritionally virtually empty; you may as well be pouring white sugar directly into your mouth.

The *second* big consideration in choosing carbohydrates is the goal of keeping your blood sugar level *as constant as possible*. This is hugely important. It partly explains why some people have very high triglyceride levels and low HDL levels and cannot lose excess weight, while others do not. It partly explains why some people become lethargic, moody, or even diabetic, including many Indians, and why other people seem always to have boundless, constant, even energy throughout their day.

This second goal—blood sugar control—is what makes the Glycemic Index so vital. If you want to control your blood sugar—and you should—then it is important to choose low-GI carbohydrates. Two decades ago, you would have been told to "choose complex carbohydrates." That advice was not bad; quite often it was right. We now know, however, that some so-called complex carbs have a high Glycemic Index! Some starchy foods like potatoes have a higher Glycemic Index than even straight table sugar! Likewise, some sweet or sugary foods that we expected to have a high GI—apples, for example—turn out to have a low GI. They break down slowly in your body and do not cause your blood sugar level to shoot up rapidly. That is why high GI versus low GI is more relevant and more accurate than simple versus complex.

In short, to maintain optimal health you need to choose carbohydrates that are (a) highly nutritious and (b) have a low GI. But that actually is not the whole story. Four plates of low-GI whole-grain rice will certainly make your blood sugar rise much more rapidly, and higher, than a single piece of sugar candy, even though the candy has a much higher GI. Why? Because of the quantities. What really matters then is the total **glycemic load** of the carbs you are eating. Glycemic load takes into account the Glycemic Index of the carb and the amount of it you ate. (Mathematically, it is the glycemic index of the food, multiplied by the amount in grams, divided by 100).

This means you can control blood sugar two ways: Either by choosing low-GI carbs and/or by restricting the quantities you eat. The worse choice, then, is to consume a low-nutritional value, high-GI carbohydrate in great quantities—for example, drinking several bottles of Coca Cola, or wolfing down a large plate of white rice. The high glycemic load this creates will raise both your blood sugar and your triglycerides, and the large number of empty calories will further be converted to fat if you do not exercise it off within the next day or two. In addition, high-GI foods lower your HDL level and make your pancreas release copious amounts of insulin, putting you at risk for diabetes if this becomes a pattern. Finally, after raising your blood sugar very high, high-GI foods often bring it down very low because of all the insulin you released, making you feel hungry again.

Did you know...
An average cup of boiled rice contains 170 calories, Japanese sticky rice contains 155 calories, sushi rice contains 350 calories, and Mexican rice contains 400 calories. A cup of ghee rice contain 450 calories.

Foods with high glycemic load per typical serving include rice, breakfast cereals, and potatoes (see Table 5.12). Many Indian foods too have high glycemic loads per serving. Choose foods that have a medium or low glycemic load (below 20) such as brown rice, lentils (*dhals*), beans, and green plantain. *Uppuma*, a popular south Indian dish made of *rava* (semolina), is very low in glycemic load per serving (below 10). The glycemic load of rice varies greatly: jasmine and white rice are very high; parboiled and brown rice are relatively low. Note that one serving of cooked rice is half a cup, and that the recommended servings of carbohydrates is only six to eight a day for anyone weighing under 200 pounds.

High-fructose corn syrup
Although high-fructose corn syrup has a low glycemic index of just 20, it is not recommended because of its low content of fiber and other nutrients. It along with alcohol and refined carbohydrates are considered empty calories.

Pizzas and candy bars such as Snickers have medium glycemic load because of their high-fat content. However, they are inappropriate diet choices because of their high saturated fat content. Additional information on Glycemic Index can be found at www.glycemicindex.com.

Choosing appropriate carbohydrates

The National Academy of Sciences Institute of Medicine recommends a minimum intake of 130

Net Carbs versus Glycemic Index
Some diet experts—of the Atkins™ school of thought, for example—advocate the use of the number of net carbs per serving as the criterion for making your carbohydrate dietary choices. It is a variation on the "calorie counting" approach, but in this case it is "carb counting." Net carbs are calculated by taking the total carbohydrate content of a serving of a particular food and subtracting the grams of indigestible fiber, sugar alcohol, and glycerine that are in it, because your body does not metabolize these so they do not count in terms of calories. Net carbs tries to count only the "active carbs" in a food.

Although net carbs gives you a sense of the "caloric density" of the food, which is clearly helpful, it does not capture how quickly your body will digest and absorb that food, and hence how rapidly your blood glucose level will rise. That is what makes Glycemic Index so powerful: GI captures the idea that different carbs affect your blood sugar to different degrees. Most nutritionists therefore believe that Glycemic Index and Glycemic load are better ways of identifying the quality and quantity of carbohydrates you should eat. The best approach is to make fruits, vegetables, and whole grains the foundation of your diet, watch the overall quantities you eat, avoid highly processed foods, and engage in physical activity everyday.

Table 5.12. The Glycemic Index and glycemic load of common foods

	Glycemic index	Serving size (g)	Carbohydrate per serving (g)	Glycemic load
High Glycemic Load Foods				
Millet/Ragi	104	70	50	52
Jasmine Rice	109	150	42	46
Idli	77	250	52	40
Pongal	68	250	52	35
Dosai	77	150	39	30
Poori	70	150	41	28
Parboiled rice	48	150	36	26
Potato	85	150	30	26
Breakfast cereal	81	30	26	24
Chapathi	76	60	30	23
Basmati rice	58	150	38	22
Sweet potato	61	150	25	21
Medium glycemic load foods				
Instant noodles	47	180	40	19
Spaghetti	68	220	27	19
Brown rice (S. India)	50	150	33	16
Barley	43	150	37	16
Banana	53	170	25	12
Black eyed beans	42	150	30	13
Tapioca	70	250	18	12
Sweet Corn	59	80	18	11
Low glycemic load foods				
Prunes	29	60	33	10
Lima beans	32	150	30	10
Pinto beans	39	150	26	10
Plantain, green	38	120	21	8
Uppuma	18	150	33	6
Split peas	32	150	19	6
Lentils	30	150	17	5
Beet root	64	80	7	5
Cantaloupe	65	120	6	4
Yogurt	36	200	9	3
Chickpeas	10	150	30	3
Kidney beans (rajmah)	13	150	25	3
Green peas	39	80	7	3
Carrot	47	80	6	3
Soy beans	15	150	6	1

Source: Enas. Ref 5.9

grams of carbohydrates, or 26% of a 2000-calorie diet. For most adults who need to lose weight or avoid a weight gain, and for whom a 1200-calorie diet is therefore recommended, this translates into 80 grams of carbs a day. Carbohydrate intake should not exceed 300g a day, especially if you have high triglycerides. In the US, carbohydrate intake has increased by 126 grams over the past four decades, with high-fructose, high-GI corn syrup constituting 10% of those calories.

The situation in South Asia is parallel but slightly different. Instead of focusing more on vegetables and fruits, many Indians consider *rotis* and rice as the main course of a meal. Vegetable and meat dishes, often prepared as curries, merely facilitate the consumption of "the main course." Typically, a particularly tasty meat—or vegetable-based curry results in greater consumption not of the meat or vegetables but rather of the main course (rice or *rotis*).

Let's look at this from the viewpoint of glycemic index and load. The overall goal in selecting carbs, besides maximizing nutritional content, is to keep your blood sugar constant by controlling your glycemic response to the foods you eat, through: (a) choosing predominantly low-GI carbohydrates and (b) lowering your glycemic load by limiting your overall intake. As we have seen, however, rice and wheat products, such as *rotis*, tend to have higher glycemic indices and loads. They should be consumed in moderation, particularly by people who have a predisposition toward insulin resist-ance, such as many Asian Indians. Indians can dramatically reduce their high triglyceride and blood sugar levels—and their risk of diabetes—by partly replacing rice and *rotis* with fruits, salads, and raw or stir-fried vegetables, and by adding appropriate amounts of protein to their diet. This risk of diabetes is the subject we will now turn to.

Glycemic load and diabetes

During the 20th century in the US, a rising intake of refined, highly processed, high-GI carbohydrates (such as those containing large amounts of corn syrup), and less and less consumption of fiber, paralleled another trend: the rising prevalence of type 2 diabetes. Recent studies suggest that glycemic load *powerfully predicts* the development of prediabetes and diabetes. The opposite also holds true: a high intake of fiber and of low GI-foods protects against diabetes, particularly in individuals with metabolic syndrome, because it helps them control their blood sugar. Some studies also suggest a significant decrease in the risk of colon and breast cancer.

It's All in the Label
When you shop for whole-grain products, read the label. It should clearly say "whole," otherwise it is not a whole-grain product. Stone-ground, a coarse form of grinding, usually leaves the germ intact, but that still does not mean the entire grain is there.

High glycemic load is in fact a major contributor to high triglycerides and diabetes among Indians. *See* Figure 5.2. If you have diabetes or a family history of metabolic syndrome and diabetes, you should limit your carbohydrate intake to 40% of your daily calories (120 grams for a 1200-calorie diet).

Whole-grain foods—another pillar of a healthy diet

Whole-grain foods are good examples of medium to low glycemic foods. They are also high in fiber, minerals, and antioxidants. In a large study involving 43,000 men over a 12-year period, the risk of diabetes was reduced by 40% in those with highest intake of whole grains compared to the lowest intake. A whole grain includes every edible part of the grain: the bran (outer shell), the germ (the innermost part), and the endosperm (the largest part). Using modern technology to refine the grain—for example, to produce white

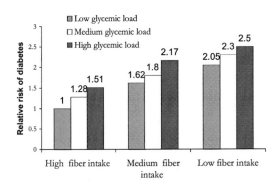

Figure 5.2. Relative risk of developing diabetes according glycemic load and fiber intake. Low glycemic load in this study was below 143 and high glycemic load above 165; Low fiber in this study was below 2.5 g and high fiber above 5.8 g. Source: Salmeron, J. Ref 5.39. *Reproduced with permission*©The American Medical Association.

bread instead of whole wheat bread—leads to the loss of highly beneficial micronutrients, anti-oxidants, minerals, phytochemicals, fiber and much of the germ. Refined grains, often bleached as well, contain mostly starch and are devoid of many vitamins and essential fatty acids.

When you shop for whole-grain products, read the food label. It should clearly state the word "whole." If it says "enriched," it is not a whole grain. Even "stone-ground wheat" is not whole grain unless it says "stone-ground *whole* wheat." "Whole" is the operative word. Another consideration is sugar: Several breakfast cereals contain whole grains, but avoid them if they have large amounts of sugar. Just 2% of the 150 pounds of wheat flour consumed per person in the US is whole-grain. The current average intake of whole grains among Americans is less than ½ a serving per day. This is likely to be true for Indians as well.

The 2005 USDA Dietary Guidelines call for three daily servings of whole-grain foods. Like any good foods, overconsumption of whole grains is not recommended; it can result in weight gain, metabolic syndrome, and eventually diabetes.

Oats

Finally, that there are many whole grains besides wheat and rice. Dozens of research studies have shown that eating oatmeal everyday reduces the risk of heart disease by lowering cholesterol levels. Oatmeal essentially acts like a broom. The water-soluble fiber in oatmeal binds to cholesterol in the small intestine and "sweeps" it out of the body, preventing it from becoming absorbed into your blood. The evidence for this is so strong that, in 1997, the FDA allowed whole-oat food manufacturers put this health claim on their food labels.

Emerging research suggests that oatmeal may have cardio-protective benefits beyond its soluble fiber content and cholesterol-lowering ability. Antioxidants such as tocotrienols and avenanthramides, which are unique to oats may also slow down atherosclerosis and endothelial dysfunction. Like other high-fiber foods, the fiber in oats also give it a high "fullness factor," keeping you feeling full longer and thereby assisting in weight management. The benefits of oatmeal are found largely in whole-grain oat products, not the "instant" kind. Cooking stone-cut, whole-grain oatmeal the old-fash-

Table 5.13. Common sources of whole-grain and refined foods

Whole-grain foods: eat these	Refined foods: limit or avoid these
Brown rice and wild rice Oatmeal Pasta Whole grain or dark bread Popcorn Wheat germ Bran Cooked cereals Whole-grain breakfast cereals Other grains such as buckwheat	White rice Most Pancakes and Cakes Sweet rolls, Donuts White bread, English muffins, Muffins Waffles Biscuits Pizza Refined-grain ready-to-eat breakfast cereals Appam, Dosa, Idli

Source: Fung, TT. Ref 5.12. Jacobs, DR. Ref 5.24.

Are Organic Foods Any Healthier For You? Many people are concerned about the harmful effects of pesticides and potential benefis of organic foods. To date, there is no convincing evidence that organic foods are any safer or more nutritious than conventionally produced foods.

ioned way is superior to the instant, one-minute variety. For more information on the benefits of oats, see for example the "Ask the Nutritionist" section of the Quaker Oats website www.quakeroatmeal.com.

Fruits and vegetables

Indian diabetics are **often afraid** that eating fruit will raise their blood sugar. Many are unaware that fruits in general have low glycemic loads. Here is a quick sample of glycemic loads, based on a 3oz or 100g portion of selected fruits. Anything under 20 is considered a medium glycemic load; anything under 10 is low. The USDA 2005 Guidelines have increased the recommended daily intake of fruits and vegetables from nine to 13 servings (5-6 cups for a person consuming 2000 calories a day). In addition to their delicious, fresh natural taste, fruits and veggies are low in glycemic load and caloric density. This means you can eat a lot of them and not jeopardize your weight management program. Some vegetables actually have a GI that is not all that low, but because vegetables have a lot of bulk and fiber, in effect the overall *glycemic load* you get from them is low because you tend not to eat a large amount of them in terms of calories. So you can usually eat a large plate of vegetables without driving up your blood sugar to unhealthy levels. Carrots, for example, have a relatively high GI (46) but a low glycemic load of only 18 per serving, because they contain only 4 grams of carbohydrates per serving. In addition, many fruits and vegetables protect your DNA from damage from oxidative stress. You cannot overload on fruits and veggies. They are packed with hundreds of nutrients and other beneficial components, as shown below:

Glycemic load per 3 oz or 100 grams of fruit	
Banana	12
Grapes	8
Kiwi fruit	8
Pineapple	7
Apple	6
Pear	6
Watermelon	5
Orange	5

1. **Phytosterols** $_x$
   These plant sterols inhibit the absorption of cholesterol and lower your blood cholesterol level. Foods rich in phytosterols include barley, almonds, cashews, peanuts, sesame seeds, sunflower seeds, corn, and whole wheat.

2. **Antioxidants**
   Antioxidants protect your DNA from damage from oxidative stress and prevent oxidation of LDL, which is what makes LDL cholesterol dangerous. Antioxidant-rich foods include deep-green leafy vegetables, such as spinach and kale. Colored vegetables such as green, red, and yellow pepper are also rich sources of antioxidants when eaten raw. Red pepper has the highest total antioxidant activity, followed by broccoli, carrot, spinach, cabbage, yellow onion, celery, potato, lettuce, and cucumber. Onions that have the most intense taste have the strongest antioxidant effects.

3. **Dietary fiber**
   Fiber is an indigestible complex plant carbohydrate that has no calories because the body cannot absorb it. High-fiber foods thus tend to be low in calories. Fiber has many health benefits, including reducing your risk of diabetes and heart disease. Most high-fiber fruits and vegetables have a mix of soluble and insoluble fibers, and both types are important. **Soluble fibers** are so called not because they dissolve in water but because they absorb water and form a gel in your digestive tract. This enables them to lower your LDL cholesterol, without raising triglycerides or lowering HDL. **Insoluble fibers** do not form gels, but they promote the smooth functioning of bowels and help you to avoid higher glycemic foods by making you feel full. Psyllium husk, one of the highest natural sources of soluble fiber, is approximately 70% soluble fiber, while wheat bran contains mostly insoluble fiber. Oat bran is about 7% soluble, yet has well-known cholesterol-lowering effects.
   The primary source of insoluble fiber is whole-grain products such as 7-grain bread and other whole-grain breads. One serving (½ a cup) of whole grain oats has 2 grams of soluble and 2 grams of

insoluble fiber. Other foods high in fiber include apples, peaches, raspberries, tangerines, broccoli (raw), Brussels sprouts, cabbage, carrots (raw), cauliflower (raw), spinach, zucchini, black-eyed peas, kidney beans, and lima beans.

4. **Blood-thinning factors**

When you are shaving and get a small cut, it stops bleeding within a few minutes because platelets, a component of blood, form a clot. Some people, however, have blood that undergoes abnormally excessive clotting, and this is associated with heart attacks. Consuming two to three tomatoes and kiwi a day are associated with decreased clumping of platelets.

Legumes

Beans and legumes (for example, dhals? and other pulses) are great sources of fiber, protein, vitamins, and phytochemicals. Canned beans that are cooked and ready to serve are ideal for salads, in addition to making curries. Some people prefer to soak dry beans overnight and pressure-cook them. Bean soups are great for winter months. Note that the glycemic load of some bean soups can become very high if they are cooked too long, because this breaks down the fiber in them.

Sweeteners

In addition to designing your nutritional program around low-GI, high-fiber, high-nutrient fruits, veggies, and whole grains, it is important that you restrict the amount of sugar you eat, because too much sugar can throw off your nutritional program. Here are some sugar substitutes:

Sugar alcohols

Sugar alcohols, also know as polyols, are ingredients used as sweeteners and bulking agents. Many of these have names ending in "itol": for example, mannitol, sorbitol, xylitol, and lactitol. They occur naturally in foods and come from plant products such as fruits and berries. These sugar substitutes provide fewer calories (about a half to one-third fewer calories) than regular sugar. Sugar alcohols are not chemically broken down into glucose. They therefore cause less of a rise in blood sugar than regular sweeteners. They are found in many hard and soft candies, chocolate bars, cookies, and ice cream. Common side effects include gas and diarrhea, particularly in children.

Non-calorie sweeteners

Unlike regular sweeteners such as high-fructose corn syrup, non-calorie sweeteners contain virtually no calories or carbohydrates. They include aspartame (Equal), saccharin (Sweet 'n' Low), sucralose (Splenda), acesulfame-k (Nutrasweet), and neotame. Saccharin is 300-500 times sweeter than sugar, and Splenda is 600 times sweeter than sugar. They come in packet and granular forms. One packet of Splenda is as sweet as two teaspoons of sugar.

Table 5.14. Nutrient values of selected vegetables

Vegetables	Serving	Calories	Carbs (g)	Sugar	Dietary fiber (%)	Potassium	Vitamin A (% DV)	Vitamin C (% DV)
Potato	1 medium (148g)	100	26	3	3	21	0	45
Tomato	1 medium (148g)	35	7	4	1	10	20	40
Onion	1 medium (148g)	60	14	9	3	7	0	20
Carrot	7 inch long (78g)	35	8	5	2	8	270	10
Celery	2 stalks (110g)	20	5	0	2	10	2	15
Sweet corn	1 ear (90g)	80	18	5	3	7	2	10
Broccoli	1 stalk (148g)	45	8	3	5	15	15	220
Cabbage	1/12 head (84g)	25	5	3	2	5	0	70
Cucumber	1/3 medium (99g)	15	3	2	1	5	4	10
Bell Pepper	1 medium (148g)	30	7	4	2	8	8	190
Cauliflower	¼ head (99g)	25	5	2	2	8	0	100
Leaf lettuce	1 ½ cups (85g)	15	4	2	2	7	40	6
Sweet potato	1 medium (130g)	130	33	7	4	10	440	30
Mushroom	5 medium (85g)	20	3	3	1	9	0	2
Green onion	¼ cup (25g)	10	2	1	1	2	4	8
Green beans	¾ cup (83g)	25	5	2	3	6	4	10
Radish	7 medium (85g)	15	3	2	0	7	0	30
Squash	½ medium (98g)	20	4	2	2	7	6	30
Asparagus	5 spears (93g)	25	4	2	2	7	10	15

Source: USDA. Note the low calorie values and high dietary fiber content of these vegetables.

Sugar-free foods

Claims on food labels indicating "sugar-free" or "made without sugar" do not mean they are carbohydrate-free or calorie-free foods. Many of the sugar-free foods can be very high in carbohydrates and glycemic load. Food sweetened with no calorie sweeteners may or may not have calories and carbohydrates, depending on the ingredients other than the no calorie sweetener. Foods, such as diet soda, diet gelatin, and many powdered drink mixes are virtually calorie free. It is important to read the food labels to understand the ingredients of these foods.

KEY · POINTS · IN · A · NUTSHELL

- ♥ Different carbohydrates have different effects on HDL, triglycerides, and blood sugar levels.
- ♥ Glycemic index and glycemic load are nutritional terms that describe the quality and quantity of carbohydrates in a food.
- ♥ High glycemic load is an important contributor to high triglyceride and diabetes among Indians.
- ♥ Fruits and vegetables are low in glycemic load but high in valuable micronutrients, antioxidants, and dietary fiber.
- ♥ The recommended intake of fruits and vegetable is 9-13 servings (5-6 cups) per day
- ♥ Whole-grain products are great sources of micronutrients and insoluble fiber.
- ♥ Lentils and beans are also low in glycemic load and high in fiber and protein.
- ♥ The recommended daily carbohydrate intake is 35-50% of your total calorie intake.
- ♥ Indians predisposed to metabolic syndrome and diabetes should limit their glycemic load by restricting their carbohydrate intake to 40% of their daily calories (120 grams for a 1200-calorie diet)

5.6 ► Healthy Protein Choices

Not long ago, boxing trainers would instruct their prize fighters to eat huge slabs of rare steak in the weeks and days before a fight, on the belief that high amounts of protein would build up their muscles and improve their performance. Who can forget the scene in the film "Rocky" when Rocky Balboa (Sylvester Stallone), training for an upcoming fight, breaks half a dozen raw eggs into a glass and, to the horror of his fiancée, drinks them down in one go? Today, we know that even pure vegetarians (vegans) can get all the protein they need from plants. Some of the most heavily muscled animals—elephants and gorillas, for example—eat nothing but plants, after all.

Proteins, nevertheless, do constitute the body's building blocks, and protein deficiency continues to pose serious health risks in many developing countries. That means it is possible, but not always easy, to find and add high-quality proteins to a diet. Even in the western world, which suffers from protein excess rather than deficiency, there are pitfalls waiting to ensnare you: Mercury poisoning from certain types of fish, for example. Or high levels of fat in certain cuts of meat. Or vitamin B_{12} deficiency for those who want to eat only plant sources of protein. In short, like fats and carbohydrates, some proteins sources are better than others.

Yet another challenge is figuring out the right amount of protein to eat, since neither protein excess nor deficiency is healthy. The amount you actually need is less than 2oz a day, which you can get from, for example, 6 to 8oz of meat or fish. The average Indian non-vegetarian, for example, eats only a small amount of animal protein, perhaps one-fourth that of the average American. You should aim to eat *enough* protein, not necessarily *high* protein. Besides the body's proper functioning, eating protein has another benefit: because protein molecules are more complex than carbohydrate molecules, it takes your body longer to digest them. Proteins therefore have a higher *fullness factor*. They leave you feeling satisfied longer.

This section explains how vegetarians as well as nonvegetarians should choose proteins in a balanced diet. The discussion is organized around the four major sources of proteins: meat and eggs, fish, dairy, and plants. Beyond being good sources of protein, lean meat and fatty fish have beneficial effects on LDL and triglycerides. Low-fat and non-fat dairy products, egg whites, lentils, legumes, nuts, and soy are also good sources of protein.

▶Meat and eggs

Some proteins are more "complete" than others. Let's see what this means: Proteins are made up of amino acids. There are 20 common amino acids, and the human body is unable to manufacture nine of them. This means we need to get these nine essential amino acids from what we eat. Non-plant sources of protein—meat, fish, dairy, and eggs—have large amounts of all the essential amino acids. They are considered particularly complete, high-quality proteins. In addition, lean white meats such as turkey breast and skinless chicken breast are very good sources of niacin, vitamins B_6 and B_{12}, iron, phosphorus, and zinc.

Note, however, that many animal sources of protein come with modest to high amounts of fat. The actual protein content of meat, for example, is only about 20% of its total weight. Not all of the meat fat is saturated (bad) fat, however. All animal sources of protein contain roughly one-third cholesterol-*raising* saturated fat, one-third cholesterol-*neutral* saturated fat, and one-third cholesterol-*lowering* monounsaturated fat (*see* Table 5.8, in section 4. The actual amount of saturated fat and cholesterol depends on the species and the cut of meat. A diet rich in poultry has been shown to reduce LDL by 24% and triglycerides 13%, if you stick predominantly to skinless white meat. A Harvard University study has shown substituting half a breast of chicken for one cup of rice can reduce the risk of abdominal obesity and metabolic syndrome. Wild game such as venison is low in fat and high in protein. Egg whites are an excellent source of protein; they contain zero fat and zero cholesterol. All the fat and cholesterol in an egg are in the yolk.

If you eat beef, consider "loin" or "round" cuts. They are the leanest. "Lean" and "select" cuts tend to be low in cholesterol-raising saturated fat. Avoid portions that say "prime" or "rib"—these are the fattiest, with the highest marbling (fat distributed within the meat itself that cannot be removed by trimming). Whether you are eating beef, pork, lamb or chicken, it is advisable to trim any visible fat before cooking. It is also advisable to supplement animal protein with plant sources of proteins, which we will discuss shortly.

▶Fish

Fish, particularly dark-meat, oily fish such as salmon, tuna, sardines, mackerel, and catfish, is an excellent source of protein and omega-3 fats (*see* Chapter V, Section 4). Broiled, grilled or baked fish can reduce your cardiac risk by 25 to 35%. In contrast, fried fish or fish sandwiches actually increase your cardiac risk by 25%. Frying fish not only destroys the omega-3 fats but also generates trans fat. Diets high in fish have been shown to improve one's lipid profile. In one study, they reduced LDL by 16% and triglycerides by 28%. Like meat, proteins make up approximately 20% of the weight of most fish. Because of its high omega-3 content and lower levels of saturated fat, many nutritionists consider fish to be a superior source of protein than meat.

Studies have linked the consumption of some fish—such as swordfish, shark, king mackerel, tuna steaks, tilefish, Chilean Sea bass, and certain kinds of salmon—to health risk from ingesting methyl mercury or PCB (polychlorinated biphenyls). Mercury accumulates over the lifetime of larger, long-lived fish that eat other fish, whereas PCBs are found in fish living in polluted waters. The FDA and other experts have disputed the claim that consumption of farmed Atlantic salmon may pose health risks that may

Table 5.15. Classification of fish by omega-3 content of fish

	Omega-3 content	Types of Fish
Dark-meat (fatty) fish	High	Salmon, tuna, halibut, lake trout, mackerel, sardines, herring, and bluefish
Light-meat fish	Medium	Pike, cod, perch, haddock, trout, catfish, sole, snapper, flounder, swordfish, and whitefish
Shellfish	Lowest in omega 3 and high in cholesterol	Shrimp, lobster, crab, crawfish, abalone, mussel, oyster, scallop, squid, and octopus

Table 5.16. Major sources of proteins

Protein source	Serving size	Grams of Protein	Total Calories
Chicken	1 breast filet (6 oz)	30-40g (1.0 to 1.4 oz)	250 to 300 kcals
Fish	1 filet (6 oz)	30-40g (1.0 to 1.4 oz)	180 to 220 kcals
Dhals	1 cup	18g (0.6 oz)	220 to 260 kcals
Beans, cooked	1 cup	16g (0.6 oz)	200 to 240 kcals
Tofu, extra firm	½ cup	10g (0.4 oz)	90 to 100 kcals
Soy burgers	2 patties	25g (0.9 oz)	200 to 250 kcals

Source: www.nal.usda.gov/fnic/foodcomp
Note that the protein is 20% of the total weight of the chicken or fish.

exceed the beneficial effects of fish consumption. Salmon contained no more than 50 parts per billion of PCB, far lower than the FDA standard of 2000 parts per billion.

Certainly there are many fish that do not pose any health risk. These include flounder, farmed rainbow trout, clams and shrimp. Other fish are fine to eat in moderation— approximately once in a week. These fish include cod, farmed cat fish, mahi mahi, wild salmon, tilapia, and canned chunk tuna. So there is no need to shun fish to avoid toxins. Frying fish is ill-advised.

▶ Dairy products

Dairy products are good sources of protein. A cup of milk has about 8 grams of protein. I urge you to choose low-fat (below 1% fat) or fat-free versions of dairy products. Many Indians, like blacks, do not digest dairy products well. They have mild indigestion and gas problems, which may be an indication of lactose intolerance. Your doctor can check for lactose intolerance if you have any such symptoms. Low-fat yogurt, cottage cheese, and soy milk are good options for such individuals.

Is a calorie the same as a kcal?

The term "calorie," as used in this book, is strictly speaking inaccurate. A calorie is actually an energy unit from physics or chemistry defined as the energy needed to heat a gram of water by one degree Celsius. In contrast, the dietary Calorie, written with an uppercase C, measures how much energy you get from a food. A dietary Calorie is actually 1000 calories (or kilocalorie) in the physics or chemistry sense. That is why you sometimes see the abbreviation "kcal," which means kilocalorie.

To avoid confusion, in this book we ignore the classic scientific definition of calorie and use "calorie" to mean just the dietary Calorie. So, a dietary Calorie = 1000 calories = kilocalorie (or kcal), but we will just call it a plain old calorie. Now, food tastes much better that way.

▶ Plant sources of protein

Unlike animal sources, vegetable proteins do not contain any harmful saturated fat. Protein sources for vegetarians include legumes and beans, soy products, whey proteins, dairy protein – low or nonfat yogurt, cottage cheese, or milk. Beans and legumes (dhals and other pulses) are also great sources of protein, vitamins and phytochemicals. Soy proteins, (such as from tofu veggie burgers), have been shown to reduce the risk of heart disease, and the FDA has permitted food manufacturers to put this health claim on the labels of foods that provide more than 25g of soy protein daily.

How much protein do you need?

The normal daily requirement of protein is 0.8g/kg of body weight or 15% of total calories consumed. This translates into approximately 40g (1.4oz) of protein for a 50kg (110 pounds) Indian woman and 50g (1.8oz) of protein for a 60 kg (130 pounds) Indian man. You can get this amount by eating about 6oz of fish or meat per day. Most vegetarians can get this amount of protein through generous servings of legumes (such as beans and dhals), soy, and low-fat dairy choices. A typical soy burger contains 9-12g of soy proteins (see 5.16).

Some people need more protein. For example, children and adolescents need a higher intake of protein because they are at an age of significant physical growth. People with metabolic syndrome and diabetes may also benefit from raising their the protein intake to up to 25% of their daily calories, but not more than 100g/day (3.5oz, or double the recommended daily allowance), to prevent and control blood sugar and triglycerides. Some protein is converted into carbohydrates in the body without any adverse effects on insulin, blood sugar, or triglycerides. Even higher amounts of protein are acceptable, as long as it comes from legumes and other plants sources, such as peas, beans, and soy.

KEY · POINTS · IN · A · NUTSHELL

- ♥ Proteins, the body's building blocks, take longer to digest in your body, so they make you feel fuller and leave your feeling satisfied longer.
- ♥ Proteins should make up about 15% of your daily calories, which translates to less than 6-8 ounces of, for example, meat or fish for the average Indian.
- ♥ Protein intake up to 25% of your daily calories (2.5 oz. / 75g) is permissible, if most of it is from plant sources.
- ♥ If your diet is carbohydrate-heavy, substituting half a chicken breast for one cup of rice can reduce your risk of developing abdominal obesity and metabolic syndrome.
- ♥ Most meats are important sources of vitamins, minerals, and healthy fat (monounsaturated fats) as well as protein. Remember, however, that animal protein usually comes mixed with high levels of fat, especially saturated fat.
- ♥ Choose lean meat or skinless poultry and limit intake to less than 5oz per day.
- ♥ Nonfat and low-fat dairy products, such as skim milk, are excellent sources of protein.
- ♥ Excellent plant sources of protein include beans, legumes, and soy products.
- ♥ Fish ranks among some of the best protein you can eat, because it often comes with cardioprotective omega-3 fats.
- ♥ Consume two fish meals (8 to 10oz) per week. However, avoid frying fish because this destroys many of its benefits.

5.7 ▶ Designing a Prudent Nutritional Program

W e are now ready to discuss ways in which you can design your own personalized comprehensive nutrition program, one that is customized to your needs, lifestyle, budget, and tastes. Let's begin with a basic observation: There are dozens of trendy diets out there that emphasize one food category at the expense of another—low-fat diets, low-carb diets, high-protein diets, even rice-only diets. Any diet can make you lose weight in the short run, if you follow it rigorously enough. The problem is the long run: In the long term, very, very few people have the power—and the narrowness—to follow an unbalanced diet. Why? Because your body was not made for it, and at some point, you can no longer fool your brain into thinking that you are getting all the nutrients you need. The result is open rebellion.

The philosophy underpinning the Prudent Nutrition Program is to have balanced meals that contain appropriate amounts of proteins, carbs, and desirable fats. Besides balancing, however, the Nutrition Program lays emphasis on the *quality* of the proteins, carbs and fats you eat. The truth is that a tremendous difference exists between really exceptional proteins, carbs and fats that are packed with antioxidants, phytochemicals, minerals, vitamins, and cardioprotective nutrients, and run-of-the-mill foods that contain large amounts of cholesterol, trans fats, refined high glycemic index carbs, and proteins laden with saturated fats.

Nutrient and caloric intake in the US population

It takes a certain amount of deliberate, strategic thinking to ensure that you are selecting great proteins, carbs, and fats—and passing over the empty or even harmful calories that we often mindlessly reach for when we go food shopping without an intentional plan. Experience has shown that people tend to fail when they simply let hunger and their eyes determine what they choose to eat. When I started out to write this book, I initially called my nutrition program the *Prudent* Nutrition Program, for that particular reason. You need to allow your rational mind to play a central decisional role, not just your stomach.

What does this mean in practice? If means, for one thing, that designing a successful nutrition program usually requires particular planning steps, such as deciding what you will eat for an entire week, based on your preferences and medical conditions, perhaps even purchasing most of this food ahead of time.

Table 5.17. The American Diet: Average Daily Calorie and Nutrient Consumption in the US, by Gender

	Average	Men	Women
Total calories per person per day	2146	2475	1833
Percentage from protein	15	15	15
Percentage from carbohydrates	52	51	53
Percentage from fats	33	33	33
Total fat, in grams	81	97	67
Percentage of daily calories from saturated fat	11	11	11
Saturated fat, in grams	28	33	23
Dietary cholesterol (in milligrams)	265	307	225

Source: American Heart Association. Ref. 1.01.

You have probably heard the advice: Don't go grocery shopping when you are hungry because it encourages impulse buying rather than rational purchasing. Similarly, raiding the refrigerator when you are famished encourages impulse eating rather than balanced eating. Instant gratification—the principle upon which the entire diet industry, not to mention much of western life, is founded—is not the right approach to healthful eating. Eating is an important part of our lives not only as biological creatures but also as social beings in community. Take a little time to do it right, and your body and brain will reward you with years of optimal service.

If impulse buying and impulse eating are unhealthy, so is falling back on the same old conventional ways in which many families have prepared meals in our culture: Deep frying everything. Overcooking vegetables. Relying on sugar and salt rather than exploring the use of fresh, tasty aromatic spices. All three practices rob dishes of nutrients.

It is important to eat a wide range of foods including whole grains, legumes, fish, fruits, and vegetables. Indian cuisine offers a much larger variety of vegetable—and fruit-based options for both vegetarians and non-vegetarians than many Indians realize. Try out different combinations of foods to help you reach your overall health goals, but read the food labels in the grocery aisle. They provide much of the information you need to select healthy foods and avoid enticing-looking but unhealthy choices. Nuts, for example, are packed with nutrients, but then again, they are also dense in calories, which means restrict your intake to small quantities. Don't avoid nuts, but don't overeat them, either. This applies to dozens of other great foods. In addition, don't skip meals in an effort to lose weight, and start your day with a nutritious breakfast, which is the most important meal of the day.

There is a wise saying: You can't put on the new unless you first put off the old. As a first step—especially for people who are comfortable with radical breaks, or who derive motivation from the idea of a brand-new beginning, such as a New Year's resolution—I recommend that you remove all unhealthy foods from your fridge and kitchen. These include foods that contain partially hydrogenated oils or vegetable shortening such as banana chips, potato chips, deep-fried snacks such as samosas, crispy foods such as fried pappads, and high-fat dairy products. It is best to plan a weekly shopping list. I suggest that you plan your meals for the whole week prior to shopping. Typical items in your shopping list should include:

- **Low-fat or non-fat dairy products:** Yogurt, cottage cheese, skim milk or 1% milk
- **Bread/tortilla:** Low-carb choices (50 to 70 calories per serving), whole-grain bread, rye bread
- **Rice/flour:** Choose whole-grain (brown) or parboiled rice and whole-grain flour.
- **Sterol-based margarines:** Smart Balance, Take Control, and Benecol
- **Healthy cooking oils:** High mono-unsaturated oils such as olive oil and canola oil. Use for sautéing; avoid deep frying
- **Salad dressing:** Extra-virgin olive oil or low-fat dressings

- **Vegetables:** Green/red leaf lettuce, baby spinach, colored vegetables (green, red, yellow, orange peppers), tomatoes, most vegetables such as eggplant, bitter melon, cabbage, cauliflower, broccoli (excellent for sambar).

- **Fruits:** apples, pears, grapes and mangos whatever is in season

- **Legumes:** Kidney beans, navy beans, soya beans, garbanzo beans, and lentils

- **Proteins:** Lean meats, fish, particularly fatty fish, and skinless chicken breast. Stick to sirloin or tender loin cuts if you shop for beef

- **Vegetarian proteins:** Tofu, tempeh, and veggie "soy" burgers

- **Nuts:** Cashew, peanuts, almond, pistachio, walnut, and pecan

Food labels

Food labels can help you choose foods that provide the right amounts of carbohydrates, fats, protein, and fiber, and that are not too high in total fats per serving, saturated fat, refined sugar, cholesterol, and sodium (salt). Figure 5.3 depicts a typical food label. Take a moment to look at it. Let me say from the outset that analyzing food labels may seem impossibly tedious, but persist. Once you have scrutinized a couple of dozen labels, learned what the numbers mean, and know what you should buy and what to avoid, you will not have to do this over and over again. There is only one learning curve! You don't have to re-read the label on a bottle of olive oil, for example, to remember that what is in it is good for you. It will become second nature to you.

The first thing to notice in the "Amount Per Serving" section, *top half,* is the number of grams of saturated fat, listed under total fat. The amount of *saturated* fat you eat is much more critical than the amount of total fat or even cholesterol that you consume. So choose foods with the least amount or proportion of *saturated* fat compared to *total* fat in a serving. One cup of chocolate fudge sundae contains 340 calories out of which 160 calories come from fat. The sundae contains 9 grams of saturated fat – almost all the daily fat allowance for an adult woman.

Pay attention nevertheless to the cholesterol figure, listed next. Six ounces of beef, lamb and pork contain about 150 mg of cholesterol and two eggs contain about 560 mg of cholesterol.

Sodium intake is also critically important, particularly for those with pre-hypertension and hypertension. Note that the total recommended daily intake of sodium, whether on a 2000 or 2500 calorie a day diet, is now 2300 milligrams—about one teaspoon. Three pieces of chicken from a fast-food restaurant may contain as much as 1200-1500 mg of sodium.

Next comes total carbohydrate. Pay special attention to the number of grams of dietary fiber and sugars. You want the first to be high and the second to be low. Both slow-cooked oatmeal and instant oatmeal have about 27 grams of carbohydrate per serving, but the instant variety has nearly 12 grams of sugar compared to 1 gram in slow-cooked oatmeal. Also, the amount of soluble fiber is double (2g) in the slow-cooked version. I recommend that you always choose slow-cooked oatmeal over instant for that reason. The government has not so far required food companies to place the food's glycemic index on the label, but choosing foods low in sugar and high in dietary fiber is a moderately good

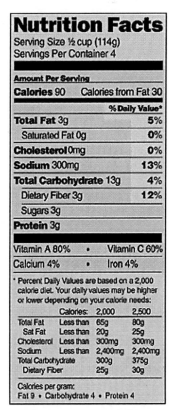

Figure 5.3. A typical food label. Focus on reducing your intake of saturated fats and sodium. Plan your carbohydrate and protein intake as per your meal plan. The percentages indicated are for a 2000 calorie a day diet. Reduce these by half if you weigh less than 200 pounds.

What does Partially Hydrogenated Mean?

A molecule of saturated fat and a molecule of unsaturated fat have exactly the same number of carbon and oxygen atoms. What makes saturated fat particularly harmful to you, and unsaturated fat beneficial, is the difference in their number of hydrogen atoms. Saturated fats are, well, *saturated* with *hydrogen* atoms. (When you think of saturated fats, it may help to think of the hydrogen bomb.) The hydrogen atoms in saturated fats are what make them solid at room temperature and give them a long shelf life. That same stability is the reason why they also stay in your arteries forever, creating waxy plaque that blood cannot push through.

To make trans fats, companies "hydrogenate" vegetable fat—meaning, they add hydrogen atoms to it—and turn it into artificial saturated fat. That is why candy bars can sit on a food shelf, or in your arteries, for months or years without change. Anything that germs do not like to eat, you should not eat either.

Trans fats are found not only in donuts, Danish pastries, commercial cakes, and chips, but in huge quantities in **fried chicken**, French fries, and anything deep-fried. They are also found in margarines and shortening—but not in the new generation of cholesterol-lowering margarines or in high-quality shortening such as Spectrum Naturals Organic Shortening, which is trans-fat free and non-hydrogenated.

Bear in mind, finally, that animal fats—butter, whole milk, pork, beef, lamb—contain tiny amounts of trans fat, but not in particularly significant quantities. Remember too that all fats contain both saturated and unsaturated fat; some just contain more of one than the other. Beef, for example, is about two-fifths (good) mono-unsaturated fat, but about 50% saturated fat. Olive oil is about 86% unsaturated and 14% saturated. Coconut oil, palm oil, and palm kernel oil are extremely high in saturated fat, even higher than butter.

approximation for low glycemic index. You can also make a list of low glycemic index foods for yourself, using in the information in Section 5 of this Chapter.

Besides limiting intake of protein sources that have too much saturated fat mixed in—such as certain cuts of meat—protein intake is not a such major issue for non-vegetarians, but it may be for many vegetarians. Two soy burgers typically contain about 10-12 grams of protein.

Trans fat content will be required on food labels beginning in 2006, although certain food companies are already including it on their labels. You can tell if a food has trans fats in it by looking at the List of Ingredients just below the Nutrition Facts label and looking for the words "hydrogenated" or "partially hydrogenated." See box, *alone side*, on hydrogenated oils.

Low-fat foods

By definition, low-fat foods can contain no more than 3g of fat for every 100 calories of serving. For example, a serving of 200 calories can have up to 6g of fat (54 calories). Low-fat food is not necessarily heart-healthy. Many low-fat foods contain loads of sugar, which raise blood levels of triglycerides and sugar. If you think about it, even ice cream can be "low fat" if you keep adding sugar to it, because the proportion of fat will decline as that of sugar rises. The best food choices are therefore low in fat *and* low in refined sugars. That is why fruits, vegetables, whole grains, and lean proteins are such a vital part of nutrition. They achieve both of these important *subtractive* goals: low sugar and low fat. But in addition, they achieve a ton of important *additive* goals.

Meal times

Consistent meal times are very important. Why? Two reasons: One is to associate specific times of the day with eating, and the rest of the day with not eating. This cuts down on the temptation to engage in mindless gratuitous eating at odd times. Second, eating at regular intervals helps to keep your blood sugar level as constant as possible by evening out your pancreas's release of insulin. This reduces cravings, mood swings, and energy lulls. Try not to have a gap of more than 4-5 hours between meals, less if you have diabetes. Start your day with breakfast (see Appendix C for a Daily Meal Plan). If you eat breakfast at around 7:00 am, consider a small mid-morning snack around 10:00. If lunch is around noon, consider a small, mid-afternoon snack around 4:00 or 4:30. Have dinner at least three to four hours before bedtime. If you have been watching your calories throughout the day, as you should, consider a light snack, glass of milk, or glass of soy milk before you go to bed.

Leverage the best in Indian cuisine

People the world over love going to Indian, Thai, Japanese, and Chinese restaurants. Why? People find Indian and other Asian spices particularly appealing. The cholesterol-lowering powers of garlic may be debatable to some, but besides great taste, there are several health-promoting aspects of the Indian diet. The variety of vegetables and legumes in Indian cuisine is astonishing. *Kootu*, a common Tamilian dish, blends lentils with steamed vegetables. *Poriyal* or *pugath* (North Indian) is steamed vegetables with sautéed spices. *Avial*, another common South Indian dish, is made with yogurt and a variety of vegetables. In Kerala, *avial* is loaded with coconut, but this delicious dish can be prepared without coconut. Sudesh's favorite South Indian dish is *pesserettu*—whole green dhal pancakes rich in lentils and fiber (see Appendix D). Apart from some mughalai dishes that float in ghee and butter, most non-vegetarian dry dishes are good sources of low-fat foods.

> **Tea's cardio-protective benefits**
> Tea is believed to lower the risk for heart disease because it is rich in flavonoids, which are powerful antioxidants. Green tea, Yerba maté, and rooibos have the highest levels of antioxidants.

The worst way of cooking *pappad* is deep-frying it, especially using oils that have been used several times previously, as discussed in Section 4 of this Chapter. Instead of frying, you can grill *pappad* and get the crunchy texture without the fat. Microwaving for 10 to 15 seconds on each side is another healthy way of cooking, but this does not eliminate its high salt content.

Coconut oil is the most concentrated source of saturated fat, even more concentrated than butter, *ghee*, pork, or sirloin steak. Those who simply cannot cook without coconut oil should consider using low-fat coconut products, similar to low-fat milk and low-fat cheese. Coconut meat, after all the milk has been removed (*peera* in Malayalam), is rich in fiber and will not increase your saturated fat intake. Limit rice to less than one cooked cup (2 servings at a time), and use whole-grain (brown) rice or parboiled rice instead of white rice to reduce its glycemic load. Limit your consumption of *chapathis* and *rotis*, especially those made of *maida*. A *roti* or *chapathi* with ghee is a whopping 250 calories! Consuming nuts up to 30g (1oz) per day can be a substitute for unhealthy food choices.

Watch your salt and sodium intake: Americans consume a lot of salt, more than double the daily requirement. Processed meats, chips, pretzels, canned soups, salted nuts, and pickles tend to be loaded with salt. Indians, on the other hand, tend to add liberal amounts of salt to their food while cooking. Either way, a high intake of salt results in hypertension, which promotes heart disease and stroke. One of the first things a person with high blood pressure should do is reduce their salt intake.

Drink water like mad: If you replace soda (soft drinks) with water and drink plenty of it, you will be amazed at the reduction in your hunger. You may feel weak if you are severely dehydrated. If it is practical, you should carry a bottle of water with you everywhere you go. Many athletes have a simple test to check their level of hydration. They examine the color of their urine stream: clear or pale yellow urine indicates good hydration (although taking vitamin supplements can turn it bright yellow). Water also prevents constipation when you increase your intake of fiber.

Moderate amounts of coffee and tea are okay: Although drinking a lot of caffeine (not one or two cups of coffee) can raise your blood pressure and anxiety level, most studies have not associated drinking coffee or tea with heart attacks, although one study showed that drinking six to seven cups of unfiltered coffee a day for six weeks increased LDL (bad) cholesterol levels by on average 33mg/dL. Daily consumption of one to two cups of coffee or tea appears to be safe. While coffee has no actual benefits, tea on the other hand has been associated with a lower risk for heart disease because it is rich in flavonoids, a powerful family of antioxidants that have numerous cardioprotective and other health benefits. Green tea, Yerba maté, and rooibos (caffeine-free South African red bush tea, pronounced *ROY-bus*) have the highest amounts of antioxidants, but white teas and black teas also have antioxidants, though not as much. The Chinese and Japanese, the world's greatest tea drinkers, tend not to add sugar, milk, or creamers. There are claims that adding milk and sugar to hot tea takes away the cardiac benefits of drinking tea, but this is not strongly substantiated.

Table 5.18. Some common problems and their suggested solutions

You find the food unappealing	Be adventurous. Try out different spices, dishes and foods
You feel hungry all the time	Your diet may have too high a proportion of high glycemic index carbohydrates. Increase in small steps your intake of healthy proteins and fats and low glycemic index carbs. (See Chapter V, sections 4, 5 and 6)
You are gaining weight	Check your total calorie intake as well as the relative proportions of proteins, fats and carbs in your diet. Review how much physical activity you are getting
You have low energy and seem to succumb to colds and sniffles	Eat more fruits and veggies. Your immune system may be compromised because you are not getting enough of the vitamins, minerals, and other health-promoting substances found in raw fruits and vegetables

Troubleshooting your nutrition program

You should begin to see the positive benefits of the Prudent Diet within two to three weeks of following it. However, fine-tuning this program to your specific taste and needs may take months. Common problems with this diet, and their suggested solutions, are outlined below. Eating food is normally a multi-sensory experience. Make sure that you enjoy the richness and fullness of the foods by eating a variety of foods. For example, try fruits and vegetables of different colors and tastes, since they provide different types of nutrients essential to your body.

Assignment: Meal plan and times for the week: Review this sheet before you go shopping for groceries.

Day of the week	Your current food choices and meal times	Your Prudent Nutrition Plan and planned meal times (Ensure that you have a meal or snack every 4 to 6 hours)
Weekdays (Mon to Fri)	Breakfast Lunch Dinner Snacks	Breakfast Lunch Dinner Snacks
Weekends (Sat, Sun)	Breakfast Lunch Dinner Snacks	Breakfast Lunch Dinner Snacks

KEY · POINTS · IN · A · NUTSHELL

♥ Plan and purchase your food for a whole week based on your meal plan.

♥ Food labels provide the necessary information you need for determining healthy choices.

♥ Eat a variety of foods including whole grains, nuts, legumes, fish, fruits, and vegetables.

♥ Do not skip meals, and always start your day with a nutritious breakfast.

♥ Indian cuisine offers a wide variety of vegetable and fruit-based options.

♥ Try out different combinations of foods to help you reach your overall health goals.

♥ The daily caloric intake should have the following proportions: carbohydrates 40-50%, fats 25-35% and the remainder protein. Examples: 50-25-25, or 40-30-30.

♥ Limit your saturated fat intake to no more than 7% of your total calories. This translates to less than 10 grams for most Indian men and women, who weigh less than 200lbs.

5.8 ▶ Physical Activity: The Other Half of the Equation ▶

Perhaps the greatest difference between the lives of people a century ago and today is the sedentary nature of contemporary life. Elevators, cars, television, washing machines, and deskbound jobs have deprived billions of people of the daily physical activity that would have been a natural part of their lives even just a few decades ago. Many modern cities are now so car-based that even walking to the post office or the corner grocery story has become inconvenient, even dangerous. There *is* no corner grocery store. Approximately 70% of the American public can now be classified as sedentary, meaning that they sit down most of their waking hours. This figure may be even higher among South Asian Indians—and if not, it is quickly catching up. The *couch potato*—with remote control in one hand and bag of chips in the other—has become a universally recognized human sub-species.

> **Did you know...**
> *The relative risk of developing heart disease from physical inactivity is comparable to the risk associated with high cholesterol, hypertension, or cigarette smoking.*

Yet regular moderately vigorous exercise, especially when combined with weight loss and a Prudent diet, can substantially reduce your risk of coronary heart disease and heart attack. Regular physical activity, even as little as 30 minutes a day, improves cardiovascular health by preventing the development of heart disease, or by allowing people who do have heart disease to enjoy a better quality of life. Indeed, encouraging physical activity has become a major goal of preventive medicine. Approximately 12% of premature deaths in the US can be attributed to physical inactivity. The relative risk of developing coronary heart disease associated with physical inactivity ranges from 1.5 to 2.4. This, according to the American Heart Association, is comparable to the cardiac risk associated with high cholesterol, hypertension, or cigarette smoking.

Yet hundreds of millions of Indians now live sedentary lives. If you are having nagging pangs of guilt that your life is increasingly looking like that of the above-described couch potato, increasing your daily physical activity will offer you a vast spectrum of benefits, summarized toward the end of the section. Suffice it to say for now that regular physical activity will:

- reduce your risk of heart disease
- reduce your risk of various chronic degenerative diseases
- slow down the onset of age-related functional decline and disability

As we will also see, staying physically active daily can be as much fun as you choose to make it. It does not matter much what type of exercise you do, as long as it burns enough calories and suits your age, health condition, skill level, and schedule. Explore different options and choose activities you enjoy and that fit into your lifestyle and schedule. This will give you the motivation to sustain that activity the rest of your life, without having to think too much about it.

This section is designed both to help inactive people to change their ideas about the subject of exercise and fitness, and to help the active to fine-tune their fitness program to achieve maximum benefit from it. We will first discuss *what* physical activity means and whether it is the same as exercise, then address *why* you should do it—in other words, the cardiovascular and non-cardiovascular benefits you can expect from it.

COMPONENTS OF A PHYSICAL ACTIVITY PROGRAM

A balanced physical fitness program has three components, each of which should be done several times a week, with not more than a few days elapsing since the last time you engaged in it. Just as a stool must have at least three legs in order to stand, all three components are indispensable. They are:

- **Cardiovascular** exercises, also called aerobic exercises
- **Resistance** training, also called weight training or strength training
- **Flexibility** exercises

Let's look at each.

Component One: Cardiovascular exercises

Cardiovascular exercises—or cardio exercises, for short—are designed to improve your cardiovascular system by raising your heart rate for an extended period, forcing your heart to become stronger by pumping harder. Also called aerobic exercises, one working definition of a cardio exercise is any rhythmic activity that enables you to maintain an elevated heart rate for longer than twenty minutes. This can include walking, running, swimming, biking, racquetball, tennis, basketball, hiking, and other sports, but gardening and housework can also count toward this category if the work is intense enough. Note that "aerobics"—which combines rhythmic leg lifts, dance moves, and abdominal work—is just one example of the general category of aerobic or cardiovascular exercise. There are three aspects of cardio exercise to which you need to pay attention, often abbreviated by the acronym **F.I.T.**

- Frequency   – how often you do it
- Intensity   – how vigorously you do it
- Time   – how long you do it

Learning how to balance and adjust these three variables—decreasing one and increasing another as need be—is critical to a successful cardio program.

i. Frequency: Compared with either the intensity of exercise or the amount of time you spend doing it, the consistency with which you stay physically active daily or almost daily, week in and week out, may be the most important factor in reducing your risk of heart disease and heart attack. Heart-healthy physical activity is somewhat like eating, sleeping, breathing, or shaving. No single meal, or sleep, or breath, or shave could ever be so perfect or complete that it saves you from having to do it again for several days. What is important is doing it consistently, and often. You should be physically active at least **five** and preferably **seven** days a week.

Naturally, if you had a particularly physically demanding day—if you raced, for instance—you should take off a day or two to recover. If you plan to take part in competitive events such as a five kilometer race, you should have at least one day off for complete recovery.

ii. Intensity: That said, how intense should your cardiovascular activities be? How much exercise do you need? That depends partly on your goal—whether it is simply disease prevention, weight loss, weight maintenance, or achieving a competitive-level of fitness. For example, to achieve weight loss, you need to focus on lower-intensity exercise over a longer duration because higher-intensity exercise consumes relatively more carbohydrates, while lower-intensity exercise burns more fat. To attain a higher level of fitness or a sculpted body, you will need to raise frequency, intensity, or time, or all three. If your goal is simply to prevent cardiovascular disease, however, all you need to do is to engage in moderately vigorous activity almost daily.

The Casual versus Vigorous Debate: In fact, surprisingly little exercise is required to meet the minimum recommendations made by the Centers for Disease Control (CDC) and the National Institutes of Health (NIH) for disease prevention. On the other hand, beware of articles and websites that claim, with the same glibness of diet books, that all you have to do to stay healthy is to engage in a leisurely walk in the park

with the dog every other day. Despite claims that casual, light exercise confers the same cardio-protective health benefits as more vigorous activities, a recent, large, longitudinal study in Wales found that *moderately vigorous* activities such as jogging, swimming, hiking, or brisk walking for an hour at a time were associated with a reduced death rate from heart disease. In contrast, the study, which followed nearly 2,000 men aged 40 to 64 for 10 years—252 of whom died during the study period, mostly from heart disease—found no evidence of a similar association between the risk of dying from heart attacks and *light or moderate* physical activity such as bowling, golf, walking at a normal pace. (*See* "The Exercise Intensity Debate: Major Support for the Healthful Life Views and Recommendations" (July 2003) http://healthfullife.umdnj.edu/archives/exercise_archive.htm.)

> **What Exactly is Pilates?**
> Created by a German athlete Joseph **Pilates**, once a sickly child, Pilates has become a popular form of exercise in gyms and fitness centers around the world. Pronounced *pi-LAH-tees*, it consists of a series of conditioning exercises done mainly on a mat, either sitting or lying down.
>
> Pilates combines stretching, strengthening and breathing and focuses on core strength, posture, awareness of the spine, and flexibility. It is essentially a low-stress, low-injury approach to building strength and flexibility, and developing balance. Check your local YMCA or health club for classes and times.

While leisurely walking for example is certainly better than nothing, there is evidence that low-intensity activities do not produce substantial health benefits, although the debate is ongoing. The consensus within the medical community is much broader that *moderately vigorous* exercise which has an intensity level of 3 to 6 METs—such as brisk walking that makes you sweat—is associated with significant reductions in the risk of coronary heart disease. (*See* Tables 1.22, 1.23, 1.24, and 1.25 for a range of activities that correspond to an intensity level of 3 to 6 METS.)

Your age is another factor in determining the appropriate level of intensity. Many exercise physiologists and physicians have speculated that, while younger people need to engage in at least *moderately vigorous* activity, less strenuous activities may have health benefits for seniors over the age of 60 or 65. The larger point is that many people underestimate their capacity for exercise, believing they are too frail or too old to start. Others, by contrast, push themselves too hard, heightening their risk for overuse injuries. The discussion below will show you how you can tell if you are exercising too hard or too little.

Measuring intensity: Once you have decided on your goals, and thus how intense your aerobic activity needs to be, how can you tell how intense any specific activity is? Intensity is measured in three ways:

- how fast your heart is beating
- how hard the activity *feels* to you or to most people
- how much energy or oxygen your body is consuming during that activity

The first way of measuring intensity is based on heart rate. The second is a subjective scale based on a person's own perceived level of effort (also called RPE, or rate of perceived exertion).

Table 5.19. Basic Exercise Prescriptions for Different Health and Fitness Goals for Older Persons (adapted from Federal Exercise Guidelines)

Fitness Dimension	Goal: Disease Prevention	Goal: Basic Health	Goal: Fitness
Cardiovascular capacity	Accumulate 30 minutes of physical activity most days	Large-muscle repetitive exercise or equivalent sports activity; 20 minutes, 3 times a week	Aerobic exercise or equivalent sports activity; 40-60 or more minutes, 4-6 times a week
Strength	Include weight-bearing activity	"Core four" or equivalent program, 8-12 or 12-15 repetitions at challenging weights, one set, twice a week; Pilates work	Balanced whole-body free weights or machines, 8-12 repetitions each to reach functional failure, 2-3 times a week; Pilates work
Flexibility	Maintain your range of motion by bending and stretching in daily activities	2-4 stretches after activity, 1 repetition, hold each stretch for 30 seconds	6-10 whole-body stretches before and after activity, 1-2 repetitions

Source: www.physsportsmed.com/issues/1999/10_15_99/kligman.htm. For a vast collection of articles on issues ranging from personal fitness, nutrition, and heart disease to aging, weight control, injury prevention and women's health, as well as an extensive index of sports medicine groups, physicians and clinics, visit the sports medicine website www.physsportsmed.com/index.html.

The third approach, developed by physiologists, is expressed in terms of Metabolic Equivalents (or METs). Determining intensity is important, so let's look briefly at each of these three.

a. The heart rate method: The first way of estimating the intensity of your workout is designed to keep your heart rate within a certain "target" range for an extended period. It uses your fitness level (as reflected in your resting pulse) and your age.

How do you know what your Target Heart Rate should be? Here is one widely used formula. Let's assume you are aiming for a "moderately hard" level of intensity, which many sports medicine experts define as 60-85% of your Maximum Heart Rate, or MHR. (Note that opinions differ: The American College of Sports Medicine defines "moderate activity" as 55-69% of your MHR, "hard exercise" at 70-89% of your MHR, and "very hard exercise" as 90% or higher. The CDC defines "moderate intensity" physical activity as 40-60% of your MHR and "vigorous intensity" activity as 70-85% of MHR. For this calculation, we will use 60-85%.) Let's say you are 48 years old, with a heart rate of 62 when you are resting.

How to Take Your Pulse

Briefly stop exercising. Turn your wrist over. Feel for the pulse in the radial artery. It runs on the underside of your wrist near the thumb. Using the tips of your index and middle fingers, press lightly on this artery. Count the heart beats for 15 seconds and multiply it by four. Count the first heart beat as "zero." not "1."

The heart rate method requires wearing a simple, lightweight heart rate monitor such as from Acumen, Cateye, Polar, Reebok, or Timex. They cost $40 and up, but the less expensive models are equally accurate. It consists of a plastic belt-like transmitter you wear around your chest, which sends your pulse readings to a special "watch" worn on your wrist. Many can be set to beep if your heart rate falls outside your target range—e.g., 120-140 beats per minute. Gym fitness machines often have a heart monitor attached. Several sporting websites sell heart rate monitors. Examples: www.polardiscount.com, www.roadrunnersports.com or www.heartzones.com. Visit Google and type in "heart rate monitor." For a review of different models, visit the superb comparative review site Consumer Search, which reviews other reviews and summarizes the best results: www.consumersearch.com/www/health_and_fitness/heart_rate_monitors.

Step One: Find your Maximum Heart Rate by subtracting your age from 220 for men. 220 - 50 = 170. Now, subtract your resting heart rate (62) from your MHR (172). 170 - 62 = 108. This is known as your "heart rate reserve." The maximum heart rate formula for women is 226 - age.

Step Two: Determine the lower end of your Target Heart Rate range by finding 60% of 108, and adding your resting heart rate to it. 108 x 0.60 = 65. 65 + 62 = **127**. This is the low end of your Target Heart Rate range.

Step Three: Repeat this, this time for the higher end of your Target Heart Rate range, using 85% instead of 60%. 108 x 0.85 = 92. 92 + 62 = 154. We can round this to **155**.

Done! Your Target Heart Rate range is **128-155** beats per minute.

Fine-tuning: There are obviously sub-ranges within this overall range, depending on your particular goal (weight loss, fitness, disease prevention, competition) and whether you are aiming for "optimal" exercise this week or just "minimal" exercise because you are very busy.

Disadvantages: *of this method* For some people, an age-based Target Heart Rate range may be misleading because it is based on the "average" person. In reality, your physiological age differs from your chronological age, depending on your health history, fitness level, genes, and lifestyle. Some exercise physiologists therefore feel that, especially as people age, the formula for predicting their Maximum Heart Rate may be off by as much as 15 or 20 beats per minute. In addition, your Target Heart Rate range can change as your become fitter and healthier. So to some degree, you need to go on how strenuous the activity feels, not just what your heart rate is.

There are other practical considerations. You may find it hard taking your own pulse especially during exercise, you may not own a heart rate monitor; or the machines in your gym may not have any, or you may be taking medications that affect your heart rate. What can you do then? There is another way.

b. The Perceived Level of Exertion method

A second way of measuring intensity is by how hard the activity feels. This may at first sound vague, but it can be a surprisingly useful and accurate estimate of intensity. The Borg Rating of Perceived Exertion scale—or RPE scale, for short—was developed by Gunnar Borg to describe the level of perceived effort an activity requires, on a scale of 6 to 20, as reported by the participant. "6" means absolutely no exertion. "9" corresponds to very light exercise, like walking slowly. "13" would be exercise that feels "somewhat hard" but not so hard that it makes you think about stopping soon. It feels fine to continue it. A "17" on the RPE scale represents very hard

Table 5.20. Heart Rate Ranges for Different Age Groups (resting heart rate assumed = 62)

Age	Max. heart rate	85%	80%	70%	60%
20	200	179	172	159	145
25	195	166	160	137	117
30	190	171	164	152	139
35	185	157	148	130	111
40	180	162	156	145	133
45	175	149	140	123	105
50	170	154	148	138	127
55	165	140	132	116	99
60	160	145	140	131	121
65	155	132	124	109	93
70	150	137	132	124	115
75	145	123	116	102	87
80	140	128	124	117	109

or very strenuous exercise that leaves you feeling very tired after several minutes. You have to really push yourself, even if you are healthy and in good condition. "19" is "extremely strenuous," for most people the most strenuous exercise they have ever experienced. "20" represents absolute maximal exertion—Muhammad Ali in the 14th round against Joe Frazier. Nothing could possibly be harder.

The advantage of the Borg approach to judging intensity is that it captures your own feeling of effort and exertion, based on your own appraisal of how you honestly feel. You should print out the Borg Scale and have it handy so you can rate your perception of exertion the next time you are engaged in aerobic activity. The idea is to combine all your sensations of physical stress, effort, and fatigue, your total feeling of exertion, not focusing on just one factor such as shortness of breath, muscle fatigue, amount of sweat, or pain in one area of your body. Then look at the scale and choose the number that best describes how your feel. The goal is to find out what a "12" or "13" feels like for you, then use it as a tool to estimate intensity, no matter what you are doing.

Table 5.21. Heart Rate Ranges for Different Age Groups (resting heart rate assumed = 62

0-6	No exertion at all; lying in bed or reading a book
7-8	Extremely light
9-10	Very light; walking slowly across the room in no hurry
11-12	Light; strolling in a park. You can still sing while doing this activity.
13-14	Somewhat hard. Beginning to perspire. You can carry on a conversation if you try. This intensity range may offer the most benefit with the least amount of risk
15-16	Hard; it is now difficult to carry on a conversation in complete sentences
17-18	Very hard or very heavy; it would take a high level of concentration and willpower to continue at this level for another 10 or more minutes
19	Extremely hard, or very, very heavy
20	Maximal exertion

How intense is enough What level should you aim for? If your goal is at least cardiovascular disease prevention, as it should be, and you are reasonably healthy, aim at activity that feels "somewhat hard" (12-14 on the RPE Scale). If you are young, consider 13-15. If you are older, 11-13. As you improve, increase intensity gradually. Back off if it starts to feel "hard" or "very hard" (15 and above). Here are some other subjective signs you can use:

- Moderately vigorous exercise should leave you feeling warm and should make your skin moist after 10-20 minutes. Overall, it should make you feel the way you do when you walk briskly for 30 minutes

- You should be breathing hard through your nose, but you should not feel a great urge to have to

Table 5.22. Recommended Exercise Intensities, in METS, by Age Range

Your Age	METs (moderate)	METs (hard)	METs (very hard)
20-39	4.8-7.1	7.2-10.1	over 10.2
40-64	4.0-5.9	6.0-8.4	over 8.5
65-70	3.2-4.7	4.8-6.7	over 6.8
80 and over	2.0-2.9	3.0-4.25	over 4.25

breath through your mouth

• If exercise leaves you feeling exhausted for several hours afterward, you are exercising too hard, too long, or possibly too often

• If you can talk very easily all the way through the activity, it is probably not vigorous enough; if you cannot talk at all, it is probably too intense

According to Borg (1998), and reported by the CDC, there is a fairly strong correlation between your heart rate during physical activity and your perceived exertion rating multiplied by 10. Your RPE may therefore be a fairly good estimate of your heart rate. For example, a level-13 intensity activity suggests that your pulse is around 130.

c. Metabolic Equivalents (METs)

A third way to define intensity—originally developed by physiologists but useful for non-medical people as well—is through the measure called the MET. Short for Metabolic Equivalent, one MET is the energy it takes to sit quietly for one minute doing nothing. (It is actually measured by the amount of oxygen you consume during that time, which is about 3.5 milliliters per kilogram of body weight.) Walking at 2mph requires an energy expenditure of to about 2.5 METs; 4mph requires about 4.5 METs. Playing tennis (doubles) is approximately 6 METs. Any cardiovascular activity that requires 4-6 METs of energy is considered moderate intensity. Vigorous activity corresponds to more than 6 METs. However, depending on the age and physical fitness of the person, these values may vary significantly. For example walking at 3 miles per hour (4 METS) is considered light for a 20-year old healthy person but represents vigorous intensity for a 80 year old person.

Knowing how many METs an activity requires also tells you how rapidly you will burn calories. To calculate this, you just need to know your weight in kilograms (which is your weight in pounds divided by 2.2), and include a simple conversion factor (3.5/200). The formula is:

Calories burned = (MET value of the activity) x (your weight in kilograms) x (duration of activity in minutes) x 3.5/200

For example, running at 6mph has an intensity level of 10 METs. If a 110 pound (50 kg) woman ran at 6mph for an hour, she would burn: 10 METs x 50kg x 60 x 3.5/200 = 525 calories.

How many METs should you aim for? Again, this depends on your goals, health history, and age. The American College of Sports Medicine has developed a set of recommended intensities by age. Most people should aim for activities of "moderate" intensity or perhaps the low end of "hard" if you are quite fit and

Table 5.23. MET Value Table A: Common Activities Ranked by Intensity, in METs

METs	Selected Common Activities
1	Resting quietly, watching TV, reading
1.5	Eating, writing, desk work, driving, showering
2	Light moving, strolling, light housework, light gardening, light work (bartending, store clerk, assembling, filing), walking around at work at 2 mph (in office or lab area)
2.5	Pushing a stroller with a child, walking the dog, walking downstairs, cooking, shopping, somewhat heavier gardening or yard work
3	Level walking (2.5 mph), cycling (5.5 mph), bowling, golf using a cart, heavy housework, scrubbing floors, washing the car, washing windows, mopping, moderately vigorous playing with children, sweeping outside the house, vacuuming, picking fruit or vegetables
4	Walking (3 mph), cycling (8 mph), doubles tennis, raking leaves or the lawn, planting shrubs, weeding the garden, heavy yard work, masonry, painting, paper hanging, moderately heavy lifting, moderately heavy farm work
5	Walking (4 mph), cycling (10 mph), ice or roller skating, digging in the garden, vigorous gardening, painting, carpentry, cleaning gutters, laying carpet, using heavy power tools
6	Walking (5 mph), cycling (11 mph), singles tennis, splitting wood, shoveling snow, using heavy non-powered tools such as shovels, picks and spades
6.5	Loading and unloading truck (standing); moving heavy objects; heavy farming work
7	Jogging (5 mph), cycling (12 mph), basketball
7.5	Walking downstairs or standing while carrying objects about 75-99 lb
8	Running (5.5 mph), cycling (13 mph), vigorous basketball
9	Competitive handball or racquetball
10	Running (6 mph)

Source: Adapted from Compendium of Physical Activities. Ainsworth, BE. Medicine and Science in Sports and Exercise. Volume 25, p.713 (1993) and volume 32, S498 (2000). http://healthfullife.umdnj.edu/archives/METsWork.htm

have other goals beyond just disease prevention. Other classifications you come across may describe "moderate intensity" as "moderately vigorous."

The overarching point is that, unless you are over 80, you should aim for activities that have a MET intensity of at least 3 and preferably closer to 5 or 6. The fastest speed at which you can walk and talk at the same time—often called "the walk-talk test"—typically represents an intensity of 4 or 5. These recommendations are for men. For women, average values are 1 to 2 METs lower than for men.

A MET Value Table—a list of common activities ranked by their intensity in METs—can help you set exercise goals by enabling you to calculate how many calories you will burn if you participate in a particular activity. Bear in mind that the MET values for various activities are approximate averages based on testing hundreds of people. Actual energy consumption will vary from person to person. As you can see from the tables below, however, almost any activity will make you consume much more energy than remaining sedentary.

Integrating the Three

Now that we have looked at heart rate, the RPE (perceived exertion) scale, and METs, a safe suggestion is for you to use all three methods as sources of guidance, finding the middle ground where they offer slightly divergent directions. The Centers for Disease Control defines "moderately intense" activity as:

- an activity with an RPE of 11 to 14
- an activity that consumes energy at the rate of 3 to 6 METs, or
- an activity that burns 3.5 to 7.0 calories a minute, depending on your weight and fitness level

If you cannot currently achieve any of this, do less, but by all means avoid being sedentary.

Table 5.24. MET Value Table B: Common Activities Ranked Alphabetically, in METs

Activity	MET Value
Aerobics: general	6
Aerobics: high impact	7
Aerobics: low impact	5
Bicycling: > 20 mph, racing	16
Bicycling: 12-13.9 mph, moderate	8
Bicycling: 16-19 mph, racing	12
Bicycling: leisure	4
Calisthenics: push-ups & sit-ups, vigorous	8
Circuit resistance training	8
Golf: carrying clubs	5.5
Golf: using power cart	3.5
Jogging: general	7
Running: 10 mph (6 min. mile)	16
Running: 5 mph (12 min. mile)	8
Running: 6 mph (10 min. mile)	10
Running: 7 mph (8.5 min. mile)	11.5
Running: 8 mph (7.5 min. mile)	13.5
Running: 9 mph (6.5 min. mile)	15
Skiing: cross-country, vigorous effort	14
Skiing: downhill, light effort	5
Skiing: downhill, vigorous effort	8
Skiing: general	7
Stretching, yoga	4
Swimming: backstroke-general	8
Swimming: breast stoke-general	10
Swimming: butterfly-general	11
Swimming: laps-freestyle-vigorous	10
Tennis: doubles	6
Tennis: singles	8
Walking: <2.0 mph-very slow	2
Walking: 2.0 mph-slow	2.5
Walking: 3.0 mph-moderate	3.5
Walking: 4.0 mph-very brisk	4
Water aerobics	4

Source: American College of Sports Medicine, Position Stand, Recommended Quantity and Quality of Exercise for Development and Maintenance of Cardiorespiratory and Muscular Fitness and Flexibility in Healthy Adults.

iii. Time: The third important dimension of an effective cardiovascular activity program is deciding how long you should exercise: Too short, and you will not derive maximum benefit from it. Too long, and it will begin to wear you down, leaving you feeling tired at the end of it rather than energized. The 2005 US Government Dietary Guidelines recommend 30 to 90 minutes of exercise per day, depending upon your weight, your age, and the activity. Start with 15 to 20 minutes of exercise a day, increasing this by 5 to 10 minutes a day every week until you build it up to the optimal duration. Note that this time does not include the warm-up and cool-down period. You should start out any exercise by warming up for 5 to 10 minutes at an RPE intensity of 3 to 4, gradually increasing it to 7 to 8, then to 11-14 during the exercise itself. A cool-down period of similar length is also required at the end. Here are recommendations based on the goal you set:

- To reduce your risk of heart disease, exercise **30** minutes a day, 5-7 days a week
- To prevent weight gain, exercise **60** minutes a day, 5-7 days a week

The Best Way to Lose Weight

Exercise physiologists are united on one thing: To lose weight, you should emphasize *low-intensity, long-duration* exercise. Why? Because burning fat simply takes **time**. This is why no reputable diet authority ever recommends crash diets—because fat does not respond well to lifestyle changes over a matter of days. But it does respond, and respond very well, to changes that take place over a period of weeks and months. To get those stubborn pounds off, work out at a level that you can comfortably maintain for a longer period of time, because the most important factor for losing weight is the duration of the activity.

•　To lose weight or reduce your waist size, exercise **90** minutes a day, 5-7 days a week

Ninety minutes a day may sound excessive, but it is often not appreciated that to lose one pound of fat (3500 calories), you need to walk about 35 miles. As we discussed under "Intensity," weight loss literally takes "time." It is best achieved by focusing on lower-intensity activities (4-6 METs rather than 7-8 METs) and doing them for a longer duration, because higher intensity activities burn relatively more carbohydrates, while lower-intensity activities burn relatively more fat. Think of carbohydrates in your body as the kindle in a fire place, fats as the thick, oily log, and intensity as the heat of the flame. If you turned up the heat very high, all you will do is burn the kindle off very quickly. To burn the log, you need a slow steady burn over a long period of time. That is how your body burns fat. Very vigorous exercise, of course, will naturally burn both more carbs and more fat per hour than moderate exercise simply because it is more intense, but it will burn off relatively more carbs than fats, while less vigorous activity will burn off relatively more fat.

For cardiovascular disease prevention, however, both the duration and the intensity of exercise offer significant benefits. For example, walking more than 3 hours a week at 20 minutes a mile can reduce heart disease risk by 30%. In contrast, walking more than 10 hours a week at 15 minutes a mile can reduce heart disease risk by more than twice, 63%. Researchers have also found that endurance training significantly raises your HDL levels and lowers your triglyceride levels. Thus, although most of your aerobic training should be at lower intensities, particularly for weight loss, other significant benefits can be achieved by performing aerobic workouts at higher intensities for shorter times. Indeed, aerobic instructors often guide their students through "interval training" that includes high-intensity aerobic activity done over a period of a minute or less. High intensity aerobic exercise is like "strength training" for the heart. It improves its pumping power (ejection fraction), maintains or increases the flexibility of your coronary artery walls, and improves your ability to withstand and survive a major coronary event.

A real-world example of high-intensity exercise would be a 155-pound man exercising to a heart rate of 150 beats per minute for 30 minutes on a treadmill, three times per week, expending approximately 350 calories per session.

Reviewing our **F.I.T.** formula: How should you combine **Frequency**, **Intensity** and **Time** into an effective fitness program? The first priority to focus on is frequency. Our bodies typically have a lower tolerance for very *intense* exercise or *long* exercise sessions than for high *frequency*. Most healthy people could probably walk an hour everyday at 3 or 3.5 miles per hour 7 days a week, because even though the frequency is high and the time is moderately high, the intensity is low. Far fewer people could walk *1.5* hours a day at *5* miles per hour for even 6 days a week. Our low tolerance of intensity when combined with long duration is one reason marathoners cannot race every week. Similarly, low tolerance of high intensity is why even the best racehorses need

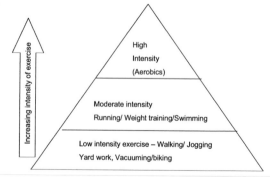

Figure 5.4. Physical Pyramid. This graph shows that you can fulfill your physical activity needs either by spending a larger fraction of time doing lower-intensity activities like gardening, or a smaller fraction of time doing higher-intensity activities liking aerobics, or a mix of the two. High-intensity workouts for short periods increase your metabolic rates, strengthen your heart's ability to withstand cardiovascular stress, and tone your muscles more quickly, while lower-intensity activities minimize your risk of injury and burn more fat. See comments on pyramid at beginning of Section.

two weeks to recover from the Kentucky Derby (which takes only a couple of minutes!) to race again in the Preakness, and some are even made to skip the Preakness entirely and race in the Belmont. Intensity exacts a high cost in recovery time.

In short, endeavor to stay active at a *frequency* of 5-7 days a week, mostly at moderate *intensity*, and adjust *duration* according to how energetic or tired you feel or how many other commitments you have. Play around with all three variables to discover what works best for you. This means that, in balancing Frequency, Intensity, and Time, you need to find out what your own natural tolerance is for each of the three, and mold your aerobic exercise program to fit this balance—gradually adjusting it as your fitness level improves, or as you notice that you may be pushing too hard.

Component Two: Strength training

There is, especially among women, a misconception that strength training—also called weight training or resistance training—will give them bulging muscles. Of course, this is what some people want—particularly men. But strength training with light to moderately heavy weights will not make your muscles bulge. It will only tone and shape them. Bulging, bulky muscles can be obtained only by lifting weights that are so heavy that you can perform no more than 8-12 repetitions at a time. Women, if you can perform 15-20 repetitions, you are safe.

Why should you do strength training? For one thing, you lose muscle mass as you age. In addition, muscle toning lowers your blood pressure, decreases your insulin resistance, and helps you burn excess fat because your muscles use more energy. Finally, by toning your muscles, strength training reduces your chances of injury if for instance you slip and fall, and even reduces the chances that you will fall at all.

How do you do it? Resistance training consists of either lifting free weights or using machines; the latter is preferred for safety and ease of use, but moderately light free weights can be very useful because they exercise a greater range of muscle groups than do machines. Resistance training classes and coaching are readily available in most fitness clubs and at your local YMCA. Muscle toning can also be done through calisthenics—strengthening exercises done without equipment, such as squats, push-ups and knee bends—or using inexpensive equipment such as stretch bands and handheld weights.

Circuit training is an excellent way to simultaneously improve mobility, strength and stamina. The circuit training format uses a group of 6-10 strength exercises (using different machines or "stations") that are completed one exercise after another virtually without stopping. Each exercise is performed for

Physical activity versus exercise

How intense does the cardiovascular component of your fitness program need to be? As we have seen, it depends on your goals, but let's cut to the chase here: Many people are put off by the notion that, for a fitness program to be any good, it must be done at a very high intensity. The truth is that a low-intensity aerobic exercise, done everyday or almost everyday for half an hour to an hour, may not get you to the next Olympics, but it is all you need for heart disease and diabetes prevention, and often all you need for weight maintenance. More than two decades ago, Sophia Loren's personal physician gave her excellent advice when the Italian actress asked him what she should do for exercise. He told her, "Just walk briskly everyday for one hour." She has been doing that ever since.

The key is to think in terms of "physical activity" rather than "exercise." For many, the word exercise conjures up negative images of monotonous, sweaty, grunt work. But physical activity need not feel like endless torture. Sure, it can be intense if you feel up to it, but it can also consist of daily recreational or occupational activities that simply get you moving-including dancing, mowing the lawn, vacuuming, and walking. In fact, anything that elevates your heart rate, gets you to use your muscles, and leaves your skin slightly moist qualifies as beneficial physical activity.

Of course, exercise—meaning a relatively demanding, structured physical activity that you do to raise your cardiovascular fitness—can achieve certain goals more quickly than simply staying active on a day-to-day basis, including weight loss, strength, endurance, and flexibility. But the important thing to bear in mind is that you should not feel you have no options if for some reason you cannot do higher-intensity aerobic exercises or simply hate them.

a specified number of repetitions or time period before moving on to the next exercise. Circuit training is really weight training that has an aerobic, pulse-elevating effect.

How often should you do it? Devote 2-3 days a week to weight training. More often will not give your muscles enough time to rebuild, because weight training works by breaking down the muscle fibers. Less often will only take you back to square one each time, because you lose too much muscle strength in between sessions.

How much weight should you lift? The rule is to aim for what exercise physiologists call *muscle fatigue*. That is, use a resistance setting or weight that is heavy enough that, after lifting it a certain number of times—let's say 12—you cannot complete another lift without losing your form. After how many repetitions should you achieve muscle fatigue?

- For muscle toning, **12-15** repetitions, 1-2 sets
- For improving strength, **8-12** repetitions, 1-2 sets
- For maximum bulk, **6-8** repetitions, 1-3 sets

Using the middle target—8-12 reps for strength—as an example, as you improve and can complete 12 repetitions relatively easily, increase the weight so you can do only 8, and start all over again. Older adults should aim to achieve muscle fatigue using slightly lower resistances and slightly more repetitions. Finally, don't hold your breath while lifting. Breathe normally.

Component Three: Flexibility exercises

It is highly important to stretch. Stretching increases tendon flexibility, improves joint range of motion and function, and enhances muscular performance by preventing cramps and muscle tears. A good time to stretch is at night just before you retire or after a warm-up; but the very best time to stretch is after exercising because your muscles are warmed up the most and they can stretch maximally. Of course, stretching after a warm-up, after you exercise, and before you go to bed cannot hurt. You can also perform simple neck and shoulder stretches any time during the day. Unlike strength training, you can and should stretch everyday.

Make sure that you breathe normally while stretching. Do not bounce; you can cause muscle cramps or tears. Simply hold the stretch for 10 to 30 seconds. Don't try to overstretch; it should not feel painful; the sensation should simply be a warm tingling feeling. Consult your physician if any consistent pain or injury develops. Don't stretch when your muscles are cold, for example, before a warm-up. Many gyms have charts on the wall that show you how to stretch, and these can also easily be obtained on the internet or in a bookstore.

Yoga adds another dimension to stretching. A product of Indian civilization that has been practiced for thousands of years, yoga is a practical spiritual science that does not belong to any particular religion. Performing **yoga asanas** involves specific body poses with associated breathing exercises and stretching. Different yoga asanas combine stretching and isometric contraction directed at specific muscle groups and specific organs. For example, padma-asana (the lotus position) facilitates relaxation, concentration and ultimately, meditation. The posture creates a natural balance throughout body and mind. When the knees are stretched enough to remain in the padma-asana position without discomfort, the posture creates a feeling of effortlessness and ease that soothes the nervous system and quiets the mind. Besides stress reduction, yoga has been shown to have other cardiovascular benefits. For example, some small studies have shown that it can improve endothelial function. Endothelial dysfunction is a hallmark of atherosclerotic vascular disease. Many gyms and health clubs now offer yoga classes.

Putting it all together: Designing your own program

As with nutrition, you should develop a physical fitness program that delivers the best benefits for you. Be patient. Such a program may take months to develop. As with food, try a variety of activities to find out what you enjoy and can perform year-round. Enjoyment translates into motivation and long-term sustainability. If you like going to the mall, join a walking program at your favorite mall. Depending on your interest, consider aerobics classes, biking, swimming, tennis, and other forms of physical activity. Join a weekend hiking club if you live in an area close to mountains and trails. Many hiking clubs in major cities have internet sites, and they are good places to make new friends. If you have a friend, office colleague, or spouse who is also interested in exercise, choose an activity that both of you enjoy. If you like watching TV, consider watching your favorite program as you exercise on your treadmill or stationary bike. Household activities such as yard work, mowing the lawn, and vacuuming can count to your aerobic hours per week if they are vigorous enough. So can shoveling snow, but on the other hand, it can be dangerous if you are not in the best of shape.

Fitness among the Young
Sedentariness among children and teenagers has become a major public health concern. A low level of fitness in young adults is associated with the development of cardiac risk factors, leading to heart disease in middle age and beyond. These associations, often mediated through metabolic syndrome and obesity, are modifiable by improving fitness.

THE BENEFITS OF PHYSICAL ACTIVITY

Why become physically active? Moderately vigorous activity, especially when combined with a heart-healthy diet, offers a vast range of benefits, both cardiovascular and non-cardiovascular. Some of its main benefits are summarized here:

Fitness and wellness

Recent studies suggest that *being fit is even more important than avoiding being fat.* Obese fit persons, the evidence suggests, have less risk of heart disease and diabetes than lean but unfit individuals. In several studies, a low-fat, low-calorie diet without exercise failed to lower LDL levels. In contrast, physical activity, including just heavy household work, is one of the most effective ways to raise your HDL level. A rule of thumb is that walking 10 miles a week for 10 months can increase your HDL by 10%. Exercise's beneficial effect on triglycerides is even greater than on HDL because it literally makes fat melt away.

This, of course, is not a justification to ignore obesity. Rather, it highlights the importance of staying active even if it does not immediately lead to weight loss. But the fact remains that even a modest weight gain can have substantial adverse effects. For example, a gain of 15 to 25 pounds after age 18 is associated with a doubling of your risk for dia-

Table 5.25. Benefits of a regular physical activity program

Cardiovascular Benefits	Non-cardiovascular Benefits
• Reduces your risk of heart disease and coronary events such as heart attack • Increases your chances of surviving a heart attack by improving your stamina • Strengthens the heart muscle and raises its pumping power (ejection fraction) • Slows down progress of atherosclerosis, including in postmenopausal women (especially high-intensity or long-duration exercise) • Slow the progress of endothelial dysfunction • Appears to increase the flexibility and dilating capacity of your coronary arteries • Prevents or controls dyslipidemia by increasing your HDL levels, and decreasing your triglyceride levels (particularly longer-duration exercise) • Increases the particle size and thus effectiveness of your HDL cholesterol • Lowers your blood pressure independently of its weight loss effect • Prevents or controls diabetes by decreasing insulin resistance (promoting entry of glucose into cells), thereby helping you use energy more efficiently and lowering your blood sugar • Helps promote weight loss, and prevent weight gain and abdominal obesity • Protects against unwarranted blood clotting by thinning your blood	• Reduces depression • Promotes a sense of well-being, self-confidence, and positive self-image • Can improve your concentration • Reduces stress and enhances relaxation partly through the release of endorphins • Can prevent the onset of Parkinson's disease • Increases your energy level and improves sleep • Strengthens your immune system, raises white blood cell count, and increases your ability to fight off infections, including colds • Increases muscle strength and flexibility • Reduces your likelihood of falls and fractures by increasing bone density and improving your balance • Reduces your risk of colon cancer • Raises your basal metabolic rate by increasing lean muscle mass, making you burn more calories even when not exercising • Can prevent the onset of osteoarthritis

betes and heart disease. These findings support the importance of maintaining a constant body weight throughout adult life.

This, however, means regular long-term physical activity, because age-related increases in weight and waist circumference are closely related with decreasing physical activity. Regular exercise burns calories and raises basal metabolic rate, so that the body needs more calories to function. It builds up lean muscle mass, increasing your body's ability to utilize body fat as energy. So although it is true that you must walk about 35 miles to burn off the 3500 calories in a pound of fat, in actuality aerobic exercise keeps "working" long after you have returned home and taken your shower, because of its effect on your basal metabolic rate. You keep burning more calories even after you stop exercising.

Another reason to stay active is the blood-thinning effects of exercise. Small blood clots are continuously formed and dissolved in the body. Physical activity has remarkable effects on blood viscosity, coagulation, and fibrinolysis (dissolving of blood clots). It decreases the levels of your blood clotting-related factors and improves the reactivity of your platelets, the tiny blood cells that initiate blood clots, thereby preventing blood clots. Part of the cardiovascular benefits of physical activity may be due to its effects on blood.

Both animal and human studies demonstrate that exercise can slow down atherosclerosis and, in some cases, actually reverse its effects. How effectively exercise does this appears to depend on the duration and intensity of the exercise regimen. In some studies, 90 minutes of moderate-intensity exercise before a meal produced a 25% increase in endothelial function and a 25% decrease in triglyceride levels. How immediately can you expect a fitness program to begin to inhibit atherogenesis if you have heart disease? A 2005 study suggests that exercise not only has long-term benefits but may also have immediate benefits for people with acute coronary disease.

The influence of physical activity on coronary events was demonstrated among the 10,000 adults participating in the Prospective Epidemiological Study of Myocardial Infarction, or PRIME (see Appendix B). This major study was prompted by the observation that, despite their geographic proximity, France and Northern Ireland have a *four-fold* difference in heart disease risk—in favor of France. It has often been theorized that the low rates of heart disease among the French can be traced to their generous consumption of alcohol. More recent studies such as PRIME suggest that greater physical activity among the French contributes more to their low heart disease rates than does alcohol intake.

Yet another cardiovascular benefit of exercise is that it seems to increase the dilating capacity of your coronary arteries by making the walls more flexible and stretchable. This may be one of the pathways through which fitness helps to counter the effects of atherosclerosis and prevent heart attacks. A 1993 study at Stanford Medical School found that, compared with inactive men, the coronary arteries of well-trained, middle-aged distance runners demonstrated a much greater dilating capacity in response to nitroglycerin. Their arteries expanded twice as much as those of the non-runners.

Non-cardiovascular benefits

As Table 5.25 (*above*) shows, the benefits of exercise extend far beyond improvements in lipoprotein levels, blood-clotting functions, and cardiovascular risk reduction. Both high-intensity and low-intensity aerobic exercises are very effective in reducing emotional stress and fighting depression. Besides the more shapely, sculpted body it can give you, exercise causes your body to release hormones called endorphins that promote a sense of well-being. Adding a healthy nutrition program to physical activity has a strong synergistic effect in improving your physical and mental well-being.

FINE-TUNING YOUR FITNESS PROGRAM: DO'S AND DON'TS

▶ *Do* follow your physician's recommendations on physical activity. This is strongly recommended. An exercise treadmill stress test can detect any hidden heart disease. Physicians often advise this test for sedentary individuals with multiple risk factors who want to start a moderate- or high-intensity exercise program.

This is particularly important for men over 40, women over 50, especially if they have been sedentary.

▶ *Do* exercise in your zone of comfort and gradually increase the activities. Be aware of any signs of discomfort and muscle pain, and consult your doctor if the pain persists. It is essential to remember that, like too little exercise, too much exercise can be counter-productive. Consistent soreness in muscles, prolonged fatigue, or difficulty sleeping at night are symptoms of overtraining.

▶ *Do* take a few days off and restart at a lower intensity. Increasing frequency, intensity, or duration too quickly can also lead to exercise-related injuries and a depressed immune system because you are taxing your body too heavily. Increase intensity over a period of weeks rather than days. Increase duration gradually—5-10% per week.

▶ *Do* incorporate a warm-up and a cool-down period of at least 5-10 minutes into your exercise routine. This may be as simple as walking at an easy pace for 5-10 minutes before and after a run. Start slowly. Don't race toward your Target Heart Rate. Remember to stretch after you have warmed up and/or after your cool down.

▶ *Do* schedule in at least one outdoor activity per week during the colder months, as long as the temperature is more than 20°F. Being outdoors helps you to fight off seasonal depression (the winter blues).

▶ *Do* dress to keep your body warm and dry in chilly weather, especially when the wind chill factor is high. Apply these four principles:

- Avoid cotton. Wear wool or polyester-based clothing such as Thermax or fleece, which keep you warm and dry by wicking sweat away from your body.
- Layer. Wear several thin layers of clothing rather than a few very thick pieces. Thin layers trap warm air around your body.
- Don't overdress. You will end up over-sweating and becoming cold. You should feel a bit on the cool side the first 10 minutes or so.
- If you want your hands and torso to stay warm, cover your head! You lose up to 50% of your body heat through your scalp. Wear a winter cap and add synthetic fiber gloves. Visit a site such as www.llbean.com for a more extensive discussion of how to dress for cold-weather exercise.

▶ *Do* wear thin, loose-fitting, breathable, light-colored clothing when it is very hot, and take it easier. Stop if you start feeling light-headed or dizzy or your chest begins to feel too tense.

▶ *Do* check the weather on your TV or on www.weather.com for air quality before heading outdoors, not only for temperature and humidity but also pollen count and the UV (ultraviolet) index. Avoid exercising when the UV index is "very high." Overexposure to UV radiation damages skin and raises your risk of skin cancer.

▶ *Don't* exercise within 1.5 hours of eating a main meal.

▶ *Don't* exercise outdoors when it is very humid and over 90°F or the UV index reads "very high." Avoid dehydration. Drink a lot of fluids before, during, and after aerobic exercise, even if you are not thirsty. Dehydration raises the concentrations of various substances in your blood, which can force your heart to work harder.

Other tips before you get started

Walking and running: Bicycling and swimming both provide excellent cardiovascular benefits, but the weight-bearing nature of walking or running provides a greater stimulus for bone mineral deposition than do cycling or swimming. Swimming, however, is better tolerated by people with joint limitations.

Shoes and injury: Walking requires little in the way of specialized equipment. Running, however, requires appropriate running shoes to prevent injuries such as runner's knee and iliotibial band syndrome. This is particularly true if you are flat-footed and you over-pronate, meaning that your feet turn inward as the toes leave the ground. If you are an over-pronator, it is imperative that you wear motion-control running shoes. It may even be necessary to visit a podiatrist and add orthotics to your shoes. Many health insurance plans cover orthotics.

Cross-training: A cross-training program is an effective compromise among several options. It mixes exercise modes within any given week or within a single session. It also helps to prevent boredom, conditions more muscle groups, and reduces the risk of overuse injuries. To train different muscle groups, mix and match a variety of aerobic exercises. Run on Mondays and Fridays, use the elliptical cross trainer on Tuesdays and Thursdays, and bike or play badminton the remaining days.

Weights: If weight loss is a goal, but you just cannot see yourself doing anything more strenuous than walking, consider adding weights to intensify your workout. Walking with weights will let you burn more calories without going any faster. You can use a pair of dumbbells (hand weights), wear a weighted vest, or wear ankle weights. Along with more rapid fat burning, the first two options will also give you an upper body workout—useful because walking does little for your upper body. With hand weights, arm movement is critical. Don't just carry the weights; pump your arms rhythmically, driving your elbows back as if you were punching the air. A set of three pairs of vinyl- or neoprene-covered dumbbells (e.g., a 2lb pair, a 3lb pair, and a 4lb pair) should cost no more than $40.

A weighted vest is a sleeveless, snug-fitting nylon vest designed to carry up to 30 pounds of weight, usually in one pound increments, properly distributed around your upper body. Made by companies such as Xvest, Uni-vest, and Walk-vest, they cost $60 and up. One advantage over hand weights is that a vest leaves your hands free to carry a bottle, wipe away sweat, or blow your nose. Visit a sporting goods store that carries weights so you can try them out for feel. However, you can also order weights over the Internet. In all three cases—hand weights, ankle weights, or vest—start with lighter weights and work your way up, building up your time gradually as well.

SAMPLE WORKOUT (based on Six Days of Activity per Week)

Day of week	Activity
Sunday	45 to 60 minutes of walking outdoors at 15 minutes a mile pace.
Monday	OFF - Stretch at night after light warm-up.
Tuesday	30 minutes of yoga and circuit training. Stretch at night.
Wednesday	30 min. of treadmill walking at 5° incline. Or 30 min. stationary cycling or elliptical cross trainer. Includes 5 min. interval training at level 16-17 on RPE scale (anaerobic activity). Stretch at night
Thursday	20 minutes of circuit strength training, 20 minutes of yoga. Stretch at night.
Friday	30 min walking, indoor cycling, rowing machine, or elliptical cross trainer. Stretch at night.
Saturday	30 min walking, indoor cycling, rowing machine, or elliptical cross trainer. Stretch at night.

PLANNING A FITNESS PROGRAM

First, what are your goals? Decide upon them from the various goals discussed in this section:

Fitness Planning Chart

Fitness Component	Type	Frequency	Duration	Intensity
Cardio-respiratory activity	_____ _____	number of days a week	minutes	heart beats per min _____ METS or RPE level
Strength	Free weights Machines	days a week	minutes _____ number of sets	no. of repetitions to muscle fatigue
Flexibility	Stretch exercises	days a week	number of seconds _____ no. of repetitions	Always keep below your threshold of pain
Balance and agility	_____ _____	days a week	no. of minutes	

□ Weight loss □ Weight maintenance □ Reduction of abdominal obesity □ Prevention of heart disease □ Achieving a more sculpted body □ Building muscular strength and bulk □ Achieving a competitive-level of fitness

Next, what is your plan? To achieve your goals, I recommend setting up a written schedule for physical activity for a week at a time at least.

Remember the following simple guidelines:
>If you have been relatively sedentary, you may not be able to start out at the level you want. But you can reach it if you set manageable intensity and duration targets.
>It is a good idea to set minimum baseline levels. For example, at least 10 miles of walking a week, at least 30 minutes a day, for at least five days a week. Distinguish between *optimum* and *minimum* levels of exercise; do the **minimal** when you are very busy or just beginning, and aim for **optimal** at other times.
>To avoid doing too much too soon, it is equally wise to set *maximum* targets for your current fitness level. For example, no more than 15 miles of running a week. Or, a maximum of 5 hours/week of cardio-respiratory activity.
>Target one or two days a week off if you perform high-intensity workouts.
>Finally, vigorous yard work such as raking leaves or mowing the lawn, housework such as vacuuming, and social activities such as lively dancing can count toward your aerobic exercise time.

TROUBLESHOOTING YOUR PHYSICAL ACTIVITY PROGRAM

Here is a list of common problems and potential solutions for your physical activity program:

Problem	Solution
You find exercise boring or tiresome	Try alternate physical activities until you find something you enjoy doing
You feel tired all the time, and you have poor sleep patterns	Decrease the frequency, duration, and/or intensity of your training. Then gradually increase it after your body adapts to the changes
You are gaining weight	Increase the frequency, duration, and/or intensity of your exercise sessions; review your calorie intake
You have become more prone to injuries, sprains and other physical ailments	Reduce the frequency, duration, and/or intensity of your workouts
You have become more prone to colds and infections	Reduce the frequency, duration, and/or intensity of your exercise. Make sure you are eating 9-13 servings of fruits and vegetables.

KEY · POINTS · IN · A · NUTSHELL

♥ Regular physical activity is integral to a healthy lifestyle.

♥ The three pillars of physical activity are cardiovascular (or aerobic) exercise, strength (or resistance) training, and flexibility exercises.

♥ For disease prevention, your fitness program should emphasize cardio-respiratory exercises done at moderate to moderately vigorous intensity, 60 to 90 minutes a day, 5 to 7 days a week. Aim to accumulate 6 to 10 hours of aerobic activity a week.

♥ To lose weight, low-intensity, long-duration activities such as long, brisk walks (55-65% of your maximum heart rate) are best, because they burn the most fat. At higher intensities, your burn more carbs.

♥ Lifelong consistency is more important than intensity and offers the best protection against heart disease.

♥ Studies of fitness versus fatness suggest that being fit may be even more important to your cardiovascular health than being trim. Both, however, are vital.

♥ The relative risk of developing heart disease from physical inactivity is comparable to the risk associated with high cholesterol, hypertension, or cigarette smoking.

♥ Among its many benefits, physical activity improves your fitness, increases bone density, and improves your cholesterol and lipoprotein levels.

♥ Sedentary individuals and those with heart disease should consult their physician and preferably get a stress test before initiating a rigorous exercise program.

♥ A short, well-defined warm-up and cool-down period loosens your muscles, dissipates lactic acid build-up from your muscles, and minimizes stress to your heart. Your heart always prefers a gradual increase or decrease in heart rate.

♥ For long-term sustainability, it is important to choose cardiovascular exercises you enjoy. To further promote compliance, decide on your goals and plan your weekly exercise regimen in advance.

♥ It is never too late to become more physically active. Start out slowly and build up to the recommended frequency, duration, and time.

Chapter VI

Controlling Hypertension, Cholesterol and Diabetes

Section 1, **Managing Your Blood Pressure**, presents a broad outline of strategies for reducing your blood pressure through lifestyle changes and medications. The section also discusses why the blood pressure goals are lower among people with diabetes and kidney disease. ◆

Preventing and controlling heart disease by lowering LDL has been one of the most important scientific discoveries of the 20th century and remains the foundation of preventive cardiology as we enter the 21st century. Section 2, **Lowering your LDL**, discusses how to lower your LDL levels through use of prescription and non-prescription medication and appropriate food choices. While lowering LDL is important for all persons, aggressive lowering is necessary for people with diabetes and heart disease. It also highlights why Indians need to be treated more aggressively. ◆

The third section, **Raising your HDL**, outlines the second most important strategy for preventing heart attacks and restenosis following coronary angioplasty and by-pass surgery. Increased physical activity is the most important strategy to raise HDL, particularly the most cardioprotective large HDL particles. This section also outlines important prescription medications and appropriate food choices to increase your HDL. ◆

Section 4, **Controlling your triglycerides**, explains the impact of high glycemic load in the Indian diet in perpetuating high triglycerides among this population. It discusses how high triglycerides can artificially lower LDL levels, leading to an underestimation of risk of heart disease. Finally, the role of different agents in lowering triglyceride levels is reviewed. ◆

Section 5, **Managing High Levels of Lipoprotein(a)**, questions the conventional wisdom of ignoring this crucial lipoprotein in the management of dyslipidemia. It presents a rational approach to lowering your lipoprotein(a)—one of the key genetic factors responsible for the malignant heart disease among young Indians. It discusses the use of safe and effective medications to simultaneously lower lipoprotein(a) and LDL and increase HDL levels. ◆

What to do about Metabolic Syndrome, the sixth section, guides the reader through the importance of poor lifestyle choices in the genesis of this syndrome and how appropriate lifestyle changes help in overcoming it. This section highlights the benefit of lifestyle changes in preventing the development of diabetes by as much as 60%. ◆

Section 7, **Cutting Obesity Down to Size**, highlights the importance of controlling obesity through a combination of caloric restriction and increased physical activity to achieve and sustain healthy weight loss. Section 7 also examines the limitations of popular weight loss diets. Finally, the section discusses potential use of prescription medications to supplement your weight loss efforts. ◆

The last section, **Living with Diabetes**, presents important strategies to control and manage diabetes. It highlights the ABCs of diabetes management-control of A1C, blood pressure and cholesterol. Several categories of prescription medications are discussed. ◆

6.1 ▶ Controlling Your High Blood Pressure

High blood pressure is one of the most important and common risk factors for stroke, heart attack, and kidney disease. The strict control of blood pressure is largely credited for the dramatic decrease in stroke experienced in the latter half of the 20th century. Most strokes occur in people whose blood pressures is untreated, or undertreated. For many patients adequate control of blood pressure may make the difference between living many more healthy years, or spending those years recovering from a debilitating stroke or heart attack.

Managing high blood pressure usually requires both lifestyle changes and medications – one complementing the other. Although safe and effective medications exist, lifestyle change is the first step, especially for those with **prehypetension**. The magnitude of blood pressure reduction achievable with lifestyle changes is similar to that of taking three different medications. Worldwide, blood pressure control remains dismally low, despite the effectiveness of lifestyle changes and the availability of medications. People with high blood pressure and diabetes or kidney disease typically need two or more medications in addition to lifestyle changes. This Chapter discusses the various strategies for controlling blood pressure.

Lowering your blood pressure can dramatically reduce your chances of having or dying from a stroke and heart disease. It can slow the progression of kidney damage (nephropathy) and eye damage (retinopathy). Every day that you spend living with higher-than-normal blood pressure puts a strain on your heart, forcing it to work harder pumping blood through your arteries and it also accelerates atherosclerosis.

In clinical trials (usually done over a period of five to 10 years), control of blood pressure reduced the incidence of stroke by 35 to 40%, heart attack by 20 to 25% and heart failure by 50%. The 70% reduction in stroke rates observed in the US in the last century is largely credited to advances in the prevention, detection, and control of blood pressure. If you have been diagnosed with prehypertension (a systolic pressure of 120 to 139) or hypertension (systolic above 140), you really need to invest in a portable blood pressure measuring device. Blood pressure measuring devices that fit over your finger are not very accurate and are not recommended. Self-inflating blood pressure monitors that use a cuff which fits over your wrist or around your upper arm and give you an automatic readout are fairly accurate, easy to use, and cost between $50 and $100.

A Word about Terminology

Throughout this book, the term Indian refers to people who trace their origin to the Indian subcontinent—meaning Bangladesh, India, Pakistan, and Sri Lanka—including those who now live abroad but originate from one of these four countries. "Indian" in this context is ethnically interchangeable with "South Asian," "Indo-Asian," or "Asian Indian." The term thus excludes native Americans but includes more than people from the nation of India.

Measurement Units: As is conventional, blood glucose levels, triglyceride levels, and cholesterol levels are stated throughout this book in milligrams per deciliter (mg/dL). Blood pressure is stated in millimeters of mercury (mmHg).

Historic perspectives of hypertension treatment

In the 1940s, hypertension was common, yet only very severe and malignant hypertension was treated. Malignant hypertension refers to severe uncontrolled blood pressure above 250 mmHg and associated with eye or kidney damage. In those days, the treatment was often worse than the disease. The only available treatment was rigid salt restriction. If that did not work, the next step was sympathectomy (disruption of the sympathetic nervous system which controls heart rate and blood pressure) and adrenalectomy (removal of the adrenal gland). Such radical surgeries were limited to the most extreme cases. Most of the patients who had such radical surgery were not able to stand-up let alone live a normal life. In the past 60 years,

A blood pressure above 140/90 mm Hg constitutes hypertension when it is being measured at the doctor's office but because people are typically less nervous while at home, anything above 135/85 measured at home constitutes hypertension.

nearly 100 medications have become available to control blood pressure within the optimum range with few or no side effects.

Section 1 Managing High Blood Pressure Lifestyle changes

If you suffer from hypertension or prehypertension, you should make appropriate changes in your lifestyle right away, not only to control your blood pressure but also to reduce your need for medications or the amount you have to take. A diet low in salt and high in fruits, vegetables, and low-fat dairy products is the foundation of lifestyle changes in hypertensive people. Early adoption of these strategies, along with prevention of weight gain or maintenance of weight loss, can substantially reduce the risk of developing prehypertension and its progression to hypertension. Several studies indicate that a low-salt diet also helps to keep your arteries flexible. Contrary to common belief, *stress or tension* has no significant role in the development of chronic high blood pressure. However, a reduction in severe, sustained stress can lower blood pressure.

Did you know....
American alcohol drinks are 50% larger than European or Indian drinks. One American drink is 1½oz or 45ml of hard liquor 12oz or 350mL of beer, or 4oz or 120mL of wine. Two American drinks contain as much alcohol as three European or Indian drinks

The benefit of lifestyle changes was clearly demonstrated in the Dietary Approaches to Stop Hypertension (DASH) Study. This program promoted a healthy life at many levels by incorporating increased physical activity, reduced salt intake, weight loss, moderation of alcohol intake, and increased potassium intake. The DASH diet is high in fruits, vegetables, and low-fat dairy products and low in fat and cholesterol. This program effectively lowered blood pressure. Other dietary factors, such as a greater intake of protein or of monounsaturated fatty acids, may also reduce blood pressure.

Salt and blood pressure

There is no known benefit from overconsumption of salt. Since genetic factors may influence the impact of salt on your blood pressure, salt-sensitive people derive greater benefit from reducing salt intake than do others. In the US, 75% of the sodium intake comes from added salt in processed foods. Avoiding pickles, salty soups, and other foods that contain more than 400mg of sodium per serving is helpful. However, reducing sodium intake is all but impossible for those who live on processed foods, which are loaded with sodium.

The human diet has evolved from one that was once high in potassium and low in sodium to one high in sodium and low in potassium. Your potassium intake should be higher than sodium. Increased potassium intake can lower blood pressure and the risk of a stroke. The major sources of potassium include beans (highest), potato skins, winter squash, spinach, papaya, banana, apricot, artichoke, and raisins. The use of light salt, which contains half sodium and half potassium, may help increase your potassium intake while lowering your sodium intake.

Alcohol and blood pressure

Regular consumption of small amounts of alcohol has many beneficial effects. However, excessive alcohol consumption is an important cause of high blood pressure. Alcohol consumption should be limited to no more than two drinks per day; week-

Table 6.1. Effect of lifestyle modifications on blood pressure

Modification	Particular Steps to Take	Systolic Blood Pressure Reduction
Weight Reduction	Maintain normal body weight (a body mass index, or BMI, of 18.5-24.9 points)	5-20 points for every 22 pound weight loss
Nutrition program	Eat a diet rich in fruits, vegetables and low-fat diary products with reduced content of saturated and total fat	8 to 14 points
Sodium reduction	Limit your dietary sodium to no more than 100 mmol per day (2.3g sodium or 6g sodium chloride)	2 to 18 points
Moderate physical activity	Engage in regular aerobic physical activity such as brisk walking at least 30 minutes a day most days of the week	4 to 9 points
Reduction of alcohol consumption	Have fewer than two drinks per day in most men and less than one drink per day in women and lighter-weight men	2 to 4 points
Total		25 to 30 points

ly intake should not exceed 14 standard drinks for men and nine for women. Recently, it has been shown that only one drink per week is enough to provide cardiac protection.

Other dietary factors

Heavy consumption of coffee (more than five cups a day) can increase blood pressure by five points, and also increases C-reactive protein levels. Daily consumption of four capsules of omega-3-based fish oil has been shown to lower blood pressure by 2 mm Hg. Most fish oil capsules contain 1000 mg of fat of which only 300 mg is the beneficial omega-3 fat. Cod-liver oil is mostly fat with *small amounts of omega -3*. In all, a comprehensive set of lifestyle interventions can reduce your blood pressure by more than 25-30 points, as shown in Table 6.1 More importantly, such a reduction in blood pressure would be similar to that obtained from taking two medications, and would correspond to a 50% reduction in cardiac risk.

Table 6.2. Common diuretics

Drug	Dosage per day
Hydrochlorothiazide	12.5 to 50 mg
Chlorthalidone	12.5 to 25 mg
Indapamide (lozol)	1.25 to 2.5 mg

Medications to control your blood pressure

Although the cause of elevated blood pressure is unknown in more than 90% of cases, this no longer poses a problem for effective management. Though lifestyle changes should be vigorously pursued, patients should not be denied medications if optimum blood pressure is not reached with the former. There are several classes of blood pressure medications currently used. Blood pressure lowering is synergistic when drugs with different mechanisms of action are used in combination. People with systolic blood pressure above 160 will require two or more medications. This is also true for those whose hypertension is complicated by diabetes and/or chronic kidney disease. Diuretics are considered the mainstay of treatment for hypertension in the US, but not in Europe. As the name indicates, they work on the kidney and flush excess water and sodium from the body through urine.

Table 6.3 Common beta-blockers

Drug	Dosage per day
Atenolol (Tenormin)	25 to 100 mg
Metoprolol (Lopressor, Toprol)	50 to 100 mg
Nadolol (Corgard)	40 to 120 mg
Propanalol (Inderal)	40 to 80 mg
Carvedilol (Coreg)	12.5to 50 mg
Labetalol (Normodyne, Trandate) (combined alpha and beta-blocker)	200 to 800 mg

The ASCOT Study (See Apendix B) completed in 2005 shows that diuretics may be inferior to other medications. These medications may be a poor choice for Indians because of their tendency to produce diabetes. It is often used as a second drug by most physicians.

Beta-blockers reduce the heart rate and the heart's output of blood. Beta-blockers not only lower the blood pressure but also relieve chest pain and prevent heart attack in people with coronary heart disease.

Calcium channel blockers are very effective in controlling blood pressure. These agents prevent calcium from entering the muscle cells of the heart and blood vessels, resulting in relaxation of the heart and blood vessels. They reduce the need for angioplasty and bypass surgery by relieving angina (see Chapter I, Section 1). These agents are also effective in reducing the risk of stroke. Certain calcium blockers (nifedipine) also preserve kidney function better than diuretics.

Table 6.4. Common calcium blockers

Drug	Dosage per day
Diltiazem (Cardizem)	120 to 540 mg
Verapamil (Calan, Isoptin)	120 to 360 mg
Amlodipine (Norvasc)	2.5 to 10 mg
Felodipine (Plendil)	2.5 to 20 mg
Isradipine (Dynacirc CR)	2.5 to 10 mg
Nifedipine (Adalat, Procardia)	30 to 60 mg
Nisoldipine (Sular)	10 to 40 mg

Angiotensin Converting Enzyme (ACE) Inhibitors and Angiotensin II Receptor Blockers (ARBs) confer protective effects on heart and kidney. ACE, under normal conditions, converts angiotensin I to angiotensin II, which constricts blood vessels. ACE inhibitors block the conversion of angiotensin I to angiotensin II, thereby relaxing the blood vessels and widening the lumen. In addition, ACE inhibitors also decrease the breakdown of bradykinin, and the accumulation of bradykinin may produce annoying dry cough in many patients using this medication. Angiotensin II binds to receptors on smooth muscle cells of the heart or blood vessels, causing constriction of these vessels.

Table 6.5.Common Angiotensin Converting Enzyme (ACE) inhibitors

Drug	Dosage per day
Benazepril (Lotensin)	10 to 40 mg
Captopril (Capoten)	25 to 100 mg
Enalapril (Vasotec)	2.5 to 40 mg
Fosinopril (Monopril)	10 to 40 mg
Lisinopril (Prinivil, Zestril)	10 to 40 mg
Perindopril (Aceon)	4 to 8 mg
Quinapril (Accupril)	10 to 40 mg
Ramipril (Altace)	2.5 to 20 mg
Trandolapril (Mavik)	1 to 4 mg

ARBs inhibit this binding to receptors, leading to relaxation of blood vessels and widening of the lumen. Ace inhibitors are good for patients with diabetes and kidney disease, as well as for some heart attack survivors. The ARBs are as effective as ACE inhibitors and may have fewer adverse effects, such as coughing.

Chronic Kidney Disease (CKD)

More than 24 million American have chronic kidney disease (CKD) and the majority are unaware of it, because symptoms (fatigue, nausea, generalized itching) are absent until the disease is far advanced. Anemia (low blood count) may be an *early sign* of CKD. CKD is a complication of high blood pressure and/or diabetes in up to two-thirds of cases. Most people who suffer from diabetes also suffer from hypertension. The usual definition of CKD is a creatinine level above 1.3 mg/dL in women and above 1.5 mg/dL in men. Under the new guidelines, CKD includes reduced Glomerular Filtration Rate (GFR) (below 60 mL/minute) and albuminuria (more than 300 mg/day). GFR measures how much blood the kidney can filter and how quickly it can remove waste products. . People with healthy kidneys have a GFR more than 120 mL/minute. Loss of protein in the urine is called albuminuria, and is often the first sign of kidney damage. Patients with diabetes or chronic kidney disease should aim to keep their blood pressure below 130/80 mm Hg - lower than that recommended for the general population.

Table 6.6. Common Angiotensin Receptor Blockers (ARBs) and their dosage

Drug	Dosage / day
Candesartan (Atacand)	8 to 32 mg
Eprosartan (Tevetan)	400 to 800 mg
Irbesartan (Avapro)	150 to 300 mg
Losartan (Cozaar)	25 to 100 mg
Olmesartan (Benicar)	20 to 40 mg
Telmisartan (Micardis)	20 to 80 mg
Valsartan (Diovan)	80 to 360 mg

The rule of halves

Just 30 years ago, about half of Americans with high blood pressure were unaware of its presence. Of those who were, only half were on treatment, only about half were able to control their hypertension adequately. Over the past 30 years, the number of Americans who are aware of and successfully treating and controlling their blood pressure has increased from 12% to 30%. However, this Rule of Halves has changed little, if any, in Europe, India, and most other countries.

Hypertension awareness and treatment

Many physicians, even in major medical centers are lackadaisical in the use of effective medications to control blood pressure. In a study of very high risk patients with heart disease and hypertension, more than 80% of the patients received antihypertensive therapy, but only 34% had their blood pressure under control (see Table 6.7.). The rate of successful control of blood pressure may be even lower among Indians. The possible reasons for this include the failure on the part of the physician to prescribe sufficient medications, and the reluctance of patients to take multiple medications and make the necessary lifestyle changes.

Currently two-thirds of patients are not meeting the goal of successful management. The national goal in the US is to increase the proportion of patients achieving their blood pressure goal to 50%. The treatment goal is to bring blood pressure below 140/90 in most patients monitored in the doctor's office, or below 135/85 if you monitor your blood pressure at home.

Table 6.7. Hypertension awareness, treatment and control.

Unaware of hypertension	30%
Aware but not treated	11%
Aware and treated but not controlled	25%
Aware and treated and controlled	34%

Source: Chobanian, AV. Ref 6.9 Note: One in three Americans is unaware of their high blood pressure and only one in three are treating and controlling it.

KEY · POINTS · IN · A · NUTSHELL

♥ The 70% decrease in stroke in the past 50 years is credited to advances in the control of blood pressure.

♥ Lifestyle changes can have an effect on blood pressure comparable to taking three different medications.

♥ Systolic blood pressure can be lowered by as much as 25 to 30 points by lifestyle changes.

♥ A diet low in sodium and high in fruits and vegetables is the foundation of dietary modification to control blood pressure.

♥ As little as one alcoholic drink per week is enough to provide cardiac protection and more than two drinks per day may raise the blood pressure.

♥ Safe and effective medications with few side effects are available to control high blood pressure.

♥ People with very high blood pressure (more than 160 systolic), diabetes, or kidney disease usually require two or more medications.

♥ Three out of 10 persons in the US have their high blood pressure under control, but this is seen in only one out of 10 persons worldwide.

6.2 ▶ Lowering LDL: Step 1 in Preventive Cardiology

Lowering LDL is the foundation of preventive cardiology. One of the major medical advances of the 20th century was reducing the risk of developing and dying from a heart attack in all populations by one-third by lowering LDL levels, irrespective of the cholesterol level. The 21st century is likely to see this increased to a two-thirds reduction as result of availability and use of more aggressive LDL-lowering therapy. Statins such as Lipitor and Crestor are currently the most effective agents in lowering LDL. Both lifestyle and medications are needed for adequate control of high cholesterol. This Chapter focuses on non-prescription and prescription medications and lifestyle changes for the control of LDL levels. Many Indians suffer from mixed dyslipidemia (cholesterol disorders), characterized by high LDL cholesterol, high triglycerides, and low HDL. Options to deal with low HDL and high triglycerides will be discussed in subsequent sections. At present, we will focus on lowering high LDL.

How much you reduce your risk of heart disease by lowering your LDL levels depends on two things: how aggressively you lower your LDL, and how old you are when you begin therapy. A 10% reduction in LDL results in a 10% reduction in cardiac events in five years Long-term or lifelong reduction of LDL results in substantially greater benefit – as much as a 90% reduction in cardiac risk with a 30% reduction in LDL (Table 6.8.).

Table 6.8. Benefits of early, aggressive, and lifelong LDL reduction on cardiac risk as a function of age and degree of LDL reduction.

Age (in years)	Cardiovascular risk reduction	
	10% LDL reduction	30% LDL reduction
Below 40	50%	90%
40 - 50	40%	80%
50 - 60	30%	70%
60 - 70	20%	60%

Source: Law, MR. Ref. 6.35. Note that the benefit is greatest if the treatment is aggressive, and secondly, if it is started before age 40. Note also that aggressive (30% reduction) treatment yields even larger benefits, comparatively, than starting early in life. The best strategy is to combine the two.

Driving down LDL

Several studies in the past five years have clearly demonstrated the safety and benefit of lowering the LDL to below 70. In the TNT Study (see Appendix B), many who received Lipitor 80 mg/d had LDL below 30 for years without any adverse effects. The 2004 interim report of the National Cholesterol Education Program (NCEP) have set an optimum LDL level as 40 that corresponds to non-HDL cholesterol of 70. Since achieving these optimum levels are *not realistic* at this time, this report did not recommend achieving these levels. However, an interim optional *LDL goal below 70* and non-HDL cholesterol below 100 was set for very high risk patients.

Since the risk of heart disease and its complications are *substantially higher* in Indians, an even more aggressive goal is appropriate for them. High levels of triglycerides (often found in many Indians) artificially decrease LDL levels. A 300 mg /dL increase in triglyceride decreases the LDL levels by 60 mg/dL leading to underestimation of risk and a false sense of security. The non-HDL cholesterol reflects the true risk in these people. For this reason, I suggest that all Indians should also meet an additional non-HDL cholesterol goal as shown in Table 6.9.

Table 6.9. Cholesterol and LDL goals for Indians with and without heart disease or diabetes

	Known heart disease or diabetes	No known heart disease or diabetes
LDL	Below 60	Below 100
Non-HDL cholesterol	Below 90	Below 130
Total cholesterol	Below 120	Below 160

Non-prescription therapy for lowering LDL

LDL levels can be lowered by as much as 40% with therapeutic lifestyle changes (Table 6.10.). Each of these strategies lowers LDL to the same degree as doubling the dose of a statin from 20mg/day to 40 mg/day. While these options do not need a prescription, I suggest that you discuss them with your physician.

Dietary cholesterol and trans fats

The cholesterol intake should also be reduced to less than 200mg per day. Two egg yolks contain 560mg/of cholesterol, whereas 6 oz of beef, lamb and pork contain 150 mg cholesterol. Most of the cholesterol in the poultry is in the skin, and wings and some in the dark meat As discussed in Chapter V section 4, minimizing your intake of trans fat is crucial to lowering your LDL and improving your HDL.

Soluble (viscous) fiber

Daily consumption of 5-10 g soluble fiber can lower your cholesterol level by 5%. Whole grain oats and oat bran are excellent sources of soluble fiber and are strongly recommended as part of your daily nutrition plan. Beta-glucan is the primary component responsible for the cholesterol lowering that occurs with soluble fiber in oats. The amount of beta-glucan fiber needed for this cholesterol lowering effect is about 3g per day. Note that "instant" and "fruit flavored" oatmeal are not recommended, as they contain significant amounts of sugar. However, "old-fashioned" oatmeal (rolled or steel-cut oats) can be cooked in a microwave. Another good source of soluble fiber is psyllium husk. India dominates the world market in the production and export of psyllium, and the US is the largest importer of this herb. Three good sources of this husk are:

- Cereals such as Kellog's All-Bran Buds (half a cup of cereal) a day
- Metamucil, one tablespoon in a glass of water or juice a day
- Sat-isabgol (powdered psyllium husk packaged in India), one tablespoon a day

Psyllium has 14 times as much soluble fiber as oat bran. All Metamucil products contain the same amount of psyllium husk: 3.4g per dose. However, dosage amounts differ by version because the sweeteners and flavorings used in each Metamucil product vary in volume. The dose of Metamucil is one tablespoon for sugar-sweetened

Low-saturated fat

Saturated fat is the strongest determinant of high LDL. The most important dietary modification to lower cholesterol is to reduce the intake of saturated fats to less than 7% of the total calories. This corresponds to about 10 g of saturated fat per day for a 1,200 calorie diet. Foods rich in saturated fat include meat (beef, lamb, pork, bacon, sausage, ribs, skin of poultry), high-fat dairy products (butter, ghee, cheese, ice cream, full-fat milk), and commercial bakery products (cakes, biscuits, cookies, donuts and rusk). Although vegetable oils are generally low in saturated fat, tropical oils such as coconut oil, and palm oil are very high in saturated fats (see Chapter V Section 4).

varieties and one teaspoon for varieties with non-calorie sweeteners (aspartame) or six capsules. Be sure to drink adequate water with these fiber supplements. Six doses of Metamucil per day (3.4 g of soluble fiber) has been shown to lower LDL by 7%, which is similar to increasing the dose of Zocor or Lipitor from 20mg a day to 40mg a day.

Medicated margarines

If you use margarine or sandwich spreads, you may want to replace these spreads with plant sterol-based margarines. These margarines serve two purposes:

Table 6.10. The extent of LDL lowering with non-prescription options

	Target and/or daily dose	Decrease in LDL
Saturated fat intake	Below 7%	10%
Dietary cholesterol intake	Below 200mg	5%
Soluble fiber intake	5 to 10g/day	5%
Plant sterols/stanols	1 to 3g/day	5%
Soy protein intake	25g/day	5%
Nuts (Almonds) intake	50g/day	5%
Body weight decrease	11 lbs	5%
Total LDL reduction	All changes	40%

Source: Enas, EA. Ref. 6.12.

a) They contain plant sterols, which are very similar to cholesterol in structure and therefore actually block your body's absorption of cholesterol from food

b) They provide healthy polyunsaturated and monounsaturated fats

Two well-known brands of such margarines are Take Control and Benecol. Two to three servings of these margarines per day can decrease LDL by 10 to 15%. Both of these margarines can be used for cooking – sautéeing and baking. Benecol is also available as a soft gel capsule. One serving equals one tablespoon of spread or two soft gel capsules. Take Control, made from soy, can be added to vegetables, bread, potatoes, etc.

Soy proteins

Foods rich in soy protein offer a good alternative to meat, poultry, and other animal-based products. FDA has allowed a health claim on food labels stating that a daily diet low in saturated fat and cholesterol and containing 25g of soy protein may reduce the risk of heart disease. To qualify for the health claim, foods must contain at least 6.25g of soy protein per serving. The principal benefit is through lowering of cholesterol.

Nuts

Substituting 50 g almonds, walnuts (or most other nuts) for other fats can reduce LDL by 8%-12%. Macadamias and hazelnuts also have an LDL-lowering effect. Care must be taken not to exceed the daily caloric intake, since nuts are very high in calories. One ounce of most provides almost 200 calories (see Chapter V section 3).

A 300 mg /dL increase in triglycerides decreases the LDL levels by 60 mg/dL, leading to underestimation of risk and a false sense of security. The non-HDL cholesterol reflects the true risk in these people with high triglycerides.

Body weight reduction

As mentioned earlier, body fat is a significant contributor to LDL level. By weight reduction, you can significantly bring down your LDL up to 5% reduction for every 10 pound weight loss (see Chapter VI Section 7)

Prescription Medications

It is often necessary to take medications for people with diabetes, high blood pressure, and high cholesterol along with making lifestyle changes. It is a mistake to consider the need for medication as "a failure of lifestyle modification." In some persons, medications may be the only way to change the effects of genetics.

However, medications alone are not sufficient – continued lifestyle changes are important to maintain their benefits. Without such changes, you may have to take double or triple the number of medications for the rest of your life. By continuing to follow the "Prudent Nutrition Program" and an active lifestyle, you will be able to take the lowest dose of these important medicines.

Statins

Statins (such as Lipitor and Zocor) have now become the medication of choice for lowering LDL. Because of the overwhelming importance of this class of medication in the prevention and treatment of heart disease, a separate section is devoted to them (Chapter VIII, Section 1).

Table 6.11.The effect of LDL-lowering medications on cholesterol, triglycerides and HDL ((statins are discussed in Chapter VII, section 1)

	Dose range (mg)	LDL (%)	HDL (%)	TG(%)	TC (%)
Bile acid sequestrants (resins)					
Cholestyramine (Questran)	1-6 packets	15-30	3-5	May increase	10-25
Colestipol (Colestid)	1-6 packets (2-16 g)	15-30	3-5	May increase	3-5
Colesevelam (Wellcol)	3,750 to 4,375mg	8-15	3-5	May increase	10-25
Cholesterol Absorption Inhibitors					
Ezetimibe (Zetia)	10mg	18	1-2	7-9	3-12

TC=total cholesterol; TG =triglycerides

Resins (bile acid sequestrants)

Resins were once the medicine of choice, before statins. Resins include Cholestyramine (Questran) Colestipol (Colestid), and the newer Colesevelam (Wellcol). These medications can lower LDL 15 to 30% by interfering with the absorption of cholesterol from food in the digestive system. Although side effects such as constipation, bloating and belching are very high, they are mostly just inconvenient, not dangerous. However, resins also interfere with the absorption of other medications, so they have to be taken two hours before or four hours after taking a resin. Now a days, the use of these agents is limited to individuals who cannot take statins because of muscle pain or abnormal liver functions.

Cholesterol absorption inhibitors—Ezetimibe (Zetia)

This is a new class of medication that, like the resins, lowers LDL by preventing the absorption of cholesterol from your intestine. It is usually given in combination with a statin when the LDL goal is not met. At the recommended dose of 10mg/day when added to a statin, Zetia produces an additional LDL reduction of 20%, but it has no significant effect on HDL.

Fibrates

Fibrates (such as Lopid, Tricor, Antara) are used primarily in lowering triglycerides, but not LDL. Lopid does not lower LDL but Tricor lowers LDL by 10%, compared to 35-65% with statins. Fibrates make small dense LDL large and less dangerous. The effect of fibrates on cardiac event reduction has been weak and inconsistent, especially in people with diabetes. Among elderly diabetics, the risk of gallstones and myopathy is high with fibrates, especially when used in combination with a statin. These agents are discussed in greater detail in Chapter VI section 4.

Niacin

At a dose of 2g/day ,niacin lowers LDL by 16% and lowers the small dense LDL (most dangerous form of LDL) by 50%. It is highly effective in increasing the particle size of LDL, which makes LDL less dangerous, and HDL particle size, which makes HDL more effective (see Chapter VIII, Section 2).

Combination therapy

It has become customary to use combination medications to treat patients with high blood pressure and diabetes, even at the start of the treatment. This is also becoming rapidly true for cholesterol management. For example, niacin can be safely combined with a statin, without increasing the side effects. An addition of 1g of niacin lowers LDL by 7%, which is similar to doubling the dose of any statin (from 20mg to 40mg/day). The addition of 2g of niacin lowers LDL by 14%, which is similar to quadrupling the dose of any statin (from 20mg to 80mg/day). Niaspan is an FDA approved niacin with fewer side effects (see Chapter VIII Section2).

Advicor is a combination of extended release niacin (Niaspan) with a statin (lovastatin) that is used to treat dyslipidemia. At the maximum recommended dose of Advicor (2000/40) this medication reduces LDL by 47%, lipoprotein(a) by 25%, triglycerides by 42%, and increases HDL by 41% (see Chapter VIII, Section 2).

Zetia can be safely combined with any statin and has LDL-lowering effects similar to increasing the dose of any statin by a factor of eight (from 10mg to 80mg/day). **Vytorin** is a combination of Zocor and Zetia. Vytorin primarily acts on LDL, which is lowered by as much as 65% with a maximum dose of Vytorin (80mg Simvastatin plus 10mg Ezetimibe).

Safety of lipid-lowering therapy

There are concerns among patients regarding the safety of many lipid-lowering prescription medicines. Your physician *always carry out tests* to monitor and ensure the safety of these medications. You should consult your physician even when using non-prescription medications, especially large doses of vitamin C and vitamin E that can drastically reduce the benefits of prescription medications.

Another issue of great importance is the timing and dosage of these medicines. You need to take your medicines correctly, and as per the instructions of your physician to maximize the benefits. Many of these medications have to taken lifelong to ensure a long and healthy life. A certain amount of discipline is essential to take these medications properly and you have to develop ways to make your medication part of your daily routine. Special care needs to be taken when you are traveling. Carrying a copy of your prescription or detailed list of medications and their dosages is the only way to insure that you continue to receive medications when you are hospitalized or traveling.

LDL apheresis

LDL apheresis is a dialysis-like treatment that removes all atherogenic lipoproteins (LDL, lipoprotein (a) etc) in the blood with minimal effect on HDL. LDL apheresis treatment is used in "emergencies" and is reserved for people with LDL above 300, or patients with heart disease and LDL above 200. It can lower LDL cholesterol levels by 80% after a single treatment lasting 4 hours. However, this lowering of the LDL is not maintained. Because most patients being treated have a metabolic defect that causes the overproduction of LDL, treatment cannot cure the underlying problem. Thus, the patient's LDL level begins to rebound after treatment, eventually returning to baseline in about two to four weeks. This treatment is usually repeated every two weeks at annual cost of $50,000.

Undertreatment and underachievement of goals

Despite the ready availability of safe and effective medications that can lower LDL up to 65%, nearly half of patients who require treatment are not receiving them, and many who are, are not getting enough medicine, so their LDL goal remains unmet. Currently less than half of patients with heart disease have their LDL goal met. The treatment deficit also applies to patients hospitalized for a heart attack. A 2005 study found that only one-third of such patients were sent home with lipid-lowering therapy.

Non-treatment and under-treatment are both widespread, but are worse in women than in men. In a study of more than 8,300 high-risk women with heart disease and/or diabetes, only one-third received recommended drug therapy and only 7% attained their recommended targets for all lipid fractions. This highlights the need for improvement of treatment for dyslipidemia in high-risk women.

Our new understanding is that atherosclerosis—the basis of virtually all heat disease—begins in childhood and progresses steadily at a rate determined primarily by your lipid levels. Yet, the current guidelines for treatment of cholesterol are **highly biased against** people without evident heart disease. For example, in persons without heart disease and fewer than two traditional risk factors, the threshold of LDL treatment is above 160 mg/dL, whereas the LDL goal in persons with heart disease is below 100 (and below 70 for very high –risk people such as those with heart disease and diabetes, or metabolic syndrome). In one recent study, on the basis of heart disease and traditional risk factor analysis, only 10% of patients would have qualified for drug treatment of high cholesterol *the day before their premature heart attack*, yet all of them qualified for such treatment the morning after. The point then is that we need to take a more proactive, preventive approach to heart disease treatment, instead of our current reactive, after-the-fact approach. In terms of human lives, economic cost, and fiscal requirements, our current approach is far more expensive.

These data clearly show that many Americans are not meeting their lipid goals. The possible reasons include cost of medication, fear of side effects by the patient, and/or reluctance of the physician to prescribe an adequate dose of the medications. There is a high chance that your LDL level is not at goal. If you r LDL is higher than it should be, you should discuss this with your physician to take additional steps to control dyslipidemia.

KEY · POINTS · IN · A · NUTSHELL

♥ Lowering LDL is the foremost priority for preventing a first heart attack or stroke and avoiding a recurrence.

♥ Combining lifestyle changes with medications are needed for adequate control of high cholesterol.

♥ LDL can be lowered by as much as 40% without prescription medications and by 50 to 65% with prescription medications.

♥ Lowering LDL by 30 points reduces the risk of a heart attack by 30%.

♥ The LDL goal is lower among Americans with heart disease and diabetes less than 100 mg/dL in people with either one of them or less than 70 in those with both of them.

♥ People with high triglycerides must also meet an non-HDL cholesterol, which is 30 points above the LDL goal.

♥ Among patients with heart disease and diabetes, LDL goal is met in less than half and non-HDL goal in less than a quarter.

♥ Many people with high LDL do not receive treatment.

♥ Goal of lipid treatment must be more stringent among Indians than other Americans due to their very high risk of heart disease.

♥ The recommended lipid goals for Indians without heart disease is similar to Americans with heart disease—less than 100 for LDL and less than 130 for non-HDL cholesterol.

♥ The recommended lipid goals for Indians with heart disease is less than 60 for LDL and less than 90 for non-HDL cholesterol.

♥ For Indians with heart disease, lowering the non-HDL levels to below 90 may more important than lowering LDL to below 60.

♥ Nearly two-thirds of Indians have high non-HDL cholesterol, even when LDL levels are not elevated.

6.3 ▶ Raising your HDL: Step 2 in Preventive Cardiology

Although statin therapy has revolutionized the management of heart disease, lowering LDL is not the whole story. Increasing your HDL level has a cardioprotective effect that is just as important for reducing the risk of a heart attack and stroke. In fact, the benefits of increasing HDL appear to be as high as or higher than lowering LDL. Most experts believe that increasing HDL levels will be the next major target in prevention and treatment of heart disease. HDL cholesterol particles go around your bloodstream acting like janitors, cleaning out junk. The larger the particle, the better. Increasing your HDL level not only slows the build-up of plaque but can also produce actual regression (shrinking) of existing plaques. A diet high in carbohydrates and low in fat decreases HDL, while a diet high in monounsaturated fats (such as meat, avocado, nuts, olive oil, canola oil) increases the HDL level. Exercise increases the cardioprotective large HDL-particle. In contrast, alcohol increases the less cardioprotective small HDL. This Chapter discusses the various strategies available to increase the HDL. Niacin is the most effective agent in raising the HDL and is discussed in Chapter VIII section 2 because of its outstanding importance.

Major causes of low HDL

- Heredity (40% to 60%)
- Elevated triglycerides
- Physical inactivity
- Diabetes
- Cigarette smoking
- Diets rich in refined carbohydrates and trans-fats
- Certain blood pressure medications ((diuretics, beta blockers etc.)

Indians and dysfunctional HDL

Unlike other populations, Indians have both quantitative and qualitative abnormalities of HDL, which render them highly susceptible to heart disease. Low HDL (below 40mg/dL) is found in more than half of all Indian men and women around the globe, compared to 30% of American men and 15% of American women. As discussed earlier, recent guidelines have increased the cut point of low HDL to below 50 in women. In the CADI Study (see Appendix B), 70% of Indian women had low HDL by this new criterion; in fact, low HDL was three-to five times more common than a high cholesterol level. It appears that a low HDL level is the most common risk factor among Indian women.

In addition to low levels of HDL, Indians also have a dysfunctional kind of HDL, necessitating a higher target goal. HDL particles can be broadly classified into large and small HDL particles. The protective effect of HDL is confined to the large particles, which correlate with longevity better than the absolute HDL levels. Currently there is no consensus about the role of small HDL particles with some studies suggesting less protection, while other studies showing no protection at all. Some studies even suggest an increased risk of heart disease with small HDL particles (see Chapter VII Section 3)

Increasing your HDL level

In epidemiological studies, a 1% increase in HDL translates into a 3 to 4% reduction in cardiovascular risk, whereas a 1% decrease in LDL results in only a 1% reduction in the cardiac risk. In clinical trials a 7% increase in HDL produced a 21% decrease in cardiac events and trials are underway to evaluate the benefits of increasing HDL by 25-75%. Significant increases in HDL levels can be achieved by making appropriate changes to nutrition and physical activity and taking appropriate medications.

Lifestyle factors that raise HDL

- Physical activity
- Weight loss
- Diet high in
- monounsaturated fats
- Fish oil containing omega-3 fatty acids
- Small amounts of alcohol
- Smoking cessation

Physical activity and weight loss

Physical activity can significantly increase HDL, particularly the most cardioprotective large HDL. Walking or running 12 to 14 miles a week (4 to 5 hrs), or burning 1200 to 1400 calories per week will raise your HDL levels by 10% in 10 months. You can increase your HDL by 30% or 10mg/dL by running 30 miles per week. Endurance training, such as marathon running, can markedly increase the HDL, and more than half of marathon runners have HDL above 60mg/dL.

The effect of exercise is raising the HDL is determined to a large extent by the level of triglycerides. The effect is minimal in persons who have a combination of very low HDL (below 25mg/dL) and low triglycerides levels (below 100mg/dL). On the other hand, the benefit is greater when triglyceride levels are elevated as seen frequently in the setting of metabolic syndrome. Thus, regular endurance exercise training may be particularly helpful in Indians among whom low HDL frequently occurs as the most common component of metabolic syndrome (see Chapter III, Section 7). HDL levels increase 1 to 2mg/dL for every seven to 10 pounds weight loss. Much of the temporary weight loss achieved through crash diets is due to water loss rather than fat loss, and does not result in increased HDL levels.

Medications that raise HDL
• Niacin
• Statins
• Fibrates
• Estrogen (for women)
• Dilantin
• Alpha blockers
• CETP inhibitor
• HDL mimetics or artificial HDL
• Apo A Milano

Diet and HDL

A diet high in total fat raises HDL levels, but the type of fat consumed is critically important, since the wrong fat can actually increase the cardiac risk. Although a diet high in saturated fat raises the HDL level, the increase in LDL with this diet is *two to three times highe*r than the increase in HDL, resulting in a net increase in the cardiac risk. A diet rich in monounsaturated fat is best: it increases HDL level without raising LDL. Such diets include meat, avocado, nuts, olive oil, and canola oil.

Although meat in general is high in saturated fat, lean meat has less saturated fat and more monounsaturated fat. Furthermore, approximately half the saturated fat in most meats is stearic acid that *does not raise cholesterol* levels. In other words, meat contains approximately one-third cholesterol raising saturated fat, one third cholesterol neutral saturated fat (stearic acid) and one third cholesterol-lowering monounsaturated fat. High intake of polyunsaturated fat lowers both HDL and LDL levels and is less desirable than monounsaturated fat.

Alcohol and HDL

Moderate consumption of alcoholic beverages can increase HDL levels by approximately 10%; however, this increase is mostly in the small HDL (less cardioprotective) type. Alcohol also increases triglyceride levels. Due to its problem with addiction and automobile accidents, I do not recommend alcohol as a medical treatment to raise HDL (see Chapter V Section 3).

Medications and HDL levels

Several medications are available to raise HDL but only three of them are used in clinical practice. These medications vary in the effects of various HDL subclasses and apoproteins.

Statins are used primarily for lowering LDL and are discussed in Chapter VIII Section 1. These medications also raise HDL by 5 to 10%. Statins differ in their ability to raise HDL; it is greater with Crestor and Zocor. However, statins do not adequately treat low HDL. Nonetheless, the cardiac risk reduction in patients taking statins is greater among those who also have low HDL than normal or high HDL levels.

Fibrates are used primarily for lowering triglycerides. Ironically their benefit is primarily due to a modest increase in HDL than a decrease in triglycerides. However, fibrates generally increase the less cardio-protective small HDL particles and are inferior to niacin, which increases the cardioprotective large HDL particles.

Niacin preferentially increases HDL 2 and LpA-I particles (see Chapter VIII Section 2). Niacin is the most effective medication in raising HDL. At a dose of 2g per day, it increases HDL by more than 40% and the

Indians and triglycerides

Many Indians live on a high carbohydrate diet, consisting of large amounts of rice and bread. Even those who are not on a high carbohydrate diet often end up consuming very high amounts of carbohydrates when advised by their doctor to go on a low-fat diet to control dyslipidemia. Most physicians and patients fail to recognize that a high carbohydrate diet can substantially lower HDL and increase triglyceride levels. In fact, a large proportion of low HDL and high triglycerides among Indians can be traced to their dietary practices.

most cardioprotective large HDL by 200%. [Because of the overwhelming importance of niacin in raising HDL among Indians, an entire section is devoted to it (see Chapter VIII, Section 2).]

Estrogens increase HDL by a substantial 25% but also make it dysfunctional. As a result, the overall the risks from estrogen therapy outweigh the benefits in most women. The only exception appears to be those with high lipoprotein (a) levels.

Other medications on the horizon

The coming decade is poised to witness a dramatic increase in people's HDL levels. The promising agents include Apo A Milano, and CETP inhibitor (Torcetrapib) and HDL mimetics. Many of these agents can raise HDL by 100% and also produce reversal of heart disease without influencing the LDL levels. These medications are not available for use and are not yet approved by FDA.

Table 6.12. Common medications that increases levels of HDL and its subclasses

Medications	HDL	HDL 2	HDL 3	Apo AI
Statins	+5 to 10%	+5 to +30%	-5 to +5%	-5 to +5%
Fibrates	+10 to 15%	-5%	+5 to +30	-5 to +5
Niacin	+25 to 50%	+50 to 200%	-5 to +5%	+5 to +30%

Treatment goals for HDL

The NCEP has not set a target HDL level to date. However, the American Diabetic Association has set an HDL goal of 45mg/dL for men and 55 for women with diabetes. The American Heart Association's goal for women is 50mg/dL. In view of Indians' dysfunctional HDL and other metabolic abnormalities, I recommend an HDL level of 60mg/dL for Indian men and women, particularly those with heart disease, diabetes, metabolic syndrome or lipoprotein(a) excess.

KEY · POINTS · IN · A · NUTSHELL

♥ Raising HDL can reduce the risk of heart disease as effectively as lowering LDL.

♥ The higher the HDL the lower the cardiac risk.

♥ Low HDL is found in more than half of Indian men and two-thirds of Indian women.

♥ A diet high in carbohydrates and low in fat can decrease your HDL; one high in monounsaturated fats can increase it.

♥ Exercise increases the large cardioprotective HDL, whereas alcohol increases the less cardioprotective small HDL.

♥ Indians have small dysfunctional HDL and therefore require a higher level of HDL than other populations.

♥ A reasonable HDL goal is 45 mg for men and 55 for women and 60 for Indian men and women.

♥ Fibrates increase HDL levels by 5 to 30% but most of the increase is not in the large cardioprotective fraction.

♥ Niacin, the single most effective agent in raising the HDL, can increase it as much as 40%; it can increase the large cardioprotective HDL by nearly 200%.

SECTION 4 ▶ Controlling Your Triglyceride Levels – The Ugly Cholesterol   231

6.4 ▶ Controlling Your Triglyceride Levels – The Ugly Cholesterol

Triglycerides come from the food we eat as well as from being produced by the liver. Triglycerides are the major form in which fat is stored in the body and is transported in the blood, serving as the backbone of many types of lipids (fats). A high triglyceride level is associated with a heightened risk of heart disease when it is accompanied by at least some elevation of non-HDL cholesterol. High levels of triglycerides make LDL smaller, denser and hence more atherogenic. Indians have higher levels of triglycerides than whites. A diet very high in glycemic load (refined carbohydrates) can markedly increase triglyceride levels. Exercise, weight management, and a diet low in glycemic load are effective in lowering triglycerides. Fibrates and omega-3 fatty acids (found in fish oil) are effective triglyceride-lowering agents. Statins are also highly effective in lowering triglycerides and are the drugs of choice in most people with triglycerides below 500. The magnitude of triglyceride lowering with statins is similar to their LDL-lowering ability. This Chapter considers the various options for controlling a high triglyceride level.

Table 6.13. Classification of triglycerides (mg/dL)

Optimal	Below 130
Normal	130 to 149
Borderline high	150 to 199
High	200 to 499
Very High	500 and above

Triglycerides levels of among Indians

Triglycerides levels among Indians in the US are about 30 to 60 points higher than whites. In a study of young Indian and white medical residents working in the Cook County Hospital (and often eating the same cafeteria food), fasting triglyceride levels were twice as high in Indians (174 versus 86mg/dL). In India, the average triglyceride levels is 155 in women and 165 in men. About 40% of Indian men and women have levels exceeding 150 and 60% have levels above 130. In whites, triglyceride levels correlate highly with obesity. This appears to be less prominent in blacks and Indians.

Triglycerides and small dense LDL

Although a triglyceride level of 150 mg/dL is considered normal, several studies indicate that the optimal level may be below 130mg/dL. A strong relationship exists between triglyceride level, HDL level, and a the size of LDL particles. Increasing triglycerides and decreasing HDL levels result in the formation of small, dense, and more dangerous LDL particles. A triglyceride level above 130 and/or a triglycerides-to-HDL ratio above three is highly predictive of small, dense LDL. These numbers can be used as a quick-and-ready, inexpensive test for identifying high-risk individuals with small, dense LDL. These two simple and inexpensive measures also identify overweight individuals at high risk of developing heart disease who would benefit from weight reduction.

Artificial lowering of LDL and underestimation of risk with high triglycerides

LDL levels may markedly *underestimate the risk* in people with high triglycerides. As discussed earlier, total cholesterol consists of antiatherogenic HDL, atherogenic LDL, and VLDL (very low density lipoprotein). LDL level is usually *calculated* from the levels of other lipids, because direct measurement of LDL is time-consuming, expensive, and unnecessary. However,

Table 6.14. Artificial reduction in LDL in persons with high triglyceride levels.

	Case 1 (low TG)	Case 2 (high TG)	Case 3 (high TG low TC)	Case 4 (high TG and high TC)
Total Cholesterol	200	200	150	250
HDL	40	30	30	30
Triglycerides	50	350	350	350
VLDL	10	70	70	70
LDL	150	100	50	150
Non-HDL cholesterol	160	170	120	220
Cardiac risk	2+	3+	1+	4+

Source: Enas, EA. Ref. 6.13. TC= total cholesterol TG = triglycerides. Note that artificial lowering of LDL may give a false sense of security to these persons (Compare case 1 and case 2). Although the triglyceride levels are similar in cases 3 and 4, the cardiac risk is four times higher in case 4 because of the high levels of non-HDL cholesterol.

both calculated and direct measurements of LDL are inaccurate when triglycerides are above 400mg/dL and/or if the person has not been fasting for 8-12 hours prior to the test.

In people with triglyceride below 400, VLDL is usually estimated as 20% of the triglycerides. An increase of triglycerides of 300 (from 50 to 350) is associated with a 60-point increase in VLDL. This in

Did you know...
Unlike very high cholesterol, a very high triglyceride level (above 500) is **not associated with** an increased risk of a heart attack. Most of the risk for heart attacks and stroke occur in people with triglycerides that are 130 to 300 mg/dL and not in those with very high levels. The cardiac risk from high levels of triglycerides primarily depends on the level of non-HDL cholesterol. Since most Indians have high triglycerides, non-HDL cholesterol level may be a simple and more accurate predictor of heart disease than LDL. Until definitive data on Indians become available, a **non-HDL cholesterol goal** of below 130 in people without heart disease or diabetes, and below 100 in those with these two conditions, seem prudent.

turn results in a spurious 60-point decrease in LDL, disqualifying many patients from needed drug treatment based on LDL criteria, as shown in the Table. 6.14. The true risk in such patients can be identified by calculating the non-HDL cholesterol as discussed below.

Patients 1 and 2 have similar levels of cholesterol but different levels of triglycerides. Although patient 2 has a 50 points lower LDL level, his or her cardiac risk is actually higher than patient 1 as evidenced by higher non-HDL cholesterol (to be discussed shortly). In addition, patient 2 is likely to have small, dense, and thus more harmful LDL than patient 1. Patients 2, 3 and 4 have similar triglyceride levels (350) but different levels of cholesterol and cardiac risk. The cardiac risk is lowest for patient 3, high for patient 2 and highest for patient 4. The true risk in these patients is best reflected by the non-HDL cholesterol.

Non-HDL cholesterol

As discussed earlier, non-HDL represents all the atherogenic lipoproteins. It is calculated by simply subtracting HDL from total cholesterol (non-HDL cholesterol = total cholesterol minus HDL). LDL level correlate closely to the non-HDL cholesterol level when triglycerides are below 150, but the correlation is lost when triglycerides exceed 150. Non-HDL cholesterol is a more accurate predictor of risk in people with elevated triglycerides, such as those with diabetes or metabolic syndrome. Since most Indians have high triglycerides, non-HDL cholesterol may be a simple and more accurate predictor of heart disease risk than LDL in populations, including Americans, Europeans and Hawaiians. Non-HDL cholesterol is a very good surrogate for Apo B, the core protein component of all atherogenic lipoproteins. Several studies confirm a strong correlation between Apo B and heart disease. Apo B is the protein component of atherogenic lipoproteins including LDL, IDL, VLDL and lipoprotein(a) (see Chapter VII, Section 2).

Until definitive data on Indians become available, a non-HDL cholesterol goal of below 130 in people without heart disease or diabetes, and below 100 in those with these two conditions seem prudent. Non-HDL cholesterol **is** a major determinant separating atherogenic **dyslipidemia** (high cardiac risk) from high triglycerides (low cardiac risk) as shown in table 6.15.

Lowering your triglyceride level

Markedly high triglyceride levels (greater than 500 mg/dL) can cause inflammation of the pancreas (pancreatitis). This is a medical emergency since acute pancreatitis has a mortality approaching 50%, with most survivors developing diabetes. Therefore, these individuals need to be treated aggressively with low fat diets and multiple medications. Strategies for lowering triglycerides include reducing the glycemic load of what you eat and cutting back on alcohol consumption.

Table 6.15. Differences between very high triglycerides and atherogenic dyslipidemia

	Atherogenic dyslipidemia	Very high triglycerides
Triglycerides	Below 500mg/dL	Above 500mg/dL
Non-HDL cholesterol	Above 100mg/dL	Below 100mg/dL
Cardiac risk	High	Low
Non-cardiac risk (pancreatitis)	None	High

Normally, your triglyceride level can drop within four to six weeks with appropriate diet, exercise, and omega-3 supplementation (see Table 6.16).

Table 6.16 Strategies for reducing triglycerides

Lifestyle	Medications
• Reducing your glycemic load • Limiting or eliminating alcohol • Weight loss • Regular exercise	• Fibrates • Fish Oil Capsules • High-dose Statins • Niacin • Combination of statin, niacin and fish oil capsules

Reducing glycemic load

A major contributor to high triglycerides in Indians is a high glycemic load (diet very high in carbohydrates (see Chapter V, Section 5). The danger is even greater if one eats all or most of one's carbohydrates in a single meal late in the evening. This practice is common among Indians, who often tend to skip breakfast and even lunch. *Rice and Roti* are staples of the Indian diet among those living inside and outside India with some variation. *Roti* is used more among northern Indians whereas rice in southern Indians. Roti is usually made of refined flour and provides up to 50% or more of the daily consumption of calories for many Indians, due to its high *volume of consumption.*

Reducing or eliminating alcohol

Although consuming small amounts of alcohol has many benefits, including raising HDL, it is associated with a marked increase in triglycerides in some individuals. Alcohol use should be eliminated if simply reducing your consumption of it fails to normalize the triglyceride level.

Regular exercise and weight loss

Triglycerides melt with exercise even if you do not lose weight, but the benefit is greater if you also achieve weight loss. A weight loss of 10 pounds or 5% of body weight is associated with up to a 50% reduction in triglycerides. Removal of fat with *liposuction,* however, does not affect triglyceride levels. In contrast, bariatric surgery can normalize triglycerides in six months. These procedures, however, are not therapeutic options for lowering triglycerides.

Omega-3 polyunsaturated fats and fish oil capsules

The three major omega-3 fats of importance are EPA (eicosapentaenoic acid) and DHA (docosahexaenoic acid), and ALNA (alpha linolenic acid). Omega-3 fish oil capsules, available without a prescription, usually come in 1g doses, but contain only 300 mg of DHA and EPA combined. A 30% reduction in the triglyceride level can be achieved with three grams of omega-3 fats (contained in 9 capsules of fish oil). Fish oil has the added advantage of a mild laxative effect: the only drawback is a fishy aftertaste if it is taken as a liquid rather than as a capsule. Although fish oil does not lower LDL, fish in general has several cardioprotective benefits including a 30 % reduction in the incidence of sudden death., consumption of fish alone is usually not sufficient to lower triglyceride levels.

Statins and triglycerides

It is often not appreciated by most doctors and their patients that statins are very potent triglyceride-lowering agents. The effect of statins on triglycerides vary from less than 15% in people with normal triglycerides (below 130) to more than 50% in patients with high triglycerides (more than 250). In other words, an effective dose of a potent statin (Crestor, Lipitor, or Zocor) that lowers the LDL by 50% also lowers triglycerides by 50% (1:1 ratio) as a bonus. Fibrates are effective in lowering very high triglycerides to less than 500mg/dL, when non-HDL cholesterol becomes the next primary goal of treatment. The NCEP has not set a specific goal of triglycerides below this level. Statins are clearly superior to other medications in lowering non-HDL cholesterol. Most recommending agencies, including the NCEP and the American Diabetic Association, recommend a statin over a fibrate, when triglyceride levels are below 500. Although Tricor has a variable effect on LDL, this agent and other fibrates are weak in lowering non-HDL cholesterol. If you are taking a fibrate and your non-HDL cholesterol is not at the desired goal level, you should check with your physician to see if statin drugs would be more appropriate in your particular case.

The FDA has approved a prescription form of omega-3 fatty acids (Omacor) for treatment of very high triglycerides. Each 1g capsule contains 840 mg of omega-3 (465mg DHA and 375mg of EPA) which makes it three times more potent than the average over-the-counter fish oil capsules. Omacor is useful in the treatment of high triglycerides both by itself and in combination with statins. Omacor has reduced cardiac mortality by 20% in clinical trials of patients with heart attack. Among patients with triglycerides ranging from 200 to 500, 4g of Omacor a day decreases triglycerides by more than 45%. Omacor also lowers small, dense LDL. It does not have any deleterious effect on LDL or HDL. The decrease in triglycerides is similar in both diabetics and non-diabetics.

Table 6.17 Muscle syndromes associated with lipid –lowering therapy

Type	Criteria
Myopathy	Any muscle complaint related to the use of lipid lowering drugs
Myalgia	Muscle pain without serum creatinine kinase (CK) elevation
Myositis	Muscle pain with serum CK elevation — 10 times the upper limit of normal (usually more than 2000)
Rhabdomyolysis	Muscle damage with CK elevation 10 times the upper limit of normal usually more than 20,000 plus elevated creatinine and dark urine (due to myoglobin)

Fibrates

Fibrates are effective triglyceride-lowering agents, especially when triglyceride levels exceed 500. The available preparations in the US are gemfibrozil (Lopid) and fenofibrate (Tricor Antara). Fibrates also increase LDL particle size from dense to more buoyant. The efficacy of fibrates in reducing the risk of stroke or heart attack is weak, scanty, and inconsistent. Although gemfibrozil (Lopid) reduced coronary events in people with low HDL, other fibrates such Tricor and bezafibrate (not available in the US) failed to produce reduction in coronary events. However Tricor has been shown to produce angiographic regression of coronary atherosclerosis, but not coronary event reduction. Lopid is neutral on LDL levels, but Tricor may lower LDL and non-HDL cholesterol levels by 15%- much less than with statins .

Table 6.18. Incidence of rhabdomyolysis with statin and fibrate combination

Single Drug Therapy	Incidence /100,000	Combination Therapy	Incidence /100,000
Lipitor	5	Lipitor +Tricor	224
Zocor	5	Zocor+ Lopid	187
Pravastatin	none	None	none
Tricor	0	Tricor + Lipitor	168

Source: Graham, DJ. Ref. 6.18.

Serious side effects - myopathy and rhabdomyolysis

Myopathy refers to any muscle complaint related to the use of statin, fibrates or other lipid-lowering drugs. The risk of gall stones and myopathy is high with fibrates, especially when used in combination with a statin (see Chapter VIII, Section 1). Myopathy occurs at a rate of 1-5 per 1000 patients treated with statins. Compared with a statin alone, the risk is increased sixfold with fibrates. Gemfibrozil (but not fenofibrate) increases the blood level of many statins leading to dangerous toxicity. Complications from fibrates are higher in small-framed elderly persons with diabetes and kidney disease.

Why fast before testing for triglycerides?
Triglyceride levels remain elevated for several hours following a meal, especially one that is high in fat, refined carbohydrates, or alcohol. It is advisable to fast 8-12 hours (no calories) before testing for triglycerides. Alcohol also should be avoided 2 to 3 days before testing for triglycerides.

Rhabdomyolysis

Rhabdomyolysis is a rare but very serious form of myopathy. There is a breakdown of skeletal muscles which causes pain and weakness. In some cases, kidney failure and death can occur. Brown or dark-colored urine, due to the presence of myoglobin released from damaged muscles, is a strong indication of impending kidney failure. In a randomized placebo-controlled trial involving statins, the rate of rhabdomyolysis was one in 20,000 for statins and one in 33,000 for the placebo (dummy pills). The risk of rhabdomyolysis is increased with older age, female sex, diabetes, kidney or liver disease. A recent study involving 252,000 patients showed a **30-to-40-fold increase in rhabdomyolysis** with a combination of Tricor (fenofibrate) and statins, compared to statin alone (See also Chapter VIII, Section 1).

In diabetics, statins are used frequently with a fibrate to control both cholesterol and triglycerides. However, the risk of rhabdomyolysis is high in elderly diabetic patients receiving both statin and fibrates (see Figure 6.1).

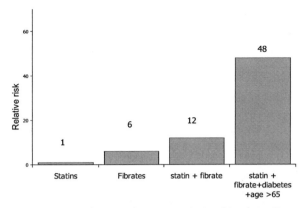

Figure 6.1. Relative risk of rhabdomyolysis with statin, fibrate and combinations of the two. Note that the risk of severe muscle damage such as rhabdomyolysis sixfold higher with fibrates. The risk is increased to 48-fold when these two drugs are given together in elderly diabetics. Source: Graham, DJ. Ref. 6.18.

KEY · POINTS · IN · A · NUTSHELL

♥ Triglyceride levels among Indians are higher than in all other populations despite their low rates of obesity and alcohol consumption.

♥ An important cause of high triglycerides among Indians is high glycemic load—from generous consumption of refined carbohydrates (rotis, white rice etc.).

♥ In people with high triglycerides, LDL level may underestimate the cardiac risk.

♥ Non-HDL cholesterol level is the primary determinant of heart disease risk in persons with a high triglyceride level.

♥ My recommendation for non-HDL cholesterol for Indians is less than 130 in the absence of diabetes or heart disease and less than 100 in the presence of either one of them.

♥ A triglyceride level of more than 130 and/or 3 times higher than HDL makes LDL particle smaller, denser, and more atherogenic.

♥ Fibrates and omega-3 fatty acids (fish oil) are effective triglyceride-lowering agents.

♥ High dose statins are highly effective in lowering high triglycerides and non-HDL cholesterol by 50% or more.

♥ Exercise and body weight loss are very effective in lowering triglycerides.

♥ Alcohol consumption may increase triglycerides levels especially if consumed in large quantities.

6.5 ▶ Managing High Levels of L-P-Little-a

As discussed in Chapter III, Section 2, lipoprotein(a) is a genetic cousin to LDL cholesterol that is far more atherogenic (promotes plaque buildup) and thrombogenic (triggers blood clots in an artery) than LDL cholesterol. Genetically inherited, elevated lipoprotein(a) is strongly associated with massive heart attacks and strokes even among people who are taking statins to lower their cholesterol and who have few or no other risk factors. When other risk factors such as low HDL, high LDL, high triglycerides, diabetes, or smoking *are* present, high Lp(a) magnifies their harmful cardiovascular effects, creating a synergy among them. It also stimulates arterial re-narrowing in heart patients who have had a narrowed artery widened through balloon angioplasty or the placement of a stent (see Key Points in a Nutshell at the end of Chapter III, Section 2 for a quick review of Lp(a)'s clinical and other characteristics). People with high Lp(a) and high cholesterol need to take both niacin and a statin. In this Chapter, you will learn strategies for lowering your Lp(a) and LDL cholesterol, while raising your HDL cholesterol.

Rationale for lowering Lp(a)

Few doctors test for or treat Lp(a) *per se*. Many physicians who are treating a patient's high cholesterol, even quite aggressively, simply ignore high Lp(a) levels even when a proactive patient has discovered it through an advanced test they *paid for themselves*. Yet in my experience, patients with high levels of Lp(a) disproportionately visit hospital cardiac care units and catheterization labs. As discussed in Chapter III, several studies, along with my own extensive personal experience, suggest that elevated Lp(a) is a powerful determinant of coronary artery renarrowing following balloon angioplasty or bypass surgery, often necessitating several more cardiac procedures.

Can Lp(a) be treated with statins?

Studies on the effects of statins on Lp(a) have produced conflicting results: Some show an increase in Lp(a) levels, others show a decrease, and most show no significant effect. Yet the most common approach to managing high Lp(a) is to lower the patient's LDL with statins *without attempting* to lower Lp(a) itself, a strategy based primarily on small studies of patients with few heart attacks or cardiac deaths. As a cardiologist who has tested and treated more than 1,000 patients with high Lp(a), I find that lowering LDL alone is inadequate in reducing risk.

Other statin studies conducted in the last 15 years show that statins reduce coronary events and deaths in only about one-third of patients—*even when* their LDL cholesterol level is lowered to below 70, which is extremely low. One-third means that **two out of every three coronary events are not prevented by the use of statins.** In the 4S Study, the use of a

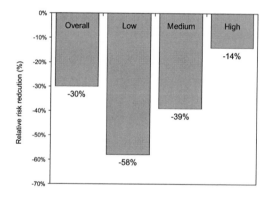

Figure 6.2. Differences in reduction in deaths with Zocor, a statin, as a function of Lp(a) levels, in the Scandinavian Simvastatin Survival Study. The overall reduction in death with Zocor was 30%. Note that the reduction in deaths was double in those with low lipoprotein(a) and half in those with high lipoprotein(a). Source: Berg, K. Ref. 6.5.

statin reduced cardiac risk in only one-sixth of patients when they had both high LDL and high Lp(a). In other words, **five out of six deaths** and heart attacks were not prevented by lowering cholesterol in people with high Lp(a). This is simply not acceptable, especially since safe, reliable, relatively inexpensive, FDA-approved medications are available to lower Lp(a) levels. An ideal approach is to treat LDL, HDL, and Lp(a) simultaneously with the combination of statins and niacin.

LOWERING YOUR LP(A)

► Things you can do yourself

As mentioned in Chapter III, exercise and weight loss do not lower Lp(a), which is unusual for a lipid, but avoiding deep-fried foods, pastries, donuts, commercial cakes, and other foods that are very high in trans fats can help significantly. Alcohol and almond lower your Lp(a) levels slightly.

▶ Things to ask your doctor about

Three treatments known to reduce Lp(a) are **estrogen**, **niacin**, and LDL **apheresis**. It is difficult to design a clinical trial to measure the precise efficacy of each of these, because they all affect other lipoproteins and thus produce several simultaneous effects. Nevertheless, the benefits of lowering Lp(a) appear to be enormous. Let's review each:

▶ Hormone replacement therapy (HRT)

Lowering Lp(a) through estrogen-based hormone replacement therapy can result in a substantial reduction in recurrent coronary events, according to a large study involving 2,763 postmenopausal women with heart disease. HRT, however, worked better in women with high levels of Lp(a). *First*, they saw greater reductions than those who had low Lp(a) to begin with, and with the greater reductions (defined as more than 9mg/dL) came a 54% reduction in recurrent heart attacks. Roughly, **each 1% reduction in Lp(a) produces a 6% reduction in heart attack risk**—a substantially greater reduction ratio than can be obtained from lowering LDL, which results in only a 1% reduction in risk. *Second*, women with high Lp(a) levels did not experience any increase in heart attacks while receiving HRT. In contrast, women who already had low levels of Lp(a) had a substantially higher risk of heart attacks **with** HRT, compared with not receiving HRT at all. HRT therefore carries some risks of its own, and the FDA has not approved HRT for lowering Lp(a). The risk-benefit ratio of lowering Lp(a) with HRT in women with high Lp(a) levels deserves more study.

Did You Know… Reducing your Lp(a) level by 50% following coronary angioplasty reduces arterial renarrowing by 50%.

▶ Apheresis

Apheresis is a very expensive procedure that removes harmful lipoproteins such as LDL cholesterol and Lp(a) from the body (*see* Chapter VI, Section 2). Lowering Lp(a) with niacin and apheresis has been shown to reduce artery renarrowing after angioplasty by up to 50%. The high expense and short-term effects of apherisis limits is use to extrem situations.

▶ Niacin

Currently, niacin is the only FDA-approved lipid-modifying agent that significantly reduces Lp(a), and it does so effectively and safely. Niacin's effect is dose-dependent, with 2 grams a day producing about a 25% decrease, and 4 grams a day about a 38% decrease, according to studies. Besides lowering Lp(a), however, niacin improves all the lipoproteins and is presently the most potent drug for raising HDL, which further inhibits the action of lipoprotein(a). In the Coronary Drug Project, taking 3 grams of niacin a day for 5 years reduced heart attacks by 27%, stroke by 26%, the need for bypass surgery by 47%, and long-term mortality by 11%, compared to a placebo. A more in-depth discussion of niacin's many benefits is provided in Chapter VIII, Section 2.

"Biochem 101"
Niacin is a broad spectrum agent that, besides lowering Lp(a), improves all the other lipoproteins, particularly raising HDL. Raising HDL, by itself, further protects against the action of Lp(a).

Treating other effects of high Lp(a) with niacin and statin

Elevated Lp(a) has now been linked to a number of pregnancy complications, including recurrent miscarriages. Snehalatha Chettiar, a 34-year-old Indian, was referred to me for management of her elevated Lp(a) and cholesterol. I was particularly struck when she mentioned that she felt depressed from having had several miscarriages. I prescribed high-dose statins and niacin for her. Within three months, Snehalatha's LDL had fallen by 60% to below 70, and her Lp(a) by 75% to below 40. Because the safety of statins and niacin during pregnancy has not been fully established, she was advised to stop taking the medications a month before attempting to become pregnant. Snehalatha not only became pregnant the very next month but carried the pregnancy to full-term and delivered a healthy seven-pound baby. I evaluated her four weeks before delivery and again four months after. She is presently back on these medications, with plans to go off after six months to become pregnant again. This case illustrates the value of testing and treating young women with a history of miscarriages for Lp(a) excess.

High Lp(a) has also been implicated in other pregnancy complications, including endometriosis, fetal growth retardation, heart attack during pregnancy, and HELLP syndrome (**H**amolysis, **E**levated **L**iver enzymes, and **L**ow **P**latelets.) Chronic kidney disease requiring dialysis is another consequence of high Lp(a). It is reasonable to evaluate all of these patients for Lp(a) excess and treat them with niacin if necessary.

KEY · POINTS · IN · A · NUTSHELL

♥ Although many physicians still approach, and treat, Lp(a) as if it were just LDL cholesterol, studies such as the landmark 4S Study show that LDL-lowering medications such as statins are not, by themselves, adequate in reducing the risk of recurrent heart attacks and death in patients who have high levels of LDL as well as high Lp(a).

♥ In studies where statins such as Zocor benefited heart patients with Lp(a), the statin worked far better among those participants who had low levels Lp(a), but less well among those with high Lp(a).

♥ Even among persons on statins who have brought their LDL level to within the recommended goals, lipoprotein(a) can trigger recurrent heart attacks that may result in death.

♥ Risking heart attacks and deaths by treating only LDL cholesterol is therefore unacceptable, especially now that safe, inexpensive FDA-approved medications such as niacin are available to lower Lp(a).

♥ Ideally, physicians should treat high LDL, low HDL, and high Lp(a) simultaneously, using both statins and niacin to counter all three, especially since these three risk factors reinforce one another synergistically.

♥ Among post menopausal women, in general, the risk of estrogen-based Hormone Replacement Therapy (HRT) may outweigh the benefits and is not recommended. However, in those women patients with high Lp(a) levels HRT can reduce both Lp(a) levels and recurrent coronary events. In those with low Lp(a), the risks of HRT is particularly high.

♥ What Lp(a) is, and why it is such a dangerous cardiovascular risk factor, are covered in Chapter III, Section 2.

6.6 ▶ Managing Metabolic Syndrome

Metabolic syndrome, formerly called insulin resistance syndrome, is a condition marked by large waistlines, borderline cholesterol abnormalities (high triglycerides, low HDL small dense LDL), prehypertension and/or prediabetes. The components and the importance of the syndrome are discussed in detail in Chapter III Section 7. The presence of metabolic syndrome doubles the risk of heart disease and triples the risk of diabetes. Studies in the past decade have shown that most of the devastating complications of metabolic syndrome, particularly the development of diabetes, are *almost entirely preventable*. Physical inactivity and obesity, particularly abdominal obesity, are the driving force behind metabolic syndrome. The best way to treat metabolic syndrome is to keep it from developing in the first place. Therapeutic lifestyle changes are, therefore, the primary weapons against it (box). In this section you will learn how to delay or postpone the development of heart disease and diabetes if you have metabolic syndrome.

High glycemic load and metabolic syndrome

The quality of the carbohydrate is as important, if not more important, than the quantity. Fruits and vegetables are low in glycemic index and load and high in *soluble fiber*. Whole grain products are also healthy carbohydrates that are high in *insoluble fiber* and other nutrients. Foods with low glycemic index (slowly digested and absorbed without causing a sharp spike in blood sugar) and low glycemic load (high in healthy carbohydrates and low in unhealthy carbohydrates (see Chapter V section 5) are the foundation of dietary modifications. The Prudent Nutrition Program described in Chapter V Section 7 and appendices C and D need to be rigorously followed by individuals with metabolic syndrome. Significant reduction in body fat, blood sugar and blood pressure can be achieved by following a prudent diet low in glycemic load and calories.

> **Therapeutic lifestyle changes (TLC) for managing metabolic syndrome**
> - Diet modification - low glycemic load
> - Increased physical activity
> - Body weight management
> - Increased fitness levels
> - Control of blood pressure
> - Control of dyslipidemia
> - Control of high triglycerides
> - Controlling insulin resistance
> - Controlling blood sugar
> - Prevention of diabetes

The usual intake of carbohydrates among Indians is typically more than 60-70%of daily calories. Carbohydrate intake should be reduced to approximately 40% the total caloric intake in persons with metabolic syndrome–lower than 50 to 60% recommended for general population. For a 1,200 calorie daily diet, this corresponds to about 480 calories or below 120 g carbohydrate (and 150g for a 1,500 calorie diet). This might require an increase in the intake of protein and healthy fats. The lower carbohydrate intake can be accomplished by partially substituting rice and *rotis* with salads for lunch or dinner. Replacing one cup of rice with one-half breast of chicken or a soy burger is an excellent choice to reduce abdominal obesity and lower the triglycerides among Indians and other populations.

Nuts are excellent sources of *healthy fat* and protein. As discussed earlier, nuts are powerhouses of nutrients, including fiber, vitamins, minerals, phytochemicals and antioxidants. A small handful of nuts (corresponding to an ounce, or 28 gm) is the recommended daily allowance. This contains about 150 to 200 calories and therefore must be balanced by reducing a similar amount of calories from other meals during the day.

Fish is another healthy source of fat and proteins. It contains the healthy omega-3 fatty acids and does not contain the unhealthy saturated fats found in meat. Virtually all the benefits of fish are lost by frying, as is customary among Indians.

Physical activity

Physical activity lowers insulin and blood pressure levels in persons with metabolic syndrome. Approximately 70% of the American public can be classified as sedentary. This figure may be even higher in Indians. A minimum of three to four hours per week of regular physical activity is required to maintain good health (see Chapter V, Section 8). Regular physical activity is particularly helpful in reducing abdominal obesity and triglycerides, and increasing HDL.

> **The price of metabolic syndrome**
> This is an expensive disorder that accounts for $4 of every $10 spent on prescription drugs. The annual prescription cost for people with metabolic syndrome is $4,116, more than four times the amount spent on drugs for people without metabolic syndrome, according to 2005 report based on a study of two million patients. Metabolic syndrome is considered to be one of the country's top five health problems.

Prevention of diabetes in people with metabolic syndrome is the *newly discovered benefit* of physical activity. In a five-year follow-up of more than 20,000 male participants of the Physicians Health Study (see Appendix B), men who exercised at least once per week had a 36% lower risk of developing diabetes compared with those who exercised less frequently–those exercising five times a week having a greater benefit. This inverse relation of exercise to risk of diabetes was particularly pronounced among overweight men. Increased physical activity is a promising approach as a primary prevention of diabetes.

Cardiorespiratory Fitness

Cardiorespiratory fitness provides a strong protective effect against death from heart disease in people with metabolic syndrome. The benefit of fitness is double in persons with metabolic syndrome, as compared to healthy individuals. On the other hand, among people with metabolic syndrome, unfit persons have a threefold higher risk of death than fit persons.

Fitness versus fatness
Among people with metabolic syndrome, the benefit of fitness appears to be greater than the dangers of obesity. Obese individuals who are fit have half the death rate of normal weight individuals who are inactive. Current evidence suggest that fit and fat may be better than unfit and lean. Of, course it is best to be fit and lean.

Weight Management

Most people gain 20 to 50 pounds of weight after the age of 18, and consider it to be normal. Recent studies suggest, however, that any weight gain after age 18 is associated with metabolic syndrome. Body weight management includes prevention of weight gain from age 18, and maintenance of optimal body weight once weight loss is achieved. We all know that virtually all persons who undergo special weight reduction programs such as crash diets succeed more than 90% of the time, but virtually all of them regain the weight within a few weeks or months. The more radical the weight loss, the greater the rebound weight gain. Since obesity is associated with greater metabolic abnormalities, care should be taken to prevent further weight gain by individuals who are of normal weight. Table 6.19 provides three different **Action Levels,** irrespective of body weight.

Action Level 1 indicates desirable waist and weight and the need to for continued balance in the physical activity and caloric intake. Action Level 2 indicates *abnormal* accumulation of fat and the need for reduction in weight and waist size. Action Level 2 corresponds to the criteria of metabolic syndrome and very high risk for diabetes and heart disease among Indians. Ideally, one should strive toward the cut-point recommended for Action Level 1, or at the least, prevent further weight gain. Of note, Action Level 3 indicates *markedly increased* risk and the need to lose at least 10 pounds of weight and two inches off one's waist.

Table 6.19. Cut-points for weight management action

	BMI	Waist size	
	Men and women	Men	women
Action level 1	21	32 inches (80 cm)	28 inches (70 cms)
Action level 2	23	36 inches 90 cms	32 inches (80 cms)
Action level 3	25	38 inches (95 cms)	34 inches 85 cms

Reducing abdominal obesity

There are a plethora of machines advertised on television and other media to "reduce stomach fat in just two to four weeks." However, no scientific data exist on the merits of these machines. No machine can target fat in just one specific area of your body. It is your body itself that decides on its own where it will take fat off as you lose weight. I recommend a combination program of increased physical activity (at least 60 minutes daily) and healthy nutrition (calories reduced by at least 500 calories/daily). Physical activity should be a combination of aerobic exercise and resistance training. A simple rule of thumb is to burn calories equal to *three 3 times the weight* in pounds for those with abdominal obesity or metabolic syndrome. This corresponds to 450 calories per day for a person weighing 150 pounds (see also Section 7: Overcoming obesity).

Controlling blood pressure

A blood pressure level above 130/85 mm Hg is one of the diagnostic criteria for metabolic syndrome. Aggressive lifestyle modification can prevent the development of true hypertension (See section 1). Antihypertensive drugs should be used to lower the blood pressure to less than 130/80 in persons with metabolic syndrome and/or diabetes. Diuretics and beta blockers can worsen insulin resistance and dyslipidemia and the dose of thiazide diuretics should be kept relatively low. Beta blockers were not previously used in people with diabetes or metabolic syndrome because of fear of aggravating blood sugar. Recent studies have shown that certain beta blockers, such as Coreg, are highly beneficial, and do not adversely affect blood sugar control. Ace inhibitors improve insulin sensitivity and may be particularly useful in controlling blood pressure and preventing diabetes.

Reducing high blood sugar

The range of blood sugar in people with metabolic syndrome is usually between 100 and 125mg/dL. However, metabolic syndrome is commonly found in people with diabetes (80%) and prediabetes (50%). Blood sugar, when elevated, should be lowered to maintain a fasting glucose of below 100 mg/dL) and an AIC below 6.5%. A1C is a measure of the blood sugar control over the preceding three months (see section 8 of this Chapter).

Table 6.20 Estimated reeducation in coronary events over 10 years by treating three major risk factors to optimum levels in people metabolic syndrome

	Coronary event reduction	
Reduction of selected risk factors to optimum levels	Men	Women
Systolic blood pressure to below 120	-28%	-45%
Reducing LDL to below 100	-46%	-38%
Raising HDL above 60	-51%	-51%
Optimal levels of all three factors	-81%	-82%

Source: Wong, ND. Ref. 3.59. Note that raising HDL to 60 has a greater benefit than lowering LDL to 100.

Control of dyslipidemia

The dyslipidemia in metabolic syndrome consists of high triglycerides, low HDL, and elevated small dense LDL. Dr Nathan Wong and associates at the Heart Disease Prevention Program, from the University of California, Irvine, CA estimated the coronary events that are preventable by treatment of lipids and blood pressure in patients with metabolic syndrome. Among Americans aged 30 to 74 years *without diabetes or heart disease,* 8 million men and 9 million women are estimated to have metabolic syndrome. Coronary events over a period of 10 years were estimated by Framingham algorithms. Events that could be prevented by statistically "controlling" blood pressure, LDL, and HDL cholesterol to either normal or optimal levels according to national guidelines were calculated. They estimated that approximately 1.5 million men and 0.45 million women, if untreated, would develop coronary events in 10 years. Lowering the LDL to less than 100 would reduce the coronary events by 46 % in men and 38 % in women. What was most striking was that elevation of HDL to **above 60 mg/dL** resulted in preventing coronary events by 51% in men and women. Optimization of all 3 risk factors resulted in preventing coronary events by 81% in men and 82% in women (See Table 6.20) Thus, most coronary events in patients with metabolic syndrome may be prevented by optimal control of lipids and/or blood pressure with intense lifestyle modification and multiple medications as necessary.

Table 6.21 Differences in the impact on lipids with the use of Actos and Avandia, medications with potential use in metabolic syndrome.

	Pioglitazone (Actos)	Rosiglitazone (Avandia)
Triglycerides mg/dL	-52	+13
HDL mg/dL	+12	
LDL mg/dL	+12	+21
LDL particle concentration (nmol/L)	-50	+110
LDL particle size (nm)	+0.46	+0.33

Source: Goldberg, RB. Ref. 6.16.

Niacin and statin combination therapy is very effective in controlling atherogenic dyslipidemia. Niacin, particularly in combination with a statin, has been found to be effective in improving atherogenic dyslipidemia and reducing coronary events (see Chapter VIII, Section 2). Chapter VIII provides an in-depth discussion on statins (section 1,) and niacin (section 2).

Rimonabant

It is a new class of medication that reduces the rate of metabolic syndrome by half. This medication has been shown to reduce waist size by 4 inches, reduce body weight by 20 pounds, increase HDL by

27% and decrease triglycerides by 11%. This appears to be a promising agent which may become available by prescription soon. In several studies lasting two years, the percentage of patients with any serious adverse effects or discontinuations due to adverse events was similar to those who were given a placebo (dummy pill).

Insulin sensitizers

A new class of medications called insulin sensitizers (thiazolidinediones or TZDs) is effective in controlling blood sugar in diabetic patients. The two medications available in the US are Actos and Avandia. They also have favorable effects on triglycerides, HDL levels, and fat distribution (see Table 6, 21).

TZDs also slow the progression of gestational diabetes (diabetes developed during pregnancy) to **full-blown diabetes.** The usual rate of progression from gestational diabetes to diabetes is 50% in 10 years or 5% per year. Weight gain is a common side effect of TZDs and caution is advised for patients with, or at high risk of, heart failure. Several studies are underway to ascertain the safety and efficacy of these mediations in preventing the progression of metabolic syndrome to diabetes.

Heart Smart Tips

Clinical trials in Sweden, China, Canada, Finland and the US have clearly demonstrated that the progression of metabolic syndrome to diabetes could be prevented in 50% to 60% of cases by the adoption of a healthier lifestyle and/or medications. The greater the risk of diabetes, the greater is the benefit from more intense lifestyle modification. Several medications have also been shown to prevent diabetes, but they are less effective than aggressive lifestyle modification.

Preventing diabetes: Lessons from Diabetes Prevention Program

Metabolic syndrome is a prediabetic state, even in the presence of a normal blood sugar level. As mentioned before, the term "prediabetes" is used when your fasting blood sugar level is between 100 and 125mg/dL. Persons with prediabetes progress to diabetes at a rate of 6 to 11% per year, with 60% developing diabetes in five to ten years. The risk of developing diabetes is higher with metabolic syndrome than it is with prediabetes. People with prediabetes and metabolic syndrome are at high risk for heart disease and have a marked increase in the number and severity of cardiac risk factors.

The Diabetes Prevention Program—a study of 3,234 individuals people with prediabetes, the majority of whom also had metabolic syndrome (see Appendix B) clearly demonstrated the ability to delay or prevent diabetes in people with prediabetes (impaired glucose tolerance or IGT).

The participants were randomly assigned to receive *intensive lifestyle intervention*, metformin, or dummy pill. Annual assessment of blood pressure, lipids, electrocardiogram, and cardiac events was undertaken. This study demonstrated a greater reduction in the development of diabetes with lifestyle modification, which was nearly double the benefit of medications. For example, the drug metformin reduced the development of diabetes by 38%, whereas lifestyle modification reduced the development of diabetes by 58%.

Ramipril, an ACE inhibitor used in the treatment of high blood pressure and heart failure, is another medication that has been shown to reduce the development of diabetes (34%). Precose has also been shown to reduce the development of diabetes by 30%. Studies are underway to evaluate several other medications in the prevention of diabetes.

In short, the complications of metabolic syndrome such as the development of diabetes and heart disease can be drastically reduced by intense modification of lifestyle directed at increasing fitness and decreasing fatness. Medications directed at blood pressure and dyslipidemia are often necessary in addition to lifestyle changes.

KEY · POINTS · IN · A · NUTSHELL

♥ Although many physicians still approach and treat Lp(a) as if it were just LDL cholesterol, studies such as the landmark 4S Study show that LDL-lowering medications such as statins are not, by themselves, adequate in reducing the risk of recurrent heart attacks and death in patients who have high levels of LDL as well as high Lp(a).

♥ In studies where statins such as Zocor benefited heart patients with Lp(a), the statin worked far better among those participants who had low levels Lp(a), but less well among those with high Lp(a).

♥ Even among persons on statins who have brought their LDL level to within the recommended goals, lipoprotein(a) can trigger recurrent heart attacks that may result in death.

♥ Risking heart attacks and deaths by treating only LDL cholesterol is therefore unacceptable, especially now that safe, inexpensive FDA-approved medications such as niacin are available to lower Lp(a).

♥ Ideally, physicians should treat high LDL, low HDL, and high Lp(a) simultaneously, using both statins and niacin to counter all three, especially since these three risk factors reinforce one another synergistically.

♥ Among post menopausal women, in general, the risk of estrogen-based Hormone Replacement Therapy (HRT) may outweigh the benefits and is not recommended. However, in with high Lp(a) levels HRT can reduce both Lp(a) levels and recurrent coronary events. In those with low Lp(a), the risks of HRT is particularly high.

♥ What Lp(a) is, and why it is such a dangerous cardiovascular risk factor, are covered in Chapter III, Section 2.

6.7 ▶ Cutting Obesity Down to Size

The CDC estimates that nearly two-thirds of Americans are overweight and one-third are obese. Obesity is an epidemic and has become the second leading cause of preventable death, surpassed only by tobacco use. Overweight and obesity are primarily due to an imbalance between energy intake and energy output. Most people become obese primarily because they eat more than they "burn." In some people, there are other factors, such as heredity and psychology. Obese people eat not only to relieve hunger, but also for other reasons: stress, tension, anxiety, loneliness, depression, anger and boredom. The best way to lose weight and overcome obesity is through healthy eating combined with regular physical activity that produces a calorie deficit. However, most obese individuals underestimate their caloric consumption and overestimate their energy expenditure by as much as 50%. Burning 3,500 kcal requires walking slowly for 35 miles or taking about 75,000 steps. General nutritional guidelines appear more adapted to the prevention and control of lesser degrees of obesity. Those with severe obesity (BMI more than 30) may require counseling by a dietician and even the use of appropriate medications. This section discusses strategies for preventing and overcoming obesity.

A diet low in calories, glycemic index and glycemic load (see Chapter V section 5) can help you achieve and sustain weight loss in the long run. Paying attention to glycemic index which more accurately gauges a person's blood sugar response to foods and subsequent weight gain has far more scientific merit than the net carb count recommended by Atkins™ diet.

Healthy weight loss

One *need not get to* the ideal body weight to derive substantial benefit. A 5 to 10% decrease in body weight can lower various risk factors by 50% or more. A healthy weight loss is one to two pounds per week and requires an energy deficit of 3,500 to 7,000 calories per week. Virtually all who lose weight too quickly or too drastically put on all the lost weight and some additional weight within weeks or months of the original weight loss. Note that a weight loss rate that exceeds two or three pounds/week is probably due to loss of muscle and water – both of which are not desirable for your long-term fitness goals. If you make big changes resulting in a big decrease in weight, the *rebound* is also bigger and quicker. Gradual, comfortable, sustained weight loss is better. If you eat 100 less calories per day than you burn, you will lose about 1 pound per month. That is about 12 pounds per year.

> **Did You Know...**
> The United States now has more ex-smokers than current smokers, but it took 30 years to see this behavioral change in tobacco use in the US population, and another 20 years to realize the benefit of such a change. Similarly, it may take as many years to change behaviors to reduce obesity and to realize its benefit on a national scale. But you should not wait until all Americans become slender to begin your own healthy lifestyle.

Crucial role of caloric restriction, serving size and food labels

Everything is "supersized" these days. Within the last two decades calories per portion have increased dramatically in the US. For example a can of soda 20 years ago had 85 cal; today it has approximately 250 cal. An order of French fries used to contain 25 cal; now a regular order exceeds 600 calories. The portion sizes of many drinks have also increased dramatically in the US. Over the years, the serving size of soft drinks has increased from 6oz to 20oz and even up to 64oz. The average American consumes 500 calories more per day now than they did 30 years ago. There is no reason to suspect Indians to be consuming any fewer amounts of calories.

The calorie measure used commonly to discuss the energy content of the food is actually a kilocalorie—the amount of energy required to the temperature of 1kg of water by 1° centigrade (from 15° to 16° C).

The recommended daily sugar intake for a person on a 2000 calorie diet is 10 teaspoons, or 40g. That is the amount present in one 12oz soft drink. A rough rule of thumb is to consume only 10% of your calories from added sugar, which corresponds to 30g or 7 teaspoons of sugar for a 1,200 calorie diet.

I do not recommend calorie counting. I do, however, suggest that you increase foods that are low in calories, and decrease foods that are high in calories. However, for those of you who revel in the use of computer spreadsheets, it may be beneficial to examine your current diet and contrast it with the recommendations of the "Prudent Diet" (see Chapter V section 3).

Food labels provide all necessary information. The first step is to examine serving size and calories per serving size for each food item. Sometimes, the serving size offered in these labels can be very misleading. For example, a serving of potato chips is only "12 pieces." How many people really do stop after eating just 12 chips? Many people can actually empty a whole bag in one sitting.

Most weight loss diets emphasize the quality of the food and virtually ignore the quantity of the food, particularly the caloric intake. Studies have shown that a reduction of 500 to 1,000 calories/day (3,500 to 7,000 kcal per week) from the usual intake is necessary to efficiently achieve a healthy weight loss. Overweight people may need up to **one-half fewer calories** to maintain their weight than do people of normal weight people. This is because the excess fat they carry does not need calories to maintain. It is important to realize that weight loss is impossible with caloric restriction alone and must almost always be combined with increased physical activity for it to be sustainable in the long run. Since most Indians weigh less than

Table 6.22 Recommended calorie intake for healthy weight loss

Body weight (pounds)	Suggested daily calorie intake
150 to 199	1,000 to 1,200
200 to 249	1,200 to 1,500
250 to 300	1,500 to 1,800

Source: Klein, S. Ref. 6.32.

200 pounds, the average caloric requirement is only 1,000 to 1,200 calories/day.

Physical activity

Even though Americans are eating more, the obesity observed in the US is really driven more by reduced physical activity than by increased calorie intake. At least one hour of physical activity is required for those who need to lose weight.

The amount of physical activity should be in proportion to your weight and waist size (see box). For example, if you weigh 150 pounds, you need to burn about 300 calories daily, equivalent to walking about three miles per day. As mentioned before, losing a pound of fat requires burning 3,500 calories. You can achieve this within a week by reducing your dietary intake by 500 calories per day or increasing your physical activity by 500 calories per day. Doing both will result in losing two pounds of weight a week. Here are some tried-and-tested strategies to initiate and maintain a regular exercise regimen:

1. Incorporate multiple short (10 to 15 minutes) bouts of activity (e.g. brisk walking) in one day. You do not need to do it all at once. They all add up.
2. Avoid long-term sedentary activities during your leisure time (e.g. watching hours of television or endlessly playing computer games).
3. Utilize simple exercise equipment at home (for example, a treadmill).
4. Add regular exercise to your daily schedule (e.g. brisk walking, jogging, swimming, biking, golfing, team sports, gardening, yard work).

Increasing the intensity of physical activity can reduce the duration of exercise. For example an average person weighing 150 lbs burn 300 calories by waking slow at 2 mph but burns 600 calories by jogging or running.

Rule of thumb for portion sizes

Tooth pick	100mg of cholesterol
Finger tip	One teaspoon
Thumb tip	One tablespoon
Thumb	One ounce of cheese or meat
Cupped hand	One ounce of nuts
Palm minus fingers	4 ounce of poultry fish or meat

Physical activity levels (in steps) equivalent of various foods and drinks

Type and amount of food	Number of Steps
One cup of stuffing or dressing	7,000
One cup of candied yams	7,800
6 ounces of roasted turkey	5,500
8 ounces of red wine	3,300
1 slice of pumpkin pie	5,300
1 slice of homemade pecan pie	1,600
12oz can of carbonated soft drink	3,000
8oz whole milk (150 kcal)	3,000
20oz fruit drink (280 kcal)	7,500
20oz ice tea (223 kcal)	7,000

Step counting

Experts recommend that people take about 10,000 steps a day, which is about five miles of walking. A mile is about 2,000 to 2,500 steps, depending on your stride, and you burn about 100 calories per mile. An additional 10,000 steps would lead to a-pound-a-week weight loss, which translates to 50 pounds in a year. However, most people take fewer than 3,000 steps a day. And one need to take 7,500 steps to burn 280 calories contained in 20oz of fruit drink. An inexpensive pedometer (less than $5.00) can help you track your steps throughout the day.

Popular Weight loss diets: Truth and consequences

About 26% of Americans are trying to shed weight at any given point. People use various forms of diet, particularly high protein diets, for rapid weight loss. The most popular diets include the Atkins™ diet (high protein- carbohydrate restricted), Ornish diet (the low-fat high carbohydrate,

Did You Know...
The amount of calories you should burn a day in exercise depends upon your weight and waist line. It is usually a multiple of your weight in pounds, as shown below.
• Normal weight person - **two times** your current weight in pounds.
• Abdominal obesity - **three times** your current weight in pounds.
• Overweight and obese person - **four times** your weight in pounds.

Energy expenditure

Activity	cal/hr
Martial arts	750
Cycling	710
Skating	600
Running/jogging	600
Jumping rope	600
Swimming	500
Aerobic	475
Racquet ball	460
Weight lifting	440
Brisk walking	440
Dancing	330
Gardening	330
Walking slow	300

the Zone™ diet, the South Beach™ diet, and the Weight Watchers™ program. Each has some merits and followers.

Low carbohydrate high protein diets

Millions of Americans have jumped on the high *protein bandwagon*. These diets recommend limiting complex and simple sugars, causing body to oxidize fat to meet energy requirements. A drastic reduction in carbohydrates also leads to reduction in caloric intake. Weight loss diets differ significantly with regards to carbohydrate, protein, and fat content and nutritional balance. High protein/low carbohydrate diets such as the *Atkins diet* tend to overly restrict some of the most healthful foods, such as vegetables, fruits, whole grains, and legumes. This diet recommends two weeks of extreme carbohydrate restriction followed by gradually increasing the carbohydrates to 35 g/day. Furthermore, this diet tends to be high in saturated fats and cholesterol. Such diets often result in rapid weight loss during the first weeks of participation, but are virtually impossible to follow over the long term.

People feel less hungry after a protein meal than a carbohydrate meal and that can help weight loss. However, a high protein diet can lack in nutritional luster and cannot deliver vitamins, minerals, fiber, and other nutrients that are found in fresh fruits, vegetables and whole grains. However, those following the high protein diet have decreased from 9% in 2004 to only 4% in 2005 leading to bankruptcy of the company.

When you eat food high in protein, the digestive system breaks it down into amino acids and dumps urea, a waste product, into the blood stream. A high protein diet increases the load on the kidneys and worsens the kidney function in people with kidney disease. More than 20 million Americans have kidney disease, and most of them do not know it. Another 20 million Americans with diabetes have a high risk of developing kidney disease.

Common Weight Loss Diets

High protein low carbohydrate	
The Atkins diet	68% fat, 27% protein, less than 35 g carbohydrates per day Only 20 g carbohydrates in first two weeks; 40 to 60 g for maintenance
Protein Power	54% fat, 26% protein, 16% carbohydrates
The Zone diet	30% fat, 40% protein, 30% carbohydrates (This is also glycemic index diet)
Glycemic index diets (focuses on low glycemic index foods.)	
South beach diet	High-protein, low-fat, low-carbohydrate diet that focus on low glycemic index foods (eliminate refined carbohydrates)
Zone diet	Focus on low glycemic load carbohydrates
High carbohydrate diets (very low fat diet)	
Ornish diet	10% fat,20% protein,70% carbohydrates Exclude nuts, and avocado, all oils,(except 3 g/d of flaxseed or fish oil)
Pritkin diet	Less than 10% fat, 15-20 % protein, remainder unrefined carbohydrates
Low calorie commercial diets	
Weight Watchers	Features an exchange diet (Points system based on type and amount of foods consumed).
Jenny Craig	Prepackaged and pre-portioned meals in frozen or shelf-stable formats
Medifast	Meal replacement shakes, bars and other packaged foods
Nutrisystem	Prepackaged meals available over the internet

Source: Dansinger, ML. Ref. 6.11.

Very low-fat diet (high in carbohydrate)

The very low fat diet typified by the *Dean Ornish Diet* appears to be the exact opposite of the Atkins Diet. The allowed fat intake is less than 15% of daily calories (typically 10%), with an equal distribution of saturated, monounsaturated and polyunsaturated fats. Eggs and dairy are permitted. It has a prevention diet for people without heart disease and a reversal diet for those with heart disease. The adherence to this diet is as low as that for the Atkins diet– 50% in one year.

Glycemic Index diets

These diets allow carbohydrate consumption as long as they have low glycemic index. As discussed in Chapter V section 5, the glycemic index is measure of the blood glucose response to a particular carbohydrate. The higher the peak in blood sugar increase, the higher is the glycemic index value. The low glycemic index foods cause a low rise in blood sugar. The glycemic load is the product of the glycemic index and total dietary carbohydrates, providing a useful measure of the total glycemic effect (per day). A glycemic load diet increases hunger and blood sugar leading to an increased risk of obesity, diabetes, and heart disease. An elevated post prandial (following the food) blood sugar causes oxidative damage and endothelial dysfunction (see Chapter III section 1) and formation of blood clots. Several large prospective studies have shown an increase in triglycerides, decrease in HDL and a high risk of diabetes with high glycemic load-three features which are present almost universally among Indians.

Obese people tend to underestimate the caloric intake by 50% and over estimate the energy expenditure by 50%.

The *South Beach Diet* restricts carbohydrates initially and restricts high-fat, meat and dairy products. Unlike the Atkins diet, the South beach diet encourages lean protein, such as fish and poultry and allows olive oil as a source of mono and polyunsaturated fats.

The *DASH Diet* is rich in fruits, vegetables, and whole grains and low in salt, and recommended by the National Institute of Health as an overall eating plan to prevent and control risk factors such as high blood pressure, cholesterol, and diabetes (See Section 1) .

A Tufts University study compared the effects and sustainability of four of these diets (The Atkins, Ornish, Weight Watchers, and Zone diets) in 160 adults with BMI 27 to 42 and one known cardiovascular risk factor. The overall dropout rate was 42%, with even higher rates of dropping out with carbohydrate restriction or fat restriction diets. Nearly 50% dropped out of the study by 12 months in two groups (50% for the Ornish diet, 48% for the Atkins diet) and more than one-third in other two groups (35% for the Zone diet, and 35% for Weight Watchers). This study has clearly shown that long-term dietary adherence is tough, no matter what the diet. The most common reasons cited by people for withdrawing was either that the diet was too strict to follow or the amount of weight loss was not sufficient.

A more effective strategy is to abandon the concept of "weight loss diets" and introduce small changes in eating and lifestyle that result in small, but sustainable amounts of weight loss and improved cardiovascular fitness.

The study also compared the amount of weight loss and its impact on cardiovascular disease risk reduction. It showed that small amounts of weight loss (approximately three pounds in total) could be achieved with each of these diets in patients who were compliant (who stuck to the diet). Only about 10% of the people in each group lost more than 10% of their initial body weight. In each group, there were significant decreases in cardiovascular risk factors associated with weight loss. The cardiac risk improvement was directly proportional to the amount of weight loss and was similar among the diet groups.

Despite what one might read in the press, no single diet surpassed the others in overall benefit. When it comes to weight management, there is no "one-size-fits-all" solution. This study suggests that the diet should be tailored and matched to individual preferences. A more effective strategy is to abandon the concept of "weight loss diets" and introduce *small changes in eating* and lifestyle that result in small, but sustainable amounts of weight loss and improved cardiovascular fitness.

Maintenance of weight loss

Virtually all diet programs are successful in inducing weight loss, but are dismal failures in helping the dieter keep the weight off. Losing weight and keeping the weight off are two different processes. Close attention to energy balance is required to maintain the weight loss and prevent weight gain.

Tid bits

The National Weight Control Registry (NWCR) is the largest study of individuals successful at long-term maintenance of weight loss. It is an observational study to assess the factors associated with sustained weight loss. To be eligible for this registry, individuals must have maintained at least a 30-lb weight loss for a year or more. Of the initial 3,000 persons the average reported duration of weight loss was six years. The average weight loss was **66 lb** or a decrease in 10 units in body mass index. The common denominator in these persons was that almost all of them restricted caloric intake and increased caloric expenditure. It is worth highlighting that less than 1% consumed a very low carbohydrate diet (less than 24% of the calories).

Obesity medications

Medications are recommended for those with BMI above 27 if life style modification fails to achieve the desired results. Orlistat (Xenical) is an effective agent that reduces dietary fat absorbtion by 30% by inhibiting the activity of intestinal lipase. The average weight loss in one year is 13 pounds (5%) for obese people. Such treatment has been shown to reduce blood pressure by 10 mm Hg, LDL by 8%, and waist girth by 3 inches. Meridia (sibutramine) is another FDA-approved drug for the treatment of obesity.

As mentioned earlier, evidence is mounting that a new class of medication called Rimonabant not only helps people quit smoking but also helps them lose weight and markedly improves dyslipidemia.. This is a novel category of drugs known as "Selective Cannabinoid Receptor Blockers." The recently discovered endocannabinoids are a system of receptors and chemical messengers believed to play a role in weight regulation and lipid metabolism. Stimulation of the cannabinoid receptors produces craving for palatable foods; rimonabant blocks the pleasure centers in brain associated with this craving. This drug has been shown to help people quit smoking and not gain weight after quitting. Unlike other medications that often lose effectiveness after a few months, rimonabant has helped trial participants maintain weight loss for up to three years on clinical trials. A large study involving more than 3,000 patients followed for two years has shown dramatic benefits, as depicted in box above.

Dramatic weight loss with Rimonabant
• Weight loss of 5% in 63 % of patients.
• Weight loss of 10% in 33% of patients.
• Waist reduction of three inches on average.

Lessons from bariatric or "gastric bypass" surgery

Bariatric surgery is an effective treatment for morbid or severe obesity, a condition promoted by genes that cause people to store fat as hedge against starvation. They probably eat more than they need to. Bariatric surgery is usually restricted to those with BMI more than 40 or more than 35 for people with added complications such as hypertension and diabetes. This surgery involves bypassing the stomach (90%) and gastric banding (9%). About 20 million Americans may qualify for bariatric surgery for weight loss. If the current trends continue, gastric bypass surgery may soon overtake coronary bypass surgery as the most common surgery in the US.

A recent study of bariatric surgery analyzed the results of 22,000 patients in 20 countries with a mean age of 39 years; 80% were women. The surgery produced a mean weight loss of 61% (90 pounds) and were able to keep it off at the end of five years. The benefits were dramatic and included a decrease in triglycerides by 80 mg/dL and cholesterol by 30 mg/dL. The vast majority of patients with hypertension, diabetes, dyslipidemia or obstructive sleep apnea experienced significant improvement or complete resolution. Similar benefits can be obtained without surgery if the same amount of weight is lost through lifestyle changes. Since every 22 pounds weight loss produces a 5 to 10 point decrease in blood pressure, a 90 pound decrease in weight translates to a 20 to 40 point decrease, equivalent to combination therapy involving three or four medications.

Table 6.23 Benefits of weight loss with bariatric surgery.

	Significant improvement	Complete resolution
Hypertension	79%	62%
Diabetes	85%	77%
Dyslipidemia	70%	Not reported
Obstructive sleep apnea	95%	86%

Source: Buchwald, H. et al, Ref. 6.07.

Bariatric surgery should not be taken lightly and should be considered as a last resort treatment option. For example, for patients with a BMI above 40 and who have failed to achieve their weight loss goals through diet and exercise (with or without adjunctive drug therapy). There are significant risks involved with this surgery, and the data presented above should not be construed as a recommendation for this procedure. Laparoscopic gastric band bypass has also been shown to be effective, with fewer risks and less benefits than gastric bypass surgery.

KEY · POINTS · IN · A · NUTSHELL

- ♥ A recommended, sustainable rate of weight loss is no more than 1 to 2 pounds per week.
- ♥ A calorie deficit of 3,500 to 7,000 kcal per week is required for such a weight loss.
- ♥ A calorie deficit is best accomplished with a combination of calorie restriction and exercise.
- ♥ Burning 3,500 kcal requires activities such as walking 35 miles or taking about 75,000 steps.
- ♥ The recommended daily intake for people weighing below 200 pounds who want to lose weight and keep it off is 1,000 to 1,200 kcal/day.
- ♥ Obese people underestimate their caloric intake and overestimate their caloric expenditure by 50%.
- ♥ Maintaining weight loss is as important as initial weight loss for overcoming obesity.
- ♥ Medications and surgery are available for people with severe obesity, whose response to intense lifestyle modification is inadequate.

6.8 ▶ Living Healthy With Diabetes

Current medical practice can control most of the complications of diabetes, especially heart disease, yet 80% of diabetics today die from heart disease. Most diabetics are unaware of their high risk for this fatal complication. Aggressive lifestyle modification can delay the need for, and reduce the dose of, medications. Early detection and aggressive treatment can retard the natural progression, and delay most of the complications; that is, the earlier the interventions, the greater the benefits. Blood sugar control protects against eye, nerve, and kidney complications associated with diabetes, but not necessarily death from heart attack. On the other hand, controlling blood pressure and cholesterol do have powerful protective effects against heart attack and stroke. As a result, lower blood pressure and cholesterol targets have been set for diabetics.

More than any chronic disease, diabetes is a disease of self-management. Lifestyle changes in the form of appropriate nutrition and regular physical activity can make a significant impact on a diabetic's health. With medical nutrition therapy and physical activity, many diabetics can live a normal life and can do almost anything, include running marathons! Medicine dosage can be reduced or even eliminated, depending on the degree of lifestyle change the person undertakes. This Chapter discusses the various strategies for reducing the heightened risk of heart disease among diabetics.

> **"Biocom 101"**
> A1C is the other name for glycated hemoglobin which is a measure of the glucose irreversibly combined with the pigment hemoglobin found in red blood cells. A1C level is the most important measure of glucose control for the past 120 days in diabetic patients. A1C makes it easier to monitor control of blood sugar over a longer period of time. Approximately 75% of diabetic patients do not know about this test, let alone its importance.

The ABCs of diabetes care

The importance of controlling dyslipidemia and blood pressure in diabetes is highlighted the ABCs of diabetic control popularized by American Diabetic Association and CDC:

A - A1C control (see box)
B - Blood pressure control
C - Cholesterol control

The other goals are outlined in Table 6.24. These goals are readily achievable with lifestyle changes and appropriate medications. However, only

Table 6.24 Key strategies to manage diabetes: the ABC approach

Parameters to control	Goals
A1C	Below 6.5
Fasting blood sugar (FBS)	Below 110
Post-prandial blood sugar (PPS)	Below 140
Blood pressure	Below 130/80
LDL	Below 100
Physical activity	60-90 minutes/ day or 3,500 calories/ week
Waist size men	Below 36 inches (90cm)
Waist size women	below 32 inches (80cm)
Institute preventive therapy for heart disease	Aspirin and other medications
Metabolic syndrome (present in 80 to 90% of diabetics)	See Chapter VI, Section 6
Atherogenic dyslipidemia (present in 80 to 90% of diabetics	See Chapter VI sections 3 and 4

7% of diabetic patients reach the first three major goals blood pressure below 130/80, LDL below 100, and AIC below 6.5%. If you are diabetic, I strongly recommend that you work closely with your doctor to achieve these goals. In addition to controlling your diabetes, you will significantly reduce your cardiac risks as well.

A1C and home blood glucose monitoring

All diabetics who intend to live a long and healthy life with minimum complications should monitor glucose levels at home. Medicare and most other insurance programs provide coverage for this monitoring. Tight control of blood sugar reduces the risk of diabetic complications, especially to the eyes, kidneys, nerves, and possibly heart. Regular testing of blood sugar helps keep A1C under control. An elevated A1C level suggests inadequately controlled blood sugar, which is associated with a high risk of complications. The higher the blood sugar, the higher the A1C level, even if your blood sugar is not high enough to be diagnosed as a diabetic. Approximately 75% of diabetic patients do not know about this test, let alone its importance. Checking A1C every three to four months can help detect complications at an early stage. The relationship between A1C and blood sugar is shown in Table 6.25.

The American College of Endocrinologists and the European Policy Diabetic Group recommend an A1C below 6.5%. The landmark United Kingdom Prospective Diabetes Study (UKKPDS – see Appendix B) has clearly demonstrated the relationship between A1C and diabetic complications. Reductions in A1C were associated with significant reductions in diabetes-related complications (see Box). Risk reductions were observed for both cardiovascular and noncardiovascular complications, ranging from 14% for heart attack to a 37% reduction in complications related to eyes, kidneys, and nerves, for every 1% decrease in AIC. These benefits highlight the importance of controlling A1C for most diabetics. Note that the benefit of lowering blood sugar is less pronounced for cardiovascular disease and more substantial for non-cardiovascular diseases.

Any reduction in A1C is likely to reduce the risk of complications, with the lowest risk being in those with A1C values in the normal range (below 6.0%). Recent studies clearly show the risk of heart disease begins with A1C level *as low as 5.0%.* Therefore, preventive efforts need be considered, not just for those with established diabetes but also for those with **A1C of more than 5.0%.** Studies are currently underway to test the benefit of maintaining A1C below 5.0% and blood sugar below 100 mg/dL in people with prediabetes.

Reduction in diabetic complications with every 1% reduction in A1C values.
• 21% reduction in diabetic complications
• 21% reduction in deaths related to diabetes
• 14% reduction in heart attack
• 24% reduction in cardiovascular complications in men
• 28% reduction in cardiovascular complications in women
• 37% reduction eye, kidney, and nerve complications

Medical nutrition and activity therapy

The main aim of medical nutrition therapy is to replace, reduce, or restrict a patient's caloric intake to remove the blood sugar challenge inherent in high carbohydrate diets. Everyone who wishes to avoid a heart attack or diabetes should follow the Prudent Nutrition Program outlined in this book. This diet is also the recommended diet for patients with diabetes, and meets all the guidelines issued by major recommending agencies. This diet is rich in fruits, vegetables, healthy fats and proteins, with minimal saturated fats, sodium and refined carbohydrates. It is designed to control blood sugar levels and improve cardiovascular fitness. Most of the fruits available in the US are low in glycemic load and recommended for diabetic patients. Medical nutrition therapy alone reduces A1C levels by 1-2 percentage points.

In 2005, the Joslin Diabetes Center in Boston announced the publication of new nutrition and physical activity guidelines for people with diabetes and those at high risk of diabetes (from being overweight or obese). The aim of

Table 6.25 Correlation between A1C and average blood sugar

A1C%	6	7	8	9	10	11	12	13
Fasting blood sugar	135	170	205	240	275	295	310	345

the guidelines was to recommend dietary and physical activity targets to improve insulin sensitivity and cardiovascular health. These guidelines recommend that approximately 40% of a person's daily calories from carbohydrates; 25 to 30% from protein; 30 to 35% come from fat, as summarized below.

This is a significant change from the Center's previous recommendations that promoted a higher carbohydrate intake. The 40% of calories from carbohydrates should total **no less than 130 g daily**. Among diabetic persons, lowering the intake of saturated fats is perhaps the most important dietary modification to reduce the risk of heart disease. Replacing saturated fats with monounsaturated fats may be more effective in lowering

> "Mild" diabetes "borderline diabetes" or "a touch of" diabetes are truly misnomers since blood sugar is only one of the components that greatly increase the risk of heart disease. In fact, LDL and HDL levels are more important than blood sugar in the development of heart disease among diabetics.

both blood sugar and cardiac risk than replacing saturated fats with refined carbohydrates (typically white rice, *rotis,* and bread).

The best sources of healthy carbohydrates are fresh vegetables, fruits, beans and whole grains. Whole grain foods are preferable to eating pasta (unless it is made from whole grains), white bread, white potatoes, and low-fiber cereals. Ironically, sweet potato has a lower glycemic index than a white potato. Fiber intake should ideally be 50g per day, a minimum of 20 to 35g per day is recommended. High-fiber foods include fruits, vegetables, nuts, seeds, legumes and whole grain cereals and breads. Fiber supplements are also available.

The 30 to 35% of daily calories fat should come mostly from mono and polyunsaturated fats, such as olive oil, canola oil, nuts, seeds and fish, especially those high in omega-3 fatty acids such as salmon, tuna, mackerel, lake trout, herring and sardines. Foods high in saturated fat such as beef, pork, lamb, and high-fat dairy products (cream cheese, whole milk) should be eaten only in small amounts. Foods high in trans fats such as fast foods, commercially baked goods, crackers, cookies, and hard margarines should be avoided. Most hard margarines are made of hydrogenated fats, which are high in trans fats. Cholesterol intake should be less than 200mg daily in people with an LDL ("bad") cholesterol above 100.

Approximately 20 to 30% of a person's total calories should come from protein. Anyone with signs of kidney disease should consult their physician before increasing the daily amount of protein intake. Scientific data reveal that eating more protein helps people feel "full" and thus causes people to eat fewer calories overall. Proteins also help to maintain lean body mass during weight loss. Examples of proteins include fish, skinless chicken or turkey, nonfat or low-fat dairy products, and legumes such as kidney beans, black beans, chick peas and lentils. Currently, sufficient data does not exist for the broader use of organic products, as they are more expensive and less available.

Tid Bits
Scientific data reveal that eating more protein helps people feel "full" and thus causes people to eat fewer calories overall. Protein also helps to maintain lean body mass during weight loss.

Weight loss guidelines

Eating smaller portions, modest carbohydrates, and slightly more protein with careful selection of fat, protein, and carbohydrate sources is recommended if you are overweight or obese and have diabetes or pre-diabetes and have normal kidney function.

Most diabetics are overweight and do not engage in recommended levels of physical activity. Diabetics need to increase physical activity to prevent weight gain and to achieve healthy weight loss. Increased physical activity can also reduce blood sugar and the need for medications and/or insulin. A target of 60 to 90 minutes of physical activity of moderate intensity, most days of the week, with a minimum of 150 to 200 minutes/week is encouraged. It should include cardiovascular activity to burn calories, stretching to maintain flexibility, and resistance activities to maintain or increase lean body mass. Examples of this include walking, biking, swimming, and dancing. The ability of your body to burn fat is based partly on the amount of lean muscle present.

Diabetic medications

Currently, about 20% of diabetics are managed with diet only. Recent studies show that those controlled only with diet fare worse than other groups, and have the **lowest rates of goal achievement.** This is because these patients do not visit the doctor regularly until they have a major complication.

Table 6.26 Proportion of Americans with diabetes receiving various forms of treatment

Treatment Strategy	Percentage
Diet only	20%
Oral agents only	53%
Insulin only	16%
Oral agents plus insulin	11%

Hypoglycemia

The blood sugar goal for diabetics is below 100 mg/dL before meals and below 140 mg/dL two hours after a meal. Many medications can produce **hypoglycemia** (low blood sugar below 70 mg/dL). It occurs when there is too much insulin and not enough glucose in the blood. If left unrecognized and untreated, hypoglycemia can become severe, leading to coma and death. This happens if the diabetic patient does not eat enough carbohydrates or if they miss or delay a meal. Doing more physical activity than usual or taking too large a dose of diabetic medication or insulin can also bring about this condition.

Hypoglycemia is unusual with medications such as Glucophage, Actos, Avandia, and Precosc. It is more common among those who use medications that increase the amount of insulin released from the pancreas. These medications include sulphonylureas, which are sold under the brand names Amaryl, Glucotrol, Diabeta, Micronase, and Glynase. Starlyx, Prandin, and insulin shots also produce these effects.

Common foods used to treat hypoglycemia

- Three or four glucose tablets
- One dose of glucose gel
- One half cup of juice, any type
- One half cup of regular soda, not sugar-free
- One tablespoon of sugar, honey, or syrup
- Six to seven hard candies
- One fruit roll-up
- One serving of crackers

Since the brain uses mostly glucose for energy, the first symptoms are related to abnormal functioning of the brain in the form of inability to think clearly and headaches. Other symptoms may include sweating, shakiness, increased hunger, blurred vision, dizziness, sleepiness and mood changes. The symptoms vary from person to person.

Hypoglycemia is usually treated with 15g of carbohydrates. A second dose of 15g of carbohydrates is taken if the symptoms do not disappear in 15 minutes. If symptoms persist, a third dose of 15g of carbohydrates can be taken after another 15 minutes.

Medications to manage diabetes

Several classes of medications are available to treat and manage diabetes and reduce its complications (see Table 6.27). Each of these medication groups is discussed below.

Insulin sensitizers

The emphasis on initial therapy for diabetes has been shifting from secretagogues and alpha-glucosidase inhibitors to insulin sensitizers such as metformin and the thiazolidinediones (TZDs). Insulin sensitizers are a class of agents which reduce insulin resistance without affecting insulin secretion. In addition to lowering blood sugar, these agents have multiple effects on lipid metabolism, reducing cardiovascular risk. The insulin sensitizers include metformin and TZDs.

Metformin is an antidiabetic agent that improves insulin sensitivity, reduces hepatic glucose production, and thereby improves the fasting plasma glucose. Its anorexic properties (loss of appetite) may help produce modest weight loss. Metformin can lower blood sugar by 60 mg/dL and A1C by two percentage points. At a dose of 2,000 mg a day, metformin lowers LDL by 10%, decreases triglycerides by

15%, and increases HDL by 5%. Among people with prediabetes, it also reduces the risk of diabetes.

TZDs (brand names Actos and Avandia) are medications approved for lowering blood sugar in diabetes. TZDs improve insulin sensitivity, allowing the pancreas to work less and possibly rest. A unique advantage of TZDs is that they redistributes the body's fats to where it really belongs - from atherogenic abdominal fat (Apple-type fat accumulation) to less dangerous fat in hips and thighs (pear-shaped fat accumulation).

Beyond controlling blood sugar, these agents also have a significant effect on diabetic dyslipidemia, the driving force for heart attack in diabetic patients. Actos has a greater effect on dyslipidemia than Avandia. In one study, Actos decreased triglycerides by 12% and increased HDL by 8%, almost as good as that obtained with Tricor (fenofibrate). Actos also produces substantial regression of atherosclerosis, whereas other antidiabetic medications have not shown such regression. Typically, Avandia increase LDL and triglycerides. Both shift the LDL particle size from the dangerous small dense LDL to less atherogenic larger particles. Recently, Avandia was shown to reduce restenosis following coronary angioplasty. A troublesome side effect of TZDs is weight gain, which can be reduced by taking Glucophage concurrently.

Table 6.27. Classes of medication to control blood sugar in diabetes.

Category	Mechanisms and comments
Oral agents	
Secretogogues	
Sulphonyl ureas (Glucortol, Diabeta, and Amaryl Glynase)	Stimulate pancreas release more insulin. Limitation: risk of hypoglycemia
Meglitinides (Prandin, Starlix)	Works similarly to sulphonyl urea and has a short duration of action Limitation: risk of hypoglycemia
Insulin sensitizers	
Biguanides Metformin (Glucophage)	Inhibits production/ release of too much glucose from the liver Makes muscle cells more sensitive to insulin Weight loss; avoid in kidney disease
Thiazolidendiones (Actose, Avandia)	Make muscle cells more sensitive to insulin
Other oral agents	
Alpha glucosidase inhibitors (Precose, Glycet)	Delay the breakdown of carbohydrates into simple sugars No weight gain or hypoglycemia
Combination medication (Avandamet)	Metformin and Avandia combination Controls the blood sugar without risk of hypoglycemia. Additionally, reduces insulin resistance.
Insulin	Always needed in type I diabetics Many type II diabetics require insulin 10 to 15 years after diagnosis

Currently, TZDs are used late in the natural history of diabetes, just before starting insulin. Emerging evidence suggests that TZDs may be better used early in the course of diabetes, to prevent the progression of metabolic syndrome and prediabetes to diabetes. TZDs are one of the few agents which can provide rest to an exhausted pancreas, thereby extending the life span of this vital organ. Several studies are underway to evaluate the role of TZDs in preventing the progression of metabolic syndrome to diabetes and, secondly, in cardiac risk reduction with a target A1C goal of 6% (ACCORD).

New drug on the horizon

Several studies (RIO-Europe, RIO-North America, RIO-Lipids and RIO-Diabetes) completed in 2004 and 2005 suggest that rimonabant, a new and potentially effective medication for the treatment of drug addiction and obesity-related disorders, is also effective in controlling diabetes and improving dyslipidemia. See table 6.28

Insulin therapy

Insulin therapy is initiated when oral agents fail to restore blood sugar to a desired level before and after meals. By lessening the body's reliance on insulin produced by the pancreas, and enhancing the sugar uptake in the muscle, exogenous insulin lowers blood glucose levels, thus allowing the beta cells to rest. Remember that "beta cells" are the ones that secrete insulin. Body weight usually increases slightly with improved control of the blood sugar, because calories consumed are used rather than expelled in urine. In many cases, insulin is given along with oral agents.

Aggressive control of blood pressure

High blood pressure is found in up to 60% of diabetics and the combination is associated with a doubling of cardiac risk compared to those with diabetes alone. The recommended blood pressure level in patients with diabetes is below 130/80. Several studies have clearly demonstrated substantial risk reduction with tight control of blood pressure in diabetics. More aggressive blood pressure control reduces stroke and diabetes-related mortality even further among diabetics than among non-diabetics. Tight blood pressure control in patients with hypertension and type 2 diabetes achieves marked reduction in the risk of deaths related to diabetes and complications of diabetes. Most diabetics with hypertension will require two or more antihypertensive medications to achieve their blood pressure goal.

Medicines that affect the renin angiotensin system (ACEIs and ARBs) are the drugs of choice because of their additional protective effect against heart and kidney disease. Although beta blockers were traditionally avoided in diabetics (due to adverse effects on lipids and blood sugar), the newer non-selective beta blocker Carvedilol (Coreg) has been shown to increase insulin sensitivity and improve HDL and triglyceride levels. Unlike other beta blockers, which cause vasoconstriction, Coreg causes peripheral vasodilatation and has antioxidant properties (see Chapter VI, Section 1).

Table 6.28. Beneficial effects of Rimonabant 20 mg

	Change
Weigt loss in lbs	22
Waist loss in inches	2
Weight loss of 5% or more	63%
Weight loss of 10% or more	33%
Decrease in A1C	0.7%
Increase in HDL	25%
Decrease in triglycerides	9%
Decrease in metabolic syndrome	41%

Control of diabetic dyslipidemia

At a given level of cholesterol, the risk of heart disease among diabetics is three- to fourfold higher. In fact, the risk of heart disease among diabetics in the lowest quintile (lowest 20%) of cholesterol levels is higher than non-diabetics in the highest quintile (highest 20%) of cholesterol levels. Diabetic dyslipidemia consists of high triglycerides, low HDL, and a preponderance of small dense LDL and high non-HDL cholesterol. The first priority in diabetic dyslipidemia is to bring LDL below 100 mg/dL and non-HDL cholesterol below 130. The 2005 ADA guidelines recommend an LDL goal of below 70 in those with heart disease and diabetes. The ADA also recommends triglycerides levels to be below 150; HDL more than 55 for women and more than 45 for men. In view of the heightened risk, I recommend an LDL of below 70, non-HDL cholesterol of below 100, triglycerides of below 130, and an HDL level above 60 for Indians (both men and women) with diabetes. Aggressive treatment with statins, niacin and omega-3 fatty acid supplementation is recommended to reach these goals.

Non-HDL cholesterol is a better predictor of risk than LDL in diabetic patients. Both the ADA and the NCEP recommend keeping the non-HDL cholesterol as the secondary target, and statins as the first-line of therapy. However, combination therapy using fibrates or niacin with statins is often required to correct multiple lipid abnormalities (HDL, LDL, triglycerides and non-HDL cholesterol.). The benefits are greater and risk lower when niacin is added to a statin, than with the addition of fibrates. Such therapy has been shown to be safe and highly effective in the management of diabetic dyslipidemia. Management of very high triglycerides is discussed in section 4.

Aspirin therapy

People with diabetes have a heightened tendency for blood clots (vulnerable blood) (see Chapter I, Section 1). This risk can be reduced by taking aspirin. The American Diabetic Association recommends aspirin for diabetics if they have heart disease, or at least one additional risk factor such as high blood pressure, cholesterol or smoking. In spite of this recommendation, many diabetics do not take aspirin; one-third of diabetics with heart disease and two-thirds of diabetics with cardiac risk factors are not using aspirin. Low-dose "baby" aspirin (81 mg) may not be sufficient in many patients with diabetes. Check with your doctor if a full dose (325 mg) is better for you.

Diabetes, angioplasty, and bypass surgery

Despite recent medical advances, such as new drug-eluting (that is, drug-releasing) stents, outcomes for diabetic patients after angioplasty and stents are still significantly worse than for non-diabetic patients. This underscores the need for aggressive medical management and lifestyle changes to avoid the need for these last-resort procedures (see Chapter VII, sections 5 and 6). The appropriate use of medication along with earnest, proactive modifications of lifestyle such as physical activity and healthy nutrition can help reduce the complications of diabetes, including heart attack, stroke, and heart failure.

KEY · POINTS · IN · A · NUTSHELL

♥ More than 80% of diabetics die from heart disease and its complications.

♥ Most diabetics are unaware of their very high risk of heart disease.

♥ Aggressive, proactive lifestyle modification can delay the need for, and reduce the dosage of, medications.

♥ The priorities of diabetes management are controlling their ABCs: A1C, Blood pressure, and Cholesterol.

♥ A1C is the single best measure for the control of blood sugar over the preceding three months.

♥ Blood sugar control protects against eye, nerve, and kidney diseases.

♥ Controlling blood pressure and cholesterol protects against heart attack and stroke and the goals are lower in diabetics than nondiabetics.

♥ Blood pressure goal is 130 mm Hg in diabetics.

♥ The lipid goals for Indian diabetics are: LDL below 70, non-HDL cholesterol below 100, triglycerides below 130, and HDL above 60.

♥ Most diabetics, particularly Indians will require medications to control dyslipidemia.

♥ Early use of TZDs can postpone the need of insulin for several years.

Chapter VII

Taking Heart: Living with Heart Disease

Section 1, **How to Assess Your Risk of Heart Disease**, presents a semi-quantitative self-assessment to determine your risk of heart disease incorporating both traditional and emerging risk factors. Depending on your level of risk (low, medium, high and very high), recommendations for appropriate action steps are given. ◆

Section 2, **Advanced Lipid Tests,** discusses types of commercially available advanced blood tests to evaluate the more atherogenic and antiatherogenic subclasses of LDL and HDL and the new international standard for measuring lipoprotein(a) accurately. This section also discusses the utility of measuring Lp-PLA-2, Apo E, high sensitivity-CRP and homocysteine. Recommendations for the type and nature of tests suitable for typical situations are also outlined. ◆

The third section, **Diagnosing Heart Disease,** outlines the standard and research methods for early detection of heart disease, years before you have any symptoms. Advantages and limitations of commonly used diagnosis techniques such as treadmill tests, ankle brachial index, echocardiogram, heart scan, calcium score, and coronary angiogram are discussed. ◆

Section 4, **After a Heart Attack, What Now?** explains the importance of aggressively treating those who have survived a heart attack, since they have a heightened risk of a repeat heart attack as compared to the general population. Lifestyle issues, tight control of blood pressure, lipids and other cardioprotective steps are outlined. ◆

Section 5, **Life after Bypass Surgery** focuses on the fact that bypass surgery does not cure heart disease. People who have undergone coronary bypass surgery remain at high risk for heart attack, stroke and death. This section outlines the various steps to identify and control the traditional and emerging cardiac risk factors after such procedures to minimize the chance of a future heart attack and need for repeat surgery. ◆

Living with Angioplasty and Stents, the sixth section, guides the reader through important aspects of coronary angioplasty and stents—common procedures to dilate clogged coronary arteries. Causes of restenosis and possible strategies to minimize the need for repeat procedures are discussed. ◆

The last section, **Reversing Heart Disease: Can It Be Done?** reviews the current research in arresting the progression of atherosclerosis by lowering LDL and achieving regression by increasing HDL. While regression is achievable, it is really not necessary to live a long and healthy life without a heart attack. ◆

7.1 ▶ How to Assess Your Risk of Heart Disease

Among people without known heart disease, the risk of developing disease can be categorized as low, medium, high, and very high. People with diabetes are considered to be *heart disease risk-equivalent* – meaning that they are to be treated as though they have heart disease even in the absence of symptoms and diagnosis of heart disease. Those who have been diagnosed with heart disease have a **3-10 -fold higher risk** of having a coronary event such as heart attack compared to those without known heart disease. Diabetics with diagnosed heart disease are at extremely high risk of recurrent heart attacks.

Among individuals *without heart disease* or diabetes, the Framingham Risk Score (which uses five traditional risk factors) is the yardstick to measure and categorize ten year risk. However, the actual cardiac risk in Indians is at least double that predicted by the Framingham model. This section provides a more accurate way of gauging the risk for Indians by incorporating many emerging risk factors and risk markers.

Several studies have shown that the traditional risk factors fail to fully explain the excess burden of heart disease among Indians. Studies in the UK have shown that the actual risk is 80% to 140% higher among Indians than that suggested by using the Framingham Risk Score, as well as other prediction models in Europe. Using the Framingham model, one study has just reported a simplified correction for improving the accuracy of the risk estimation among Indians *in the United Kingdom*. The study found the following four modifications to traditional risk factors:

- *Age: add 10 years*
- *Weight: add 40 lbs*
- *Systolic blood pressure: add 50 mmHg*
- *Cholesterol level: add 108 mg/dL*
- *Total cholesterol/HDL ratio: add 1.7*

> **A Word about Terminology**
>
> Throughout this book, the term Indian refers to people, who trace their origin to the Indian subcontinent—meaning Bangladesh, India, Pakistan, and Sri Lanka—including those who now live abroad but originate from one of these four countries. "Indian" in this context is ethnically interchangeable with "South Asian," "Indo-Asian," or "Asian Indian." The term thus excludes native Americans but includes more than people from the nation of India.
>
> **Measurement Units:** As is conventional, blood glucose levels, triglyceride levels, and cholesterol levels are stated throughout this book in milligrams per deciliter (mg/dL). Blood pressure is stated in millimeters of mercury (mmHg).

No similar adjustments for predicting heart disease among Indians in the US are available. Manisha Chandalia from Dallas, has shown that an Indian 5'8' tall and weighing 160 lbs has the metabolic abnormalities similar to a American of the same height but weighing 200 lbs. This suggests that Indians need to add approximately 40 lbs to his or her weight to better estimate the obesity related risk. Table 7.1 provides a guide to predict your level of risk for heart disease and heart attack by incorporating both traditional and emerging risk factors. Unlike Framingham point score (Table 7.2), this point score model takes into consideration the available data on the cardiac risk from emerging and traditional risk factors.

Categories of heart attack risk

Total up the 13 scores. The higher the number, the higher is your risk. This scoring system is based on my experience and review of scientific literature and awaits validation.

Low risk

Those with a score below 20 are considered to be at low risk and generally enjoy a long and healthy life, provided they do not get lackadaisical about proper nutrition and regular exercise. The large Chicago Heart Association Detection Project in Industry Study of 3,000 women aged 18 to 39 who were followed for 30 years has demonstrated the benefits of having a low-risk status at a young age. This low risk was characterized by blood pressure less than 120, cholesterol below 200, BMI below 25, no diabetes, and no smoking. Only 20% of the study population had low risk status. These low risk women had a 90% lower rate of death from heart attack and all other causes. They had *double the quality of life*, half the average yearly health care costs, and the lowest need for medications.

Moderate risk

Those with a score 20 to 49 are at moderate risk. having high levels of lipoprotein(a) and homocysteine levels with or without metabolic syndrome also puts you in this category. Measurement of lipoprotein(a) and homocysteine is particularly important if you have a personal or family history of premature heart disease. Measurement of C-reactive protein (CRP) is particularly recommended in people with obesity, metabolic syndrome and diabetes. Each of these emerging risk factors (common among Indians) can *double the risk* ascertained from traditional risk factors; the risk is increased *four-fold* with any two of these risk factors and *eight-fold* with all three: lipoprotein(a), homocysteine, and CRP.

High risk

If your score is 50 to 100, you are at high risk. Irrespective of your scores, you are considered to be in the high risk category if you suffer from diabetes or heart disease. This is also true of those with chronic kidney disease, peripheral artery disease, carotid artery narrowing, stroke, or mini-stroke. The benefits of aspirin outweighs the risk in people of this category

Table 7.1. Risk prediction score for heart disease among Indian men and women

Risk Factor	If you are	For men, add	For women, add
Age	25 years or younger 25 to 34 35 to 44 45 to 55 55 to 64 65 to 75 Above 75	0 +2 +4 +6 +8 +10 +12	-2 0 +2 +4 +6 +8 +12
Total Cholesterol in mg/dL	Below 120 120 to 159 160 to 199 200 to 239 240 to 279 Above 280	0 +1 +3 +6 +10 +12	0 +1 +3 +6 +10 +12
HDL in mg/dL	Above 80 60 to 79 50 to 59 40 to 49 30 to 39 Below 30	-3 -1 +2 +4 +6 +8	0 +1 +3 +6 +8 +12
Triglycerides in mg/dL	Below 130 130 to 200 200 to 299 Above 300	0 +2 +2 +3	0 +3 +3 +4
Systolic blood pressure	Below 120 120 to 129 130 to 139 140 to 159 Above 159	0 +1 +2 +3 +4	0 +1 +2 +3 +4
Smoking	Age- 20-39 Age -40-49 Age -50-59 Above 60	+8 +5 +3 +1	+10 +8 +5 +2
Family history of diabetes	Yes No	+2 0	+2 0
Parental history of heart disease Sibling history of heart disease	Yes No Yes No	+2 0 +4 0	+2 0 +4 0
Waist size	Below 32" 32 to 35" 36 to 39" Above 40"	-2 +1 +4 +10	0 +4 +8 +12
C-reactive protein (CRP) mg/L	Below 11 to 3 3 to 10 Above 10	0 +2 +4 +5	0 +2 +4 +5
Homocysteine mmol/L	Below 10 10 to 15 16 to 20 Above 20	0 +3 +5 +10	0 +3 +5 +10
Lipoprotein(a)	Below 15 15 to 29 30 to 49 50 to 75 75 to 99 Above 100	0 +3 +10 +20 +25 +30	0 +3 +10 +20 +25 +30
Urine microalbuminuria mg/dL	Above 300	+5	+5
Blood creatinine mg/dL	1.5-3.0 Above 3.0	+5 +10	+5 +10
	Total score		

Table 7.2. Cumulative point scale for estimating 10-year CHD risk in men and women (Framingham point scores)

Age	TC (age 40-49 y)	TC (age 50-59 y)	Smoker
20-34 = -9/-7 35-39 = -4/-3 40-44 = 0/0 45-49 = 3/3 50-54 = 6/6 55-59 = 8/8 60-64 = 10/10 65-69 = 11/12 70-74 = 12/14 75-79 = 13/16	<160 = 0/0 160-199 = 3/3 200-239 = 5/6 240-279 = 6/8 ≥280 = 8/10	<160 = 0/0 160-199 = 2/2 200-239 = 3/4 240-279 = 4/5 ≥280 = 5/7	(age 20-39 y) No = 0/0 Yes = 8/9 (age 40-49 y) No = 0/0 Yes = 5/7 (age 50-59 y) No = 0/0 Yes = 3/4

Systolic Blood Pressure			HDL-C
Treatment:	No	Yes	≥60 = -1/-1
<120 =	0/0	0/0	50-59 = 0/0
120-129 =	0/1	1/3	40-49 = 1/1
130-139 =	1/2	2/4	<40 = 2/2
140-159 =	1/3	2/5	
≥160 =	2/4	3/6	

Total points: <0 0 1 2 3 4 5 6 7 8 9 10 11 12 13 14 15 16 ≥17 18 19 20 21 22 23 24 ≥25 (men)

10-y CHD risk (%):   <1 1 1 1 1 1 2 2   3 4 5   6 8   10 12 16 20 25 ≥30

<1 1 1 1   1 2 2 3   4   5   6 8 11 14 17 22 27 ≥30 (women)

CHD = MI or coronary death

Source: NCEP, ATP. III. Ref. 6.43.

Highest risk

You are in the highest risk category if your score is above 100 or you have both diabetes and heart disease (prior heart attack and/or bypass surgery/angioplasty). This is discussed in greater detail in Section 4 in this Chapter.

Table 7.3. Risk of heart attack according to your score

Your score	Risk Category	Comments
Below 20	Low	Excellent. Keep up your good lifestyle. It will keep you from falling into a high risk category in the future.
20 to 49	Medium	Good. Increase lifestyle changes to get you into the low risk category.
50 to 100	High	Intensify your lifestyle changes and consult your cardiologist for appropriate medication.
Above 100	Very high	Request your physician to write down the various goals and ascertain the reasons why your goals are not met.

KEY · POINTS · IN · A · NUTSHELL

♥ In people without heart disease, the risk of developing a heart attack can be categorized as low, medium, high, and very high.

♥ Aspirin is recommended only for people with medium or higher risk.

♥ People with diabetes **or** heart disease are at a high risk for heart attack and stroke.

♥ Those with both diabetes **and** heart disease are at the highest risk for heart attack and death.

♥ The targets goals for treatment of blood pressure and cholesterol are lower in high risk individuals, lower still for highest-risk persons.

♥ The Framingham Risk Score significantly underestimates the risk for heart attack among Indians.

♥ When using the Framingham Risk Score for Indians, adding 108 mg/dL to cholesterol, 50 mmHg to blood pressure, 40 pounds to weight, and 10 years to age or doubling the 10-year calculated risk can provide a better estimate of the cardiac risck.

7.2 ▶ Advanced Lipid Tests

"The good doctor knows what tests to do and when to do it. But the very good doctor knows what not to do and when not to do it." Herbert L Fred.

As discussed in detail Chapter II, LDL increases the risk of heart disease whereas HDL plays a protective role. The standard lipid profile measures total cholesterol, triglycerides, and HDL *but not LDL, which is* calculated from these three figures. LDL and HDL can be further categorized through advanced lipid testing as either small- or large-particle. Small LDL particles are much more dangerous than large-particle LDL. Similarly, the cardioprotective effect of HDL is largely limited to large-particle HDL. Small HDL particles are associated with less cardiac protection. Some but not all studies indicate that small HDL particles may actually promote and accelerate atherosclerosis. Women, in general, have larger HDL particles than men and this contributes to their lower risk, at least at younger ages. Indians in general have smaller HDL particle size and have less of the cardioprotective large HDL. People with a family history of premature heart disease benefit the most from advanced lipid testing. Individuals with premature heart disease, unexplained heart disease, repeat angioplasty, or bypass surgery are also candidates for advanced lipid testing. This Chapter addresses the merits, limits, and uses of advanced lipid testing.

The predominance of small dense particles is also called atherogenic phenotype, which is different from atherogenic dyslipidemia. The former is a characteristic feature of the latter and is common among people with diabetes and metabolic syndrome.

LDL subclasses

Not all LDL particles are created equal. LDL particles are broadly classified as pattern A, pattern B, or pattern AB. LDL pattern A is large and less atherogenic; pattern B is small, dense, and more atherogenic. Pattern AB particles are intermediate in both in particle size and atherogenicity. Smallest LDL particles are correlate strongly with rapid and severe progression of heart disease. Most individuals have both small and large subfractions of LDL, but the proportion may vary. People who have a preponderance of small dense LDL have a *three- to four-fold* higher risk of heart disease than people with large buoyant LDL, especially if the total LDL particle numbers are also high.

> **Poor man's test for small dense LDL**
> A fasting triglyceride level above 130 mg/dL and a triglyceride/HDL ratio of more than three identifies individuals with a preponderance of small dense LDL particles.

Blacks, in general, have larger LDL particle size, even after adjustments are made for triglycerides levels. Although Indians are thought to have a higher proportion of small dense LDL, several studies from the CADI Research group using three different methods have failed to confirm this. Berkeley HeartLab classifies LDL into seven different subclasses with the three large LDL particles being less dangerous than the four small, dense LDL particles and LDL IVb being the smallest and most atherogenic subfraction. In normal individuals without dyslipidemia the average small dense LDL level is below 30 mg/dL, which is usually 30% of the total LDL. However, an individual with 100 mg/dL of LDL may have more than 30 mg/dL small dense, LDL if the triglyceride level is elevated (more than 130). The opposite applies when the triglyceride level is low. Recent report studies in the Quebec Cardiovascular Study has somewhat dampened the enthusiasm for determining LDL particle size because the increased risk observed during the first seven years of follow up among people with small dense LDL disappeared during the next seven years of follow-up.

National Cholesterol Education Program (NCEP), which provides up-to-date guidelines for cholesterol testing and treatment, has published three successive guidelines. Each of these guidelines targets LDL as the primary focus of treatment. It is worth highlighting that NCEP does not recommend the direct measurement of LDL, since the calculated value is accurate and more than adequate in most clinical situations and patient care. It is very difficult to justify measuring LDL subclasses in all persons, when none of the recommending agencies advise even direct measurement of LDL level. However, the presence and preponderance of small dense LDL can be calculated from the standard lipid tests with an accuracy exceeding 85%.

LDL particle number

Recent studies suggest that the number of LDL particles (reported in nmol/L) may be more important than the quantity of LDL (normally in mg/dL). The LDL particles are "counted" by Nuclear Magnetic Resonance. The LDL particle number is approximately 11 times higher than LDL quantity reported as mg/dL in people without significant dyslipidemia but may be 12 times higher in people with metabolic syndrome or diabetes (Table 7.5). The disparity between LDL cholesterol concentration and the number of LDL particles can be explained by abnormal LDL composition.

Non-HDL cholesterol

In clinical practice, non-HDL cholesterol is an excellent surrogate for LDL particle number (Chapter II Section 3 and Chapter VI Section 4). Non-HDL cholesterol calculation does not involve any expense and is accurate even in a non-fasting state.

Table 7.4. Interrelationship between LDL, Apo B, LDL particle number and non-HDL cholesterol goals

LDL (mg/dL)	Apo B (mg/dL)	LDL particle number (nmol/L)	Non-HDL cholesterol
70	60	800	100
100	90	1100	130
130	110	1300	160
160	130	1400	190

It is unlikely that persons with low levels of non-HDL cholesterol and triglycerides levels would have an abnormally high number of LDL particles. Both LDL particle number and size can be brought to low risk categories by maintaining:

- Non-HDL cholesterol below 100 mg/dL
- Triglycerides below 130 mg/dL
- Triglyceride to HDL ratio less than three

From a therapeutic point of view, statins are the most effective medication in lowering LDL, lowering both large and small particles. Similarly, niacin is highly effective in increasing the average size of LDL, rendering it less atherogenic and increasing the size of HDL, thus rendering it more cardioprotective.

Table 7.5. Lipoprotein subclasses and their importance to cardiac risk

Tests	Significance
LDL subclasses	Smaller LDL particle confer a three fold risk as compared to larger LDL particle Triglycerides /HDL ratio above three and/or triglycerides above 130 mg/dL are fairly accurate in predicting the presence of small dense LDL.
LDL particle number	Better predictor of risk than LDL levels Non-HDL cholesterol above 100 identifies high LDL particle number.
Apolipoprotein B	Apolipoprotein B is the major protein associated with LDL High levels confer high risk for the development of heart disease Non-HDL cholesterol provides a reasonable estimate of Apo B
Apolipoprotein AI	Apolipoprotein AI is the major protein of HDL Low level confers increased risk HDL provides a reasonable estimate of Apolipoprotein AI
HDL subclasses	Cardiovascular protection highest with large particles and least with small HDL particle Conditions that contribute to a preponderance of small dense LDL also contribute to small dense HDL (worthwhile test for Indians)
Lipoprotein(a)	Needs to be measured, especially for Indians
Homocysteine	Needs to be measured, especially for Indians
Lp-PLA2 (PLAC)	High level (more than 310 mg) confer a two-fold risk
Insulin	Highly variable result and normal values are not established
Chlamydia	Treatment not successful - only of research interest at this stage
Fibrinogen	Recommended in selected individuals only
Apoprotein E Genotype	Limited use in identifying people more responsive to diet and less responsive to statins.

HDL subclasses

There are five different sizes of HDL particles (Table 7.5.). As with LDL, bigger is better for HDL. Large HDL is common in women and in persons who exercise regularly, but not in those who drink alcohol excessively. Regular exercise and niacin are the best strategies for raising your proportion of large HDL. The 2b subfraction of your HDL is the largest and most cardioprotective. An HDL sample with a 2b fraction below 20% is considered low and predicts high risk of heart disease, even when the overall HDL level is normal. Dr. Superko and I have reported low HDL 2b to be present in more than 90% of Indians, including those with normal HDL levels.

Several recent studies have suggested that small HDL particles not only lack the protective properties of large HDL, but may actually promote and accelerate atherosclerosis – properties similar to that of small dense LDL. These properties include increased risk of development, progression, and severity of heart disease. Furthermore, small dense HDL often coexists with small dense LDL and small dense lipoprotein(a). This combination is highly dangerous and appears to be particularly common in Indians.

Indians and small dysfunctional HDL

Dr. Bhalodker and I have published several reports that show significantly smaller HDL particle sizes among Indian men and women as compared to that from the participants of the Framingham Heart Study. We found that HDL particles among Indians were smaller than in whites. At a given level of HDL, Indians have less of the more cardioprotective large HDL and more of the atherogenic small HDL particles as shown in Figure 7.1. A decrease in the number of large HDL particles combined with an increase in the number of small HDL particles result in dysfunctional HDL which may not be reflected in the HDL level. Even Indians with normal total HDL have

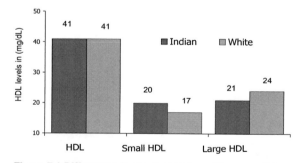

Figure 7.1 Differences in small-particle and large-particle HDL between Indians and whites. Although the overall HDL levels are not different, Indians have less of the cardio-protective large HDL. Source: Bhalodker, N. Ref. 6.6.

small dysfunctional HDL that may not be evident without advanced lipid testing. The role of small HDL particle in the excess burden of heart disease among Indians is currently being investigated. Although large HDL is cardioprotective, abnormally large HDL particles, resulting from severe abnormalities in CETP gene, also result in dysfunctional HDL with less of the cardioprotective HDL 2b.

The HDL particle can also be fractionated into various subclasses by quantitative two dimensional gel electrophoresis. Large alpha 1 particles are the most protective fraction by this method. This generally corresponds to HDL 2b measured by other methods. Increase in the alpha 1 HDL level was associated with less progression of coronary stenosis in the HATS study (see Appendix B). Atorvastatin has been shown to increase alpha 1 HDL by two dimentional gradient gel electrophoreses. However, this test is not commercially available.

Apolipoprotein B (Apo B)

Apo B is an essential component of LDL Apo B interacts with specific LDL receptors located on cell surfaces in many tissues, including the liver, and to remove LDL particles from the circulation.

Table: 7.6. Relative probability (RP) of having a heart attack for those in highest vs lowest quintile

Individual variables	RP
LDL	1.62
Apolipoprotein A-1	1.75
Total cholesterol	2.08
HDL	2.32
Apolipoprotein B-100	2.50
Non-HDL cholesterol	2.51
High-sensitivity CRP	2.98
Lipid ratios	
Apo B-100 to apo A-1	3.01
LDL-C to HDL-C	3.18
Apo B-100 to HDL-C	3.56
Total cholesterol to HDL-C	3.81

Source: Ridker, PM. Ref. 7.46.

Apo B represents all the atherogenic lipoproteins contained in LDL, VLDL, and lipoprotein(a). Several studies have shown Apo B to be a better predictor of heart attack than LDL. As mentioned above, non-HDL cholesterol has been shown to be a fairly accurate surrogate for Apo B.

Apo AI, and Apo B/Apo AI ratios

Apo AI is the primary protein in HDL and is considered responsible for most of the protective effects of HDL. Many experts believe Apo AI may be a better protector against heart disease than HDL. This ratio of Apo B to Apo AI represents the ratio of total atherogenic to antiatherogenic lipoproteins. It is perhaps the single best measure of atherogenic risk. In the INTERHEART study, this ratio was 0.85 in people with heart attack and 0.80 in people without heart attack. A ratio of total cholesterol to HDL (TC/HDL) is a reasonably accurate surrogate for the Apo B/Apo AI ratio (see Chapter II, Section 8).

Total cholesterol HDL ratio

In a large prospective study of initially healthy US women, the authors compared individual lipid measures, lipid ratios, and CRP as predictors of CV events. Subjects included 15,632 healthy women aged 45 or older, enrolled between November 1992 and July 1995, and followed over 10 years for the occurrence of cardiovascular events. The adjusted risk ratios for future cardiovascular events in the top versus bottom quintiles, for each variable measured (individual lipid variables and lipid ratios), and have been adjusted for age, smoking status, blood pressure, diabetes, and body mass index are summarized in Table 7.6.

This data supports the use of standard lipid measurements, rather than apo A-1 and B-100, in primary risk detection. Non-HDL cholesterol and the ratio of total cholesterol to HDL were as good as or better than apolipoprotein fractions for predicting cardiovascular events. High-sensitivity CRP added prognostic information beyond that conveyed by all lipid measures. While differences between apo B-100 and non-HDL-C may be of biological

> **Large HDL and longevity**
> A gene closely associated with HDL level and size (CETP gene) has been recently shown to influence longevity. In one study, the lipid profile of Askenazi Jews, who have exceptional longevity, was compared with that of the participants of the Framingham Heart Study, who had an average life span. There was no difference in total cholesterol, triglycerides, LDL, and HDL levels. However, these Jews with exceptional longevity had significantly larger HDL particles due to a polymorphism (favorable modification) of the CETP gene. This phenotype is also associated with a lower prevalence of hypertension, cardiovascular disease, and metabolic syndrome. This study suggests that lipoprotein particle sizes are an important inheritable factor influencing longevity.

VAP II (Atherotec) directly measures *Lp(a) cholesterol,* which is usually one-third that of the Lp(a) mass. Lp(a) cholesterol above 7 mg/dL may be considered high and corresponds to a Lp(a) mass of 20 mg/dL

interest, this data does not support the use of apolipoprotein B-100 in primary risk detection because non-HDL-C can be calculated by subtracting HDL-C from total cholesterol at no incremental cost beyond that for usual lipid evaluation.

Lipoprotein(a)

Lipoprotein(a), or Lp(a) for short, is one of the powerful predictors of premature heart disease (see Chapter III, Section 3). Lp(a) testing is strongly recommended for people with a family or personal history of premature heart disease. Testing for Lp(a) is also recommended for people who have undergone **repeat coronary angioplasty, stent, or bypass surgery**. High levels are found in more than 40% of Indians and correlate highly with their malignant heart disease at young age. Lp(a) levels **cannot be calculated** or inferred from the standard lipid tests and should be measured *in all Indians* (other than senior citizens) being evaluated for heart disease risk.

Accurate measurement of lipoprotein(a) is critically important, **but not all** commercially available methods are accurate. Lipoprotein(a) is usually expressed as **lipoprotein mass** which includes protein, cholesterol, and other components. Most labs measure lipoprotein(a) mass, whereas other labs measure lipoprotein(a) cholesterol or lipoprotein(a) protein. Therefore, it is not unusual to find a **three-fold difference in results** when the same blood is analyzed by different labs using different methods. There are 34 different isoforms of lipoprotein(a) depending primarily on the size of the apo a particles. The smaller ones are associated with the greater risk, but the Lp(a) levels may be artificially low, when it uses a method affected by particle size. Unfortunately most of the commercial labs use such methods leading to **inaccurate results.** This problem is likely to be resolved shortly because a new international standard (ELISA) has been developed and approved by the National Heart, Lung & Blood Institute and the World Health Organization. This method is to be incorporated by all future commercial test kit makers to ensure the accuracy of the test. Do make sure that your blood test is done by a lab that uses a method that confirms with the new international standard.

A level above 30 mg/dL is generally considered abnormal when lipoprotein(a) is measured and reported without specific mention of protein or cholesterol. However, recent studies indicate the risk from lipoprotein(a) begins at a level above 20, particularly in Indians. VAP II (Atherotec) directly measures *lipoprotein(a) cholesterol,* which is usually one-third that of the lipoprotein(a) mass. Lipoprotein(a) cholesterol above 7 mg/dL may be considered high VAP and corresponds to a lipoprotein(a) mass of 20 mg/dL. The University of Chicago measures lipoprotein(a) as protein and the recent special report from NIH also suggest measurement of lipoprotein(a) protein. As a result, the new international standard will specify reporting of lipoprotein(a) in nmol/ L. Liposcience has adopted this new method with a cut-point of less than 75 nanomoles for normal result.

Apo E

Apolipoprotein E is a plasma protein involved in the transport of cholesterol in the blood. Apo E genotypes are genetically fixed and are present in combinations of E2, E3, and E4. Differences in apo E genotypes can affect LDL and triglyceride levels as well as a person's response to therapy with diet and medications. Apo E2/2 is found in less than 1% of the population and is associated with type III hyperlipidemia (described below). People with this genotype respond well to niacin and fibrates. These people also have greater response to exercise but lower response to diet. Apo E3/3 is the normal genotype. Apo E4/4 and E4/3 are associated with higher LDL levels and a greater response to a diet low in saturated fats. Apo E4/4 is also associated with high risk of Alzheimer's disease.

Type III hyperlipidemia

Type III hyperlipidemia is a condition in which levels of highly atherogenic lipoprotein particles, known as "remnants," are elevated, leading to an increased risk of heart disease. Remnants are lipoprotein particles that have had most of their triglycerides removed. Remnants are very high-risk particles and type III confers an eight-to 10-fold increase in heart disease risk. The liver normally removes these particles from the blood. However, they build up to abnormal levels in people with type III hyperlipidemia. The prevalence of type III hyperlipidemia in the general population is only around 0.5%, but it accounts for 3 or 4% of early heart attacks. Very early heart attacks can be seen in patients with more severe type III hyperlipidemia. The treatment is somewhat different from other forms of hyperlipidemia.

Lipoprotein-associated phospholipase A2 (Lp-PLA2)

Lp-PLA2 is a novel risk marker that is specific to vascular inflammation. Lp-PLA2 is a proinflammatory enzyme that preferentially modifies LDL to oxidized fatty acids. It is produced by inflammatory cells in the arterial intima and resides mainly on the LDL particle in the human blood. It appears to be involved in the initiation of the early stages of the vascular inflammatory process. Unlike CRP, which is a general marker of inflammation, Lp-PLA2 is not affected by other inflammatory conditions. An increased Lp-PLA2 level may enhance the atherogenicity of LDL by increasing vascular inflammation. An elevated blood level of Lp-PLA2 correlates with a two-fold risk of heart attack or stroke. In the ARIC Study (see Appendix B), among persons who have low LDL, high Lp-PLA2—either alone or in combination with high CRP—identified a subgroup with a three-fold risk of coronary events. Lp-PLA2 levels are elevated among Indians and is associated with accelerated atherosclerosis. It can be lowered by all statins and can be useful for identifying patients for more aggressive LDL targeting.

Fibrinogen

Fibrinogen is a plasma protein involved in the formation of a blood clot. A high level doubles the risk of heart disease. Niacin lowers fibrinogen.

C-reactive protein

The role of CRP and homocysteine in heart disease are discussed in Chapter II, section 4. High CRP levels among Indians correlate highly with abdominal obesity. Increased physical activity and weight loss are the preferred treatment options in people with elevated CRP. When evaluating CRP for cardiac risk assessment, the *high sensitivety* CRP or hs-CRP must be used, since it may be high when the standard CRP test is not elevated.

Who needs advanced lipid testing?
- People with family or personal history of premature heart disease or stroke.
- People with unexplained heart disease.
- People with unexplained severity of heart disease.
- People who require repeat coronary angioplasty or bypass surgery.
- People who have poor response to statins (statin resistance).
- People with chronic kidney disease.
- Asian Indians less than 65 years of age.
- People suspected of, or receiving treatment for lipoprotein subclass abnormalities.

Homocysteine

Indians have the highest levels of homocysteine of all populations. This appears to be related to dietary and nutritional factors as well as the cooking process they use. Homocysteine levels should be measured in Indians with premature heart disease and can be lowered with medications that contain adequate amounts of folic acid, B_6, and B_{12}.

International differences in cholesterol testing practices

In the US, measurement of one's cholesterol and lipid profile is recommended for everyone above 20 years of age. No such official recommendations exist in Canada or Europe. A *20% risk* of heart attack in 10 years is considered the highest risk category in the US, requiring the most aggressive treatment. In the UK the qualification to have a blood cholesterol test done was to have a *30% risk* of dying within 10 years. This has recently been reduced to a 5% risk. Both cholesterol testing and treatment are free in these countries. As result, the recommendations for testing are stringent and dictated by the brutal fact of what the **society is wealling afford** to provide all its citizens.

Where to get the advanced lipid testing?

The methodology and normal values vary from lab to lab, making both comparison and interpretation of results difficult. Lipoprotein subclasses are measured by different methods by the commercial labs. Therefore, lipoprotein subclass measurements done through different labs are not directly comparable. Moreover, significant discrepancies have been observed when the same blood is analyzed by the same lab using different methods.

Should you pay for the advanced tests?

Many managed care plans do not pay for advanced lipid testing in people *before a heart attack* and sometimes, even after a heart attack. I

List of laboratories that provide advanced lipid testing

Test Lab	Website	Remarks
Atherotech ultracentrifugation	www.atherotech.com	Provides lipoprotein(a) cholesterol, LDL and HDL subclasses and remnants as a single test and reasonable cost.
Berkeley HeartLab gradient gel electrophoresis	www.bhlinc.com	Lipoprotein(a), LDL subclasses and HDL subclasses are done separately and needs to be ordered separately.
Liposcience nuclear magnetic resonance	www.liposcience.com	Provides lipoprotein particle size and number, but the technology does not allow the measurement of the all-important lipoprotein(a).

believe paying from your pocket for certain tests may be worthwhile if your managed care plan does not cover it. The price of advanced lipid tests offered has come down drastically in the last few years. For example, you may be able to get a lipoprotein(a), homocysteine, Hs-CRP, and HDL and LDL subclasses for under $300 T. LDL, HDL and VLDL subclasses, together with an accurate measurement of lipoprotein(a) all as a single test, is also available at a very reasonable cost of less than $100.

KEY · POINTS · IN · A · NUTSHELL

♥ Total cholesterol to HDL ratio and non-HDL cholesterol concentrations are powerful predictors of heart disease but do not convey the risk imparted by small HDL particles and high Lp(a) levels.

♥ Both LDL and HDL can be categorized into small and large particles through advanced lipid testing.

♥ Small LDL particles are more dangerous than large LDL.

♥ The cardioprotective effect of HDL is primarily limited to large HDL; small HDL particle provides less protection against heart disease and may even increase the risk.

♥ In general, Indians have a smaller HDL particle size, even when their total HDL levels are not low.

♥ More than 90% of Indians, including those without low HDL have low levels of HDL 2b—the most protective HDL subclass.

♥ Lipoprotein(a) testing is strongly recommended for people with a family or personal history of premature heart disease or stroke, and for people who have undergone repeat coronary angioplasty, stent, or bypass surgery.

♥ People with premature heart disease, repeat angioplasty, bypass surgery, or a family history of premature heart disease are likely to benefit the most from advanced lipid testing.

♥ Testing for lipoprotein(a), homocysteine, and possibly hs-CRP appears to be very useful for predicting risk among Indians, in addition to conventional lipid profile.

7.3 ▶ Diagnosing Heart Disease

How can you tell if you have heart disease? The truth is that heart disease progresses silently for several decades before you develop any symptoms. Even severe heart disease may exist for many years without causing a heart attack (as happened to President Clinton). Like high blood pressure, there is no correlation between the severity of heart disease and its symptoms. Sudden death may be the very first symptom of heart disease that you get; indeed, half of all heart attacks and sudden cardiac deaths occur without offering any advanced notice the telltale symptoms such as chest pain. Fortunately, tremendous strides have been made in the diagnosis and treatment of heart disease in the past 40 years. This Chapter will discuss the tests physicians use to detect heart disease before any obvious outward symptoms of the disease, such as chest pain, a heart attack, or cardiac arrest.

Silent heart disease

Heart disease progresses at very different rates in different people, even with all other things being equal. For any given level of exposure to risk factors among several people, there will be substantial variation in the extent of atherosclerosis. For example, one person with a systolic blood pressure of 200, cholesterol of 250, and a history of 20 pack-years of cigarettes may have no blockage of the arteries. Another person with similar or lower risk factor levels may have advanced disease requiring four or five bypass surgeries.

Evidence of silent heart disease or **subclinical atherosclerosis** (atherosclerosis without observable symptoms) was noted in 40% of the participants in the Framingham Heart Study and in the Cardiovascular Health Study. This indicates that nearly one out of two seemingly or apparently healthy individuals may have atherosclerosis. Recent studies have suggested that the knowledge of the extent of subclinical atherosclerosis may improve the outcome if appropriate treatment is undertaken before the development of any symptoms.

Tests for early detection of heart disease

There are several noninvasive tests that can detect heart disease with proven efficacy, and allow preventive intervention. Generally, invasive procedures such as angiograms are reserved for patients with symptoms like chest pain. There are two kinds of diagnostic tests: those with and those without imaging. A number of them are standard tests based on proven technology; others are just emerging, research-oriented tests on the cutting edge. Both standard and emerging tests are shown in Table 7.6.

Electrocardiogram (ECG/ EKG)

An electrocardiogram (EKG or ECG) records the electrical signals of the heart. Although it is the main tool used in the diagnosis of a heart attack after one occurs, an EKG may be normal even just a few minutes before a heart attack. Thus, a normal EKG does not necessarily mean the heart is normal. It is not very useful in many people, who have an abnormal EKG from a previous heart attack or other electrical abnormalities.

Echocardiogram

An echocardiogram uses ultrasound waves to create a kind of video or

Table 7.7. Various tests for detecting heart disease

Standard tests	Research/Emerging tests
• Electrocardiogram (ECG/EKG)	• Heart scan (for coronary artery calcification)
• Exercise stress EKG	• Carotid intimal medial thickness (CIMT)
• Echocardiogram	• Positron emission tomography (PET)
• Exercise stress echocardiogram	• Hybrid PET/CT
• Holter monitor	• Magnetic resonance imaging (MRI)
• Ankle-brachial index	• Magnetic resonance angiography (MRA)
• Carotid ultrasound	
• Coronary angiogram	

moving picture of the heart. The picture is much more detailed than an X-ray image and involves no radiation exposure. An instrument that transmits high-frequency sound waves, called a transducer, is placed over your ribs near the breastbone and directed toward the heart. Like the sonar of a dolphin or a bat, the transducer picks up the echoes of the sound waves coming from your heart and transmits them as electrical impulses to the "brain" of the echocardiography machine, which then converts the impulses into moving images of the heart. Echocardiograms work well for most people and allow doctors to see the beating heart and to visualize its structures. The test is widely available and relatively inexpensive.

This test also allows for the evaluation of the left ventricle's ejection fraction, which is the fraction (percentage) of the blood that the ventricle pumps out into the aorta with each heart beat. The ejection fraction is more than 55% in healthy people. An ejection fraction below 30% indicates severe left ventricular dysfunction associated with severe heart muscle damage, heart failure, and a death rate exceeding 50% in five years (similar to many inoperable cancers).

Finally, an echocardiogram shows the size of the heart chambers and the thickness of its walls. The echocardiogram is the most sensitive test to detect **left ventricular hypertrophy**, a complication of hypertension that involves enlargement of the heart and thickening of the left ventricle and can lead to heart failure and sudden death. Echocardiograms can also determine valve function and detect pericardial effusion (abnormal collection of fluid around the heart). An echocardiogram is usually combined with Doppler studies that detect abnormal blood flow within the heart.

> **Did you know...**
> A treadmill test that turns out to be normal is often misinterpreted as a clean bill of health. A stress test is positive only when heart disease is far advanced, with severe narrowing (75% or more) of at least one coronary artery on the day of the test; those with less severe narrowing of all three major arteries may very well post a normal test. Many people have a false sense of comfort and wrongly believe that this test guarantee freedom from a heart attack in the near future. A negative stress test rules out the presence of severe narrowing requiring angioplasty or bypass surgery, but does not rule out the risk of a heart attack in the near future. Most heart attacks happen to people with mild or moderate narrowing that do not compromise the blood supply to heart. A normal stress test, therefore, is not a justification for complacency.

Exercise stress EKG

In the hands of an experienced physician, an exercise stress test can play a pivotal role in the evaluation of patients with known or suspected heart disease. You walk on a moving treadmill while your EKG, heart rate, blood pressure and breathing are monitored. Both the treadmill's speed and elevation are increased every two to three minutes, depending upon the protocol used. The most common protocol is the Bruce Protocol and is recommended for patients with average fitness and exercise capacity. The test is terminated when the person achieves the target heart rate, or sooner if severe abnormalities are noted in the cardiogram or blood pressure level monitoring.

An exercise treadmill test is one of the most powerful cardiovascular prognostic tools available. How long a person can exercise before developing chest pain, and the severity of chest pain, are the major determinants of both quality and length of life. Other predictors of high-risk status include the extent of abnormalities on the cardiogram, the time it takes for the heart rate to return to its pre-exercise level, any drop in blood pressure, and the development of dangerous ventricular arrhythmia (erratic heart beats that may indicate abnormal behavior of heart). **Heart rate recovery** (how quickly a person's heart rate falls after an exercise session) is also important. After exercise, the heart rate drops 20 beats a minute in an average person, but up to 50 beats a minute in world-class athletes.

For the results to be reliable, the person tested must be able to exercise at a level sufficient to produce more than 85% of their maximum age-predicted heart rate. The test cannot diagnose heart disease in persons with an abnormal ECG, and it is less accurate in women.

Several studies indicate that the stress test provides information that is complementary to data obtained by a coronary angiogram (described further down). One study reported that men, who had one or more risk factors and two abnormalities on exercise testing, had a five-year cardiac risk that was *30 times higher* than men with no risk factors and no stress test abnormalities. Similarly, among men with multiple risk factors, a four-fold increase in seven-year cardiac mortality is observed in those with abnormal stress test compared to normal test results.

Myocardial perfusion scan (MPS)

Myocardial perfusion scan or MPS, allows physicians to obtain very clear images of the heart and locate areas of the heart muscle that are not receiving adequate blood supply due to narrowing of the coronary arteries. MPS techniques include stress echocardiogram (discussed further down) and nuclear perfusion imaging. To obtain nuclear images, tiny amounts of radioactive materials (called "tracers") are introduced into the person's body. The tracers give off gamma rays, which can be detected by machines. **Single photon emission computed tomography (SPECT)** uses a gamma camera to detect this energy. The information detected and recorded by these machines is then analyzed and reconstructed by computers to create very clear images of the target area of the heart.

SPECT imaging also allows detection and quantification of **scar tissue** of the heart muscle. The larger the defect, the greater is the severity of ischemia and/or scar. A heart attack results in dead heart muscle and it shows up as a scar, or a fixed defect that does not change with exercise. Angioplasty and bypass surgery provide no benefit for scar tissue.

SPECT is widely available and usually reimbursed by insurance companies. It is also very accurate in helping to classify people into high risk and low risk. People with a normal scan have a low risk and usually require only medical management, whereas those with large areas of ischemia are at high risk and may require coronary angioplasty or bypass surgery. In one study, the coronary event rates were below 1% in two years among those with normal MPS. Thus, the results of MPS are important independent predictors of survival in both women and men. In some studies, the extent of ischemia on MPS was a better predictor of death than even the Gensini score (which represents angiographic severity and extent of coronary artery disease).

MPS is particularly useful for patients who are taking certain medications like digoxin, beta blockers, and estrogens, which interfere with the accuracy of EKG changes on a stress test. For those, who are unable to exercise to an adequate level, medications such as adenosine or dobutamine can be injected to increase the heart rate and simulate exercise.

Exercise capacity is a more powerful predictor of mortality than other traditional risk factors for cardiovascular disease. The prognosis (the chance of living long) is poor when the exercise capacity is below 7 METS, (discused in Chapter V section 8) or six minutes on a treadmill using a Bruce Protocol. Conversely, the prognosis is good when the exercise capacity is more than 7 METS even in the presence of known heart disease. In one large study involving 6,200 men, 1,256 deaths occurred during thirty years of follow-up. Each 1 MET increase in exercise capacity conferred a 12% improvement in survival, among both healthy people and those

Stress echocardiogram

Narrowed coronary arteries do not show up on the echocardiogram at rest. With exercise, however, if the heart is not getting enough blood, an abnormal echo image appears. A stress echocardiogram involves performing an echocardiogram before and immediately after completing the stress test. Development of new abnormal echo imagers after exercise indicates ischemia and high risk of developing a heart attack in the near future. It is also less expensive and involves no radiation. For those unable to exercise, an infusion of certain chemical agents (adenosine or dobutamine) can be used to mimic exercise. The abnormalities are then compared with results from a resting echocardiogram. Recovery images must be obtained within 60 to 90 seconds; the sensitivity drops dramatically afterwards.

Up to 60% of stress echocardiography results are nondiagnostic or less than accurate. First, good quality echocardiograms may not be achievable in about 30% of patients, especially among those who are obese or heavy smokers. Another 20% of patients are not good candidates because of the difficulty of obtaining adequate images. Finally, in 15 to 20%, the images are considered equivocal. Stress echo cardiography appears to be more accurate in predicting heart disease in women than other imaging techniques. Obtaining accurate results in women is a challenge. Women often fail to exercise to their aerobic capacity and false positive EKG changes are fairly common. However, women have fewer false negative tests, which mean that a negative test reliably rules out significant heart disease.

> MPS allows measurement of the **extent of ischemia** by comparing the blood flow at rest and during stress. Ischemia signifies living heart muscle that is not receiving enough blood supply due to severe narrowing of the coronary arteries. Ischemia indicates high vulnerability to a heart attack in the not-too-distant future. Ischemia is diagnosed when the defect is reversible – that is, when it is produced by exercise and disappears at rest. The larger the areas of ischemia, the higher is the risk of death. Persons with large areas of ischemia benefit more with angioplasty and bypass surgery than with medical treatment alone. SPECT imaging appears extremely useful in identifying asymptomatic (symptom-less) diabetic patients who might benefit from bypass surgery.

Holter monitoring

A Holter monitor, which looks like a large Walkman, is a device that records the heart rate and rhythm for 24 to 48 hours, in contrast to an EKG, which records these for less than 15 seconds. Holter monitoring is usually done to evaluate the presence and severity of various arrhythmias in people with symptoms of palpitation or syncope (fainting). People are encouraged to continue their daily routines while wearing the monitor, since the device is usually less than one pound in weight and is nonrestrictive. Another use of holter monitoring is the detection of **silent ischemia** (abnormal EKG changes without chest pain) in patients with multiple risk factors. The prognosis of persons with silent ischemia is as bad as in those with painful ischemia (chest pain). The reason why some individuals do not develop chest pain with ischemia is the subject of ongoing research.

Ankle Brachial Index (ABI)

An ankle brachial index (ABI) is a very simple, inexpensive, and noninvasive test to diagnose peripheral arterial disease (PAD). This disease involves extensive atherosclerosis of the arteries that supply blood to the legs and feet. However, symptoms are absent until the disease is far advanced. ABI studies indicate that for every person with symptomatic PVD, there are at least *five without symptoms*. ABI can add significant information to traditional risk assessment. It involves blood pressure measurement in the wrist and the ankle using a handheld Doppler and reported as a ratio of systolic blood pressure at the ankle to that at the wrist. A normal ratio is 1.0 or above. An ABI below 0.90 confirms the diagnosis of preclinical disease of the lower extremities, while below 0.40 indicates severe obstruction. PVD is very common among smokers, diabetics, and those over 40. Diabetics have a *400-fold higher risk* of amputation than nondiabetics. These individuals can be identified 20 years before the development of any symptoms by this simple test. ABI has high sensitivity (that is, an abnormal test reliably identifies disease) and high specificity (that is, a normal test reliably indicates that the patient has no disease).

Atherosclerosis is a systemic disease that affects the arteries throughout the body. An abnormal ABI usually indicates severe and advanced atherosclerotic disease of coronary and/or carotid arteries (to be discussed below). In one study, severe heart disease was observed in 50%, and carotid disease in 30% of those with an abnormal ABI. In another study, those with an ABI below 0.4 had a fivefold risk of death, with 75% dying within 10 years, usually from heart disease or stroke. Thus, an abnormal ABI detects those who may lose not only a leg, but also their life in a few years time.

Carotid duplex

Carotid arteries, located in the neck, provide blood to the brain, and interruption of which causes a stroke. Carotid duplex is an ultrasound procedure performed to assess blood flow through the carotid artery to the brain. High frequency sound waves are directed from a handheld transducer probe to the area. These waves "echo" off the arterial structures and produce a two-dimensional image on a monitor. This test is very useful for detecting people at high risk of developing a stroke but may not have developed any symptoms yet.

Coronary angiogram, the invasive gold standard

The coronary angiogram has been the *gold standard* for the diagnosis of heart disease for several decades. In simple terms, a coronary angiogram is an x-ray of the coronary arteries to see if any of those arteries are narrowed or blocked with plaque. A long flexible tube (a catheter) is inserted into a blood vessel and maneuvered gently toward the heart. The physician typically numbs the area before inserting the catheter. A mild sedative is given before the cardiac catheterization and patients do not ordinarily feel the movement of the catheter within the blood vessel, even though they are awake. In a coronary angiogram, a dye is injected into the coronary arteries through the catheter. Depending on what the angiogram shows, the physician may recommend treatments such as medication, angioplasty or bypass surgery. A major limitation of angiography are that it is invasive and expensive.

RESEARCH OR EMERGING TESTS

Heart scan and coronary calcium score

Atherosclerosis of the coronary arteries is typically accompanied by calcification of the plaques, which can be measured by **EBCT** (Electron Beam Computerized Tomography) or **MDCT** (Multi-Direction Computerized Tomography). These tests, often called "heart scans," take less than 10 minutes to complete and give a good idea of the state of the patient's arteries. Heart scans are emerging as reliable options for coronary artery wall and lumen imaging. While cholesterol in the plaque cannot be visualized, the inflammation in the plaque draws in calcium, which shows clearly on these scans. Heart scans cost between $250 and $700, compared to $15,000 for a coronary angiogram. Whereas these tests identify significant disease of the proximal and mid -egments of the coronary artery, they cannot evaluate the entire artery.

To obtain the person's coronary artery calcium score (or **CAC score**), all the plaques in each artery are added. The CAC score is used as a yardstick for your coronary plaque burden, something no other test, even a stress test, can do. The higher the calcium score, the greater is the quantity of calcified plaque in your coronaries. Compared to men, women have lower CAC score.

Heart scans, however, cannot detect fatty plaques, which are more susceptible to rupturing and can lead to a heart attack. (MDCT also allows some visualization of *noncalcified plaques*). An important limitation of these scans is that about 5-10% of persons with a clean scan may develop a heart attack. CAC score correlates strongly with the severity of atherosclerosis but not with the severity of stenosis,

Did you know...

An angiogram is essentially a picture that reveals the extent of narrowing in an artery. See Color plates 3.2,3.4, and 3.5 The problem is that the major pathology of atherosclerosis lies within the thickness of the artery wall itself and not inside the hole or lumen of the artery, which is what an angiogram shows. In other words, an angiogram shows the *"hole in the donut but not the donut itself"*. The degree of narrowing or blockage revealed on an angiogram, therefore, represents only 1 to 5% of the actual amount of plaque present in the arterial wall. Most of the plaque is embedded within the wall itself. An angiogram thus only offers us a view of the tip of an iceberg. An angiogram cannot indicate the amount, shape, and composition of the plaque in the arterial walls. A person may have a large plaque encircling the entire artery but its shape may be such that it does not encroach upon the arterial lumen (See **color plates 1.3, 1.6**).

the major determinant of the need for coronary angioplasty and bypass surgery. However, CAC score is a strong predictor of future coronary events. A recent meta-analysis of studies on CAC showed the following risk of heart disease:

- Twofold risk with a CAC score of 1-100
- Fourfold risk with a CAC score of 101-400
- Sevenfold risk with a CAC score above 400
- Twenty fold risk with a CAC score above 1000

A CAC score above 400 should nearly always prompt additional evaluation, such as stress testing with MPS. Those found to have a large area of ischemia may require coronary angioplasty or bypass surgery; a very high CAC (more than 1,000) is a recognized *heart disease risk-equivalent.* Abnormal (ischemic) MPS is associated with a high likelihood of subclinical atherosclerosis by CAC, but is rarely seen for CAC scores less than 100. In most patients, low CAC scores appear to obviate the need for subsequent noninvasive testing. Patients with normal MPS, however, frequently have extensive atherosclerosis by CAC criteria.

CAC score correlates strongly with the severity of atherosclerosis, but not with the severity of stenosis, the major determinant of the need for coronary angioplasty and bypass surgery.

Carotid Intimal Medial Thickness (CIMT)

Ultrasound allows doctors to view the walls of the arteries from the outside in to see the thickening of the arterial walls as plaques accumulate. In contrast, an angiogram is like looking through a tube. It gives a tunnel-like view of the empty space, or lumen, within the artery from the inside, but not of the arterial wall, which is the site of the disease. During the long subclinical phase of atherosclerosis, arterial wall changes that lead to intimal medial thickening (IMT) occur that can be easily measured in the carotid artery (CIMT) by using ultrasound in a relatively simple way. Since atherosclerosis is a systemic disease, an increase in CIMT indicates early atherosclerosis not only in the carotid arteries but also in the coronary arteries. CIMT is increased in people with risk factors and is a predictor of cardiovascular events such as heart attack and stroke. In the Cardiovascular Health Study (see Appendix B) an increased CIMT was associated with a fourfold higher risk of a heart attack and/or stroke over the next six years. The average increase in CIMT is 0.04 mm for every 10 years of age.

Did you know...
Your CAC score can also be tracked for its increase, stabilization, or decrease, allowing evaluation of the success or failure of the treatment. In the absence of effective intervention, your CAC score may grow 30% or more per year. Risk of heart attack can be up to *20-fold higher* in people with growing score, compared to people with stable scores. Those who succeed in stopping the progression have a very low risk. As a rule of thumb, a 10% increase per year is acceptable, 20% puts you at high risk, and 30% or more at very high risk. Achieving a stable or decreasing heart scan score can be a very important goal to reduce your risk of heart attack.

Magnetic resonance imaging (MRI)

MRI is a novel, noninvasive, and safe technique that allows serial monitoring of atherosclerotic plaques over time, and constitutes a powerful *research tool* to study the progression of atherosclerosis. This method uses powerful magnets to look inside the body. Computer graphics show the heart muscle and any damage from a heart attack, and it can evaluate the disease of larger blood vessels such as the aorta. The technique can be used on most patients except those with pacemakers.

Positron Emission Tomography (PET)

A PET scan is a noninvasive nuclear imaging technique that produces three-dimensional images of the heart, brain, or other organs. A PET scan can help detect, localize, and describe heart disease. It can determine portions of the heart muscle that are still viable (living and functioning) after a heart attack. However, its use is limited by its inability to detect mild coronary stenosis (below 50% narrowing of the artery).

Noninvasive coronary angiography

Noninvasive coronary angiography is a new and rapidly developing imaging test that can identify patient's coronary plaques, supplementing the information gleaned from an ordinary calcium scan and assessment of traditional risk factors. Electron beam angiography, magnetic resonance angiography, and multi-slice (spiral) computed tomography are the promising noninvasive coronary angiographic methods to visualize severe narrowing in the coronary arteries. Multi-slice computed tomography can identify patients with both soft and hard plaques. All three methods are used clinically in certain centers with appropriate expertise. Currently, it is not an alternative to conventional X-ray angiography in all cases. Selective use of these tests may provide a cost-effective, safer, and less invasive way of identifying heart disease in patients who do not require coronary angioplasty and bypass surgery. These techniques have the potential to identify vulnerable plaques and may revolutionize the way we look at coronary artery disease by the next decade. There is the risk of bombarding patients with two to three times the ionizing radiation of a coronary angiogram but similar to that of a nuclear scan of the heart.

Intravascular Ultrasound (IVUS) and silent plaques

IVUS is a method of visualizing the plaque in the arteries by using ultrasound. Advances in IVUS have made it possible to evaluate the plaques in coronary arteries and have revolutionized our understanding of plaque behavior. Several coronary IVUS studies have shown that a coronary angiogram may give an *overly optimistic picture* of arterial health. These studies have shown that plaques within the artery walls first expand the wall outward, not inward (**Color Plate 1.2**). In other words, they push the elastic outer layer of the artery wall away from the inner wall of the artery and lumen (see Chapter I, Section 1). As a result, the lumen (the opening in the artery) remains unaffected and looks surprisingly normal until the disease is far advanced (**Color Plate 1.3**). The narrowing of the artery is only the last step in a long sequence. By the time angiography detects atherosclerotic narrowing of a coronary artery, the disease is already present in nearly 90% of the coronary arteries.

Angiographically invisible or silent plaques can rupture and produce a heart attack as the first symptom of heart disease a person ever experiences. This explains why prior warning symptoms are absent in two-third of men and half of women who have had a heart attack. IVUS studies of 30- to 39-year-old men and women who died in accidents have shown extensive plaque build-up, even though most of them had a normal coronary angiogram (see Chapter IV, Section 4). IVUS studies have also been extremely useful in evaluating the clinical significance of mild to moderately severe disease in the left main coronary artery.

Who benefits from heart scan?

Not all persons should undergo a heart scan. It is a waste of money to get a heart scan for those who already have heart disease or are at very high risk. They need the maximum aggressive treatment, regardless of the result of heart scan. Those with low risk also may not benefit in many cases. Most of the benefit is to those who are at moderate risk and who might become high risk, if found to have high CAC Scores. Early noncalcified plaques cannot be detected by a heart scan and may, therefore, give a false sense of security. On the other hand, a high calcium score can cause a lot of anxiety, unnecessary tests, and even bypass surgery, if the results are not properly interpreted.

KEY · POINTS · IN · A · NUTSHELL

♥ Electrocardiograms are the standard, accurate way of diagnosing a heart attack after it occurs, but an ECG may look completely normal even just minutes before a heart attack.

♥ Exercise treadmill tests, with or without imaging techniques, are used extensively to diagnose silent heart disease before any symptoms.

♥ An exercise treadmill test becomes abnormal only when the disease is far advanced, with severe blockage in two or three major coronary arteries.

♥ A treadmill test that turns out to be normal is not an insurance against the future risk of a heart attack.

♥ Approximately 50% of heart attacks occur in individuals who had a normal treadmill test.

♥ The coronary angiogram has been the gold standard of diagnosis of heart disease for several decades.

♥ A coronary angiogram becomes significantly abnormal only when the disease is far advanced with arterial narrowing. Early atherosclerosis is angiographically silent or unimpressive

♥ Asymptomatic atherosclerosis can be diagnosed with carotid ultrasound or a heart scan (EBCT) years before the development of any symptoms.

♥ Coronary calcium scores allow quantification of the plaque burden and the physiological age of the arteries of the person.

7.4 ▶ After a Heart Attack, What Now?

A person who has had a heart attack has a five to seven times greater risk of having a second heart attack, and three to four times greater risk of having a stroke, compared to the general population. The risk is even higher if his or her cholesterol level is elevated or HDL is low. This is also true of those who have undergone coronary angioplasty, stent, or bypass surgery. This increased risk can be substantially reduced by aggressively modifying one's lifestyle and controlling various risk factors discussed in previous Chapters. The benefit of taking daily aspirin clearly outweighs the risk in patients with heart disease. Cardiac rehabilitation can restore the functional capacity in most patients. For patients with chronic stable angina, the first priority of therapy is the prevention of a heart attack and death; the second priority is reduction of symptoms, thereby increasing the quality of life. Testing for emerging risk factors is essential in people with *premature heart disease.* This Chapter discusses the importance of aggressive treatment with lifestyle changes and medications to improve the quality and length of life in people with heart disease. You will learn why people with heart disease require multiple medications which are initiated at a much lower threshold as compared to in people with without heart disease.

In the US, nearly half of all heart attack patients receive a coronary angiogram, 31% receive coronary angioplasty, and 14% receive coronary bypass surgery. These rates are lower in the northeastern US and among blacks. The need for bypass surgery appears to be higher among Indians. These procedures may reduce the need for repeat hospitalization in the near future.

Lifestyle changes

Lifestyle changes, including increased physical activity and better nutrition, are the primary strategy for not only preventing but also controlling heart disease. The degree of change needs to be more radical in those who have already developed heart disease. For smokers, the number-one priority is to quit smoking.

Regular physical activity

At least 45 minutes of physical activity daily is strongly recommended even if you are of normal weight. Those who are overweight or obese will require more exercise. Your physician may prescribe an exercise regimen and provide the necessary guidelines. Brisk walking is an exercise virtually every cardiac patient can undertake. Several shopping malls sponsor free indoor walking programs. Walking on a treadmill at a comfortable pace is an acceptable exercise throughout the year. See Chapter V, section 8 for details of physical activity programs.

Cardiac rehabilitation

In the US, Canada, Australia and Europe, most patients are discharged on or before *the fourth day* after a heart attack. Cardiac rehabilitation programs have now become the standard extended care for people recovering from heart attacks, coronary angioplasty and bypass surgery. Most hospitals provide such services and many insurance programs cover them at least for the first three months. I strongly recommend that you make use of such programs if you are a cardiac patient. The benefits of formal cardiac rehabilitation and exercise training are well proven and include improvements in body fat and obesity, exercise capacity, and dyslipidemia. Depression (common in older persons) and hostility (common among younger persons) are also significantly improved by cardiac rehabilitation.

Therapeutic lifestyle changes through a three-month cardiac rehabilitation program significantly improve numerous cardiac risk factors, including a 40% decrease in the C-reactive protein levels (See Chapter III section 4.) For patients with stable heart disease, exercise and stress management training reduces emotional distress and improves markers of cardiovascular risk more than usual medical care alone.

Table 7.8. Therapeutic goals for selected risk factors in Asian Indians with heart disease

Cardiac Risk Factors	Goals
Non-HDL cholesterol	Below 100
LDL (mg/dL)	Below 60
HDL (mg/dL)	Above 60
Triglycerides (mg/dL)	Below 130
Lipoprotein(a) (mg/dL)	Below 20
Homocysteine (mol/L)	Below 10
Blood pressure (mm Hg)	Below 120
Fasting glucose (mg/dL)	Below 100
Waist size men (inches)	Below 36
Waist size women (inches)	Below 32

Source: Enas, EA. et al. Ref.6.13.

Nutrition Program

A balanced nutrition program rich in fruits and vegetables and low in sodium (salt) is outlined in Chapter V. Special care must be taken to ensure that saturated fat intake is below 7% of your total calorie intake, or 12g per day (see Chapter V for food labels). Dietary intake of cholesterol should be below 200mg per day. Salt intake should be below 6g a day (lower for persons with high blood pressure). I encourage you to increase your total dietary fiber intake to 25-30g a day. You can get this by consuming 9-13 servings (five to six cups) of fruits and vegetables per day and liberal consumption of legumes. Avoid prolonged cooking because it reduces the nutrient value of foods.

Heart rate reserve and target heart rate

Your target heart rate is the heart rate (or number of heart beats per minute) at which you should exercise, except during the warm-up and cool down periods. It is calculated using your maximum heart rate, your resting heart rate, and your heart rate reserve, which is just the difference between your maximum heart rate and resting heart rate. Your maximum heart rate refers to how fast your heart can beat. A standard formula for calculating this is 220 minus your age. Note that many refinements to this formula are in use and can be found on the internet. So for example, if you are 40, your maximum heart rate is 180 (220 minus 40). If you have a resting heart rate of, for example, 60, then your heart rate reserve is 180 minus 60, or 120. Your target heart rate is calculated as a range: It is 50% to 80% of your heart rate reserve, plus your resting heart rate. So for our hypothetical 40-year-old, with a heart rate of 60 his target heart rate would be between 120 (60 + 60) and 156 (96 +60). Beginners start at 50% and gradually increase up to 80% of the heart rate reserve.

Waistline management

As mentioned in Chapter III, Section 7 waist size is more important than overall weight, particularly in Indians. Targets for waist size should be below 36 inches for men and below 32 inches for women, irrespective of age and height. It is advisable to cut down on calories and increase physical activity if your waist size approaches these cut points. *Do not wait till you surpass these cut points.*

Controlling dyslipidemia

The recommended LDL level in a patient with heart disease is much lower than for someone without heart disease (see Table 7.8.). Note also that these levels, specified for Indians, are more stringent than those recommended for whites and other populations. **The LDL goal is below 60 mg/dL for Indians with heart disease** (see Chapter VI, sections 2, 3 and 4 for cholesterol-lowering options, both non-prescription and prescription-based). In a study of 1,000 patients with heart disease at the Henry Ford Hospital in Detroit, only one in two patients with coronary artery disease reached their LDL goals, even though most were on statins. Furthermore four in five *did not* meet all four of their lipid level goals. Therefore, there is at least an 80 % chance that your goals for LDL and other lipoproteins are not met. I recommend that you talk to your physician about aggressive management of these lipoproteins. Most Indians will require at least two medications (a statin and niacin) to achieve and maintain these goals.

Table 7.9. Cardiac patients who met their goals for LDL and other lipids at a major teaching hospital

Target Level (mg/dL)	% of patients meeting the target
LDL below 100	46
HDL above 40	50
Triglycerides below 150	60
Non-HDL cholesterol below 130	48
All four	20

Source: Khanal, S. et al. Ref. 6.29.

The combination of high triglycerides and low HDL levels is very common among Indians. This is often due to a high glycemic load from consumption of large quantities of carbohydrates (such as rice, *rotis* and other high glycemic index foods). You can control your triglycerides significantly by decreasing excessive consumption of these foods. Carbohydrates *should not exceed 40%* of the caloric intake in people with abnormalities of triglycerides and HDL. Vegetables and select fruits, in addition to balanced protein-rich meals, can have a positive effect on both triglycerides and HDL.

Table 7.10. Incidence of heart attack death per 1,000 person years

	incidence
No metabolic syndrome, diabetes, or heart disease	3
Metabolic syndrome without diabetes or heart disease	4
Metabolic syndrome with diabetes but no heart disease	5
Diabetes, without metabolic syndrome or heart disease	6
Prior heart disease	11
Prior heart disease and diabetes	17

Source: Malik, S. et al. Ref. 7.35.

Controlling blood pressure

As mentioned earlier, high blood pressure (hypertension) is a significant risk factor for heart disease, particularly for stroke (see Chapter VI section 1). I urge you to be proactive in maintaining your blood pressure as close to the optimum as possible (below 120/80). In addition to medications and regular exercise, controlling your salt intake can significantly reduce your blood pressure. I recommend that you invest in a good blood pressure monitor and track your blood pressure on a daily basis.

Controlling diabetes

Persons with diabetes as well as heart disease have exceptionally high rates of heart disease complications, including heart attack, heart failure, stroke, and death (See Table 7.10). If you suffer from diabetes and heart disease, I urge you to maintain blood glucose level goals as follows: Fasting (before a meal), 80-120 mg/dL; bedtime, 100-140 mg/dL. Work with your physician to ensure that your A1C is below 7%. If you are diabetic, your blood pressure should be below 120/80.

Aspirin therapy

In patients **with heart disease,** the benefit of taking daily aspirin far outweighs the risk, and is recommended for every patient who has no obvious conditions that render the patient unsuitable for its use.

For example, aspirin given daily for a *month* to 1,000 patients with an acute heart attack will help prevent 40 coronary events during that period. If the aspirin is continued for *two years,* another 40 coronary events would be prevented. Among patients with chronic heart disease, 10 to 15 coronary events would be prevented for every 1,000 patients over a period of two years. Lower doses (75-150 mg) of aspirin are as effective as high-dose (325 mg and above) regimens. Aspirin should be continued indefinitely. Plavix is an alternative to those who are unable to take aspirin or are allergic to it.

Beta-blockers

Beta-blockers are drugs known to have many favorable effects on the heart and include preventing repeat heart attacks and death. These agents also lower the blood pressure and slow the heart rate. Resting heart rate is a simple measurement with prognostic implications. High resting heart rate is a predictor of cardiovascular mortality independent of other risk factors. In a study of 24,913 patients with heart disease from the Coronary Artery Surgery Study registry and followed for 15 years, those with resting heart rate above 82 had a 31% higher death rate than those with a heart rate of below 62. World class athletes and marathon runners have rates in their 40s without the beta-blocker and explain their very low rates of heart disease.

The benefits of beta-blockers in persons with heart disease is so overwhelming that this class of medications is prescribed to all persons who have had a heart attack, unless they have conditions such as asthma that are made worse by the medication. Just 20 years ago, beta blockers were not given to patients with heart failure. Now they have become a "must use" drug in heart failure. Brand names include Lopressor, Tenormin, and Coreg.

ACE inhibitors

These medications have strong cardioprotective effects and are used in a broad spectrum of patients. They also have a protective effect against the development of diabetes, kidney disease and heart failure. ACE inhibitors are recommended in patients with heart muscle damage and reduced ejection fraction - that is, reduced pumping action of the heart (See Chapter VI section I).

Anti-depressants

Many patients and doctors are afraid to use anti-depressants following a heart attack because of an increased risk of heart attack following the initiation of such treatment. Underlying depression, not the use of antidepressants may be responsible for the increased risk of heart attack associated with taking antidepressants, according to a study released in 2005. Researchers analyzed data on the use of anti-depressants among 60,000 British patients diagnosed with a first heart attack between 1998 and 2001. The results were compared with those of 360,000 randomly selected individuals without a history of heart attack.

Management of anger, hostility, depression personality D. Many studies suggest that anger and negative handling of stress can have a powerful effect on a person's immune system and risk of heart disease. Anger management, stress reduction programs, and meditation may be useful to minimize the effect of these factors to heart disease in those prone to anger and hostility. Yoga or other stress relief methods may be helpful in some individuals. Social support through emotionally-based connections such as family, friends, religious communities, and networks of other social activities (volunteer work) can help improve a person's outlook and immune system. Pets have also been shown to have a beneficial effect on the health of the person.

The researchers found that the patients faced an increased risk of heart attack during the first month of taking an antidepressant, irrespective of the class or type of antidepressant used. In both groups, depressed patients taking antidepressants for the first time faced double the risk of a heart attack within the first seven days as compared to the people who were not taking these drugs. A similar observation of heightened risk of suicide following initiation of anti-depressants has been reported. These phenomenon have been attributed to the fact that many of the patients are at very high risk of suicide – necessitating the use of medication which takes several weeks to confer full protection. In the British study mentioned above, the most striking finding in this study was *the steep decline* of risk of heart attack with the continued use of antidepressants for more than a month. Thus, it is safe to use anti-depressants in cardiac patients with severe depression.

Other stressors

Garden-variety stress is universal and in general cannot be eliminated. Even priests and nuns, who have dedicated their life for God, are not immune to stress. There is no justification for happily employed individuals to quit their job following a heart attack. However, it has been found that healthy people with stressful jobs who work long hours, but get little satisfaction from what they do have twice the risk of dying from heart disease as satisfied employees. Those who have control over their work and derive benefit and satisfaction from hard work (12 to 16 hours a day) have no higher risk of heart disease.

Testing and controlling emerging risk factors

If your heart disease was diagnosed before age 65, you should ask your doctor to have at least two additional tests done: lipoprotein(a) and homocysteine,(see Chapter III, Sections 2 and 3). You should be aware that many insurance companies do not cover the costs of these tests. I, nevertheless, strongly recommend getting these tests done; they are worth spending your hard-earned money on.

Sexual activity

Sexual activity with a familiar partner is generally safe four to six weeks after a heart attack, angioplasty, or bypass surgery. Many medications, especially beta blockers, given after a heart attack, have adverse effects on sexual activity. Depression and anger can influence the person's interest in resuming such activity. Those who can climb two flights of stairs or walk six minutes on a treadmill (Bruce Protocol) or can carry a wet load of clothing one flight of stairs without symptoms can usually return to work and resume normal daily life, including sexual activity. Please consult with your physician prior to initiating such activity. Those who take certain heart medications such as nitroglycerine to control chest pain should not use medications for erectile dysfunction such as Viagra, Cialis or Levitra.

You should work with your physician to keep your lipoprotein(a) level below 20 mg/dL (or lipoprotein cholesterol below 7). Niacin is the only medication that lowers lipoprotein(a), and it can be taken with any statin. At the maximum recommended dose of 2g/day, it lowers lipoprotein(a) by 25% and increases HDL by 40%. (see Chapter VIII, Section 2).

Homocysteine levels in Indians are more closely related to low intake of vitamin B_{12} than low intake of folic acid. A combination of B_{12}, B_6, and folic acid is available by prescription (Metanx, Foltx, Folgard). Usually, one tablet daily is enough in people with mild homocysteine elevation (below 15 mmol/L), and two tablets daily for people with higher levels.

Medication adherence

Cardiac patients often need multiple medications. Lowering cholesterol in the blood stream and keeping blood pressure under control are key to preventing heart disease. The percentage of patients taking both drugs as prescribed declined sharply over the course of time according to a study done in 2005. Only 44% were still taking both drugs given to combat these diseases after six month. M*ore than a third* of patients (35%) stopped taking the medicine altogether and 23% were taking one drug only after six months. The heaviest fall-off was among patients who were already taking a number of other prescription drugs, perhaps reflecting the complicated task of managing several drugs at once, the study said. Patients, who are started on two drugs on the same day, were 34 percent more likely to continue taking both medications. Starting the medications at the same time or better still using combination of two medications as a single pill is likely to ensure continued use (adherence) of the medications. I urge you to take your prescribed medications religiously.

Life after a stroke

Most strokes among Europeans and Indians are the ischemic type with less than one in five being due to hemorrhage. The word "ischemic" means that oxygen flow to the brain is blocked, usually by a blood clot and fatty plaque in an artery. Brain tissue dies by the minute. Such strokes are preceded by a ministroke or "transient ischemic attacks" or TIAs. The only difference between a full-fledged stroke and a ministroke is the severity and the persistence of symptoms: A ministroke's symptoms tend to disappear on their own, typically in minutes or within one to two hours. Symptoms can last up to 24 hours, but that is unusual. Approximately 12% of stroke among Indians occur below 40 years of age.

Unlike a heart attack, strokes often appear with modest symptoms that can be easy to ignore. Occasionally there can be a headache. Typical symptoms include numbness or weakness in the face, arm or leg, often on one side. Sudden difficulty in speaking or a partial loss of vision or double vision also can arise (See Chapter I section1). The strategies for preventing recurrent stroke are similar to those outlined for a heart attack.

Checklist of questions

You should inform your physician about any allergies that you have and any other medications you are currently taking, including over-the-counter drugs, vitamins, dietary supplements, and herbal medicines. Many such products, including the so-called "natural herbs," can interfere with the efficacy of prescription medications. Recent studies suggest that supplements of vitamins C and E are not useful and may cut down the benefit of cholesterol-lowering medication by 50%. These supplements reduce the lipid optimizing effects of statins and niacin as well as increase the risk of heart attack. If you are at high risk of or have been recently diagnosed with heart disease, I encourage you to discuss your options with your physician (box).

12 questions to ask your physician

1. What is my risk of a heart attack (first or repeat): low, medium, high or very high?
2. How can I reduce my risk?
3. What additional tests might be of value in my particular case?
4. What are the target goals of my treatment?
5. Am I at goal with respect to cholesterol, blood pressure, and/or blood sugar?
6. Am I at my goal for weight and waist line?
7. If I am not at goal for these risk factors, what are the reasons?
8. What improvements in lifestyle, diet, and exercise do I need?
9. What are the recommended medications?
10. Is there any need to increase, decrease the dose of medications or add and new ones?
11. How does the benefit of medication compare with the risk of treatment?
12. What possible side-effects I should watch out for?

KEY · POINTS · IN · A · NUTSHELL

♥ A person who has had a heart attack has a five- to seven-fold risk of having a repeat heart attack, compared to the general population.

♥ The annual risk of another heart attack is 5 to 10% per year (In persons with heart disease).

♥ The risk of stroke is also increased three-to fourfold in people who have had a heart attack.

♥ The heart attack risk is similarly high among people who have had coronary angioplasty and/or bypass surgery.

♥ This risk can be substantially reduced by aggressively modifying your lifestyle and optimally controlling various risk factors.

♥ The target goals for various risk factors, particularly LDL, are lower in people with heart disease.

♥ Most heart disease patients require five or more medications to prevent further heart attacks and to prolong life.

♥ The benefit of aspirin clearly outweighs the risk in most patients with heart disease.

♥ Testing for emerging risk factors is beneficial in people with premature heart disease.

♥ Cardiac rehabilitation can improve the quality and length of life.

7.5 ▶ Life after Bypass Surgery

Coronary artery bypass graft surgery, commonly referred to as CABG (pronounced "cabbage"), prolongs life in patients, who have left main coronary artery disease or triple-vessel disease, especially when this is accompanied by impaired left ventricular function. The procedure reroutes, or "bypasses," blood flow around a clogged artery to restore blood supply to areas of heart muscle that are not receiving an adequate supply. In this procedure, a blood vessel is taken from another part of the body (usually the patient's leg) and attached above and below the clogged segment of the coronary artery. Blood flow through the newly attached vessel (the graft) serves as the detour around the blockage. Angina (chest pain), fatigue, and other symptoms caused by the reduced blood flow improve dramatically and often disappear. Most people with severe symptoms feel better and energized and return to work in a few months. CABG is one of the most common surgical procedures in the US. Until 1978, CABG was the only treatment available for severe narrowing of coronary arteries.

How fast can bypass surgery fail?

Mrs. Archana Sood received a Quintuple bypass surgery at age 60. All five bypasses failed within four weeks. She was treated with four stents (see Section 7). The stents also failed within the next four weeks with recurrence of chest pain. Mrs. Sood subsequently underwent a repeat Quadruple bypass surgery, approximately eight weeks after the first bypass surgery. The second bypass series of bypass grafts also failed and was followed by another set of four stents. Unfortunately, those stents also failed. Both her cardiologist and her cardiac surgeon refused to intervene any further, when she was referred to me by her primary physician.

Mrs. Sood was found to have very high levels of lipoprotein(a) and homocysteine, as has been true of many other cases of rapid re-stenosis following bypass surgery. Ironically, she had a very high level of HDL (62 mg/dL) that did not protect her against a heart attack. (The patient did not have the HDL subclasses determined because of problems with insurance). I have seen several cases like this requiring repeat bypass surgery and angioplasty and stents at frequent intervals. This case illustrates the importance of lipoprotein(a) as one of the few factors that can override the protective role of HDL. Mrs. Sood was treated with appropriate medications to lower her lipoprotein(a) and homocysteine levels, and has done well since then, without the need for additional hospitalizations.

Far from a cure – continuing risk of heart attacks

Bypass surgery does not cure heart disease which, in reality, is an incurable disease. It is directed at severe narrowing of coronary arteries that limits the blood supply to the heart, yet most heart attacks occur in arteries *without severe narrowing*. The risk of a heart attack after a bypass surgery remains high unless all risk factors are identified and treated aggressively. A patent (open and functioning) bypass graft can be a life saver if the patient gets a massive heart attack from a sudden blockage of a different artery. Dr. Jacob Peter—had a single bypass graft to his right coronary artery at age 45. His other arteries appeared perfectly normal on the coronary angiogram. To everyone's dismay and disbelief, he developed a massive heart attack from a blockage of his left main coronary artery the following year. The patent graft on the right coronary artery allowed some blood flow to his left ventricle. Had the bypass surgery not been done, he might have died from this heart attack. Though he survived, he was permanently disabled at the prime of his career.

Within five years of bypass surgery, 15% of the patients have angina, and 10% develop a heart attack. While most patients are motivated to make changes after a bypass, many erroneously believe that their problems have been "fixed" and continue to indulge in unhealthy habits, including smoking. The rates of these complications are double among those who continue to smoke after bypass surgery. Compared to those who continue to smoke, people who quit smoking after bypass surgery are 15% more likely to be alive and 50% less likely to have a heart attack or require a repeat bypass surgery in 10 years.

Did you know...
Coronary bypass surgery has become one of the most common surgeries in the US. More than 500,000 bypass surgeries are done annually on Americans.

The risk of a further heart attack and the need for repeat bypass surgery can be substantially reduced by enrolling in a formal cardiac rehab program and taking appropriate medications (discussed in Section 4). Many people are understandably depressed at the time of a CABG, and about half remain depressed after the surgery. Aerobic exercise as part of a cardiac rehabilitation program also helps relieve symptoms of depression.

Advances in surgery have made it possible to use arteries from the chest, leg or arm to bypass the clogged arteries with better results than employing veins for such purposes. The internal mammary artery is generally resistant to atherosclerosis even when used in a bypass graft (in stead of a vein graft) with a 90 to 95% patency (artery remaining open) in 10 years. However, I have treated several patients, who had developed stenosis of internal mammary arteries (that had been used for bypassing a diseased left main coronary artery). This underscores the importance of making lifestyle changes that reduce your risk factors.

Table 7.11. Increasing risk and decreasing benefits with first, second and third bypass surgeries.

	First Bypass	Second Bypass	Third Bypass
Death following surgery	1%	7%	25%
10-year survival (with or without a heart attack)	78%	55%	Data not available
10-year survival (without a heart attack)	65%	40%	Data not available

Source: Weintraub, WS. Ref. 7.54.
Note: Aggressive modification of risk factors with lifestyle and medications can to avoid or delay repeat bypass surgeries.

Continuing atherosclerosis and the need for repeat bypass surgery

Unlike arteries, veins are not usually subject to high pressure. Veins used for bypass therefore clog up faster than arteries due to aggressive atherosclerosis. Approximately 10% of venous grafts clog in one month, and 10 to 20% by the end of the first year. Beyond the first year, vein grafts occlude at a rate of 2-5% per year; within 10 to 15 years, more than 50% are occluded or have significant stenosis. About 10% of such patients require a second bypass surgery in five years, and 50% in 10 years.

My clinical experience suggests that restenosis following coronary bypass surgery and angioplasty is at least twice as common among Indians as among whites. Repeat bypass surgery is certainly far more common in Indians than whites. A disproportionate number of my Indian colleagues have undergone repeat bypass surgeries.

Table 7.12. Annual death rates according to the number of severely narrowed coronary arteries

Number of coronary arteries with significant narrowing	Death without a heart attack	Death from heart attack
Single artery disease	1%	2%
Double artery disease	3%	3%
Triple artery disease	6%	3%
Left main coronary artery disease	12%	2%

Left main coronary artery disease and bypass surgery

The ultimate goal of any therapy is to increase the length of life, the quality of life, or both. Bypass surgery clearly provides both in patients with severe heart disease, such as left main coronary artery or three-vessel disease with low ejection fraction. The benefit of CABG in comparison with medication therapy is directly proportional to the severity of the person's heart disease. For example, the left main coronary artery provides blood supply to more than 75% of the left ventricular muscle mass. Severe narrowing of this artery places the patient at a very high risk of sudden death but not necessarily from a heart attack (see Table 7.12). Patients with severe left main coronary artery disease, therefore, often benefit greatly from bypass surgery. In contrast, patients with one- or two-vessel disease other than left main disease usually do not derive much benefit from a bypass surgery, over and above what could be achieved with medication therapy.

"Left main" refers to that first portion of the left coronary artery (usually one inch long) from its origin in the aorta before it divides into the left anterior descending and circumflex arteries (see color plate 1). Approximately 4% of patients undergoing a coronary angiogram for chest pain have signifi-

Malignat progresion of heart dessease following CABG?

Meet Mrs. Therisamma Joseph, a nurse who has had diabetes for 20 years. She had three-vessel bypass surgery following a heart attack, which was the first clue of her heart disease. Within seven months, two of the three bypasses had failed, with a recurrence of severe chest pain and inability to walk more than half a block. A repeat coronary angiogram showed diffuse disease in key arteries (narrowing at several locations along the artery), rendering them unsuitable for angioplasty, stent, and repeat bypass surgery. Mrs. Joseph had been told that "nothing could be done" to improve her chances of survival and quality of life. She was told "to go to the emergency room" if her symptoms severely worsened's so that doctors could relieve them. She was given no hope and began preparing for imminent death.

I had the opportunity to evaluate this desperate woman. I identified the underlying problem as a combination of high lipoprotein(a), high C-reactive protein, and low HDL, in addition to long-standing diabetes. She was treated extremely aggressively with multiple medications. Today, Mrs. J can walk two hours at a stretch without any symptoms. More importantly, a repeat angiogram three years later showed no progression of her heart disease. A stress test with imaging showed no evidence of vulnerable heart muscle. Here is a case in which cardiac medications, rather than heart surgery, proved to be the solution to a heart patient's crisis.

cant stenosis (more than 50% narrowing) of the left main artery; more than half of them have severe stenosis (over 70% narrowing). The long-term prognosis of patients with stenosis of left main artery is extremely poor. The overall three-year survival rate is 50%, which decreases to 40% when the stenosis severity exceeds 70%. Recent studies show that a low level of HDL and a high level of lipoprotein (a) correlate strongly with left main disease. Left main and three-vessel disease are more common among Indians than other populations, whereas blacks have a lower prevalence of both (see Chapter I, Section 4).

Bypass surgery remains the treatment of choice for left main disease and three-vessel disease. Although a stent can be placed successfully, the immediate and long-term outcomes inferior to bypass surgery, limiting its use. Stents are now being placed in patients with two- or three-vessel disease.

Did you know... *The number of bypass surgeries done on octogenarians in the US—(80,000 a year) exceeds the total number of bypass surgeries for all ages done in India.*

Complications associated with bypass surgery

The death rate within 30 days following a coronary bypass surgery has decreased from 3% in 1994 to 2% in 2004. Mortality is only 1% in low-risk cases (for example, patients with normal left ventricular function, those younger than 65, and those having surgery as an elective procedure). Conversely, mortality is very high in the elderly, particularly those over 80. Although most octogenarians survive the surgery, their quality of life does not improve, with nearly half of them ending up in a nursing home.

Stroke is another dreaded complication of bypass surgery occurring in approximately 3% of cases. The three major determinants of stroke following bypass surgery are age above 70 (2-fold risk), repeat bypass surgery (four fold risk) and prior stroke or ministroke (five fold risk). The risk of a person undergoing bypass is 1% in those with none of these three factors but 33% in those with all three, according to the results of a nine year prospective study of 6,245 patients and reported in 2005.

Off-pump bypass surgery

In conventional coronary bypass surgery, the breast bone is split and the chest is surgically opened, which accounts for the lengthy postoperative recovery. Until recently, the heart had to be stopped for several hours to perform this procedure. The patient is put on a heart-lung machine, which provides cardiopulmonary bypass to maintain the oxygenation of the body. Recovery after surgery is usually protracted because of the slow healing of the breast bone and chest wall (four to six weeks at a minimum). Many patients develop subtle neurological deficits that interfere with intellectual work and memory. Some experts believe this to be caused by tiny blood clots during the time spent on the heart-lung machine during the surgery.

Off-pump bypass surgery was developed to overcome these shortcomings. Currently, about 10 to 25% of bypass surgeries are done without stopping the heart. In such cases, a special clamp is used to keep the artery from moving while the heart continues to beat. The patient's discharge from hospital and overall recovery is faster with off-pump procedures? two-to three days for discharge and two-to three weeks for recovery. Off-pump bypass surgery is particularly suited to women, who are more sensitive to having a midline chest scar. However, a clear advantage of off-pump bypass surgery has not being clearly demonstrated.

Bypass Surgery among Indians

Indians have a higher risk of death following bypass surgery, primarily due to the advanced nature of their atherosclerosis. In one study, Indians had almost twice the death rate of whites following bypass surgery. Other studies indicate greater rates of restenosis and need for repeat interventional procedures. In one study of patients undergoing bypass surgery who were matched for age, Indians had higher rates of diabetes than whites (39% versus 12%). On the other hand, Indians had a lower prevalence of smoking (36% versus 80%), and a lower rate of previous heart attack (47% versus 62%). More Indians had the procedure done on an *emergency basis* (43% versus 32%). As mentioned earlier, having emergency bypass surgery is a known predictor of higher morbidity and mortality. Indians are generally smaller than whites with correspondingly smaller coronary arteries, which also makes surgery more challenging and results in a poorer outcome.

Table 7.13. Mean charges and in-hospital death rate for the following the procedures

Procedure	Mean Charges	In-Hospital Death Rate
Coronary artery bypass surgery	$60,853	2.4%
Coronary angioplasty	28,558	0.9%
Diagnostic cardiac catheterization	17,763	1.0%
Cardiac pacemaker or cardioverter defibrillator	40,852	1.7%
Heart valves surgery	85,187	5.8%

Source: American Heart Association. Ref 1.01.

Health Tourism in India
Hospitals in India are wooing foreign patients for coronary bypass surgery. There are certain hospitals in India that have particularly high standards of care and are staffed with surgeons and clinicians who spent many years training and practicing in the US. A bypass surgery, including air travel, typically costs $6,000 in India, compared to $23,000 in a private hospital in the UK and $50,000-$60,000 in the US. However, post-operative complications, particularly infection, are usually higher in Indian hospitals compared to western countries. Moreover, most VIPs, including Members of Parliament and Ministers, make every effort to come to the US when they need a bypass surgery.

Coronary artery bypass surgery among Indian women

Among the 516,000 Americans undergoing CABG, only 150,000 are women. Women undergoing bypass surgery in general are more severely ill than men and have double the mortality following this surgery. Women are older, have a higher number of risk factors, particularly diabetes. Yet, the five-year mortality rates in women and men undergoing CABG surgery are similar. Women have less graft patency (lesser chance that new bypass artery remains unblocked) and symptom relief and are more prone to re-operation within the first five years following CABG surgery. Metabolic syndrome, particularly a high triglyceride level is particularly dangerous in women who undergo CABG surgery. Aggressive lipid-optimizing therapy appears to be particularly beneficial in these women before and after the surgery. Thus, bypass surgery should not be considered a complete and definitive treatment in women, as well as in men.

Coronary bypass surgery versus angioplasty

Heart patients with two or more blocked arteries live longer if they have bypass surgery than if they have their arteries cleared out with angioplasty and propped open with wire-mesh devices called stents, according to the results of a study of almost 60,000 patients treated from 1997 to 2000 published in June 2005. This is the largest and most recent study comparing the long term death rates for these two procedures. It found that patients were 33% to 56% more likely to die after angioplasty and stenting than after bypass surgery. The need for repeat procedures was also five times higher following angioplasty. The study was done when stent use was not widespread. However a carefully designed study published in August 2005 seems to indicate that the rates of death and heart attack in five years are similar when people with multivessel disease are treated with stents and bypass surgery (see Section 6).

Although the initial cost of bypass surgery is higher than that of stents, it is no higher than the total cost of angioplasty plus stents over a period of 10 years. This is because of a four-to fivefold higher need for repeat interventions in those who had a stent placement (see Section 6). The next section reviews the current status of the use of coronary angioplasty and stents.

KEY · POINTS · IN · A · NUTSHELL

♥ Bypass surgery clearly prolongs life in patients with severe disease, such as left main coronary artery disease and three-vessel disease, but not in most patients with one- and two-vessel disease.

♥ Coronary bypass surgery is directed at severe narrowing of the arteries that limits the blood supply to the heart, yet most heart attacks occur in arteries without severe narrowing.

♥ In most patients, bypass surgery does not reduce the future risk of heart attack unless all risk factors have been identified and corrected.

♥ Rates of heart attack and death are lower with bypass surgery than angioplasty.

♥ Death rates are similar with bypass surgery and coronary stent.

♥ Nearly 50% of people will require a repeat coronary bypass surgery within 10 years, but the chances can be reduced substantially through aggressive lipid management.

♥ Repeat bypass surgery is associated with less benefit and more complications, including death than first time bypass surgery.

♥ Complications are more frequent with successive coronary bypass surgeries.

7.6 ▶ Life after Coronary Angioplasty and Stents

When a road can no longer carry the amount of vehicle traffic that comes through it, the Transportation Department has two options for easing the traffic congestion: create a new bigger road that bypasses the original one, or widen the original road, particularly if it has bottlenecks that slow down the traffic. In cardiac terms, the first option is called bypass surgery. The blocked segment of the artery is simply bypassed with a new segment of a blood vessel taken from, for example, the patient's leg. The second option is called angioplasty. If your intuitions tell you that it is easier to widen an existing occluded artery than to graft a bypass around it, your intuitions are right. Coronary angioplasty and stent, which dilate the clogged artery rather than bypassing it, have replaced coronary bypass surgery as the most common forms of coronary artery revascularization procedures (CARP), a term that includes coronary angioplasty, stenting procedures, and bypass surgery.

More than a million angioplasties are done every year in the US, compared to half a million bypass surgeries. In coronary angioplasty, also called balloon angioplasty, a long thin catheter with a balloon at the tip is inserted through an artery in the patient's groin or sometimes arm and guided toward the heart. Once the catheter reaches the blocked coronary artery, the balloon at the tip is then blown up to dilate (open up) the narrowed part of the artery (**see Color Plate 1.8.**). Coronary angioplasty with or without a stent is highly effective in **aborting and or minimizing the damage** from an acute heart attack. In people with chest pain but no heart attack, an angioplasty is highly effective in relieving chest pain and improving quality of life, but generally does not prevent future heart attacks or extend life.

A major limitation of balloon angioplasty is the recurrence of restenosis (renarrowing of the artery at the site where the angioplasty was done). This occurs in up to 60% of patients within six months. A stent is a small ball pen spring-like piece of metal mesh, that is left in the artery to keep it propped open (**see Color Plate 1.9.**) Stenting is an extension of angioplasty and is done along with an angioplasty to prevent the artery from collapsing immediately or within a few weeks or months. Regular or bare-metal stents have reduced the rate of restenosis rate to 20-30% and the latest drug-eluting (drug-releasing) stents have further reduced restenosis rate to 5 -10%. Stents, however, have not been shown to offer any additional advantage in preventing heart attacks or prolonging life, because most heart attacks occurs at sites with only mild narrowing that are not severe enough to qualify for the procedure. This Chapter summarizes current strategies available to reduces the chances of restenosis and prevent a heart attack after angioplasty and stenting procedures.

Angioplasty and stenting are performed without surgery. The patient is never cut open. They are done by means of a small puncture through the skin. Most of these procedures are done immediately after an angiogram to locate the site of severe narrowing. PCIs are done in patients with significant blockage of one or two coronary arteries. They are not done in patients with more severe disease requiring bypass surgery, such as those with left main disease or three-vessel disease with decreased left ventricular function.

Several studies have clearly shown that bypass surgery reduces the death rate among patients with *severe heart disease.* But this is not the case for patients with *less severe heart disease,* which has shown no difference in cardiac events (heart attack) with bypass surgery, angioplasty and medication therapy. In a recent study (2004) in patients with multivessel heart disease (narrowing of two or more arteries), rates of severe chest pain, heart attack, and/or death occurred more frequently with angioplasty or stent than with bypass surgery. The need for repeat procedures is higher with coronary angioplasty than with bypass surgery. Since the long-term mortality and costs are similar to CABG, the patient and the doctor must balance the convenience of angioplasty and stent against the need of a second procedure.

Coronary angioplasty

As mentioned earlier, in coronary angioplasty, also called balloon angioplasty, a special catheter with a small balloon at the tip is advanced through the femoral artery in the thigh up into a coronary artery. When the balloon is inflated it stretches the artery, flattening and often rupturing the plaque. The procedure is painless and is usually done as an out-patient procedure. The patient usually goes home the same day and goes back to work within a week. However, as mentioned earlier, angioplasty by itself has little impact on the natural history of the patient's disease and the progression of atherosclerosis.

Complications following PCI are lowest in obese people with BMI 30 to 40 (obesity paradox). Small individuals such as Indians

Some Terms You Should Know
The first coronary angioplasty on a human was performed on September 16, 1977 in Zurich, Switzerland by Dr. Andreas Gruntzig. He later moved to Emory University in Atlanta and ushered in the era of interventional cardiology, revolutionizing the management of heart disease.

Cardiologists use the term "percutaneous coronary intervention" (PCI) to mean angioplasty with or without stenting. PCI has substantially reduced the need for bypass surgery over the past 25 years.

Coronary Angioplasty and Stents: Quick fixes but far from a cure
Angioplasty and stents are a form of "damage control." Just as a tooth extraction does not cure the underlying problem of gum disease caused by dental neglect, angioplasty and stents do not cure the underlying problem, which is the continuing progression of atherosclerosis or plaque buildup. They, therefore, have little impact on the natural history of heart disease (length of life and risk of future attacks). Many persons who undergo these procedures have recurrent problems unless they undertake fundamental lifestyle changes to reduce their risk factors.

have a greater rate of complications, which may be partially related to the small size of coronary arteries. It is worth noting that small coronary arteries do not lead to more heart attacks but only more complications following PCI.

Primary coronary angioplasty—the gold standard of treatment following a heart attack

Most heart attacks are due to a large blood clot that suddenly blocks a coronary artery that had only a mild narrowing just minutes before the catastrophe (see Chapter I section 1, **Color Plate 1.4**). Such blockages can be reopened with immediate administration of medications or angioplasty (See **Color Plate 1.8.**). Dissolving such blood clots with medication is called **thrombolytic therapy** and is practiced worldwide. People, who have had a recent surgery or stroke, may experience life-threatening bleeding and cannot be offered this therapy. Stroke is a dreaded complication of this treatment particularly in the elderly. Moreover, approximately four in 10 patients treated with thrombolytic therapy for a heart attack fail this initial treatment. Either the clot is not dissolved with this treatment or a second clot develops leading to reocclusion of the artery and recurrent heart attack upon cessation of therapy. Coronary angioplasty is often performed in such patients if facilities are available, which is not the case in the majority of community hospitals in the US and most of the hospitals worldwide.

Primary angioplasty refers to coronary angioplasty done in patients with acute heart attack *without thrombolytic therapy*. It is an effective treatment that immediately restores blood supply to heart for patients presenting to the emergency room with a full-blown heart attack. Primary PCI frequently leads to an **"aborted heart attack"** if done within two hours, and it salvages the heart muscle to prevent complications and death. Every minute of delay in primary angioplasty decreases the amount of salvaged myocardium, and increases the rate of subsequent death. A particular advantage of angioplasty is the low rates of stroke and recurrent heart attack. Compared to thrombolytic therapy, primary angioplasty is associated with a 50% reduction in stroke and two-thirds reduction in recurrent heart attacks. Thus, following a heart attack, primary angioplasty is clearly superior to thrombolytic therapy. Efforts are underway to develop regional medical centers that provide primary PCI around the clock.

Compared to thrombolytic therapy, primary angioplasty results in 50% reduction in stroke and two-thirds reduction in recurrent heart attacks. Thus, following a heart attack, primary angioplasty with or without a stent is clearly superior to thrombolytic therapy.

Did you know...
Stents, however, have not been shown to offer any additional advantage in preventing heart attacks or prolonging life, because most heart attacks occurs at sites with only mild narrowing that are not severe enough to qualify for the procedure.

In patients with stable heart disease and severe angina, coronary angioplasty is less effective in preventing heart attack and cardiac death, but it markedly improves symptoms, reduces ischemia, and raises the quality of life. Combining angioplasty with medications and appropriate lifestyle changes can also prevent future heart attacks and cardiac deaths.

Coronary stent

The initial success rate of angioplasty is more than 98% and complication rates are less than 1%. Despite these gratifying short-term results, continued narrowing of coronary arteries over several months significantly limits the benefits of balloon angioplasty. Restenosis or the recurrence of arterial blockage occurs in up to 60% of cases within six months.

The high rates of restenosis that occurs following a coronary angioplasty can be reduced by implanting a stent. A coronary stent is a small tubular device that is permanently placed in an artery to keep it open (see **Color Plate 1.9**). The major advantage of a stent over balloon angioplasty alone (usually both done together) is that a stent reduces the need for emergency bypass surgery (from 4% to 1%). Stenting can significantly reduce the restenosis rate observed with "plain-old" balloon angioplasty. In a recent meta-analysis (combined analysis of several similar studies) involving nearly 10,000 patients, coronary stenting reduced the rate of restenosis and the need for repeated angioplasty by nearly 50% to less than 25%. There was no difference in rates of death or heart attack between those treated with stenting versus angioplasty alone. Similar to balloon angioplasty, a stent does not affect the natural history of the disease, especially its progression in other arteries.

Restenosis following stent placement

Restenosis that occurs within a stent is called **in-stent restenosis.** I have been consulted by Dr. Kishore Shah, an interventional cardiologist, who has had a **"complete coronary stent jacket,"** as he puts it. He has more than **10 stents covering the entire 7 inches** of his three major coronary arteries. Mr. Varghese Benedict had a five-vessel bypass surgery following a heart attack at 53. He did well for five years and then started having recurrent chest pain, requiring a repeat angiogram. He was found to have a new coronary blockage, which was treated with a stent. Within four months, he had developed recurrent chest pain and an angiogram showed in-stent restenosis. He was treated with radiation at the site of the restenosis. However, his chest pain returned within another three months, necessitating another angiogram. This time Mr. Benedict had a new blockage at a different location, which was treated with a drug-eluting stent. His case is one of many that show that stenting is not a cure for atherosclerosis, but a temporary quick fix, as is true of balloon angioplasty and bypass surgery. Restenosis following angioplasty and stenting are shown in **Color Plate 1.10.**

> **Tid Bits**
> In 2002, an estimated 1,204,000 angioplasty procedures, 515,000 bypass procedures, 1,463,000 diagnostic cardiac catheterizations, 63,000 implantable defibrillators and 199,000 pacemaker procedures were performed in the US.

Causes of restenosis

Low HDL and high lipoprotein(a) are both powerful predictors of restenosis following angioplasty and stenting. The risk is particularly high when both of these conditions coexist. In contrast high LDL is not related to restenosis. Mr. Benedict and Dr. Shah had both of these abnormalities that could explain their need for repeat interventions. However, Mr. Benedict refused to take the appropriate dose of medication until after multiple stent placements. Niacin is highly effective in lowering lipoprotein(a) and raising HDL, but requires at least a dose of 2,000mg per day to have any meaningful impact on lipoprotein(a). Lowering lipoprotein(a) has been shown to reduce restenosis by 50%. Mr. Benedict has done well since he started taking the recommended medications at higher doses without ever missing a single dose. The therapeutic use of niacin is discussed in Chapter VIII Section 2. As discussed earlier, about half of all Indians have high lipoprotein(a) and more than two-thirds have low HDL or dysfunctional HDL rendering them highly vulnerable to restenosis and repeat interventions.

Some studies have shown that a high level of homocysteine is also associated with a high risk of restenosis. Clinical trials are underway to demonstrate the benefits of lowering homocysteine. In the meantime, it is advisable for Indians who have had coronary interventions to have their lipoprotein(a) and homocysteine levels evaluated and if high, brought under control, under the supervision of a physician or cardiologist. The FDA has approved several drugs (for example, Foltx and Folgard, Metanx) that lower homocysteine.

Subacute thrombosis or non-sudden development of blood clot is a dreaded complication of stent. As a foreign body placed in the artery, the stent stimulates a cascade of reactions promoting blood clot particularly in the first six months, until the stent becomes covered by normal endothelial cells. This risk is increased among smokers and can be reduced with blood thinners such as Plavix (see Chapter VIII Section 3). Even though the risk of thrombosis (blood clot) has been substantially reduced in those taking Plavix, this condition is associated with a mortality rate as high as 50%. Coronary stent thrombosis appears to be more common among Indians.

Sometimes, acute stent thrombosis occurs within days of stent placement. Henry Sebastian, a Chicago resident, had a heart attack upon arrival in India to attend his brother's funeral. He was unable to attend the funeral since he required immediate hospitalization. Upon returning to Chicago, he sought a second opinion from me. He had an uneventful balloon angioplasty done at a world-class hospital. In spite of this, he required a stent implantation the same day as the angioplasty due to recurrent severe chest pain and signs of an imminent heart attack. Unfortunately, the stent developed thrombosis within 24 hours. His cholesterol was only 160 mg/dL. He was found to have low HDL and high lipoprotein(a),- which probably accounted for his blood clot. Prompt medical treatment of these factors allowed him to stay healthy for many years without further interventions.

> Did you know...
> Drug-eluting stents have no significant impact on the risk of future heart attacks, which is similar to balloon angioplasty and non-medicated stents. Stents by their very nature do not affect the development of new blockages at different locations.

Drug-eluting stents

In-stent restenosis—one of the greatest challenges in long-term patient treatment in interventional cardiology. I have seen several patients, who required up to 20 stents each before turning 50 years of age before the arrival of drug-eluting stents. 2003 is remembered as the year of the drug-eluting stents among cardiologists, whereas 1997 was the year of the non-medicated, bare-metal stent. As discussed before, in-stent restenosis occurs in 10 to 50% of patients who receive bare-metal stents. Balloon angioplasty is the first-line treatment option for in-stent restenosis. Yet, the results have been disappointing, with a recurrence rate above 40%. The new drug-eluting stents have further reduced the restenosis rate by more than 90%. Functioning a bit like a time-release capsule, drug-eluting stents are coated with powerful medications that are released over several months to prevent restenosis (reblockages). For now, US patients and physicians have two safe and extremely effective kinds of stent for prevention of in-stent restenosis. These are Sirolimus-eluting CYPHER stents and the Paclitaxel-Eluting TAXUS stents.

Drug-eluting stents have no significant impact on the risk of future heart attacks, which is similar to balloon angioplasty and non-medicated stents. Stents by their very nature do not affect the development of new blockages at different locations. The average cost of a drug-eluting stent is $3,200 per stent, $2,200 more than an uncoated stent in the US. Since the average patient requires more than one stent, the estimated average net additional charge is $4,400 per patient. Currently, 800,000 patients receive stents in the US a year. Drug-releasing stents were used in 87% of coronary interventions in last three months of 2004. The initial high cost of a drug-eluting stent may be offset by the reduced need for repeat coronary angioplasty.

Complications of coronary angioplasty

Kidney failure is a common occurrence after coronary angiogram and PCI. This is the third-leading cause of in-hospital acute renal failure. Patients with chronic kidney disease and diabetes are especially prone to this complication.

The elderly have a higher rate of complications and mortality following coronary angioplasty and stent. In a recent study (2004) of nearly 3,000 octogenarians, the overall mortality, following PCI was 4%. However, the mortality was seven times higher (14% versus 2%) in those who had this procedure done as an emergency, following a heart attack, compared to those who had it done for stable angina. Mortality was also higher in those with decreased ejection fraction and/or diabetes. Although death following angioplasty and stenting is uncommon in contemporary practice, four factors have recently been identified as strong predictors of death. The risk of *death* increases from 0.2% when none of these risk factors are present to 9% when all four are present. These factors are:

- Heart attack within 14 days of the procedure
- Elevated creatinine level or chronic kidney disease
- Involvement of two or more coronary arteries
- Age above 65 years

Coronary angioplasty and Quality of Life

As mentioned earlier, the primary benefit of coronary angioplasty in patients with stable angina is not preventing heart attack, but improving quality of life. The latter is a broader concept than mere alleviation of symptoms. It includes the effect of the disease process on the person's ability to function and enjoy life in multiple dimensions, including its physical, emotional, and social aspects. This is particularly important in the US, where patients and their doctors are unlikely to tolerate persistent angina (chest pain). In fact, one of my patients refused to take any nitroglycerine tablets, even though he had one bypass surgery and five stents at three different times in the past 10 years. Before the last stent, he had chest pain occurring predictably on the eighth hole of his golf game and demanded to have a fifth angioplasty and stent. He wanted to enjoy the game just like his friends and colleagues without the help of **nitroglycerine**.(This is a medication usually given under the tongue in persons suffering from angina/chest pain; see Chapter VIII Section 3).American patients are increasingly fond of quick fixes like angioplasty and bypass surgery and reluctant to take the necessary medication and make the all important changes in lifestyle.

> **Coronary angioplasty and symptom relief**
> The higher the severity of symptoms before angioplasty, the greater the relative improvement in quality of life. Conversely, those with minimal symptoms have minimal improvement.

A recent study (2005) has demonstrated that the improvement in a person's quality of life depends on the severity of symptoms before the angioplasty. The higher the severity of symptoms before angioplasty—the greater the relative improvement in quality of life after PCI. Conversely, those with minimal symptoms had minimal improvement. A minority of patients with no symptoms actually had a deterioration of quality of life after angioplasty for reasons that are not clear. These studies underscore the importance of the presence of severe symptoms in patients undergoing angioplasty. Undoubtedly, angioplasty with or without stenting will remain the treatment of choice for the majority of patients with severe symptoms, but those with mild to moderate symptoms have several options.

Coronary angioplasty and future risk of a heart attack

A limitation of angioplasty and bypass surgery is that they address only the more severely narrowed coronary segments, yet most heart attacks arise from rupture of plaques that do not produce blockage of the coronary arteries severe enough to qualify for angioplasty and stent (see Figure 7.2). This explains the continuing risk of heart attack and death among these people. Most heart attack victims do not have severe arterial narrowing; they have plaques that burst, creating a blood clot. This also explains why the death rates from heart attacks are similar in the US and Canada despite a three- to fourfold higher rate of coronary angioplasty and bypass surgery in the US. However, Americans with severe heart disease have a substantially better quality of life.

Researchers conducted a meta-analysis of 11 randomized clinical trials of medical therapy versus coronary angioplasty with or without a stent in 2,950 patients. This 2005 study showed clear benefit with a 60% reduction in coronary events in those who had a recent heart attack but not in those with chronic stable heart disease. This meta-analysis shows that compared to conservative treatment with medications, coronary angioplasty with or without a stent does not offer any benefit in reducing the risk of death, heart attack, or the need for subsequent angioplasty or bypass surgery in patients with stable heart diseas, (except for patients with a recent heart attack). Some of these trials were

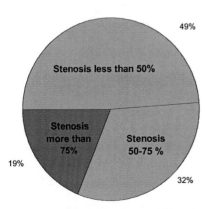

Figure 7.2. Proportion of persons who suffer a heart attack and the degree of coronary artery narrowing on a prior angiogram. The significance of these data is that only 19% of persons had severe (over 75%) narrowing before the heart attack. Source: Fishbein, MC. Ref. 7.22.

conducted before the routine use of stents, and no trial involved the use of drug-eluting stents. The available data suggest that stents may not offer any benefit other than to reduce the need for revascularization, whereas the risk of death and heart attack is not affected.

> **Did you know...**
> Coronary angioplasty and bypass surgery are done only on the more severely narrowed coronary segments. Yet most heart attacks arise from the rupture of plaques that, before the rupture, did not block the coronary arteries severely enough to qualify for bypass surgery, angioplasty, or stenting. This explains the continuing risk of heart attack and death among people who have had these procedures.

A study of 2,382 patients who had coronary angioplasty with or without a stent at Cleveland Clinic showed 951 major coronary events (defined as death, heart attack, or repeat angioplasty) in eight months. This translates into a coronary even rate of 40% per year. Those, who had metabolic syndrome, had nearly double the rate of major coronary events. Noncoronary vascular disease is another independent predictor of heart attack and death after angioplasty and stent. Noncoronary vascular disease includes atherosclerosis in other arteries, such as carotid arteries in the neck or femoral arteries in the thigh. In one study, patients with noncoronary vascular disease were twice as likely to die or to have a heart attack within one year as those who did not have disease in any other arteries.

Coronary angioplasty and future risk of repeat procedure

Coronary angioplasty is usually done for severe narrowing, but mild narrowing at other locations can progress rapidly, with recurrence of chest pain or a heart attack. A 2005 study of more than 3,000 patients found that a repeat angioplasty at a **different location** was required at a rate of 6% per year (in a new artery or a new site on the same artery), despite taking all the recommended cardiac medications. The average narrowing was 40% at the time of the first angioplasty which progressed to 84% by the time of the second PCI.

Coronary stent versus bypass procedure

A carefully designed study involving 1205 patients and published in August 2005 seems to indicate that the rates of death and heart attack are similar when people with multivessel disease are treated with stents and bypass surgery. At five years, there was no difference in mortality between stenting and surgery for multivessel disease. Furthermore, the incidence of stroke or heart attack was not significantly different between the two groups but the need repeat revascularization was fourfold higher with stents. As a result, the overall freedom from death, heart attack, stroke and repeat revascularization was lower with bypass surgery than with stenting.

Coronary angioplasty versus exercises training

Regular exercise in patients with stable heart disease has been shown to improve blood flow to the heart muscle and to retard disease progression in coronary arteries. A 2005 study compared angioplasty and stent with a 12-month program of regular physical exercise in patients with stable heart disease. The result showed a greater coronary event-free survival rate with exercise (88%) than angioplasty and stent (70%). The exercise group also had greater exercise capacity and lower healthcare costs, notably owing to reduced re-hospitalizations and repeat coronary procedures such as angioplasty and stents. This study underscores the importance of exercise training in improving the quality of life. Note that this trial was done in people with stable heart disease and may not be applicable to patients admitted with chest pain and unstable angina.

Table 7.14. Five-year outcome following bypass surgery and stent

	Stent	CABG
Number of patients	600	605
Death	8%	8%
Death among diabetics	13%	8%
Death, stroke or heart attack	18%	15%
Repeat revascularization procedures	30%	9%
Repeat revascularization among diabetics	43%	11%
Freedom from angina	80%	80%
Freedom from death, stroke, heart attack, or repeat revascularization	76%	52%

Source: Serruys, PW. J Am Coll Cardiol 2005;46:575-81.

Coronary angioplasty versus medication therapy

The benefits of angioplasty, stent and bypass surgery are immediate, but decrease over time, during which the blockages return at the same site, different sites of the same artery or a different artery. In sharp contrast, the benefits from treatment with medications are slow, but increase over time. For example, the risk of heart attack continues to decrease with increasing duration of treatment with medications. In several studies using statins to lower the LDL cholesterol, the reduction in risk was only 10% in the first year but more than 50% after the fifth year. For these reasons, combining medical treatment with angioplasty and bypass provide maximum short-term and long-term benefits. Advances in medicines, such as the use of statins and niacin, have been shown to be highly effective in preventing heart attacks as well as death, in people with and without coronary angioplasty and bypass surgery. Therefore, optimal control of risk factors, particularly cholesterol disorders, is vitally important before and after angioplasty.

KEY · POINTS · IN · A · NUTSHELL

- ♥ An emergency angioplasty, with or without a stent, can abort a heart attack, prevent complications, and even prolong life, among patients having an acute heart attack.
- ♥ The primary benefit of coronary angioplasty in people with stable heart disease is in relieving chest pain and improving the quality of life.
- ♥ Coronary angioplasty with and without a stent has limited impact on the risk of a future heart attack
- ♥ The primary benefit of coronary stenting is in reducing restenosis (re-blockage) at the same site following angioplasty that occurs in up to 60% of patients within six months.
- ♥ Restenosis is reduced to less than 25% with bare metal stents and less than 10% with drug-eluting stents.
- ♥ The risk of having a future heart attack is similar following balloon angioplasty, bare-metal stent, and drug-eluting stent.
- ♥ Both coronary angioplasty and stents do not cure the underlying condition of heart disease, which progresses in the same or different arteries requiring repeat intervention at a rate of 6% per year.
- ♥ High levels of lipoprotein(a) and low HDL levels are both common among Indians and are associated with a markedly increased risk of restenosis following coronary angioplasty and stent.

7.7 ► Reversing Heart Disease: Can It Be Done?

Atherosclerosis was once thought to be a degenerative disease process that cannot be stopped or reversed. However, autopsy studies in several countries of those who have died from starvation during famine and as prisoners of war have shown a virtual absence of atherosclerotic plaques due to forced diet-induced reversal.

More than 20 studies over the past two decades have conclusively demonstrated that atherosclerosis is an active process that can be reversed with aggressive medical treatment of a person's lipids to optimal levels. Several lines of evidence indicate that atherosclerosis progression correlates best with an increasing LDL level. On the other hand, regression or reversal of atherosclerosis correlates best with a high HDL level. In clinical practice, regression is best achieved by simultaneously lowering and maintaining LDL below 60 and increasing and maintaining HDL above 60. Such reversal has been demonstrated in coronary, carotid (neck region), and femoral (leg region) arteries using various methods. It has been found that a 1-2% regression is accompanied by a 70 to 90% reduction in risk of stroke and heart

attack. This dramatic benefit is best
explained by the stabilization of vulnerable
plaques that generally contain a large
amounts cholesterol but have less inflammatory activity and calcium. This Chapter
addresses the importance of lipid-optimizing therapy in reversing heart disease.

Vulnerable versus stable plaques

 As discussed in Chapter I, atherosclerosis is a
slowly progressive disease characterized by the
accumulation of cholesterol (primarily LDL
and lipoprotein(a)) and proliferation of smooth
muscle cell within the artery wall. Coronary
events most commonly spring from rupture of
vulnerable plaques that initially produce mild
or moderate narrowing of the artery. Upon rup-

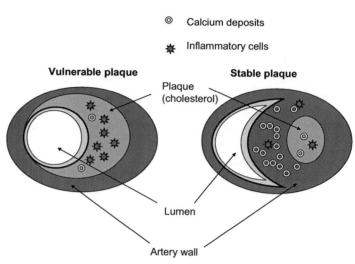

Figure 7.3 Differences between stable and unstable plaque. Also see Figure 1.7 in Chapter I section 1

ture, however, these plaques undergo a disruptive transformati ive lowering of LDL with apheresis? a dialysis like procedure that lowers LDL and lipoprotein(a) by more than 60 % in four hours . The procedure
needs to be repeated every two weeks (See Chapter VI section 2) and the cost is about $4,000 per treat-
ment or $50,000 a year. Accordingly, apheresis is not a viable option for reversing heart disease com-
pared to medications such as niacin, statins, calcium blockers, and thiazolidinediones or administering
HDL itself. Moreover, not all plaques undergo reversal. Plaques that are heavily calcified with small
amounts of cholesterol and low level of inflammatory activity are resistant to reversal.

Limitations of assessment of atherosclerosis reversal by angiogram

Earlier studies using first-generation statins used *triple-drug therapy* to achieve reversal of atherosclerosis.
In one study, intensive multi-drug lipid-optimizing therapy reduced the frequency of progression and
increased the frequency of regression of coronary atherosclerosis on repeat coronary angiogram. This was
accompanied by a better-than-expected reduction in coronary events (heart attack, death, need for coronary
angioplasty, bypass surgery etc). This regimen involved taking 20mg of lovastatin *twice a day,* 10 g
Colestipol *three times a day* and 1g of niacin *four times a day.* This study also showed that motivated
patients are prepared to take large quantities of
medication three to four times per day to avoid
cardiac catastrophe. Many of these patients did
not want to have their chest cracked open for a
second bypass surgery.

   Angiogram was the only tool available to
measure reversal for many decades, and angiographic studies conclusively demonstrated to
the skeptical medical community that reversal
of atherosclerosis is indeed possible. However,
the degree of reversal achieved was miniscule.
For example, among those treated intensively in
Familial Atherosclerosis Study (FATS, See
Appendix B) the average improvement in the
severity of narrowing per patient was 1%; only
12% of narrowed segments showed convincing

Table 7.15. Contrasting features of vulnerable and stable plaques

Vulnerable plaque	Stable plaque
Large amount of cholesterol and other lipids	Small amount of cholesterol and other lipids
No calciuml or small amount of calcium	Large amount of calcium
Thin fibrous cap overlying the lipid pool	Thick fibrous cap overlying the lipid pool
Prone to rupture	Resistant to rupture
Severe inflammation	Inflammation absent or low grade
High CRP levels	Low CRP levels
Grows outward or within the artery wall	Plaque large and grows inward
Produces minimal or no narrowing	Produces severe narrowing
Produces no symptoms of angina	Strong predictor of symptoms like angina
Strong predictor of heart attack and acute coronary syndromes	Rarely produce a heart attack and acute coronary syndromes
Not ideally suited for angioplasty and bypass surgery	Ideally suited for angioplasty and bypass surgery

regression. However, this small degree of reversal was accompanied by a surprisingly large *75% reduction* in coronary events and death. This was entirely due to prevention of progression from mild narrowing to severe stenosis. This and other studies have shown that plaques producing mild stenosis (diameter reduction less than 50%) respond more readily to lipid-lowering therapy as compared to severe narrowing (more than 50%). However, plaques with heavy calcification, irrespective of the degree of stenosis, respond poorly, if at all. We all know the soft plaque on the teeth can be removed with brushing and flossing but not the hard plaques. If these plaques are allowed to accumulate for months most of them would become calcified and not amenable to flossing. Such hard plaques require the intervention of a dentist and the use of metallic instruments. Coronary plaques behave and respond the very same way. The data, although limited, indicates that lipid-optimizing therapy may work better to slow or reverse atherosclerosis in women than in men.

> Did you know…
> Remodeling is a process by which the artery wall is reshaped by atherosclerosis and is a major determinant of the arterial lumen. Contrary to earlier beliefs, plaque progression and regression are not closely related to the size of the arterial lumen and is dependant upon the type of remodeling that occurs. A negative remodeling shrinks the arterial walls making the artery looks smaller, as happens with a spasm. On the other hand, positive remodeling causes the artery wall to expand outward making it looks larger.

Coronary remodeling and underestimation of atherosclerosis reversal

Angiography has major limitations in its ability to assess plaque progression and regression, as it only reflects changes in the inside diameter of the artery. IVUS offers unique capabilities to assess coronary atherosclerosis and plaque composition (see Section 3). These ultrasound studies have shown significant amounts of plaque build-up at various segments of arteries which look normal or near normal on an angiogram. IVUS studies have contributed substantially to our understanding of *remodeling* of the artery wall. Remodeling is a process by which the artery wall is reshaped by atherosclerosis and is a major determinant of the arterial lumen (inside diameter) Contrary to earlier beliefs, plaque progression and regression is not closely related to the size of the arterial lumen and is dependant upon the type of remodeling that occurs. A *negative remodeling* shrinks the arterial walls, making the artery looks smaller, as happens with a spasm. On the other hand positive remodeling (see Chapter I section 1) causes the artery wall to expand outward making it looks larger. Negative remodeling is more common with stable plaque and positive remodeling is more common in vulnerable plaque. HDL levels have an important role in the type of remodeling. Low HDL is associated with a negative remodeling, whereas high HDL levels produces positive remodeling.

Lipid-optimizing therapy can produce significant regression of plaque volume, without reflecting it in the lumen size of the artery. Positive remodeling that occurs with vulnerable plaques is sometimes replaced by negative remodeling upon treatment that transforms a vulnerable plaque to a stable plaque. This reversal of the positive remodeling process results in a paradoxical decrease in the lumen diameter. In short, coronary angiogram may underestimate the true extent of regression of atherosclerosis. This phenomenon explains why angiographic regression often lags behind improvement in coronary risk reduction. This observation has led to the search for other tests to measure regression and reversal of atherosclerosis.

Regression of atherosclerosis assessed by intravascular ultrasound (IVUS)

Lipid-optimizing therapy not only changes the plaque volume, but also changes its composition. It decreases the lipids in the plaques, making it stable and less prone to rupture. IVUS studies have shown that lowering LDL to below 80 mg/dL is associated with only arresting the progression as opposed to achieving regression, which requires substantial increase in HDL as well. IVUS is likely to emerge as the "gold standard" in the study of atherosclerosis progression-regression over the next few years. However, IVUS is invasive and expensive and, therefore, not suitable for large clinical trials to demonstrate regression.

Regression of atherosclerosis assessed by carotid intimal medial thickness (CIMT)

Measurement of carotid intimal medial thickness (CIMT) is safe, noninvasive, and inexpensive and can be repeated at frequent intervals, as discussed in Section 3. CIMT offers several advantages over angiography. Atherosclerosis is a disease of the arterial wall and CIMT measures the thickness of the arterial wall, rather than the inside diameter of the artery (or lumen). Studies in the past decade have clearly demonstrated an association between CIMT and coronary atherosclerosis. Unlike angiography, CIMT is capable of detecting almost all cases of early atherosclerosis and lipid-rich plaques that are vulnerable to rupture.

Several studies have shown that *lipid-optimizing therapy* slows progression and promotes regression of atherosclerosis assessed by CIMT. The Arterial Biology for the Investigation of the Treatment Effects of Reducing Cholesterol (ARBITER) found that the use of 80mg of atorvastatin a day that achieved aggressive lowering of LDL to *as low 76mg/dL* was associated with significant CIMT regression, compared with results obtained with less aggressive reduction of LDL (to 110mg/dL). The ABIRTER II Study found that *progression continued* in people who had their LDL lowered to below 90, clearly underscoring the need to lower LDL further (see Appendix B). This study for the first time also demonstrated the benefit of raising HDL with niacin (Niaspan) in arresting the progression of atherosclerosis (see Chapter VIII Section 2).

Table 7.16. Treatment option for reversing heart disease

LDL lowering with statins	Best for preventing progression
HDL raising with niacin	Best for achieving regression must be combined with LDL lowering
Combined LDL lowering and HDL raising	Achievable through with statin niacin combination therapy
Apo A Milano	Supercharged HDL not approved or available for treatment

Progression and regression assessed by Electron Beam Computerized Tomography (EBCT)

Progression and regression of atherosclerosis can be evaluated by EBCT, repeatedly and noninvasively (see Section 3). The role of EBCT in tracking disease progression is the subject of ongoing studies. EBCT is more useful in assessing *progression rather than regression,* since it quantifies the calcified plaque which does not undergo regression. An EBCT study of 163 diabetic patients (average age 65 years) showed that all subjects had calcified plaques in their coronary arteries with a high calcium score of 636, although none of them had any history of heart disease. Only six patients had no calcified plaques. During a follow-up of 27 months, there was a significant progression of plaques at a rate of 20% per year among people not treated with lipid -optimizing therapy. The rate of progression was reduced to 10% per year in those receiving statin therapy.

HDL raising, Apo A-1 Milano and "medical angioplasty"

Virtually all studies showing impressive regression involved not only lowering LDL, but also raising the HDL. Statin/niacin combination therapy has consistently been shown to improve both angiographic and clinical outcomes. It appears that increasing a person's HDL level may bring about more effective regression of atherosclerotic plaques than lowering their LDL. The best results are obtained by simultaneously **lowering LDL and raising HDL to a one to one ratio.** Opening the narrowed coronary artery wider, achieved by substantive regression with optimum control all lipoproteins by medications may be called **medical angioplasty.** This not only dilates the narrowed segment but the entire length of the coronary arteries as well as all other arteries in the body.

Apo A-1 Milano is a supercharged genetic variant of Apo A1 itself, which is the principal apo protein of HDL. It was identified in about 40 inhabitants of Limone sul Garde, a small town in rural northern Italy. These individuals had extraordinarily low HDL levels. It was expected that these people would have very high rates of heart disease because of this deficiency of "good" cholesterol. Instead, they seemed to be protected from heart disease and enjoyed longer lives than usual. Dr. P. K. Shah has done pioneering research on *Apo A Milano* and invented this unique protein. The gene responsible for this mutant protein has been cloned. The administration of genetically engineered Apo A-1 Milano has been shown to produce marked regression of atherosclerosis in cholesterol-fed rabbits, without changing the rabbits' cholesterol levels.

A study was also done in humans using a recombinant Apo A-1 Milano/phospholipids complex (ETC-216). Intravenous administration of five doses of this complex at one-week intervals produced significant regression of coronary atherosclerosis, as measured by IVUS. Of note, the same investigator in another study was unable to produce regression of atherosclerosis with 80mg of Lipitor given for 18 months. I expect Apo A-1-based treatment to open the door for medical angioplasty in the next decade.

Rapid progression of atherosclerosis is a strong predictor of early heart attack, whereas regression of atherosclerosis confers a low risk of heart attack. In short, regression of atherosclerosis is possible but not necessary to live a long and healthy life. Only lipid rich vulnerable plaques are amenable to regression which requires both lowering of the **LDL to less than 60 mg/dL and increasing the HDL to more than 60 mg/dL**. In addition, diligent attention should be paid to maintaining optimal levels of all other risk factors including body weight and waist line.

> **Did you know...**
> Regression of athero-sclerosis is possible but not necessary to live a long and healthy life. Only lipid-rich vulnerable plaques are amenable to regression which requires maintaining LDL below 60 mg/ dL and HDL above 60 mg/dL.

KEY · POINTS · IN · A · NUTSHELL

- ♥ Atherosclerosis continues even when your LDL level is maintained below 80 mg/dL.
- ♥ Rapid progression of atherosclerosis is a strong predictor of early heart attack, whereas regression of atherosclerosis confers a low risk of heart attack.
- ♥ Advances in medical treatment have made it possible to reverse atherosclerosis both in coronary and in other arteries.
- ♥ Increasing a person's HDL level is more effective in reversing heart disease, whereas, lowering LDL is effective in preventing progression of atherosclerosis.
- ♥ A combination treatment involving both niacin that increases HDL and statin that decreases LDL is more effective in producing regration that either agent alone.
- ♥ Regression of atherosclerosis is possible but not necessary to live a long and healthy life.

Part Three

Further Issues

Chapter VIII

Heart Medications and Devices

Sections 2 and 3 of Chapter VI, respectively, introduced you to the powerful cardiovascular benefits of lowering your LDL cholesterol and raising your HDL. Sections 1 and 2 of Chapter VIII build on that, offering further details about two outstanding but relatively new medications: statins and niacin. Statins, a new class of anti-cholesterol drugs that are safer than aspirin, have ushered in what is quickly turning out to be a revolution in the treatment of heart disease—quite possibly on par with the introduction of antibiotics after World War II. *Section 1*, **Statins: Those Underused Wonder Drugs,** discusses how statin therapy works, how it affects atherosclerosis, why it promotes plaque stabilization, and what makes statins so promising for such a wide range of patients. The section also tells you about their possible side effects, what dosages are optimal, and the promise statins hold for treating illnesses beyond heart disease. Finally, the section presents evidence suggesting that statins are especially potent when taken by members of certain ethnic groups, including Indians and Japanese, and that they are particularly effective when combined with other lipid-improving medications such as niacin. ◆

Section 2, **Niacin: A Powerfully Effective HDL Booster,** is about the remarkable benefits of niacin. The vital importance of having high HDL has not received quite the same medical or media coverage as that of lowering LDL cholesterol. Yet, a number of the high-risk, low-heart-disease paradoxes that we saw in the ethnic populations we examined in Chapter 4, Section 2 *(The Complex Interplay of Ethnicity and Heart Disease)* point directly to HDL's powerfully protective functions, and are best explained by them. Statins are most effective lowering LDL. Niacin specializes in raising HDL. The two together complement each other like rice and curry. Section 2 discusses niacin-statin and other combination therapies in greater detail than did Section 1, summarizing the results of some very promising recent major studies that have shown not only atherosclerosis inhibition but reversal.

Despite its pronounced effect on HDL, niacin, which is really vitamin B3, is a broad-spectrum medicine that has a favorable effect not just on HDL, but on all the other lipoproteins—LDL, VLDL, and triglycerides. It is also the only drug presently available that reduces your blood level of Lp(a), the powerful heart disease risk factor with which many Asian Indians are born. The section discusses how to manage niacin's side effects, such as the temporary sensation of skin flushing, and explains in clear, simple language the essential differences between regular immediate-release niacin, no-flush niacin (avoid it), sustained-release niacin (don't take it), and best of all, extended-release niacin or Niaspan. It ends with a summary of practical do's and don'ts for treating physicians, who desire to optimize niacin's benefits for their patients. ◆

Section 3, **Other Medications and Devices,** summarizes what you need to know about the most important prescription heart medications, particularly anticoagulants such as Coumadin and Panwarfin, and the antiplatelet medications such as aspirin and Plavix. This is followed by a discussion of nonprescription medicines—including nutritional supplements like vitamins and minerals, antioxidants, garlic, and fish oil supplements—and their potential effect on cardiovascular health. Many people swear by vitamin and other nutritional supplements. While remaining open-minded that some supplements may help, the section stays with the scientific evidence, drawing on formal studies and meta-studies to evaluate some of the claims made by vendors of dietary supplements. Using harm-benefit analysis, it compares the option of getting your antioxidant and other trace minerals from a healthy diet to that of obtaining them from supplements, and cautions about the possibility of harmful interactions with prescription drugs you may be taking.

The section brings the same level of scientific scrutiny to assessing the burgeoning field of Complementary and Alternative Medicine, Ayurvedic medicine, and herbal medications. It points out that many of the natural herbal concoctions used in these healing systems often contain high levels of toxic heavy metals such as arsenic, lead, and mercury that can become lethal through chronic overexposure. Finally, Section 3 presents an overview of the most commonly used cardiac devices, pacemakers, implantable cardioverter defibrillators (ICDs), and devices used in cardiac resynchronization therapy and enhanced external counter pulsation (EECP). ◆

A Word about Terminology

Throughout this book, the term Indian refers to people who trace their origin to the Indian subcontinent—meaning Bangladesh, India, Pakistan, and Sri Lanka—including those who now live abroad but originate from one of these four countries. "Indian" in this context is ethnically interchangeable with "South Asian," "Indo-Asian," or "Asian Indian." The term thus excludes native Americans but includes more than people from the nation of India.

Measurement Units: As is conventional, blood glucose levels, triglyceride levels, and cholesterol levels are stated throughout this book in milligrams per deciliter (mg/dL). Blood pressure is stated in millimeters of mercury (mmHg).

8.1 ▶ Statins: Those Underused Wonder Drugs

A S WE SAW in Chapters 1 and 6, high levels of LDL (or bad) cholesterol in your blood are strongly associated with atherosclerosis—the accumulation of plaque in the linings of your arteries. When this fatty buildup occurs in your coronary arteries, it greatly magnifies your risk of angina (chest pain) or a heart attack if a large plaque or blood clot from a ruptured plaque obstructs an artery, starving the heart muscle of oxygen.

The medical world has been abuzz with excitement over the introduction of statins, a new family of powerful yet safe anti-cholesterol medications that have the potential of dramatically reducing the incidence of heart disease and mortality from coronary and vascular events. It would not be an overstatement to say that the emergence of statins is one of the great success stories of modern medicine, comparable to the discovery of antibiotics for bacterial infections. In 2002, statins sales in the US surpassed $13 billion.

The benefits of statin therapy have been observed in a wide range of people—with and without heart disease, with and without high cholesterol, in both genders, and at all ages. Some statins have also been found to be safe for children, but not for women, who are or will soon become pregnant. So promising are statins that, according to WHO estimates, more than 200 million individuals worldwide, who have heart disease, stroke, or diabetes, may benefit from this new class of heart disease drugs. Currently, about 25 million patients worldwide—13 million of them in the US—are being treated with statins. Those numbers, however, are relatively small. According to the National Heart, Lung & Blood Institute, about half of the American adult population have elevated levels of total cholesterol. Statin therapy is already quietly revolutionizing the treatment of coronary heart disease; yet fewer than half of patients who need statins are currently getting them.

> The benefits of statin therapy have been observed in people of all ages and sexes—with and without heart disease, and with and without high cholestrol. Yet fewer than half of patients who might benefit from statins currently receive them, partly because physicians tend to reserve statins for their highest-risk patients.

Before continuing, however, let's put the role of statin therapy in proper perspective. Like many other medications and other clinical interventions, statins are most effective when taken in conjunction with lifestyle changes such as diet and exercise (discussed in Chapter V). Statins may well be miracle drugs poised to perform even greater wonders than antibiotics did against bacterial diseases in the se-cond half of the 20th century. Infectious diseases, however, would not have waned without the introduction of better sanitation, improved sewage systems, sterilization techniques, and other advances in hygiene. Similarly, for optimal prevention and control heart disease, statins need to be combined with personal lifestyle modifications. Just as heart disease risk factors—such as inactivity, smoking, saturated fat, cholesterol, overweight, abdominal obesity, diabetes, stress, heredity, and age—work in tandem, creating a synergistic multiplier effect on one another, so do heart disease interventions.

> The promise of statins is enormous, but just as heart disease risk factors work in tandem, so statins need to be combined with lifestyle changes for optimal benefits.

Statins and cardiac risk reduction

Statins are able to lower blood cholesterol by a third to two-thirds—for example, from 320 to 120mg/dL—in just two to four weeks. Prospective, placebo-controlled clinical trials conducted with statins and involving some 100,000 people have demonstrated over of the past 15 years that statins significantly reduce not only the risk of dying from a heart attack, but the risk of getting a heart attack by 25 to 35%, regardless of the level of the patient's cholesterol when therapy began. Unlike other cholesterol-lowering medications, the benefits of statins on stroke are equally spectacular—up to a 25% reduction in the risk of stroke. Not only do statins lessen the likelihood of developing a stroke, they also lessen its severity. Earlier studies have shown that stroke patients who are on statins both before and after their stroke are substantially more likely not only to survive it but to avoid developing a level of disability that requires living in a nursing home. Statin patients were twice as likely to survive their stroke or be discharged to their homes as those who were not taking a statin before their stroke. But a new study now suggests that even stroke patients, who were not on statins, benefit from it if medication is started immediately upon hospitalization.

How statins work

What exactly do statins do at the biochemical level? Statins lower LDL cholesterol in your blood two ways: by pulling it out of your bloodstream, and secondly, by inhibiting LDL manufacture in your liver. They achieve the second by blocking the main enzyme that controls cholesterol production in the liver, HMG-CoA reductase. This cholesterol-manufacturing enzyme happens to be more active at night. The best time to take statins, therefore, is between dinner and bed-time, so that the amount of statin in the body is highest just when the liver cell enzyme is at its most active. (Statins may also have an inhibitory effect on blood platelets, and produce other changes within the artery's inner lining.)

> Besides slowing, arresting, or reversing atherosclerosis, the cholesterol-lowering effect of statins also stabilizes **unstable** plaques, making them less likely to rupture and cause a heart attack.

It has been thought that the cholesterol-lowering effect of statins influences plaque formation, but only now are we beginning to understand how this occurs. Several studies have demonstrated that the buildup of plaque during atherosclerosis can be slowed and even brought to a standstill with statin therapy. In addition, with very aggressive statin therapy, this process can actually be reversed to some extent, but the degree of reversal is usually quite small—in the order of 1 to 2% of existing plaques, or a 1 to 2% increase in the internal diameter of a clogged coronary artery. What has surprised researchers in study after study is the 40% to 80% reduction in heart attack and death rates among statin-treated patients, compared to those given placebos. These larger-than-expected reductions in coronary events are much greater than could have been predicted from the slow-down, arrest, or reversal or the plaque buildup.

> *When statin doses are raised, the benefits also increase but at an ever diminishing rate. Side effects, however, increase at an accelerating rate.*

How can a statin's effect on cholesterol decrease heart attack and death rates so dramatically without shrinking existing plaques or increasing the internal diameter of the coronary arteries? Clearly, something else is going on other than regression, arrest, or a slow-down in atherosclerotic progression. It is now believed that, quite apart from retarding, halting, or reversing atherosclerosis, statin therapy changes the nature of some of the plaques, turning unstable vulnerable plaques into more stable ones. Plaque stabilization makes formerly vulnerable plaques much less likely to rupture and result in a blood clot that could block a coronary artery and trigger a heart attack.

> Reversing plaque buildup can be done with aggressive, high-dose statin therapy, but we now know that, usually, it is not necessary. After all, the real goal is not banishing atherosclerosis, but rather living a life free of major coronary events.

The larger implication of these findings is that reversing atherosclerosis—as attractive a goal as it sounds—is no longer as critical an objective as was once thought, because it is clear that statins achieve a powerful effect on heart attack rates through means other than reversing plaque buildup. Studies show that statins stabilize unstable plaques. In addition to this, although slowing down or even stopping the formation of new plaques is a practical and achievable goal with statin therapy, actually *reversing* atherosclerosis is another matter entirely. It requires progressively higher doses to accomplish this because, as with many other medications, when the dose is increased, the benefits increase but at a *diminishing* rate. In contrast, the side effects increase at an *accelerating* rate. Reversal can be realized, but we now know that, even among patients with fairly advanced atherosclerosis, it is not absolutely necessary because it comes at a high cost in patient effort, prescription purchases, and side effects. After all, the real goal of heart disease management is not banishing atherosclerosis, but rather being able to live free of heart attacks and other major coronary events. However this can be achieved—through therapy or lifestyle modification—should be the patient's goal, not whether atherosclerosis can be slowed, arrested, or regressed. Table 8.1 shows the effect of various statins on LDL, HDL and triglyceride levels.

Table 8.1. Effect of various statins on cholesterol triglycerides and HDL

Statins	Dosage (mg)	HDL-C: % increase	Triglycerides: % reduction	Total Cholestrol: % reduction
Fluvastatin (Lescol)	20-80	3-8	12-25	16-27
Fluvastatin ER (Lescol XL)	80	5-7	19-25	25-30
Lovastatin (Mevacor)	10-80	2-7	6-27	16-34
Pravastatin (Pravachol)	5-80	4-8	15-24	16-30
Simvastatin (Zocor)	5-80	5-8	12-34	19-36
Atorvastatin (Lipitor)	10-80	5-8	17-53	25-42
Rosuvastatin (Crestor)	10-40	8-10	10-35	33-46

Source: NCEP. Ref. 8.34.

Measured on a per milligram basis, statins vary as much as 16-fold in their ability to lower LDL and total cholesterol, as shown in Table 8.2, *below.* For example, 5mg of Crestor has the same LDL-lowering efficacy (41%) as 20mg of Lipitor, 40mg of Zocor, or 80mg of Pravachol. In general, the greatest benefit per milligram is achieved at the lowest dose. In fact, the Statins Rule of Sevens states that every time you double a statin dose, you double its cost and side effects but gain only 7% extra benefit. Example: Starting with 5mg of Lipitor, each doubling of the dose until 80mg reduces LDL by 7%, yet it doubles the side effects and the cost. Treating physicians, therefore, often find that the first few milligrams offer the biggest bang for the buck in the form of benefit-to-risk, benefit-to-cost, and benefit-per-milligram. Doctors thus find it more effective to combine a low or moderate dose of a statin with other medications, especially niacin and Zetia.

The benefits of aggressive statin therapy

Although low doses of statins work very well, aggressive statin therapy may provide even greater benefits in high-risk patients. The first generation of studies recorded LDL reductions of 25 to 35%, accompanied by a corresponding 25-35% reduction in heart attack and death rates. A logical question was whether a 50-65% reduction in LDL level would translate into a correspondingly large reduction in heart attack and death rates. Two recent clinical trials—Reversal of Atherosclerosis with Aggressive Lipid Lowering (REVERSAL), and Pravastatin or Atorvastatin Evaluation and Infection Therapy (PROVE IT)—prospectively tested and confirmed the validity of more aggressive LDL-lowering in high-risk patients.

Table 8.2. Percentage Reduction in LDL with Common Statins (daily dosages in mg)

Crestor	Lipitor	Zocor	Mevacor	Pravachol	Lescol	LDL reduction
	5	10	20	20	40	27%
	10	20	40	40	80	34%
5	20	40	80	80		41%
10	40	80				48%
20	80					55%

Source: Roberts, WC. Ref. 8.39

Both studies compared the safety and efficacy of 40mg of Pravachol to that of 80mg of Lipitor, equivalent to 320mg of Pravachol. The REVERSAL Study, which followed more than 600 patients at 34 community and tertiary-care centers in the US, administered the two statins for 18 months. The Lipitor-treated group achieved an average LDL of 79mg/dL, compared to 110 for the Pravachol-treated group. Additionally, although clear reversal was not demonstrated, the Lipitor-treated group showed complete arrest of the progression of atherosclerosis when this was measured using ultrasound.

In the PROVE IT study, which observed more than 4,000 patients, the more aggressively treated (Lipitor) group safely reduced their LDL to an average of 62mg/dL compared to 95 for the Pravachol group, accompanied by a 25% reduction in coronary events. These studies were instrumental in the issuance of new interim LDL-lowering guidelines by the NCEP. The NCEP currently recommends LDL below 70 for patients with heart disease and other high-risk factors, such as diabetes or metabolic syndrome.

Not the best thing for boosting HDL levels

Despite the remarkable LDL-lowering results achieved in studies such as REVERSAL and PROVE IT, reducing LDL is not all there is to lipid management. Case in point: In the PROVE IT study, 22% of the aggressively-treated (Lipitor) group experienced coronary events within two years. This underscores the need to address other components of dyslipidemia beyond LDL, such as low HDL and high lipoprotein(a). Statins, however, are not especially effective in raising HDL levels; the maximum increase is usually no more than 10%, compared to 10-15% when you take fibrates and 20-40% with niacin. Statins, however, do have many other benefits, including lowering uric acid, fibrinogen, and high-sensitivity CRP levels. The benefits of statins are summarized in Table 8.3.

SAFETY AND AVAILABILITY ISSUES

How safe are statins? The short answer is very safe—in fact, are 100 times safer than aspirin, an over-the-counter medication used extensively to prevent heart attacks and strokes. (Read about aspirin and its side effects in Section 3 of this Chapter). Although statins are not entirely free of side effects, their side effects are few, occasional, and relatively mild, and they have proven to be extremely safe in the vast majority of patients receiving them. No subgroup of patients has been found in whom harm from statin therapy has yet been proven. Zocor, for example, is available without a prescription in Europe, a clear testament to belief in its safety. In the US, however, the FDA has refused to make statins available over the counter. Occasional side effects involving liver or muscle toxicity have been known to occur (discussed below).

Despite their proven safety and benefits, however, many, who could benefit from statins, are not receiving them. In one British study, a person who had had two bypass surgeries in five years was nevertheless not tested or treated for high cholesterol. When the patient subsequently changed doctors, the patient's cholesterol was measured at 300mg/dL. In another study, this one Canadian, only 19% of high-risk elderly patients who had survived a heart attack were prescribed statins. In a recent US study, a lipid panel was not obtained in 42% of heart attack patients. Another study showed that approximately 20% of American patients who were eligible for lipid-lowering treatment did not receive it. This ultra-cautious use of statins is observed not only in Europe but even in the US, usually known for its more aggressive stance on treatment therapies. Taken together, these data suggest that a person with heart disease had a 40% chance of never being tested for high cholesterol, and a 20% chance of not being treated for cholesterol even after being tested.

One issue may be cost. For example, fully implementing the NCEP III guidelines on LDL-lowering could cost $500 billion a year, a third of current total US healthcare expenditure. Cost issues may be why Europeans are less aggressive in treating dyslipidemia. For example, in Norway, statins are prescribed only for patients

Statins' effect on triglycerides
The ability of statins to lower triglycerides is not fully appreciated or utilized. Although they have little impact on patients with normal triglyceride levels, among patients with high triglycerides (above 250mg/dl), statins lower triglycerides to a degree similar to their LDL-lowering efficacy. In fact, a 50% lowering of triglycerides can be achieved with high doses of statins.

Table 8.3. Pharmacological and clinical benefits of taking a statin

Pharmacological benefits	Clinical benefits
• Significantly lowers LDL • Significantly lowers triglycerides • Raises HDL slightly • Significantly decreases CRP level • Slightly lowers blood pressure • Lowers uric acid levels • Lowers fibrinogen levels	• Significantly reduced heart attack risk • Significantly reduces stroke risk • Arrests the progression of atherosclerosis • Stabilizes atheroma • Limits inflammation in atheroma • Reduces plaque thrombogenicity (i.e., its likelihood to rupture and form a blood clot) • Reduces oxidised LDL accumulation in plaque • Decreases the need for coronary angioplasty and bypass surgery

with cholesterol levels exceeding 310mg/dL. Clearly, the higher the cardiac risk, the greater the potential benefits of statin therapy, but this does not mean doctors should reserve statins exclusively for their highest-risk patients. A potentially much larger proportion of the general population would benefit from combining lipid-lowering therapy with diet and exercise, yet even some high-risk patients are not receiving statins.

Statins: How much safer are they than Aspirin?
Consider this. Studies show that for every 1000 patients with a 5% risk of heart disease, taking aspirin for five years would prevent 6 to 20 heart attacks but would cause up to two hemorrhagic strokes, and 2 to 4 cases of gastrointestinal bleeding. By comparison, taking 40ms of a statin such as Zocor for 5 years would prevent 70-100 major cardiovascular events (such as stroke and heart attack) in 1000 patients, with no risk of hemorragic stroke or gastrointestinal bleeding.

Side effects: liver functions

At high doses, statins create a 1-2% risk per year of causing usually temporary abnormalities in liver function. These are almost always reversible within 4-8 weeks after the dose is reduced, and usually disappear without your having to stop taking the medication. It is extremely unusual for statins to produce permanent liver damage. The risk of acute liver failure from statins is much lower than, for example, from medications used to treat diabetes or depression. Elevation of liver enzymes three times the upper limit of normal would nevertheless be a reason to suspend medication, if this ever occurred, and liver enzymes should be monitored in anyone taking a statin.

Contrary to common belief, the side effects are not caused by LDL levels that have become "too low" but by the *dose* used. For example, 80mg of fluvastatin lowers LDL by 35%, but increases liver enzymes and creatine kinase levels in 3% of people. By contrast, 40mg of Crestor decreases LDL by much more, 65%, yet liver enzyme elevation is found in less than 1% of people taking it.

The benefits of statins in lowering cholestrol and preventing heart disease far outweigh the small but potential risk of liver damage, even in patients who have chronic liver disease.

Statins have a stronger effect on some ethnic groups
Studies among Indians and Japanese show that statins like Zocor are up to four times as effective in these groups as they are in whites. Among Japanese, 5mg of Zocor has the same LDL-lowering effect as 20mg in whites. Blood levels of the statin Crestor have also been shown to be higher in Indians and Japanese who are taking an identical dose as white patients. This may be because they metabolize Crestor more slowly than whites, but the exact cause is still unclear. The good news, obviously, is that Indians and Japanese can take statin doses 50% to 75% lower than those typically taken by whites, resulting in fewer side effects. Differences in statin efficacy may well exist in other ethnic groups that have not yet been studied.

Of note, slight elevations of liver enzymes are common in people even if they are not taking a statin. Approximately 25% of the US population has elevated liver enzymes related to metabolic syndrome or obesity. Alcohol and psychotropic drugs are also associated with liver enzymes elevation and should be carefully evaluated before and during statin treatment. In short, the cholesterol-lowering and heart disease prevention benefits of statins far outweigh the potential but small risk of liver damage, even in patients with chronic liver disease.

Side effects: muscle soreness and damage

Myopathy, a rare side effect of statins characterized by muscle soreness and inflammation, occurs in between one in 1,000 and one in 2,000 patients. In one clinical trial, one-third of subjects receiving lovastatin had muscle soreness and elevated creatine phosphokinase (CK) enzyme. Surprisingly, one-third of those who received a dummy pill also had muscle soreness and CK elevation. Clearly, muscle soreness is a common occurrence, particularly in middle-aged and elderly people, even in the absence of taking statins.

Rhabdomyolysis (pronounced *rab-dough-my-ALL-is-is*) is a severe and even rarer form of myopathy in which some of your skeletal muscle tissue breaks down. The muscle damage leads to release of potentially toxic muscle cell components, most notably CK and myoglobin, into your blood circulation (see Chapter VI, Section 4). Darkened urine due to myoglobin may signify rhabdomyolysis. The destruction of large amounts of muscle can lead to kidney failure and death if it is not recognized and treated early.

In a randomized, placebo-controlled trial involving three statins, Pravachol, Zocor, and Mevacor, the rates of rhabdomyolysis per million person-years were 50 for statins and 30 for the placebo. For comparison, the risk from aspirin use is 100 to 400 per million users for hemorrhagic stroke and 400 to 800 for major gastrointestinal bleeding. Conditions that are associated with an increased risk of rhabdomyolysis include being older than 65, diabetes, hypothyroidism, and compromised liver and kidney functions.

You should, as a matter of course, discuss your current medications with your physician before initiating statin therapy, or any therapy for that matter. In 59% of the 601 cases of rhabdomyolysis reported to the FDA up until 2003, an additional agent was considered to have contributed to the condition.

Contrary to belief, statin side effects are not caused by LDL levels that have become "too low" but rather by the dose used.

The accompanying table lists the most common culprits associated with cases of rhabdomyolysis when taken together with a statin. The statin and co-medication pairing responsible for the highest number of reported cases of rhabdomyolysis—the statin Baycol, made by Bayer, and the anti-hypertension drug Mibefradil—have both been removed from the market, substantially reducing the incidence of myopathy. In the 601 reported cases of rhabdomyolysis, only 38 cases (6%) were fatal. The overall rate of fatalities from rhabdomyolysis with the use of statins is **one per seven million** users. This is a very low probability—lower than that of dying in a plane crash while flying from New York to LA, and **100 times lower** than the risk of dying from taking aspirin to prevent a heart attack.

Statins' Excellent Safety Record
Of the 601 cases of rhabdomyolysis (muscle breakdown) reported to the FDA up until 2003, a second drug besides statins was believed to have contributed to it in 59% of the cases. The overall death rate from rhabdomyolysis with the use of statins is just **one** per seven million users. This is a lower probability than that of dying while flying from New York to LA, and 100 times lower than the risk of dying from taking an aspirin a day.

Medications that increase the risk of rhabdomyolysis

Taking certain medications at the same time as a statin can increase your risk of rhabdomyolisis by raising the level of statin in your blood dangerously high. Typically, this happens when the other medication you are taking inhibits the activity of one of the important enzymes that helps to metabolize (break down) statin in your body. Since the inhibited enzyme can no longer metabolize statin quickly enough, your statin blood level rises substantially. One of the important statin-metabolizing enzymes is cytochrome P450-3A4, or CYP3A4 for short. Medications that inhibit CYP3A4 include Amiodorone, cyclosporine, HIV protease inhibitors, antibiotics such as Biaxin, Erythromycin, or Zithromax; and antifungal medications such as ketoconazole or Itraconazole. Taking Biaxin, for example, inhibits CYP so powerfully that it can increase your blood level of Pravachol twofold, Lipitor fourfold, and Zocor tenfold. It is thus my practice to suspend statin therapy temporarily if a patient is taking an antibiotic like Biaxin that is a CYP inhibitor. Alternatively, change the statin to one that is not metabolized by CYP-3A4, like Pravastatin.

Drug Interactions
The statin level in your blood can rise dangerously high if you take it along with certain medications (e.g., Biaxin, Lopid) that inhibits the enzyme which breaks down statins in your body.

Grape fruit juice Grape fruit juice is another potent inhibitor of cytochrome p-450 3A. Drinking more than a quart of grape fruit juice can interfere with the metabolism of many drugs, including most statins, although not Pravachol. It can increase statin blood levels toward a level approaching toxicity. A glass of grape fruit juice or half a grapefruit, however, does not seem to have any adverse effects.

COMBINING STATINS WITH OTHER LIPID-OPTIMIZING AGENTS

As stated earlier, the greatest benefit per milligram for a statin is usually achieved at its lowest dose. Low doses give the biggest "bang for the buck." Combination therapy involving a statin and something else therefore offers attractive advantages. It may allow the use of lower doses of multiple drugs rather than maximum doses of any one single drug. As noted here, however, physicians and their patients need to exercise caution when combining statins with certain other agents.

*Studies show that lipid management requires both lowering LDL and raising HDL. Statins work superbly for LDL. Niacin is ideal for HDL. **Combining** them often yields the best results.*

Statins and fibrates

You need to be careful when you take fibrates along with statins, particularly the fibrate Lopid, which raises the level of most statins in the blood. Combining statins with fibrates is associated with a several-fold increase in the risk of rhabdomyolysis, particularly in elderly diabetics (*see* Table 6.18 in Chapter VI, Section 4). One statin, Baychol, was withdrawn from the market because of an unacceptably incidence of rhabdomyolysis in people taking both it and Lopid. More than half of these cases, however, were caused by overzealous physicians misusing the statin with Lopid and disregarding specific warnings.

Statins and niacin

The FDA has approved a combination of statin and niacin (Advicor), which is safe and effective and carries no risk of rhabdomyolysis. Niacin should be considered before fibrates not only because of its lower risk of myopathy, but because of niacin's superior efficacy in raising HDL levels.

Other benefits of satins

Several recent studies, published in 2005, show that statins protect against several cancers, including colorectal, prostrate, and breast cancer. For example, in a large Israeli study involving 1953 patients, the use of statins was associated with a 47% relative reduction in the risk of colorectal cancer, after adjusting for other known risk factors. Other studies have also shown up to a 20% reduction after five years of using satins.

The next section addresses the use of **niacin**, another truly potent weapon in the arsenal of medications for treating dyslipidemia, particularly when it is combined with a statin.

Table 8.4. Cases of rhabdomyolysis while taking a statin and another medication

Co-Medication Taken	Number
Mibefradil (a blood pressure medication not longer available)	99
Fibrates	80
Cyclosporin	51
Macrolide (antibiotic)	41
Warfarin (blood thinner)	33
Digoxin (heart medication)	26
Azol fungal agents	12
Niacin	4
Other medications	6
No co-medication (statin alone)	249
Total	**601**

Source: Omar, MA. Ref 8.36

KEY · POINTS · IN · A · NUTSHELL

♥ Statins are a class of powerful anti-cholesterol drugs that are quickly establishing themselves as the pharmacological foundation of preventive cardiology.

♥ Statins substantially reduce the incidence of heart disease, reduce the risk of heart attack, stroke, and death 25% to 40%, and can reduce the need for angioplasty and bypass surgery by as much as 35%.

♥ Statins can lower LDL cholesterol by a third to two-thirds in 2-4 weeks, and raise HDL by 10%.

♥ Statins lower triglycerides by 10%, when triglycerides levels are low, and **up to 50%** when triglycerides are high

♥ By lowering blood LDL levels, statins slow down atherosclerosis. They also transform soft, unstable plaques into more stable plaques, making them less likely to rupture and trigger a heart attack.

♥ Statin therapy benefits people with and without heart disease, with and without high cholesterol, both male and female, and at all ages, including some children.

♥ Studies show that statins may be even more effective in lowering cholesterol in Indians and Japanese than in whites.

♥ Recent studies show that statins can protect against several cancers, including colorectal, prostrate, and breast cancer.

♥ Statins are even more effective as a lipid management therapy when combined with other medications, especially niacin. Several FDA-approved combinations are already on the market.

♥ Statins are **100 times safer than aspirin** because their side effects are so few and so rare.

♥ Those rare serious side effects are often due to interaction with other drugs, such as fibrates or CYP enzyme inhibitors. Muscle damage resulting in death is extremely rare.

♥ Statins may have as great an effect on public health, as antibiotics did against bacterial diseases, but not enough people who need them are getting them.

8.2 ▶ Niacin: A Powerfully Effective HDL Booster

I N 1914, US government public health physician Dr. Joseph Goldberger defied commonly-held medical opinion and theorized that the epidemic of pellagra plaguing southern states was caused not by germs but by poor nutrition and diet deficiencies. Through meticulous observations and controlled studies among Mississippi prison inmates, the 40-year-old doctor discovered that a diet rich in milk and eggs reduced the incidence of dermatitis, dementia, diarrhea, and death—the four Ds of pellagra. Goldberger never figured out what was in the diet that prevented pellagra before his death in 1929, only that germs did not cause it. A few years later, nicotinic acid, one of the B-complex vitamins, was isolated as the pellagra-preventive ingredient in this diet and renamed niacin in 1935.

The work of Goldberger and other physician-scientists early in the 20th century established the important principle that food is more than just proteins, carbohydrates and fats. Food contains powerful vitamins, trace minerals, and phytochemicals that promote cellular and biological health on multiple levels. Today, that view has birthed an entire nutritional supplements

> **Biochem 101: How Does Niacin Work?**
> Niacin works primarily by inhibiting the breakdown (or catabolism) of HDL in the liver so that more of it is available. Niacin also inhibits hepatic lipase, an enzyme that stimulates the production of small, dense LDL. Finally, niacin stimulates lipoprotein lipase, the key enzyme that breaks down triglycerides.

industry that in some ways has gone overboard—a topic discussed in the next section of this Chapter. But the fundamental principle should not be missed: food contains not just calories and fuel but also potent micronutrients. Some of these micronutrients—when isolated, concentrated, and given at high doses—assume new levels of potency that have therapeutic benefits which go beyond mere nutrition. One of these is the vitamin niacin. This section discusses what niacin is, when to use it, what to combine it with, and how to derive maximum benefit from lipid-improving therapy.

Niacin's effect on coronary risk

For daily nutritional purposes, the minimum recommended daily allowance (RDA) of niacin is just 50mg, but at high doses—500 to 2000mg—niacin is powerfully effective in treating dyslipidemia. It is a broad-spectrum agent that has a favorable effect on all the lipoproteins. But perhaps its most unique and perhaps most valuable role is its tremendous ability to raise HDL. It is in fact the most potent agent for raising HDL, particularly large-particle HDL, the most cardio-protective fraction. Raising your HDL while simultaneously lowering your LDL is far more beneficial to cardio-vascular health than just lowering your LDL cholesterol. Niacin also decreases LDL and triglycerides, and it is the only agent that effectively lowers lipoprotein(a).

Because of its beneficial effects on lipoproteins, niacin, whether given alone or in combination with a statin, significantly reduces morbidity and mortality from heart disease and reduces the rate of heart attacks by retarding, halting, or even actually reversing atherosclerosis. Several niacin-statin therapy trials have shown that this combination reduces the risk of heart attack 60% to 90%, compared to only 25 to 35% when a statin alone is used, even at the highest dose. Given alone or in combination, niacin also reduces the risk of strokes and the need for bypass surgery.

The box Above summarizes the results of the Coronary Drug Project, in which patients took 3 grams of niacin a day for five years and were followed for potential side effects for an additional 11 years, totaling 16. One surprise finding was an 11% reduction in total mortality, meaning death from all causes.

Arresting and reversing atherosclerosis: the evidence

Several studies have shown that, in combination with statins or other lipid-lowering therapy, niacin cannot only *slow down* or *arrest* atherosclerosis, but actually *reverse* it—something that even high doses of statins alone (for example, 80mg doses of Lipitor in the REVERSAL Study) have not been shown to do. Chapter VII, Section 7 discusses this in greater detail.

One reason for niacin's powerful effect on atherosclerosis is its ability to raise HDL levels. HDL actually removes cholesterol from your arteries and takes it back into the liver. A recent study, the ARBITER-2 trial, showed that atherosclerosis can continue even in people with low LDL levels, because arresting the progress of atherosclerosis requires both low LDL and high HDL. In ARBITER-2, heart disease patients who had both low LDL (below 90) and low HDL (below 40) and were on statins increased their HDL by an average of 21% after being given one gram a day of Niaspan for a year. In addition, the niacin-statin combination completely arrested their atherosclerosis, reducing coronary events by 60%. In contrast, another group who took various statins (but no niacin) showed continued progression of atherosclerosis, even though they maintained their LDL level below 90, which is very low.

Table 8.5. Available Niacin Preparations

Type	Remarks
Niacin ER: Extended release niacin (Niaspan®)	FDA-approved. Low rates of flushing (sensation of heat, and skin redness); no liver damage. Highly recommended
Regular or immediate-release niacin (niacin IR)	High rates of flushing. Multiple doses needed. Recommended
Long-acting or sustained-release (niacin SR)	High rates of liver damage. Not FDA-approved for dyslipidemia treatment. Avoid
No-flush niacin	Contains no niacin. Avoid

The niacin-statin group in ARBITER-2, incidentally, did not show evidence of atherosclerotic regression, most likely because the niacin dose they used was too small and the treatment period too short. Other studies using larger doses of niacin and over longer periods—including HATS, FATS, and CLASS—have consistently demonstrated reversal of atherosclerosis (see box below, as well as Chapter VII, Section 7 and Appendix B).

Which form of niacin has the fewest side effects?

Despite its powerful benefits, the use of niacin has not been as widespread as it should be because of worries about side effects and liver toxicity. Many of these fears, however, are unwarranted if you take the right formulation, because most the side effects are caused by particular formulations. The four available forms of niacin are summarized here. Some are far safer than others, and it is easy to distinguish between them.

Extended-release niacin (niacin ER or Niaspan)—far and away the best form

Niaspan is an FDA-approved, extended-release, prescription-only niacin made by Kos Pharmaceuticals. It is administered once-daily at bedtime. Niaspan® is as effective in improving lipoprotein levels as an equivalent daily set of niacin IR doses. At the maximum recommended dose of 2g per day, Niaspan raises HDL by 41% and decreases LDL by 16%, lipoprotein(a) by 25%, and triglycerides by 32%. A meta-analysis of Niaspan studies has shown 50% greater LDL-lowering in women than men, but no difference in the other lipoproteins.

Combined with a statin, niacin not only can slow down or arrest the process of atherosclerosis, but can actually begin to reverse it.

As discussed in Chapter VII, Section 2, lipoprotein subclasses vary in their atherogenic and antiatherogenic properties. Small, dense LDL particles are particularly atherogenic; large HDL particles are especially cardioprotective. One of the impressive facts about Niaspan is that, of the various subclasses of LDL and HDL, its effect is greatest on small-particle LDL and on large-particle HDL, the two classes that matter the most. In other words, Niaspan seems to focus most on the worst LDL and the most cardioprotective HDL, decreasing the harmfulness of the first by increasing its average size, and boosting the effectiveness of the second also by increasing its average size, especially in people who have high triglyceride levels. In quantitative terms, it increases large HDL by almost 200% and lowers small LDL by almost 50%. This is why niacin produces such a dramatic reduction in coronary events in those taking it. By contrast, fibrates tend to raise the less-protective small-particle HDL.

Niaspan's benefits
Raising your HDL while lowering your LDL is far more beneficial than simply lowering LDL. It is this **dual role** that makes niacin, whether alone or combination with another cholesterol drug, so promising.
  At the maximum recommended dose of 2g a day, Niaspan raises HDL 41% and lowers LDL 16%, triglycerides by 32%, and LP(a) by 25%. Note that its **selective** effect on large-particle HDL and small-particle LDL is even greater than these numbers suggest!

Niaspan's safety has been demonstrated conclusively in several large studies. Because it is released slowly into the bloodstream, it causes less flushing of the skin (a sensation of heat accompanied by skin redness). In addition, unlike Niacin IR which must be taken several times a day, patients find it easy to take Niaspan because it is administered just once daily, at bedtime. This convenience markedly improves adherence.

One of the strongest points in favor of Niaspan® is that it has gone through the FDA's very stringent approval process, and the FDA continues to monitor the safety and side effects of any drug it approves. The drawback is that the FDA has limited the maximum dose to 2g a day, which is in reality low. Niacin doses ranging between 2 and 12g are considered high.

As with any medicine, however, higher doses are associated with higher rates of side effects and are therefore reserved for those at exceptionally high risk, such as people with very low HDL counts and very high lipoprotein(a) levels, or people who frequently need repeat coronary angioplasty or bypass surgery.

Regular niacin (IR) — not bad, but not great

Immediate-release niacin is the standard form. A 2g dose of niacin IR lowers LDL by 14% and raises HDL by 21% and has little liver toxicity. As the name implies, however, all of it is released immediately, which can result in flushing of the skin and itching as a result of vasodilation (the sudden opening up of your arteries). Many light-skinned people turn beet red within three or four hours of taking large quantities of niacin. The benefits and side effects of niacin are both dose-dependent; the more you take, the greater the benefits and side effects. As a result, physicians gradually adjust the dose to achieve the desired effect. Besides flushing and itching, one other disadvantage of Niacin IR is that it needs to be taken three to four times a day, which many patients find inconvenient and intrusive.

Long-acting or sustained-release niacin (SR)—potentially harmful, avoid

Long-acting niacin was developed to reduce the sensation of flushing, but it can cause very serious liver toxicity, including severe, rapid liver failure and death. It is, therefore, not approved by the FDA for treating dyslipidemia and not monitored by the agency. It does lower LDL, but its effectiveness in raising HDL—one of the celebrated strengths of niacin—is low. It is deeply troubling that many patients prescribed niacin buy nonprescription long-acting niacin at health food stores because of its promise to reduce flushing and because it is often less expensive.

One of the truly impressive facts about Niaspan is that its effect is greatest on the most harmful subclass of LDL—small-particle, dense LDL—and on the most protective kind of HDL, large-particle. It boosts large HDL by almost **200%** and lowers small LDL by almost **50%**.

No-flush niacin—ineffective, avoid

No-flush niacin, widely touted to have few side effects, is one of the most expensive forms of this vitamin. It is said to contain a form of niacin (inositol hexanicotinate) that causes no sensation of flushing. However, recent studies have clearly demonstrated that it causes no flushing simply because it contains no niacin! So-called "no-flush niacin" cogently illustrates the potential pitfalls of using nutritional supplements in place of prescription medications.

Prescription niacin versus dietary supplements

I strongly discourage the use of niacin preparations sold as dietary supplements. No regulatory agency oversees the quality or toxicity of nonprescription niacin, unlike Niaspan. Many of these products have no established record of safety and efficacy and are sometimes of uncertain quality. You may not get much benefit and you risk severe liver damage. I recommend only regular niacin or—better still—Niaspan, and strongly advise against long-acting (SR) niacin, which is dangerous, and no-flush niacin, which is ineffective.

The rationale behind combination therapy

With many medications, including statins, when dosage is increased the benefits also increase but at a *diminishing* rate. Side effects, by contrast, increase at an *accelerating* rate. Thus, typically, the benefit-to-risk ratio, benefit-to-cost ratio, and benefit-per-milligram ratio all rise at a diminishing rate when dosage is raised. This means the first few milligrams often offer the biggest bang for the buck. Lower doses often form a medication's "sweet spot."

Besides the issue of diminishing benefits per milligram, medications have different strengths. Niacin, for example, is not very effective in lowering LDL, unlike statins, but it is very effective with other kinds of lipid management. Other examples: Niaspan is twice as effective in raising HDL as gemfibrozil (Lopid)— 26% versus 13%—but less potent than gemfibrozil in lowering triglycerides (30% versus 40%). Ezetimibe reduces the amount of *dietary* cholesterol your body absorbs, which is different from the way statins or niacin work. To take advantage of the diverse strengths of different medications, as well as the high benefit-to-risk that occurs at lower doses, it often makes more sense to combine several medications, each at a relatively low dose, than for a physician to prescribe one single medication at a high dose.

Combination therapy is widely used to manage hypertensive and diabetic patients, as well as other patient groups such as those who are HIV-positive. This is equally true for dyslipidemia, especially among Indians, whose lipoproteins often have qualitative and quantitative abnormalities. Because niacin is weak in lowering LDL, the principal target of dyslipidemia treatment, it is often used in combination with other lipid-lowering agents, particularly statins. Statins, on the other hand, are highly effective in bringing a patient's LDL down to as low as 60 or 70mg/dL, but the corresponding reduction they achieve in coronary events is only on the order of *25% to 40%*. It did not take long for physicians to realize that a "cocktail" of drugs that *raise* HDL as well as *lower* LDL might reduce coronary events by 60% to 90% (*see* Table 8.6). This, indeed, is exactly what studies have shown. The trend today is, therefore, to add a second drug to a moderate dose (20-40mg) of a statin.

The AIM-HIGH Study Niacin-Statin Combination Therapy Gains Momentum

In July 2005 Kos Pharmaceuticals, the makers of Niaspan® (extended-release niacin), began a major six-year study to see if combining Niaspan with simvastatin, the second most widely prescribed statin, is more effective than just taking the statin by itself in preventing cardiac events such as heart attacks and strokes in people with coronary artery disease who have low HDL and high triglyceride levels but have attained their LDL goals.

Called AIM-HIGH, the two-country, multi-center, double-blind study follows up on previous smaller studies such as HATS and ARBITER-2 that have shown that niacin-statin combinations are effective in controlling abnormal lipids; but AIM-HIGH, funded by the NIH, is the first truly large-scale study of its kind. The decision to launch it recognizes what physicians have increasingly come to believe—that lowering LDL alone is not enough to stave off cardiovascular disease. Many people with heart disease, or metabolic syndrome, or a history of recurrent heart attacks, have abnormal lipid levels and require broad improvement in their entire lipid profile beyond just reducing their bad cholesterol level. Combining Niaspan and a statin is currently one of the most promising approaches to multi-pronged lipid intervention.

In addition, the American Heart Association stated in its 2004 guidelines that, of the two sexes, women are at even greater cardiac risk than men when they have low HDL levels. To slow down atherosclerosis and reduce their risk, women need even higher HDL levels (at least 50mg/dL) than men do (at least 40mg/dL).

More and more treating physicians are becoming convinced of the efficacy of combination therapy, and the FDA has already approved Advicor, which integrates Niaspan and lovastatin. With 3,300 patients at 60 clinical trial sites, however, AIM-HIGH is larger and more ambitious than earlier studies and should be scientifically more definitive. The acronym AIM-HIGH stands for "Arterial Biology for the Investigation of the Treatment Effects of Reducing Cholesterol conducted by Walter Reed Army Medical Center."

Niacin-Statin Combination Therapy: How well does it work?

What are the most common combinations? Niacin can be combined with resins and statins to produce marked improvements in lipoprotein levels. Combining simvastatin and niacin (as in the HATS study) has been shown to partially reverse coronary atherosclerosis and reduce coronary events by 60% to 90%. A provocative finding in HATS was that taking vitamins C and E supplements partially negated the benefits of statins and niacin. Those, who took these supplements along with simvastatin and niacin, had only a 60% reduction in coronary events, compared to 90% in those, who took just simvastatin and niacin.

Diminishing Returns
A limitation of statins is that higher doses offer diminishing returns. Doubling the dose doubles the side effects (and cost) but increases the benefits by only 7%. The first 10mg of Lipitor, for example, lowers LDL by 34%. It takes the next 70mg to lower LDL by an additional 21%. Answer? Lower doses of statins in combination with other therapies such as niacin.

As mentioned in the previous section of this Chapter, the FDA has recently approved a combination of Niaspan and lovastatin for dyslipidemia, called Advicor. In one study, taking a daily dose of Advicor 2000/40—meaning 2000mg Niaspan plus 40mg lovastatin—raised HDL by 41%. It also lowered LDL by 47%, triglycerides by 41%, Lp(a) by 25%, LDL/HDL ratio by 58%, TC/HDL ratio by 48%, and CRP by 24% (see Table 8.7). No cases of myopathy were reported, and liver function abnormalities—that is, levels three times the upper limit of normal—were observed in only 1 out of 200 cases.

Data from several studies, taken together, suggest that combining 2g of Niaspan with any statin is as effective in lowering LDL as quadrupling the statin dose (from, for example, 20mg to 80mg), while combining 1g of Niaspan with any statin is, in its LDL-lowering effect, like doubling the statin. This suggests that when it is necessary to go beyond a moderately low dose of a statin, it makes more sense to add niacin to it than to increase the dose of the statin, particularly because niacin has other benefits as well.

The benefit of raising HDL has received less attention than that of lowering LDL. The reduction in cardiac risk gained by raising HDL to over 60 is estimated to be 50%. By comparison, the risk reduction from lowering LDL to below 100 is 38 to 46%. The potent effects of niacin on HDL should be particularly welcome to Indians, who tend to have low HDL.

Another study, the ADVOCATE Study (see Table 8.8), compared Advicor (lovastatin plus Niaspan) to Lipitor and Zocor, two popular statins, at different doses (20 and 40mg). The results indicate that Advicor

Table 8.6. Preventing Coronary Events: Statin Alone versus Combination Therapy

Study	Alone or in combination	Events prevented	Events not prevented
Prospective Study of Pravastatin in Elderly at Risk (PROSPER)	Statin alone	15%	85%
Myocardial Ischemia reduction with aggressive cholesterol lowering (MIRACL)	Statin alone	16%	84%
The Long-Term Intervention with Pravastatin in Ischemic Disease (LIPID) Study	Statin alone	24%	76%
Cholesterol and Recurrent Events Trial investigators (CARE)	Statin alone	24%	76%
Heart Protection Study	Statin alone	24%	76%
West of Scotland Coronary Prevention Study (WOSCOPS)	Statin alone	29%	71%
Anglo-Scandinavian Cardiac Outcomes Trial—Lipid Lowering Arm (ASCOT-LLA)	Statin alone	21%	79%
Scandinavian Simvastatin Survival Study (4S)	Statin alone	34%	66%
Aggressive Lipid-lowering therapy compared with angioplasty in stable coronary artery disease. Atorvastatin Versus Revascularization Treatment (AVERT)	Statin alone	36%	64%
Air Force/Texas Coronary Atherosclerosis Prevention Study (AFCAPS/TexCAPS)	Statin alone	37%	85%
Arterial Biology for the Investigation of the Treatment Effects of Reducing Cholesterol (ARBITER-2)	**Combination**	**60%**	**40%**
HDL Atherosclerosis Treatment Study (HATS) with vitamin C and E	**Combination**	**60%**	**40%**
HDL Atherosclerosis Treatment Study (HATS) without vitamin C and E	**Combination**	**90%**	**10%**
The Familial Atherosclerosis Treatment Study (FATS)	**Combination**	**73%**	**27%**

Source: Enas, EA. Ref. 8.11

1000/40 lowers LDL more effectively than does 20mg of Zocor, and nearly as effectively as 20mg of Lipitor—but with far superior effects on Lp(a), triglycerides, and HDL, especially the most cardioprotective portion of your HDL, large-particle HDL. Likewise, Advicor 2000/40 lowers LDL more than 40mg of Zocor does, but not as effectively as Lipitor 40mg. Again, however, Advicor 2000/40 has superior effects on several other lipoproteins besides LDL. These additional benefits suggest that it often makes more sense to combine niacin with a statin than just to raise the dose of the statin by itself.

> Several studies show that combining 1 gram of Niaspan with any statin lowers LDL an additional 6-7%. This is comparable to the lowering achieved by doubling the statin dose (e.g., from 20mg to 40mg). Similarly, combining 2g of Niaspan with a statin is comparable in LDL-lowering effect to quadrupling the statin dose: It lowers LDL by an additional 14-16% beyond statin only.

Advicor also appears to be safer and somewhat more effective than the combination of Zocor and the fibrate Tricor. In the SAFARI Study, 20mg of Zocor taken with 160mg of Tricor reduced patients' triglycerides by 43% and LDL by 31% and increased their HDL by 19%. These results are roughly comparable to those of Advicor 1000/40mg: the Zocor-Tricor combination was more effective in lowering triglycerides but less effective in lowering LDL. The Zocor-Tricor medication, however, was associated with liver function abnormalities in 3% to 4% of patients, compared to just 0.5% reported for Advicor. The liver function abnormalities with Advicor were similar to or lower than those observed with Lipitor and Zocor in the ADVOCATE study.

Note, finally, that Vytorin—a combination of the statin Zocor with another cholesterol-absorption inhibitor, Zetia—is especially effective in lowering LDL (54% in studies), although somewhat less effective in lowering triglycerides or in raising HDL. Vytorin may, therefore, be a particularly effective combination drug to prescribe to people who are genetically already predisposed to having low triglycerides and high HDL, such as African Americans and other blacks, but not Indians, who tend to have high triglycerides and low HDL.

Giving niacin to diabetics with dyslipidemia

A third to two-thirds of patients with heart disease are also diabetic or prediabetic. Until recently, physicians, therefore, tended not to treat heart disease patients with niacin for fear of increasing the blood sugar of patients who might be prediabetic. Several recent studies, however, have shown that niacin is safe for diabetics, if appropriate precautions are taken. The rise in blood sugar is in fact small, temporary, and easily managed by adjusting the person's diabetic medication.

Niacin is safe for diabetics, but how well does it work for them? The results of the Coronary Drug Project, published in 2005, show that taking 3 grams of niacin a day for five years offered similar benefits to nondiabetics as to those in the group who were subsequently found to be prediabetic or diabetic. Niacin re-

Table 8.7. Changes in Lipid Levels: Comparing Niaspan to Advicor

	Niaspan 2000mg	Advicor 2000/40
Triglycerides reduction	32%	42%
LDL reduction	16%	47%
HDL increase	24%	41%
Lipoprotein(a) reduction	25%	25%

Source: Kashyap, ML. Ref 8.23. Morgan, JM. Ref 8.32.

Table 8.8. The ADVOCATE and SAFARI Studies: Comparing the Combination Drug Advicor to Taking a Statin Alone

	LDL Reduction	Apo B reduction	Triglycerides reduction	Lipoprotein(a) reduction	HDL increase	HDL 2b (large-particle HDL) increase
Advicor 1000/40mg	-39%	-36%	-29%	-19%	+17%	+113%
Advicor 2000/40mg	-42%	-38%	-49%	-21%	+32%	+189%
Zocor 20mg	-35%	-27%	-15%	-1%	+8%	+43%
Zocor 40mg	-39%	-31%	-19%	no change	+7%	+42%
Lipitor 20mg	-45%	-36%	-30%	-2%	+4%	+24%
Lipitor 40mg	-49%	-40%	-31%	no change	+6%	+30%
Zocor 20mg + Tricor 160mg	-31%	NA	-43%	NA	+19%	NA
Vytorin 10/20 (Zetia 10mg + Zocor 20mg)	-54%	-41%	-24%	NA	+10%	NA

Source: Bays, HE. Ref 8.03. Grundy, SM Ref 8.17.

The Polypill: A Provocative Preventive Plan Based on Combination Therapy

In a provocative study published in June 2003 in the British Medical Journal, British medical scientists Nicholas Wald and Malcolm Law offered a very creative proposal: the introduction of a once-a-day combination pill, to be called the **Polypill**, that they believe could reduce coronary events by 88% and stroke by 80% in the general population. Somewhat like a multivitamin, the Polypill would have few side effects and would combine six drugs: a statin to lower LDL, aspirin to thin the blood, low doses of three blood pressure medications (an ACE inhibitor, a beta-blocker, and a diuretic), and finally folic acid to reduce homocysteine, which as we have seen is one of the emerging risk factors for heart disease.

Examining data from 759 trials involving 400,000 people, Professors Wald and Law project that if diabetics, people with cardiovascular disease, and everyone over 55 took the Polypill, it would benefit about a third of them. They would on average gain about 11 additional years of life free from a heart attack or stroke.

Whether or not the Polypill ever comes to market—studies are under way—its implications are strongly provocative. The basic idea behind it is that it makes sense to take a population-based, public health approach to heart disease. That is, it makes sense to have a disease-prevention program that focuses less on identifying only very ill individuals and offering them expensive treatments, and more on preventing cardiovascular disease across the board, even before people develop any symptoms. This can be achieved simply by concentrating on lowering people's risk factors—cholesterol, blood pressure, homocysteine, and blood-clotting function-based on what we already know about risk. It does not require testing every individual. Thus, giving the Polypill to millions of people, particularly older people, diabetics, and anyone in a high-risk group—every overweight Indian smoker, for example—would be like the drug equivalent of telling everyone to exercise, manage their weight, and eat a heart-healthy diet! One does not need to have several tests to know that prevention-oriented lifestyle modifications have a very high probability of being beneficial. The Polypill proposal, however, has run into very strong resistance from various parts of the health community.

duced their rates of coronary events and death to about the same degree. This held true even though the study used the latest, stricter definition of diabetics as people with fasting blood glucose above 126mg/dL and prediabetics as people with fasting blood sugar of 100 to 125. These were, in other words, "true" diabetics and prediabetics. Fibrates, by contrast, do not work very well for diabetics. In the BIP Study (Appendix B), taking bezafibrate did not reduce rates of coronary events and death among diabetics and prediabetics.

Managing niacin's side effects

- *Flushing and itching:* Both physicians and patients should learn what to do to reduce the unpleasant side effects of niacin such as flushing (heat and skin redness) and occasional itching. Even though these are not dangerous—flushing is just an effect of capillary dilation—they can be uncomfortable, and some people worried about what they might mean may decide to stop the medication altogether.

I tell patients in advance about the possibility for flushing when niacin is first initiated, and reassure them that, in virtually all cases, the sensation recedes in both frequency and intensity with use. To minimize flushing, nevertheless, start patients on a low dose—for example, 500mg of Niaspan or Advicor 500/20mg. I normally wait 2-3 months before increasing the dose, and after reevaluating the patient. Increase the dose gradually, up to 2000mg of Niaspan, or until all of the patient's lipid goals have been met. The full potential of niacin cannot be realized if the patient remains at the starting dose. Other rare side effects, however, can be more harmful. They include:

- *Muscle soreness and damage:* Unlike with statin-fibrate combinations, myopathy has not been a substantial problem in statin-Niaspan combinations, especially Advicor. Physicians should monitor the patient's liver functions every 3-6 months to ensure continued safety.

- *Uric acid levels:* All niacin except Niaspan can raise uric acid levels, which can lead to gout in a few individuals with a genetic predisposition to it, so your physician should check your uric acid level before starting you on niacin. People with high uric acid should take allopurinol along with niacin to prevent gout.

20 Do's and Don'ts for Doctors Who Want to Maximize Niacin's Benefits

What to give

1. Insist on prescription niacin, meaning niacin IR (regular niacin) or, even better, once-a-day extended-release niacin (Niaspan) or Advicor.
2. Warn the patient against using long-acting niacin (which is dangerous), no-flush niacin (has no benefit), or any niacin sold as a nutritional supplement.
3. Compared to regular niacin, flushing is reduced by 80% with Niaspan and 90% with Advicor.

Under what circumstances

4. When a patient has one or more of these conditions: low HDL, especially HDL2; a high proportion of small HDL; a high proportion of small LDL; high lipoprotein(a); or when a moderate dose of statins has not met the patient's LDL, triglycerides, and HDL goals.
5. When a patient has metabolic syndrome, including low HDL and high triglycerides, combine niacin with a statin.

How much to give

6. Start niacin at a low dose, increase it only gradually, and maintain or decrease the dose as long as the patient continues to find flushing uncomfortable.
7. If a patient must discontinue niacin for some reason (surgery, for example), niacin should be restarted at lower dose and gradually increased.
8. Don't forget to titrate the dose gradually, but limit Niaspan to 2 grams a day.

When to take it

9. Niacin IR is taken in 3-4 divided doses throughout the day.
10. Niaspan should be taken once nightly; advise against a morning or afternoon schedule.
11. Take low-fat snacks, low-fat yogurt, or Metamucil if Niaspan is taken at bedtime or if it is taken several hours after the dinner.
12. Regular users of aspirin should take it just before their niacin.

Flushing: What to do about it

13. Tell patients in advance about flushing of the skin and reassure them that it is a temporary, harmless effect of capillary dilation that will subside after the first few doses and disappear with continued use.
14. Remind patients that Niacin is in fact **10 times** safer than low-dose aspirin.
15. Anything that dilates arteries increases flushing: hot baths, spicy foods, MSG, caffeine, hot beverages, and alcohol, particularly red wine. These can be resumed once the body acclimates to niacin.
16. Warn against missing doses for more than a day or two; this causes flushing to resume, and with greater intensity.
17. Taking niacin after a meal, with yogurt, or an hour after a full dose of regular or chewable aspirin reduces flushing.
18. Consider switching the patient to Advicor instead of Niaspan if flushing persists.

What to avoid

19. Don't combine Niaspan and regular niacin.
20. Don't cut the Niaspan tablet or split the dose; both increase its side effects.

- *Homocysteine:* Homocysteine levels should also be checked before taking niacin. Like fibrates and some diabetic medications, niacin can increase homocysteine. People with high homocysteine can safely take niacin if they take a vitamin B-based homocysteine-lowering medication such as Foltx, Folgard, or Metanx (see Chapter III, Section 4).

- *Elevated liver enzymes:* Patients and physicians are often concerned about elevated liver enzymes in patients receiving niacin. Elevation of liver enzymes twice above normal is usually acceptable with careful mentoring, but three times normal is a reason to stop niacin. Many factors can contribute to elevated liver enzymes. Metabolic syndrome (prevalent in 25% of the population) and excess body weight (65% of the population) can both mildly elevate liver enzymes, as can alcohol. I usually advise people to stop alcohol altogether for at least six months if their liver functions are abnormal. Other individuals with elevated enzymes should be evaluated to see if diabetes or anti-depression medications are contributing to this.

- *Vasodilatory foods:* Avoid foods that dilate your blood vessels when you first go on niacin because this can magnify the flushing sensation. This means spicy foods, MSG, alcohol, caffeine, and hot beverages. Hot baths also dilate your vessels. After a few months, you can resume these as your body gets used to niacin.

KEY · POINTS · IN · A · NUTSHELL

- ♥ Niacin (vitamin B3) is a broad-spectrum agent that is very effective in treating dyslipidemia because it has a favorable effect on all the lipoproteins: HDL, LDL, VLDL, and triglycerides.

- ♥ It is the only medicine currently available that lowers lipoprotein(a).

- ♥ Niacin is the most effective agent for boosting your levels of large-particle HDL, the most cardio-protective type of HDL and lowering small, dense LDL, the most dangerous type.

- ♥ Along with its effect on lipids, niacin not only slows down atherosclerosis but induces regression of atherosclerotic plaques, thereby significantly reducing morbidity and mortality from heart disease.

- ♥ Particularly in combination with other lipid-lowering therapies such as statins, niacin can reduce the risk of heart attack, stroke, and death by 60% to 90%.

- ♥ Niacin sold as a nutritional supplement may not provide the benefits achieved with prescription niacin.

- ♥ Do not confuse extended-release niacin (Niaspan®) with sustained-release, modified-release, timed-release, or long-acting niacin. Extended-release niacin, taken once a day, is the best form of niacin by a substantial margin.

- ♥ Sustained-release, modified-release, timed-release, or long-acting niacin is potentially dangerous and should be avoided because it can cause serious liver damage. It is not FDA-approved.

- ♥ Standard (immediate-release) niacin causes the most itching and flushing of the skin, needs to be taken several times a day, and is, therefore, not as patient-friendly as Niaspan.

- ♥ No-flush niacin has no serious side effects, but tests also show that it contains no niacin.

- ♥ Flushing, a sensation of heat accompanied by skin redness, can be irritating but is harmless, and usually abates with continued use and with aspirin.

- ♥ Itching and flushing are milder with Niaspan®, an FDA-approved extended-release niacin that also does not result in liver damage, and milder still with Advicor, a niacin-statin combination.

8.3 ▶ Other Medications and Devices

The dramatic decline in cardiovascular disease in the US in the second half of the 20th century was brought on partly by advances in medications that could control cholesterol, blood pressure, and diabetes. Many of these medications have been addressed in preceding sections of this Chapter. This section highlights medications and devices not addressed before.

PRESCRIPTION MEDICINES

Anticoagulants

Anticoagulants, as the name implies, reduce the ability of blood to clot, or coagulate. In other words, they are blood thinners. Two commonly used ones are as Coumadin (warfarin) and Panwarfin (Dicumarol). Anticoagulants are often used to prevent stroke in people with atrial fibrillation, a condition where the upper chambers (atria) of the heart quiver in a haphazard way instead of pumping rhythmically (discussed in Chapter I, Section 1). As a result, the atria do not effectively pump all the blood down into the ventricles. The blood left behind can pool along the atrial walls and form clots, which can dislodge and travel out of the heart into the rest of the body. If one of these travels toward the brain and gets stuck—for instance, in the carotid artery that supplies blood to much of the brain—it can cause a disabling ischemic stroke. About 15% of all strokes are caused by atrial fibrillation—a condition that affects 2-4% of all adults older than 60 and more than 10% of those older than 80. Other conditions where blood thinners are used include a history of blood clots in the leg or lung, mechanical heart valves, dilated cardiomyopathy (where an enlarged heart cannot pump effectively), severe heart failure, and occasionally for someone who has had a massive heart attack.

Aspirin and Plavix: The antiplatelet medications

Anticoagulants inhibit clotting by preventing the liver from using vitamin K to produce clotting proteins. Antiplatelet drugs, by contrast, also prevent unwanted clotting but they do this by interfering with the normal function of platelets. Platelets are small, disk-shaped pieces of cells that clump together to form a blood to clot. When you cut yourself, platelets rush in and amass like little beavers trying to plug up a leaking dam. However, this amazing ability of platelets to clump together and do "damage control" can, in other circumstances, cause unwanted excessive clotting. This can lead to acute coronary syndrome (ACS) or cause complications during and after coronary angioplasty and stent. Since antiplatelet drugs can also interfere with *normal* clotting, dangerous bleeding can occur if they are used carelessly. Unlike anticoagulants, antiplatelet agents do not require frequent monitoring. Two common antiplatelet agents are aspirin and Plavix:

Getting Blood Thinning Right

Anticoagulants need to be monitored because you do not want your blood to become too thin. Excessively thin blood is as dangerous as excessive clotting because it can cause internal bleeding and even stroke (see also aspirin, below).

Until recently, doctors used a test called prothrombin time, or **protime**, to precisely adjust the amount of anticoagulant you need by measuring the levels of certain factors needed for clotting that are present in your blood. Protime, however, has been superseded by the International Normalized Ratio (**INR**). INR is more sensitive because it takes into account the differences in the strengths of the compounds used in this test itself.

Using an anticoagulant is a balancing act because many commonly used medications, including aspirin and Tylenol, can influence the results that protime and INR give.

Table 8.9 Minor, major, and life-threatening bleeding complications from aspirin per 1,000 people

Bleeding Category	Specific complications	Bleeding per 1,000
Major bleeding	Hemorrhagic strokes	1
	Death	2
	Requiring 4 or more units of blood	10
	Requiring 2-3 units of blood	9
	Total major bleeding	27
Minor bleeding	Not requiring blood	24
Minor and major bleeding combined		41

Source: THE CURE Study

Table 8.10 . Major bleeding complications with different dose of aspirin and Plavix per 1,000 people

Aspirin dose	Aspirin alone	Aspirin plus Plavix
Less than 100 mg	20	26
100 -200 mg	23	35
More than 200 mg	40	49

Source: The CURE Study

▶ **Aspirin** A time-tested drug that has found new uses, aspirin is the most common antiplatelet agent. Although it can be purchased without a prescription, aspirin is also the world's most widely prescribed cardiovascular medication. Some 30 million Americans, it is estimated, take aspirin daily for cardiac protection. In high-risk individuals, aspirin is associated with a 25% reduction of heart attack. It also prevents stroke and is just as good as, and safer than, Coumadin (warfarin).

• **Risks:** Although aspirin is recommended for all heart disease patients in the absence of such contraindications as a prior history of severe gastrointestinal bleeding, it has its dangers. It can cause gastrointestinal complications and bleeding, resulting occasionally in the need for a transfusion or even death. In fact, *in low-risk individuals aspirin's risks may outweigh its benefits*. Taking aspirin prevents only one heart attack in every 1000 low-risk, healthy persons, compared to 40 to 80 coronary events in every 1000 high-risk people. Studies such as a recent meta-analysis of 31 clinical trials involving 192,036 patients show that these complication rates do not vary significantly whether the dose is 75mg or 325mg. High doses (500mg to 1,500mg) are more gastrotoxic yet no more effective than small and medium doses.

• **Gender:** Women benefit less than men from using aspirin to prevent a first heart attack. The Women's Health Study, the first large trial of aspirin to prevent a first heart attack in women, nearly 40,000 women each received a dummy pill or 100mg of aspirin every other day for 10 years. There was a 24% reduction in strokes, but the results failed to show any reduction in heart attack risk (*see box*). Among women older than 65, there was a 26% reduction in cardiovascular events. Even though the women received the very small doses, however, the risk of gastrointestinal bleeding that required transfusion was 40% higher among the aspirin group than in the control group.

• **Ethnicity:** Severe intestinal bleeding and death from taking daily aspirin is not that common, but it is more common among Asians than whites. A 81mg dose may thus be more appropriate for Indians and other Asians who are at risk for heart disease.

▶ **Plavix (Clopidogrel):** Plavix is slightly more effective than aspirin in preventing blood clot as an antiplatelet agent, and is used in people who are resistant to, intolerant of, or allergic to aspirin. It is also given in combination with aspirin to those who have had angioplasty or stent placements. The downside is that Plavix costs 100 times more.

Other heart medications

▶ **Digoxin:** For much of the 20th century, Digoxin was the most common cardiac medication and considered the "vitamin of the heart." Its use waned as safer, more powerful drugs such as ACE-inhibitors and beta-blockers emerged for treating heart failure (see Chapter VI, Section 1 and Chapter VII, Section 4). Calcium blockers have also replaced Digoxin for treating atrial fibrillation. These newer agents have a wider therapeutic window and other benefits, such as lowering blood pressure.

▶ **Nitroglycerine:** Nitroglycerine dilates blood vessels, including the coronary arteries, thereby relieving chest pain caused by stable angina. This makes it dangerous to use in combination with erectile dysfunction medicines such as Viagra, Levitra, and Cialis, because nitroglycerine lowers blood pressure. It is available in the form of a spray, a paste, or a tablet you put under your tongue.

An Aspirin a Day Does it Help or Harm?
In low-risk people, aspirin's risks may outweigh its benefits. For instance, it is estimated that 100mg of aspirin taken every other day for 10 years by **1000 low-risk women** with a 10-year heart disease risk of 3% would prevent three ischemic strokes but no heart attacks or deaths. It would also cause between 0 and 3 hemorrhagic strokes and one case of serious stomach bleeding. Taken together, the overall benefit of taking aspirin regularly is thought to be somewhat harmful, except in high-risk women with multiple risk factors.

CONTROVERSIAL NONPRESCRIPTION MEDICINES

A number of nonprescription medications and supplements have drawn controversy. This subsection looks at the most important ones.

Nutritional supplements

Americans spend billions on dietary supplements, many of which are as yet unproven in large, formal clinical trials. The benefits of many popular supplements—including co-enzyme Q-10 and various Chinese and Indian herbal medicines—are yet to be demonstrated in controlled clinical trials, and their use by patients who really should be taking prescription medications is strongly discouraged. Some of them may have unintentional harmful consequences, and many can interact or interfere with prescription medications, either diminishing their effectiveness or *increasing their toxicity.*

▶ Antioxidants

Antioxidant pills are an example of the controversy surrounding supplements. Everyday, our bodies produces harmful substances called free radicals as a bi-product of normal bodily processes. Free radicals travel throughout the body and cause oxidation—meaning they add oxygen atoms to cells. Oxidation causes extensive tissue damage at the cellular level. Part of this oxidation occurs in your arteries when LDL cholesterol is oxidized. LDL oxidation is a chemical process similar to rusting, and is a key step in atherosclerosis and plaque buildup. Our weapon against oxidation is antioxidants. Antioxidants are powerful disease fighters—including heart disease—because they neutralize the free radicals that cause cellular oxidation and damage. Several vitamins and minerals are antioxidants—including vitamins A, C, and E and beta carotene.

Some but not all studies have shown the beneficial effects of taking vitamin C supplements. Numerous studies on vitamin supplementation, however, has failed to show any benefit in using vitamin E, and recent studies even indicate potential danger. A meta-analysis of 135,967 participants in 19 clinical trials undertaken between 1966 and 2004 showed an increased rate of death in those who received more than 150 units (IUs) of vitamin E per day. Among those who received smaller doses (less than 400 units), there was an excess of 16 deaths per 10,000 persons. This rose to 39 per 10,000 persons among those who received more than 400 units a day. These data suggest that the potential harm may outweigh the benefits in those taking more than 150 units of vitamin E. In principle, whether we take them as vitamin supplements or get them from a diet rich in fruits, whole grains and vegetables, antioxidants from any source should be highly protective of heart disease. In practice, however, the results are highly inconclusive about antioxidants in the form of supplements (*see box*).

By contrast, the evidence that a diet rich in antioxidant-containing foods protects against atherosclerosis and heart disease is much clearer and more convincing. Fruits, whole grains, and vegetables—particularly dark orange, red, and green leafy vegetables—contain not only vitamins

---

Nutritional Supplements versus Medications: A Crucial Difference

What's in a name? As it turns out, sometimes a lot. Federal laws give makers of **nutritional supplements** much more leeway to make unproven claims about their health benefits than if the company were marketing a **medication**. For something to earn the right to call itself a "medication" that has been proven therapeutically effective, it must pass through the FDA's strict approval processes in a lengthy, controlled trial.

By contrast, any label on any supplement can claim to be a "tonic that will purify your blood," or promise to help you lose weight in just one area of your body, reverse the aging process, cure cancer, give you energy, or improve your mental performance—all with no real scientific proof. Numerous supplements even vary in quality from bottle to bottle.

Of course, many supplements are not harmful, and some may be quite beneficial. Yet because the laws governing them are so lax, you do not necessarily know what you are getting, or getting into. Unscrupulous companies know this, and sadly, many are willing to prey on the public's desperation to grab onto dramatic but often unverified claims about anything that will help them feel or get better.

What's Wrong with Mixing Nutritional Supplements and Prescription Medications?

What's wrong? As comedian Bill Cosby rhetorically asks in the TV ads for Kodak camera film, Who knows? That is precisely the problem. Drug interactivity is a vast, complex field, and not enough research has been done in the area of health food supplements and their interactions with prescription and nonprescription medications. Many people simply take both, hoping for the best, but it is a shot in the dark.

An analogy is that of adding lemon juice to milk. Millions of tea drinkers in the West add lemon, whereas Indian tea drinkers typically add milk. From this, it might seem logical that, since both lemon and milk are good with tea, you can mix the two. Of course, you would simply end up with curdled undrinkable tea—an unexpected interaction between two independently good things.

Similarly, in the area of health-store supplements, millions are looking for the elixir of life and are willing to experiment, believe, and pay. But better safe than sorry. The real elixir of life they are looking for is what physicians have been telling patients for years: healthy nutrition, weight management, exercise, stress control, anger management, smoke-free lungs, fresh clean air, medical checkups, and careful adherence to prescription medications—if and when you need to take them.

and minerals but also flavonoids, lycopenes, and other nutrients and phytochemicals that swarm through the body, fighting disease and oxidation on several levels. In all, the evidence thus far suggests that supplements are no substitute for eating a diet rich in a wide variety of antioxidants and other disease-fighting agents, along with staying physically active, maintaining a normal weight, managing stress, and avoiding smoking. Since it is not clear whether supplements help and since some of them may actually cause harm, the use of antioxidant supplements is discouraged.

▶ Garlic

There is conflicting data that garlic can lower cholesterol and blood pressure. The active preventive ingredient in garlic is destroyed within minutes of cooking.

▶ Fish oil supplements

Fish oil containing omega-3 fatty acids can reduce the risk of sudden death by 50%, and triglycerides by 30% in people, with high triglycerides. Commercially available fish oil preparations, however, vary in quality.

Some studies show that taking vitamin C can benefit you, but many studies on vitamin supplementation have failed to show any benefit in using vitamin E, and some even indicate potential danger.

▶ Herbal medications

Like antioxidant supplements, the use of herbal and homeopathic remedies has risen dramatically in the last few decades. This poses a concern to treating physicians because of the potential for adverse interactions with prescription medications, including those for cardiovascular disorders. It is a well-known principle in pharmacology that medicines frequently interact with each other by either boosting or depressing the rate at which your body processes the active ingredient in another medicine. Insufficient data exist not only about the efficacy of some of the most widely used herbs, including echinacea, garlic, ginseng, gingko biloba, ephedra, and **St. John's Wort** (*Hypericum perforatum*).

Some herbal remedies can increase the potency of prescription drugs. Still others decrease the effectiveness of blood pressure medications, or increase blood pressure themselves. **Ginkgo Biloba**, for example, raises blood pressure when taken with a thiazide diuretic. Some herbs can deplete blood potassium, potentially leading to a fatal case of arrhythmia. **Siberian ginseng** (*Eleutheroccus senticosus*) increases the serum concentration of digoxin, leading to toxicity. St John's Wort has been found to decrease the blood concentrations of digoxin and coumadin. Some herbs interfere with tests for thyroid function, leading to mistaken diagnosis of overactive or underachieve thyroid. In addition to **coenzyme Q10's** potential interaction with warfarin, there is currently no scientifically-based evidence that this supplement prevents cardiovascular events, although many vendors are touting it as "good for the heart."

Finally, there is little public awareness of the potential for liver toxicity from herbal and dietary supplements. In a study of 20 liver transplant patients whose livers had failed, conducted at a tertiary-care university hospital, 50% of the liver failures were attributable to supplements or herbs toxic to the liver. Among them, supplement use accounted for more cases of severe liver failure than viral hepatitis. If you are taking or have taken herbal products and nutritional supplements in the past year, make sure you give a complete list of them to your physician.

COMPLEMENTARY AND ALTERNATIVE MEDICINE

Complementary and alternative medicine—or CAM, for short—embraces a broad range of treatment systems and culturally-based healing traditions—from acupuncture and yoga to chiropractic and Ayurvedic medicine; from prayer and meditation to hypnosis and biofeedback; from naturopathy and homeopathy to herbal medicine, vitamin supplements, and massage therapy. There is no agreed upon definition of CAM, but for working purposes, it can be defined as a diverse group of healthcare practices, interventions, and products that are currently not regarded as part of mainstream medicine and are neither generally available in hospitals nor taught widely in medical schools. More importantly, these practices and products generally lack the level and kind of scientific evidence of their safety and efficacy that would make them acceptable in mainstream medical practice.

As a cardiologist, I cannot endorse a majority of the methods of CAM; yet the truth is that the range of therapies is so diverse that no single sweeping statement can be made about all of them. In Section 8 of Chapter V, for example, I recommend yoga as part of a balanced physical activity program. Conventional medicine has already embraced many of the principles espoused in complementary and alternative systems, including stress reduction techniques, the emphasis on achieving a balance between nutrition, exercise and the other activities of your life, and the "holistic" idea that the body is a single, interrelated organism so that what you do to one part of it can affect other organ systems. Our medical knowledge is constantly growing; it does not stay static. Purging and blood-letting have given way to antibiotics and MRI. Even within cardiology itself, knowledge that was once considered controversial or peripheral (newly emerging risk factors, for example) gradually becomes more accepted and mainstreamed over time—if it is legitimate.

Of course, sometimes there are cultural biases and other reasons why conventional medicine resists doing more research on therapies that are widely used in other parts of the world. The overarching point, however, is that a good deal of previously "alternative" medicine is no longer alternative because conventional medicine has accepted it! Yet at the same time, mainstream medicine must continue being cautious and drawing distinctions, because wisdom from 3000 years ago is not necessarily always wisdom just because it is old. The real science underlying a practice must be identified and separated from ancillary beliefs and philosophies before it is incor-

---

Supplement Studies Range from Disappointing to Discouraging

Several studies, including a very large meta-analysis undertaken by The Cleveland Clinic and published in Lancet in 2004, have not been able to show conclusively that antioxidant vitamins and beta carotene in supplement form can reduce heart disease or cancer. The Cleveland Clinic researchers, who analyzed 15 large randomized trials of vitamin E and beta carotene supplements involving some 220,000 patients, concluded they could find no clear cardiovascular benefits to taking vitamin E supplements among any patient populations. Regarding beta carotene, they expressed concern that beta carotene supplementation was actually statistically associated with a small but significant increase in all-cause mortality and a slight increase in cardiovascular deaths. Other studies suggest that certain supplements may paradoxically act as pro-oxidants, actually promoting oxidation under certain conditions.

These are provocative findings, considering that millions of people personally spend hundreds and even thousands of dollars a year on nutritional supplements, and may feel disappointed by the conclusions. It is noted that the Cleveland Clinic meta-analysis was limited to vitamin E and beta carotene supplements, the two generally most studied antioxidants. Other studies are underway.

The point to be underscored, however, is that while abundant evidence exists that a diet naturally rich in antioxidants is highly beneficial, the evidence for antioxidant *supplements*—after numerous studies—is controversial, non-existent, ambiguous, or actually contradicted.

Complementary and Alternative Medicine
A Personal Viewpoint

I am often asked to comment on the role of complementary and alternative medicine in the prevention and control of heart disease. Clearly, there are many things we still do not understand about how the heart and body work, and how they interact with the mind. Our diagnostic and treatment paradigms are constantly expanding. There are remarkable cases, along with a vast body of anecdotal evidence, that "western" medicine often cannot explain.

As a result, there could well be preventive practices and therapeutic interventions from various traditions of complementary and alternative medicine that could some day enrich and even revise what we have learned about heart disease from conventional medicine. There are already several ongoing trials funded for example by the National Heart Lung & Blood Institute to test certain alternative therapies, and in non-cardiac medical specialties, one or two inroads have already been made.

Despite these initial forays, a true merging of the two healing traditions—if it will ever happen—is still quite far away. Because our knowledge is still so incomplete, there are at present no complementary or alternative therapies I recommend for heart disease prevention or control.

Some may regard this position as too cautious. The rationale for it is that I work in a medical specialty that does not have a great margin for error. Cardiology rarely allows you to go back and undo the harmful effects of a mistake you or a patient made in adopting an experimental approach or an untested procedure.

Our field thus tends to be conservative, cautious, rigorous, and intolerant of insufficiently tested hypotheses. To offer maximum protection to patients who have placed their lives in our hands, cardiology cannot proceed on compelling conjectures, rich traditions, or even persuasive anecdotal evidence. It must go on scientific facts as it sees them—but some of those facts may change in the future, as they have in the past.

porated into modern medicine. That process is slow, but it is ongoing.

Ayurvedic medicine

Birthed in India 3000 to 5000 years ago, Ayurvedic medicine is a comprehensive, holistic treatment system that combines yoga, aromatherapy, meditation, body cleansings, and herbal food supplements to maintain a balance of the life energies within each individual. The herbal preparations of Ayurvedic medicine are used by approximately 80% of India's one billion people and increasingly by Indians abroad, including in the US where they are sold as supplements that therefore fall outside FDA regulation. Although Ayurvedic medicines and herbal treatments are widely believed to be safe, more than an estimated one third of the 6,000 Ayurvedic supplements that exist contain harmful heavy metals. It is often purported that these medicines are "detoxified." However, a recent study of 70 of them, prompted by an unexplained seizure disorder in a child in Boston who had been taking Ayurvedic medicines, found that 14 contained toxic heavy metals such as mercury, lead, and arsenic. Some contained levels thousands of times above the limits permitted by the FDA and EPA.

Several studies show that many natural herbal supplements used in Ayurvedic and other traditional healing systems contain high levels of toxic heavy metals—such as mercury, lead, and arsenic—that could cause extensive but unrecognized harms to users after chronic long-term exposure.

In other studies in India and the UK, one-third to two-thirds of the Ayurvedic medicines tested contained unacceptably high levels of heavy metals. In addition, between 2002 and 2003 the Centers for Disease Control reported 12 cases of lead poisoning among adults, who had taken Ayurvedic medications. Traditional medicines from other countries and regions of the world—China, Malaysia, Mexico, Africa, and the Middle East—have also been shown to contain heavy metals.

Taken together, these are ominous signs. Many users of herbal medicines may unknowingly be at risk for heavy metal toxicity. The symptoms of chronic toxicity can be hard to recognize because they develop slowly and can be very similar to symptoms of other illnesses. The body cannot break down large amounts of heavy metals, so they accumulate in the soft tissues and become toxic. If you take Ayurvedic or other traditional herbal preparations and have had unexplained symptoms, discontinue them and discuss this with your physician immediately.

What are some common symptoms? **Mercury** toxicity can cause seizures and damage the central nervous system and kidneys. **Arsenic** can also damage the central nervous systems, produce inflammation in your nerves, and induce numbness, tenderness, a burning sensation, or tingling in your hands and feet. Long-term use of supplements that contain high levels of **lead** can cause nausea, allergies, mood swings, retardation, autism, dyslexia, arthritis, hyperactivity, lack of concentration, seizures, weight loss, trembling hands, muscular weakness, and paralysis in the forearms. Children are particularly sensitive to lead.

> **A Word about Terminology**
> The terms "complementary" and "alternative" medicine are often used interchangeably. In principle, however, complementary medicine refers to practices and products intended to be used *along with* conventional medicine. Alternative medicine refers to those intended to be used *instead of.*

CARDIAC DEVICES

Cardiac resynchronization therapy

Cardiac resynchronization therapy uses a specialized pacemaker to re-coordinate the action of the right and left ventricles in patients with severe heart failure. Early studies have demonstrated its ability to improve the symptoms and feeling of wellbeing of many patients with moderate to severe heart failure.

Enhanced external counter pulsation (EECP)

An EECP is a non-invasive treatment for patients who have refractory angina (chest pain) from end-stage heart disease and who therefore are not suitable candidates for coronary bypass surgery or angioplasty. Refractory angina refers to severe chest pain that is not relieved by optimal medical care. An EECP uses a special device to inflate and deflate a series of compressive cuffs that are wrapped around the patient's calves, lower thighs, and upper thighs. The cuffs increase coronary blood flow by rapidly inflating under high pressure at the end of diastole—the heart rest that occurs after every heart beat. The cuffs then rapidly deflate at the end of systole (after the heart has just finished pumping). EECPs have been shown to reduce angina and improve myocardial ischemia and quality of life in patients. Patients typically receive 35 treatments for one hour once a day over a seven-week period. EECPs have been approved by Medicare, and there is a strong demand for this treatment.

> **Watch for Potential Interactions when Taking Prescription Drugs**
> A major safety concern in taking alternative medicine products is the potential for adverse interactions with prescription medications, particularly drugs that have a narrow margin of safety, like warfarin. Herbal products that potentially increase the risk of bleeding, or may intensify the effects of warfarin therapy, include: Asafoetida, capsicum, celery, clove, fenugreek, garlic, ginger ginkgo, horse chestnut, licorice root, onion, parsley, passionflower herb, red clover, sweet clover, turmeric, borage seed oil, and willow bark.
>
> Products associated with documented reports of potential interactions with warfarin include coenzyme Q10, ginseng, green tea, papain, and vitamin E. American ginseng, for example, reduces the anticoagulant effect of Coumadin. Thus a wide range of alternative therapy products have the potential to interact with warfarin.

Implantable cardioverter defibrillator (ICD)

An ICD is a small, lightweight electrical device placed inside your body to keep track of your heart rhythm. You may be given an ICD if you have had a cardiac arrest or if you have a fast heart rhythm problem that could lead to a cardiac arrest. It is not a cure for the heart rhythm problem, but it can save your life by quickly controlling a dangerously fast heart rhythm (ventricular tachycardia and/or fibrillation). If you need an ICD, you will need it for the rest of your life. Recent studies suggest that people with severe ventricular dysfunction (meaning an ejection fraction below 35%) have a very high risk of cardiac arrest and benefit from an ICD. Medicare has recently approved this treatment, making 500,000 patients eligible for this expensive therapy (it costs about $40,000).

Pacemaker

A pacemaker is a battery-powered electronic device that is implanted just under the skin of the chest of a patient with a heart that has a "spark plug" or electrical system that is no longer functioning normally. One or two long thin wires, called leads, pass through a vein in the chest to the heart. The pacemaker electrically stimulates the heart to contract and pump blood. It keeps track of the patient's heart beat and generates small, electrical impulses when necessary to keep the heart beating at a normal speed and rhythm. Once the size of a deck of cards, today's pacemakers are the size of a small cookie.

KEY · POINTS · IN · A · NUTSHELL

♥ Unlike statins and niacin, the use of aspirin carries a small but significant risk from stomach bleeding and hemorrhagic stroke.

♥ In low-risk individuals, particularly women, these risks outweigh the benefits. In high-risk individuals with multiple risk factors, the benefits outweigh the risk.

♥ Currently, there is no evidence that taking antioxidant vitamin supplements has any beneficial effects.

♥ The liberal use of vitamin supplements can neutralize the therapeutic efficacy of many medications, particularly medicines that are used to optimize lipid levels.

♥ It is best to get all of your antioxidants, vitamins and minerals from fruits, vegetables and nuts rather than from nutritional supplements.

♥ The potential harm from taking vitamin E supplements in doses exceeding 150 IU a day outweighs its benefits.

♥ The safety, efficacy and drug interactions of herbal medicine and alternative medicine products have not been adequately researched, tested or validated. Some are implicated in heavy metal poisoning, liver failure, and bleeding complications.

♥ Like vitamin supplements, many of these products may interact with prescription medications, with a potential for serious harm and even death.

♥ People with severe ventricular dysfunction (meaning an ejection fraction below 35%) have a very high risk of cardiac arrest and benefit from an Implanted Cardioverter Defibrillator.

Appendix A ► Measuring the Impact of Heart Disease

Researchers employ a handful of different measures to quantify how much of a disease exists in a population. These measures all have different strengths and weaknesses. Some are more expensive than others; some are less subject to error than others. Regardless of whether one uses mortality rates, prevalence, the incidence rate, or the hospitalization rate, Indians all over the world turn out to have high rates of heart disease. This Appendix reviews the most commonly used measures of the impact of heart disease. The following is a quick summary of mortality, prevalence, incidence, and hospitalization rates:

1. The **mortality** rate, or **death** rate, of a disease is the estimated proportion of the population who have died from it over, for example, the past one year.
2. The **prevalence** of a disease is the population of people who are managing that disease at any given time. It offers a snapshot of the total number of people who currently have that disease in a particular population, regardless of when they first developed it. The prevalence is lower when the mortality is high, conversely, the prevalence increases as the people survive a heart attack.
3. The **incidence rate** of a disease, by contrast, refers to the number of new cases diagnosed each year. A seasonal disease such as the flu tends to have a high incidence rate because many new cases emerge each year, particularly in the winter months, but it has a low prevalence (total number) because people recover from it quickly. In contrast, a chronic, life-long disease such as heart disease or diabetes tends to have a relatively low annual incidence, but over time, it acquires high prevalence. Incidence is therefore a rate, while prevalence is a stock. If incidence is the rate at which water enters a bathtub from a faucet, prevalence is the total amount of water currently in the bathtub.
4. The **hospitalization** rate, or the number of new admissions, is a rough surrogate for the incidence rate.

COMMONLY USED MEASURES OF THE IMPACT OF A DISEASE IN A POPULATION

1. The Mortality Rate

The mortality or death rate, the most widely used measure of the overall health of a community, refers to the proportion of a population who have died from a particular disease over a given period. It is usually expressed per 100,000 persons per year. In the case of heart disease, it refers to the number of individuals dying from its complications, such as sudden death, heart attack, or heart failure. Mortality rate numbers are obtained from death certificates, which are included in the vital statistics of all developed countries and most developing countries.

Although mortality rates can readily be compiled for an entire country or population, the results are often more riddled with error than results from incidence data. Why is this? First, in gathering mortality data, the practice in most countries is not to record the ethnicity of the deceased person, only their country of origin.

Furthermore, often an undertaker, not the treating doctor, records the person's country of origin, frequently basing it merely on their last name and morphological features such as skin color, rather than consulting with the family members of the deceased. For example, a large study of neonatal deaths (deaths among babies younger than 30 days old) found a 30% error rate between the ethnicity documented on the birth certificate and death certificate.

The upshot of all this is that such errors can result in substantial overestimation or underestimation of death rates in a given ethnic group. It has been said, for example, that Filipino immigrants often enter the US as Filipinos and die as Hispanics. Why? Because many Filipinos have Hispanic-sounding last names or even just look Hispanic.

Another reason why mortality rates can be inaccurate is that crude mortality rates are not reliable when populations of widely differing ages are compared. Like inflation-adjusted prices, **age-adjusted mortality rates** make adjustments for the age differences between two populations that are being compared so that the comparisons are more meaningful. For example, India's overall population is younger than the US population. Just as you would not compare salaries from 1955 with salaries from 2005 without making adjustments for inflation and purchasing power, you would not compare mortality rates from India and the United States without adjusting for age differences, because age affects mortality rate. Another example: women develop and die from heart disease 10-15 years later than men. As a result, the death rates for women worldwide, once they are age-adjusted, are usually lower than those of men by one-third to one-half.

The important thing to bear in mind, however, is that in spite of the difficulties of gathering highly reliable mortality rates and the inaccuracies that can dodge the process, any which way you look at it, Indians emerge with some of the world's highest heart disease rates. Data from a 2004 study in California, for example, show that while death rates due to heart disease decreased 10-15% in the general population between 1990 and 2000, Indian women showed a 5% increase in deaths due to heart disease (see Chapter IV, Section 3).

Proportional Mortality Ratio

When it comes to mortality rates, there is another very useful number: It is called the **Proportional Mortality Ratio (or PMR)**. Like relative risk, PMR is a comparative figure. Unlike straightforward mortality rates, which just tells you how many people are dying from a particular disease within a specific population group, the *proportional mortality ratio* tells you how dangerous that disease is to that population group, as compared to the other things that kill people in that group. It tells you how large a contribution that disease is making to the overall death rate, and therefore how much people within a particular ethnic group should worry about this disease. Essentially, the PMR tells you how a disease *ranks* in order of importance.

The mortality rate for heart disease among Indians in the US, for example, is 50% higher than for the rest of the population. However, as compared with other killer diseases, heart disease ranks higher as a killer of Indians than in the rest of the general population, who tend to die from a greater variety of illnesses and other conditions. In fact, one major study shows that Indians younger than 45 and living in California have a PMR for heart disease *three times* higher than the rest of the state's population. This very high PMR figure tells us that compared with other population groups, Indians are dying from heart disease much more frequently than from other diseases and killers. In short, PMR is another indicator of the excess burden of heart disease compared to other causes of death.

Morbidity

Before we go on to consider the second major data collection concept, the incidence rate, let's take a brief look at another number related to the mortality rate: the morbidity rate. Morbidity refers to the effects of a disease short of death. It indicates the complications of a disease (other than death) that result in a reduced quality of life. Some of the results of morbidity include disability, hospitalization, loss of income, and medical care costs. Those who survive a major heart attack have greater morbidity than those who sustained just a small attack. Morbidity is an important concept because, while it does not result in death (mortality), it leaves you sapped of strength and vulnerable to a stream of complications.

2. The Incidence Rate

If the mortality rate measures how many people *have died* from a disease over a period of years, the incidence rate measures how many people *have been newly diagnosed* with the disease during that period. It is usually expressed per 100,000 persons per year. Researchers measuring the incidence of heart disease generally include how many

people have been hospitalized, and how many have had heart attacks, angina, or sudden death. Especially in the US, incidence also includes the number of people newly diagnosed with heart disease by coronary angiogram, as well as those undergoing coronary angioplasty and bypass surgery.

Of all the rates, incidence offers the best indicator of the need for greater preventive measures or, alternatively, the effectiveness of existing public health programs. However, because of the formidable cost of collecting incidence data over extended periods of time, incidence data are sparse in most countries, including India.

3. Prevalence

If the incidence rate estimates how many new cases of a disease have emerged over a certain number of years, prevalence tells us how many people have been diagnosed with the disease today, or at some specified point in time. Incidence studies collect data by taking a long-term view over a period of years and therefore show how the situation is changing over time. Prevalence takes a static snapshot of today. Because of this, prevalence data are useful in assessing how much medical and social care will be needed to cope with current cases.

Note that it is not so much the *prevalence* of a disease but rather its *incidence* rate that doctors and public health officials are trying to decrease. An example would help: Suppose 50% of the people in a community as HIV-positive as of today. That would indicate a very high prevalence of HIV; but what is more important is the incidence rate, which tells us *how many new cases* of HIV are being added to the list. Incidence tells us whether that 50% figure is going to increase rapidly, or slowly, or perhaps even decrease. Prevalence, by contrast, tells us the extent of the situation, and how much resources the government and medical community must commit to taking care of the ill.

The prevalence of heart disease is the percentage of the population who have survived a coronary event (meaning a heart attack, death, coronary

Commonly Used Measures of the Impact of a Disease in a Population

	Accuracy in yielding reliable data	Data collection costs	Usage within medical community	Comments
Mortality Rate	Often low	Very low	Most widely cited	Gives us a measure of a community's overall health
Incidence Rate	High	Very high	Hard to come by and thus not cited so often	Tells us how quickly new cases are emerging, and so how well a public health program is doing in preventing new cases of a disease
Hospitalization Rate	Moderate	Very low	Provides a crude substitute for incidence data	Gives us an indirect measure of the incidence of heart disease, but of course does not include those who die before reaching the hospital
Prevalence	Moderate	Moderately high	Widely cited measure	Tells us how bad things are at the current time, and thus the resources a community must commit to take care of the ill

angioplasty/stent, or bypass surgery). Mathematically, it is the incidence rate minus the death rate. Unlike incidence and mortality, prevalence is usually expressed per 100 or 1000. Note that prevalence—the percentage of people who have a disease—does not capture the number of people who have died from it. So prevalence figures can sometimes be artificially low if many people have already died from a disease that kills quickly, such as Ebola. That is one of the considerations that can potentially make prevalence figures less accurate.

Appendix B ▶ Major Heart Studies

ADVOCATE (the ADvicor Versus Other Cholesterol-Modulating Agents Trial Evaluation)

This study compared the relative efficacy of a once-daily niacin extended-release (ER)/lovastatin fixed-dose combination (Advicor) with standard doses of Lipitor and Zocor for 16 weeks. Advicor increased HDL significantly more than Lipitor or Zocor at all compared doses. Advicor also provided significant improvements in triglycerides, lipoprotein(a), apolipoprotein A-1, apolipoprotein B, and HDL subfractions. A total of 6% of study subjects receiving niacin ER/lovastatin withdrew because of flushing. No significant differences were seen among study groups in discontinuance due to elevated liver enzymes. No drug-induced myopathy was observed. Advicor 1000/40 mg was comparable to atorvastatin 10 mg and more effective than simvastatin 20 mg in reducing LDL, was more effective in increasing HDL cholesterol than either atorvastatin or simvastatin, and provided greater global improvements in non-HDL cholesterol, triglycerides, and lipoprotein(a). Advicor 2,000/40 mg lowered LDL by 42% versus 39% with the 40-mg dose of Zocor and 49% with Lipitor 40 mg/day.

AFCAPS/TexCAPS (Air Force/Texas Coronary Atherosclerosis Prevention Study)

In this study, Mevacor 20 to 40 mg daily or placebo (in addition to a low-saturated fat, low-cholesterol diet) were given to the total of 5,608 men and 997 women. These individuals had no heart disease and most of them had no cardiac risk factors. They had average cholesterol, but below average HDL. After a follow-up of five years, Mevacor reduced the incidence of a first heart attack and other coronary events by 37%. This study demonstrated the benefit of statins in preventing heart attack in people with low HDL without high cholesterol.

ARBITER Study (Arterial Biology for the Investigation of the Treatment Effects of Reducing)

This study tested the efficacy of aggressive lowering of LDL with 80 mg Lipitor, compared to moderate lowering of LDL with 40 mg of Pravachol on carotid intima-media thickness (CIMT). After 12 months of treatment, Lipitor lowered LDL to 76 mg/dL (49% reduction)

compared to 110 mg/dL in the Pravachol group (27% reduction). Lipitor, but not Pravachol, induced progressive regression of atherosclerosis. This study showed that marked LDL reduction with high dose Lipitor provides superior *efficacy for atherosclerosis regression* at one year.

ARBITER 2 Study (Arterial Biology for the Investigation of the Treatment Effects of Reducing Cholesterol)

This study was similar in design to ARBITER 1. It tested the efficacy of Niaspan 1000 mg added to heart disease patients being treated with a statin who had already achieved a low LDL level of 87 mg/dL. Addition of 1000 mg of Niaspan produced a 21% increase in HDL in one year. The addition of Niaspan to statin therapy slowed the progression of atherosclerosis among individuals with known heart disease and moderately low HDL. This was accompanied a 60% reduction in coronary events. Niacin reduces heart disease morbidity and mortality when taken either alone or in combination with statins. This study showed the additional benefit of adding niacin to a people already taking statins with well controlled LDL levels.

ARIC Study (Atherosclerosis Risk in Communities)

This is an ongoing prospective study of 14,502 Black and White middle-age adults in four different regions of the country. All participants were free of heart disease at the beginning of the study. Its main objective was to ascertain the White/Black differences in risk factors and their relationship to cardiovascular disease. This study has shown the lowest risk of heart disease occurs in women with **HDL above 80 mg/dL**. Women with HDL below 40 mg/dL have a five-fold risk compared to the former.

BIP Study (Bezafibrate Infarction Prevention)

The BIP study was a secondary prevention prospective double-blind study comparing bezafibrate, a fibrate, to placebo (fake pill). This study involving a total of 3,122 patients with heart disease and cholesterol level between 180 and 250 mg/dL, showed no reduction in coronary events. Diabetes and prediabetes were common in the BIP study participants and were predictive of a worse clinical outcome that was not reduced with bezafibrate treatment.

ASCOT BP LA (Anglo-Scandinavian Cardiac Outcomes Trial-Blood Pressure Lowering Arm)

This trial was designed to compare the outcome between those taking newer agents or standard treatment for blood pressure. The trial enrolled 19,257 hypertensive patients with at least three other risk factors. This study was terminated ahead of schedule because of the impressive benefit of Norvasc with or without Aceon (perindopril) over Atenolol with or without a diuretic. Although the blood pressure reduction was similar in both groups, there was a 10% reduction in heart attack and 14% reduction in death in the those treated with Norvasc. This study is expected to have important implications in the choice of medications in treating blood pressure

ASCOT LA (Anglo-Scandinavian Cardiac Outcomes Trial--Lipid-lowering Arm

This study aims to establish the benefits of lowering cholesterol in patients with well-controlled hypertension and average/below-average cholesterol concentrations, but without heart disease In the lipid-lowering arm of the study 10,305 hypertensive patients with no history of heart disease but at least three cardiovascular risk factors were randomly assigned to receive 10 mg atorvastatin or dummy pill. During a follow-up of 3 years, concentrations of LDL was 40 mg/dL lower in those allocated Lipitor compared with placebo. There were 116 major cardiovascular events or procedures in the Lipitor group and 151 events in the placebo group resulting in 23% reduction in relative risk. This study showed impressive benefit in lowering LDL in patients with out heart disease

Bogalusa Heart Study

This is an ongoing long-term study to determine the differences in prevalence of risk factors between White and Black children, as well as the relationship of these risk factors on the future development of heart disease as older adults. This study has shown that risk factors observed in children are strongly predictive of heart disease as young adults. It also showed that most obese children grow up to become obese adults.

BRFSS (Behavioral Risk Factor Surveillance System)

This is a state-based system of health survey established in 1984 by The Center for Disease Control and Prevention. Interviews are completed each year with more than 200,000 adults, making BRFSS the largest telephone health survey in the world. At the start of the new millennium, almost 60% of older adults without disabilities and 70% with disabilities were not obtaining a recommended amount of physical activity, which qualified for being sedentary.

CHS (The Cardiovascular Health Study)

This is an ongoing study of 4,775 adults 65 years or older (range, 65 to 98 years) and free of known cardiovascular disease at baseline in 1989 to 1990 to determine the prevalence of risk factors and their relation to cardiovascular disease in the elderly. Among other things, this study has shown consumption of fish one to four times per week was associated with a **27% lower** risk of stroke.

CADI Study (The Coronary Artery Disease in Indians Study)

This study was the first systematic study of heart disease among Indians in the US. It was commissioned by the American Association of Physicians of Indian Origin (AAPI). Unlike any other study among Indians, CADI Study participants were highly educated physicians and their family members. This study involved a total of 1,688 Indian physicians and their spouses, who attended national medical conventions of the AAPI. They had come from different parts of India, and had settled in different parts of the US. Thus, they were representative of the Indian physicians in the US, but not necessarily the overall Indian population. This study showed a **10% prevalence of heart disease** among these highly educated physicians and family members compared to 2.5% observed in the overall US population. It also showed a low prevalence of standard risk factors and a high prevalence of emerging risk factors among Indians.

CUPS (The Chennai Urban Population Study)

This is an epidemiological study involving two residential areas in Chennai in South India involving more than 1,000 adults. This study has provided valuable information on the prevalence of heart disease, diabetes, and metabolic syndrome in South India. This study showed an overall prevalence rate of heart disease of 11%. The prevalence of heart disease was 9% for those without diabetes or prediabetes, 15% for those with prediabetes, and 21% **in those with diabetes**. This study also showed a high prevalence of metabolic syndrome in the middle compared to the low income group.

CDP (The Coronary Drug Project)

This study was conducted between 1966 and 1975 to assess the long-term efficacy and safety of five lipid-influencing drugs in 8,341 men aged 30 to 64 years with previous a previous heart attack. The two estrogen regimens and thyroxine, which were first given to lower cholesterol, were discontinued early because of adverse effects. No evidence of efficacy was found for the fibrate treatment. Niacin treatment showed modest benefit in decreasing heart attack. With a mean follow-up of 15 years, nearly 9 years after termination of the trial, mortality in the niacin group was 11% lower than in the placebo group (dummy pills). Thus, niacin became the **very first** cholesterol lowering medication to show reduction in heart attack and death from all causes.

DPP (The Diabetes Prevention Program)

This study randomized 3,234 individuals with prediabetes to placebo (dummy pills), Glucophage 850 mg twice a day, or an intensive program of lifestyle modification (weight reduction of at least 7% plus moderately intense physical activity for at least 150 minutes weekly). The metformin reduced the incidence of new onset diabetes by 30% compared with placebo. This study demonstrated a **58% reduction** in the development of diabetes with lifestyle modification, which was nearly double the benefit of medication.

FATS (The Familial Atherosclerosis Treatment Study)

This study evaluated the effect of aggressive treatment of dyslipidemia in people with heart disease, high cholesterol, and elevated apo B (above 125 mg/dL). The aggressive therapy included lovastatin (20 mg twice a day) and colestipol (10g three times a day); niacin (1g four times a day). This study showed a coronary event reduction of 73%. The progression of mild narrowing of the coronary arteries to more advanced narrowing was reduced by 93%.

Framingham Heart Study and Framingham Offspring Study

The Framingham Heart Study is the oldest epidemiological study. More than 5,000 adults (every other adult in the entire village of Framingham, MA, population: ?10,000) was enrolled in 1948. They were given a detailed examination every two years, during which, various risk factors were ascertained by the most up-to-date scientific methods. All the original participants have since died; their children and spouses are now enrolled in the Framingham Offspring Study. These studies analyzed the relationship between smoking, blood pressure, high cholesterol, and other factors to heart attack, stroke, diabetes, and other diseases. More than 100 key papers on heart disease have been published in the past 5 decades from these studies. These results helprd develop the concept of cardiovascular risk factors, as well as identify all major traditional risk factors.

HATS (HDL Atherosclerosis Study)

This was a double-blind trial in 160 patients with heart disease, low HDL levels, and normal LDL levels. They were randomly assigned to receive one of four regimens: simvastatin plus niacin, antioxidant vitamins (C and E),

simvastatin-niacin plus antioxidants; or placebos. The end points were evidence of the regression and occurrence of a first cardiovascular event (death, myocardial infarction, stroke, or revascularization). This study showed Zocor plus niacin reduced the risk of heart attack and produced regression of the plaques in coronary arteries in patients with heart disease and low HDL levels. The use of antioxidant vitamin C and E partially negated the benefits.

Health Professionals Study

This ongoing prospective study involves long-term follow-up of nearly 52,0005 male health professionals (dentists, pharmacists, and optometrists, podiatrists etc.), who were free of major chronic disease, and completed baseline questionnaires in 1986. The purpose of this study was to ascertain the prevalence of risk factors and their relationship to future development of cardiovascular diseases (heart disease, stroke, diabetes, etc.) over an extended period of time. A 2005 report from this study showed a **waist size above 37 inches** may identify more people at risk of diabetes than the conventional cutpoint of 40 inches for abdominal obesity.

Heart Protection Study

This is the largest study to demonstrate the benefit of cholesterol-lowering medication in people without high cholesterol (as low as 140 mg/dL). Cholesterol lowering therapy with Zocor 40 mg/day reduced coronary events by 24%. This study helped to change the NCEP Guidelines by lowering the LDL target to below 70 mg /dL in very high risk patients. Among the more than 20,000 participants, a large representation was given for women, the elderly, and diabetics. This study showed that the overall side effects of Zocor 40 mg/ day given for a period of five years were **no higher** than those given placebo (dummy or fake pill) and helped reinforce the enormous safety record of statins (100 times safer than aspirin).

HOPE Study

This study randomly assigned 9,297 patients at high risk of cardiovascular events to receive double-blind Altase 10 mg/day or matching placebo for five years. This study conclusively demonstrated that Altase an angiotensin-converting enzyme (ACE) inhibitor reduces the risk of cardiovascular death, as well as the rate of development of heart attack, heart failure, and diabetes.

INTERHEART

This is a standardized case-control study of heart attack in 52 countries, representing every inhabited continent. 15,152 cases (heart attack patients) and 14,820 controls were enrolled. This study found that abnormal lipids, smoking, hypertension, diabetes, abdominal obesity, and psychosocial factors, account for most of the risk of a heart attack worldwide. Abnormal lipids and smoking were the strongest predictors of heart attack. A significant protective effect of consumption of fruits, vegetables, and alcohol, and regular physical activity were also documented.

Johns Hopkins Precursors Study

In this study, cholesterol levels were measured among 1,017 young men (mean age, 22 years) and followed for 27 to 42 years. The cholesterol level at age 22 was strongly associated with the risk of developing and dying from heart disease. A 36 mg/dL increment in total cholesterol, measured while in college, was associated with a two-fold increase in risk of heart attack 20 to 40 years later. This study also showed a three-fold risk of diabetes by age 45, among those who were overweight at age 25 compared to those with normal weight.

The Lipid Research Clinics Program Prevalence Study

This study showed HDL is 10 mg/dL higher in blacks than White. Despite obesity, blacks also have 40 to 50 mg/dL lower triglycerides. This anti-atherogenic lipid profile may explain the low rate of heart disease among blacks.

The Lipid Research Clinic Follow-up Study

This large study showed HDL to be a strong determinant of death among both men and women. An HDL increase of 1 mg/dL was associated with a decrease in cardiovascular death of 4% in men and 5% in women in 14 years.

MRFIT (The Multiple Risk Factor Intervention Trial)

This study examined the relationship of severity of risk factors to subsequent heart disease death in **316,099** men. One report specifically addressed the combined influence of blood pressure, cholesterol level, and cigarette smoking on death from heart disease over 12 years. Smokers with cholesterol and systolic blood pressure levels in the highest quintiles (20 percent) had heart disease death rates that were approximately 20 times higher than non-smoking men with systolic blood pressure and cholesterol levels in the lowest quintile. This study also showed men with **high grades of hostility** have double the risk of dying from heart disease than men with low hostility.

Muscatine Study

This is a study of 2,874 school children that began in 1971. Obesity in childhood was a strong predictor of adult obesity. Coronary risk factors measured in children and young adults predict the early development of coronary plaques. Adverse effects of risk factors beginning in childhood contribute to the lifetime risk of heart disease. The results of this study indicate that a child's cholesterol level is similar to his or her family members. A higher

cardiac mortality was observed among young relatives of children with high cholesterol levels. Death from heart disease was two-fold higher in male relatives and 10-fold higher in female relatives of children with high cholesterol (compared to children with low cholesterol levels). Therefore, a high cholesterol level in a child identifies families at risk of heart disease.

NAVIGATOR (Nateglinide and Valsartan in Impaired glucose Tolerance Outcome Research)

In this on-going trial, 43,509 nondiabetic persons were screened for detecting eligible patients with prediabetes to evaluate the efficacy of two medications in preventing the progression on to diabetes. Of these 9,125 had evidence of prior cardiovascular disease. Among those with prior cardiovascular disease, diabetes was detected in 24% and prediabetes in 41% after a glucose tolerance test. Of those with prediabetes, impaired glucose tolerance was two times more common (29%) than impaired fasting glucose (12%). This study confirmed the rule of 3 for presence of diabetes among nondiabetic people with heart disease - upon testing, one-third will be found to be diabetic, one-third will be prediabetic, and the remaining third will be truly nondiabetic. This trial underscores the preponderance and the significance of prediabetes and undiagnosed diabetes in people with cardiovascular disease.

NHIS (The National Health Interview Survey)

This survey provides information on the health status of the US civilian population through confidential interviews. This is the nation's largest household health survey and involves 32,374 respondents. This study has shown wide differences in the rates of overweight (BMI above 25) among Asian Americans. For men, the percentage overweight ranges from 17% of Vietnamese to 42% of Japanese, while the total male US population is 57% overweight. For women, the percentage overweight ranges from 9% of Vietnamese and Chinese to 25% of Asian Indians, while the total female population is 38% overweight. The study also showed increasing overweight and obesity with increasing duration of stay in the US.

National Health and Nutrition Examination Survey (NHANES I to III)

This is a survey of a nationally represented sample of more than 7,600 Americans. The study started in 1970 as NHANES I and is still ongoing as NHANES III. These people are periodically interviewed, examined, and blood samples drawn to ascertain the prevalence of various diseases and risk factors and its changes over decades. Data from NHANES indicate that over the past four decades, the mean systolic blood pressure has declined by 10 mm Hg, cholesterol by 30 mg/dL and age-adjusted mortality rates from heart disease and stroke have decreased by 50% and 60%.

The North Karelia Project

Finland had the unique distinction of having had the highest heart disease mortality in the world. The North Karelia Project was launched in 1972 in response to the local petition to get urgent and effective help to reduce the exceptionally high heart disease mortality. The outstanding success of this project is evidenced by a reduction in heart disease mortality of 55% in men and 68% in women in 20 years (between 1972 and 1992). The decline was even greater in those under 45 years of age. This led to a shift in the occurrence of cardiac events and deaths to older people. The average age of a first heart attack increased by 20 years, from 50s to 70s. This is in sharp contrast to the pattern in India where the age of first heart attack has decreased by more than 10 years in the last two decades. There was equally spectacular decline in stroke and cancer as a result of changes in lifestyle. Two-thirds of this decline was attributed to advances in prevention directed at the whole country. This study underscore the enormous benefits community wide prevention strategies.

NHS (The Nurses Health Study)

This is the largest and most extensive ongoing epidemiological study in the world. A total of 117,629 American female nurses aged 30 to 55 years who were free of known cardiovascular disease at baseline were enrolled. They were recruited in 1976 and have been followed continuously since. This study to date has more than 2 million person-years of follow-up, providing vital data on women. Among other things, this study showed that even a weight gain of **18 pounds after age 18** is associated with a doubling of the risk of diabetes. This study also showed daily walking was highly protective against heart disease and diabetes.

PDAY (The Pathobiological Determinants of Atherosclerosis in Youth Study)

In this study, extensive autopsy evaluation of the heart was made to determine the severity and extent of plaque buildup in the coronary arteries in nearly 3,000 persons aged 15 to 34 years dying of accidents and homicides. This study showed evidence of significant plaque build-up in **one in 6 teenagers** and increased with advancing age.

PHS (The Physicians Health Study)

This is an ongoing prospective follow-up study involving 22,071 healthy male physicians aged 40 to 84 years in 1982. The risk factors were analyzed at baseline. These physicians were followed for the development of various diseases, to ascertain the relationship of certain risk factors of heart disease. This study has shown that mortality from heart disease among the US physicians decreased dramatically from 115% to 15% of the general population between 1960 and 1990. This is clear proof that the ravages of heart disease can be reduced with appropriate preventive measures. This was also the first study to show the benefit of aspirin in reducing the risk of a heart attack in otherwise healthy adults. The latest report from the study shows that lipoprotein(a) is a *strong predictor* of severe heart disease, requiring coronary angioplasty and bypass surgery.

PRIME (The Prospective Epidemiological Study of Myocardial Infarction)

This is a prospective cohort study which included 9,133 French and Northern Irish men aged 50 to 59 at entry, without a history of heart disease. Northern Ireland and France are two geographically close countries with contrasting risk for heart disease (four-fold difference). This study showed a strong relationship between lipoprotein(a) and heart disease, which was further increased with high cholesterol levels. This study also showed that the difference in heart disease rates between these two countries was explained more with increased physical activity than with a higher intake of alcohol. In France, people consume alcohol everyday, with only a slight increase during weekends, whereas, in Northern Ireland, Fridays and Saturdays accounted for 66% of total alcohol consumption. This study showed that the Framingham Risk Score is inaccurate in both these European populations with overestimation of the risk in Southern Europeans and underestimation of the risk in Northern Europeans.

PROCAM Study (The Prospective Cardiovascular Munster Study)

This ongoing study was initiated in 1979 to determine the prevalence of cardiovascular risk factors and improve the prediction of heart disease in the German population. Ongoing data from 4,043 men and 1,333 women, ages 50 to 65 years, show that more than 50% of all diabetics have hypertension. Dyslipidemia is a more significant risk factor for heart disease than hypertension or diabetes mellitus. Triglycerides above 500 mg/dL are prevalent in 30% of all diabetics, two to three times more frequently than in nondiabetic patients. Blood levels of triglycerides, HDL, and lipoprotein(a) are sensitive indicators of increased risk of coronary events among Germans. Lipoprotein(a) excess increases the cardiac risk, especially in men with high LDL, low HDL, and hypertension.

SAFARI Trial (The Effectiveness and tolerability of simvastatin plus fenofibrate for combined hyperlipidemia)

This study evaluated the safety and efficacy of Zocor with Tricor in patients with combined hyperlipidemia (elevated triglyceride and LDL levels.) Combination therapy with Zocor 20 mg and Tricor 160 mg in patients with combined hyperlipidemia resulted in additional improvement in all lipoprotein parameters measured compared with simvastatin 20 mg monotherapy. However the benefits were less than that observed with statin niacin combination therapy.

The Scandinavian Simvastatin Survival Study

This study was designed to evaluate the effects of cholesterol lowering with simvastatin on mortality and morbidity in patients with coronary heart disease. A total 4444 patients aged 35 to 70 years with heart disease and blood cholesterol levels of 213-310 mg/dL receiving a lipid-lowering diet were randomly assigned to take double-blind treatment with Zorcor, 20 to 40 mg once daily, or placebo (fake pill). This study conclusively demonstrated the benefit of statins in reducing death. The reduction was 42% for cardiac death and 30% for death from all causes. This study helped to prove the colecterol hypothesis that high cholesterol increases the risk of heart disease by demonstrating reduction of the risk with treatment.

The Seven Countries Study

This study involved 12,763 men aged 40 through 59 years living in Europe, the US, and Japan. The principle objective of this study was to ascertain the international differences in risk factors and its relationship to cardiovascular disease. The study began 1957 and several reports on long term follow-up have been published. This study showed marked difference in heart disease rates between countries. At an identical level of risk factors Japanese had only one-fifth the rate of heart disease observed in Finland and the US.

The St. James Survey

This study in Trinidad consisted of nearly 2,000 adults who were free of heart disease and followed for a period of 10 years for the development of new heart disease. The relative risk of heart disease incidence in Indians was two times higher than whites and seven times higher than people of other ethnic origins.

SHARE (The Study of Health Assessment and Risk in Ethnic groups)

This Canadian study recruited 985 participants by random sampling and analyzed the prevalence of heart disease, traditional risk factors, and emerging risk factors. Indians, Chinese, and whites formed a third each of the total people. Indians had the highest prevalence of heart disease (11%) which was double that of whites (5%) and 5 times higher than Chinese (2%). Indians had an increased prevalence of diabetes, higher total and LDL cholesterol, higher triglycerides, and lower HDL cholesterol. Indians also had much greater abnormalities in emerging risk factors, including higher concentrations of fibrinogen, homocysteine, and lipoprotein(a). This study also showed that at a given degree of plaque build-up, Indians had double and Chinese had half the rate of heart attack compared to whites.

SCORE (The Systematic Coronary Risk Evaluation)

This is a risk prediction model developed to predict the risk among Europeans, since the Framingham Risks Score is inaccurate in this population. The SCORE predicts the 10-year risk of **cardiac death**, as opposed to **cardiac events** with the Framingham Risk Score. Furthermore, the SCORE uses two different prediction models, depending upon whether the people live in a low-risk or high-risk country. Low-risk countries include Belgium, France, Greece, Italy, Luxembourg, Portugal, Spain, and Switzerland. People living in these countries have their risk calculated using a low-risk chart separate from that used for every other European nation.

TNT (Treat New Target Study)

This study of more than 10,000 people with heart disease showed better outcome with Lipitor 80 mg/day than Lipitor 10 mg/day. The LDL was reduced to 75 mg/dL with Lipitor 80 mg and the 5 year events were 9% . The corresponding values for Lipitor 10 mg were an LDL of 100 mg/dL and coronary events of 11%. This translated into a 22% risk reduction. Adverse events were noted in 8% and 6% on those taking high and low doses respectively. The number of rhabdomyolysis was 2 and 3 cases with high and low doses, indicating high dose of Lipitor is not associated with a high risk of muscle damage.

UKPDS (The United Kingdom Prospective Diabetes Study)

This landmark diabetic study analyzed the impact of diabetes on heart disease and the difference in the benefits of various medication used in the treatment. It has clearly demonstrated the relationship between A1C and diabetic complications. This study showed that cholesterol levels and HDL levels are the two most important predictors of heart disease in diabetic patients. The blood sugar level was only the third most important predictor.

VA HIT (The Veterans Affairs Study)

In this study, 8,500 patients with heart disease were screened to identify those with low HDL. On screening 63% had HDL below 40 mg/dL compared to 13% with LDL above 160 mg/dL. These people were randomized to receive Lopid or matching dummy pills to determine the effect of raising HDL in people with low HDL. This study demonstrated that raising HDL by 1% reduces the risk of a coronary event by 3%.

WHI (The Women's Health Initiative)

This is a research program involving 161,000 generally healthy postmenopausal women designed to study the relationship of risk factors to heart disease in women. This study showed that panic attacks may be relatively common among postmenopausal women and seem to be associated with stressful life events and functional impairment.

WAVE (The Women's Angiographic Vitamin & Estrogen Trial)
This is a randomized, controlled trial of hormone therapy and antioxidant vitamins. The study involved a total of 425 postmenopausal women with angiographic heart disease. It showed that metabolic syndrome was common among postmenopausal women with heart disease and conferred an increased risk of clinical cardiovascular events.

MAJOR REPORTS AND PROGRAMS

Various government agencies and professional associations have published guidelines for prevention and treatment of heart disease, diabetes, high cholesterol, high blood pressure, etc. These agencies include, American Heart Association, American College of Cardiology, National Heart, Lung, and Blood Institute, and so on.

NCEP (The National Cholesterol Education Program)
The NCEP was initiated in 1985 to educate health professionals and the public about the dangers of high blood cholesterol as a risk factor for heart disease and about the benefits of lowering cholesterol levels to reduce the deaths from heart disease. From 1983 to 1985, the % of the public who had their cholesterol checked rose from 35% to 75%, showing that 70 to 80 million more Americans were aware of their cholesterol levels in 1985 than in 1983.

NHBPEP (The National High Blood Pressure Education Program)
This program is focused on translating research results into improved medical care outcomes and the public's

health, with focus on high blood pressure. Significant improvement in the awareness, detection, and treatment of blood pressure is credited to NHBPEP.

Joint National Committee Reports
These reports are prepared by more than 40 different medical associations and governmental agencies on the detection and treatment of high blood pressure. Seven reports have been published to date. The last report has defind optimom blood preasure to be less 115 systolic and less than 75 diastolic.

NHAAP (The National Heart Attack Alert Program)
This was initiated in 1991 to reduce morbidity and mortality from heart attack, including out of hospital cardiac arrest through educated health professionals, patients, and the public, about the importance of rapid identification and treatment of individuals with heart attack symptoms.

OEI (The Obesity Education Program)
This was initiated in 1991 by NHLBI to inform public and health professionals about the health risk associated with obesity. Obesity is not only an independent risk factor for heart disease, but also a contributor to high blood pressure, high cholesterol, and sleep apnea.

The Women's Heart Health Education Initiative
This was launched in 2001 to increase the awareness of heart disease and its risk factors among women.

The Healthy People 2010
This is a national health objective for 2010. Its objectives also include reducing the health disparities among Americans of different ethnic origins.

Appendix C ▶ Prudent Diet Meal Plans

Prudent Breakfast
Start with a healthy breakfast every morning—this is your most important meal of the day. The term "break+fast" indicates that your body has been without food for at least eight hours. A recent study found marked deterioration of blood sugar and lipoprotein levels among those who skipped breakfast compared to those who ate breakfast. In this study, total daily calories were identical for both groups.

You can get a boost in your morning energy level and your metabolism by having a healthy breakfast. If you are not used to a breakfast, consider starting out with just a glass of skim milk and an apple. Half an avocado

with lemon squeeze is another tasty way to start the day. As you increase your exercise and advance in your nutrition program, you need more healthy calories. If you are targeting to lose fat around your waist, a healthy breakfast is all the more important.

An ideal breakfast should contain healthy "fat + protein + carbohydrates". Consider having half an avocado for the fat component of your breakfast. For protein sources, consider soy protein powder mixed in your cereal. Low or no cholesterol egg mixes (Egg Beaters) are also available. A vegetable egg white omelet can be a great way to start your day. Please use a small amount of canola oil or olive oil to lightly cook your eggs in a frying pan rather than frying your eggs. Egg whites are the most easily metabolized source of proteins by our body. Boiled eggs without yolk are excellent sources of healthy proteins.

A variety of carbohydrates are available including whole grain bread, fruits, and high fiber cereals. Consider having "Sat Isabgol" with yogurt or Kellog's Bud Bran breakfast cereal. Both these sources contain psyllium husk - a rich source of soluble fiber that help reduce your cholesterol level.

Indian breakfasts such as uppuma made with 50% oat bran and 50% rava (cracked wheat) with some vegetables—peas, onions and tomatoes are very healthy too. Half a cup of low-fat or no fat cottage cheese with a bowl of fruits is an excellent way to start your day, as it provides protein and healthy carbohydrates for most vegetarians. Most traditional Indian breakfasts such as idlis, chapathis etc. have a high glycemic load.

Reducing the quantity of these foods and supplementing your breakfast with good fats and proteins will help your satiety, reduce caloric intake, and avoid fluctuations in blood sugar levels.

Prudent Snacks

The key idea behind snacks between meals is to keep your **blood sugar** even throughout the day. This is particularly important for diabetics who want to maintain their blood sugar level under adequate control. In addition, to giving you consistent energy, snacks are an ideal way to prevent you from overeating during main meal times. Good times to have a snack include mid-mornings, evenings (two hours before dinner) and at bedtime. Good snacks include a glass of low-fat milk, soy milk, low-fat yogurt, one half to one ounce (15 to 30g) of nuts, fruits such as apples and oranges. An energy bar can also make a good snack, provided the energy bar is limited in calories and "balanced" in fat, protein and carbohydrates—some energy bars are loaded in calories and sugar similar to candy bars. While samosa is a favorite Indian snack especially at the parties, it is high in glycemic load and "fat" load. Broiling rather than frying such snacks can reduce your calorie intake by 50 to 60%.

Prudent Lunch / Dinner

Traditional Indian lunches are very high in rice and rotis (very high glycemic load). A typical south Indian lunch consists of three courses of rice: with sambar, with rasam and with curd along with one or two vegetable side dishes. In such a meal, the person may consume three to five cups of rice in one meal.

A way to design a good lunch is to choose healthy proteins and fats and then add enough carbohydrates. Lean meats, soy burgers, dhals (Indian lentils) are good choices for low-fat proteins. The daily act of simply replacing 2 cups of rice (350 calories) with a generous salad (see below) and low-fat dressing (80 to 120 calories) can keep triglycerides under control. Low-carb tortillas (70 calories per tortilla) are good substitutes for chapathis and rotis made from maida (enriched flour). Typical ghee soaked chapathi contributes a whopping 200 to 300 calories to your diet and adds little to the nutritional content of your meals. Two vegetables (preferably stir fried, dry or "sookha" sabjis - vegetable dishes) are good additions to any meal. The key idea is to make rotis and rice as a side dish and increase the amount of vegetables consumed. Avoiding curries and eating steamed or sautéed vegetables reduce the temptation to feast on rice and roti. See Table below for typical daily servings of various foods.

SALADS

The traditional view of the salad to Indians evokes images of dull iceberg lettuce with a small tomato and shredded carrots. However, you can be imaginative with your salad choices. Start with the **traditional**

Typical Daily/ Weekly Serving Sizes of Various Foods

	Serving size	Number of servings
Grain	1 slice of bread 1 ounce of cereal ½ cup of cooked rice or pasta	2 to 3/day
Vegetable	1 cup of raw leafy vegetable ½ cup of other vegetable (cooked or raw) 6 ounce of vegetable juice	4 to 5/day
Fruit	A medium fruit (apple, banana or orange) ½ cup of fresh, frozen, cooked or canned fruit ¼ cup dried fruit 6 ounce of fruit juice	4 to 5/day
Milk	8 ounce of milk 1 cup yogurt 1½ounce of cheese	2 to 3/day
Meat, poultry and fish	2-3 ounces of cooked meat, poultry or fish 2 ½ ounce soy burger counts as 1 ounce of lean meat	2 or less/day
Beans	½ cup of cooked dry beans and peas	4 to 5/week
Egg	1 egg 1 egg counts as 1 ounce of lean meat	2/week
Nuts and seeds	2 tablespoons or ½ oz seeds (2 tablespoons of peanut butter, 1 ½ oz of nuts. Counts as 1 ounce of meat)	4 to 5/week
Sugar	1 tablespoon sugar 1 tablespoon jelly or jam ½ oz jelly beans 8 oz lemonade	5 per week
Fat & oils	1 teaspoon soft margarine 1 tablespoon low fat Mayonnaise 2 tablespoons light salad dressing 1 teaspoon vegetable oil	2 to 3 per day

greens (avoid iceberg lettuce because it has virtually no nutritional value); choose baby spinach, baby greens, and red leaf, green leaf, or Romaine lettuce to form a good base for your salad. Consider a variety of vegetables in season - cucumbers, green, red, yellow peppers, and carrots. Wash all vegetables with warm water before chopping them. This will remove any dirt or mud sticking to fresh vegetables and act as possible sources of food contamination.

Beans are a good addition to the salad as they add to the flavor. As discussed before, cans of pre-cooked beans—multi-bean-fava beans, garbanzo and navy beans make excellent additions to your salads. Remember to rinse out the water from these beans as they contain insoluble fiber that causes abdominal gas.

A variety of low-fat salad dressings are available to satisfy your taste. Extra virgin olive oil is one such healthy choice. Spices such as oregano and basil leaf may be added to the olive oil to enhance the flavor. Hot chili sauce or salsas can be used as healthy salad dressings. Make sure that the dressing you choose is low in sodium and low in saturated fat. In appendix D, there are some heart healthy salad recipes. A special Mediterranean salad dressing made out of extra virgin olive oil and red wine vinegar can provide a healthy dose of mono-saturated fats and antioxidants.

Salad as a meal: You can make a complete meal out of salads by choosing good protein sources such as lean meat, chicken, or fish. If you are vegetarian, you can add one to two spicy black bean burgers and some mixed beans or dhal as your protein source.

Appendix D ▶ Heart-Healthy Recipes

Sudesh's Mediterranean Salad Dressing

½ cup (8 Tbs.) extra-virgin olive oil
¼ cup (4 Tbs.) red wine vinegar
1 tsp. salt (to taste) – I use Morton Lite Salt (a combination of potassium chloride and regular salt)
½ tsp. Italian basil (dry powder)
½ tsp. dry crushed oregano leaves
½ tsp. roasted crushed red pepper
1 clove of fresh organic garlic (crushed in a garlic press)
Freshly ground black pepper to taste

Preparation
Whisk together olive oil and red wine vinegar.
Add rest of ingredients: salt, herbs, garlic and black pepper.
Whisk together until well blended.
Pour over fresh lettuce salad and toss lightly.
Allow to sit 10 min. Enjoy!
Makes enough dressing for a 3 to 4 person salad.

Sudesh's Special Salad
This is an easy, healthy salad that combines a variety of vegetables and beans. You can add lean meat such as a grilled chicken breast or two spicy veggie burgers and make a complete meal. Consider using the salad dressing above, extra virgin olive oil or any low-fat salad dressing. Adding salsa, chili and cumin powder is another option.

Prep Time: 15 Minutes
1 can (15 ounce) mixed beans, drained and rinsed
3 to 4 leaves of red leaf lettuce
1 large red pepper
1 to 2 stalks of celery stick finely chopped

2 to 3 plum tomatoes

Preparation
In a large bowl, stir together the beans, red pepper, tomatoes and celery. Add dressing and mix well just before serving. Serve over a bed of lettuce.
 Makes 4 servings

Akila's seasoned tofu
Extra Firm Tofu 1 pound
Seasoning -1/2 tsp -1 tsp (ready-made chicken masala, garam masala or curry powder)
Rinse the tofu and let the extra water drain. Pat it dry with a paper towel. Slice tofu slab into ½" long slabs and place on a non-stick frying pan on medium heat. Toast the tofu slabs on both sides until golden brown. Remove from the pan and cool it in a plate. Slice the tofu slabs to ½-1" cubes. Transfer them back to the frying pan. Sprinkle salt (remember your seasoning may have some salt in it already) and seasoning and gently mix the tofu pieces. Cook the tofu at medium heat for 10 to 15 minutes or till the raw smell of spices is gone. Serve the tofu as side dish or on a salad. Makes 3-4 servings

Note: Tofu or bean curd is a very versatile cooking ingredient since it absorbs most of the Indians spices very well. Most health foods and grocery stores carry extra-firm tofu. In many shops, you can find a low-fat version of tofu. . These "stir-fried" tofu cubes (with or without masala) can be added to most Indian curries especially saag (spinach curry) or any bean dishes such as Rajma (kidney beans) or Chole (chick peas or garbanzo beans). Most dishes that require paneer (Indian cottage cheese) can be substituted with tofu.

Akila's spicy green gram dhal pancakes

Green gram dhal – 1 cup
Green Chilies – 3-4 long pieces
Ginger – 1 inch piece
Salt – 1 tsp or to taste

Soak green gram dhal in water overnight. Rinse out and drain the excess water. In a blender, add the green gram dhal, green chilies, ginger and salt and grind to a batter. Add little water at a time to get a smooth consistent batter, which will spread like a dosai or pancake. On a medium hot griddle, spread a ladle full of batter. Cover the pancake with a lid for 30-60 seconds. Remove the lid and flip the pancake and cook the other side for 30-60 seconds. Remove and serve hot with sambar or vegetables. Makes about 7 pancakes.

Glossary

To complement your understanding of commonly used terms in the field of cardiovascular health, visit websites such as that of the American Heart Association (www.americanheart.org). The AHA also makes available several free downloadable publications to educate the public about heart disease.

Atherosclerosis: Commonly called hardening of the arteries, atherosclerosis, is a process, in which the inner layers of the artery become thick and irregular due to deposits of fat, cholesterol, and other substances called plaques. If the plaque grow large inward it can narrow the artery compromising the blood supply that results in characteristic chest pain called angina. More commonly the plaques grow outward with in artery walls and rupture without warning causing a heart attack or sudden death.

Aneurysm: A ballooning-out of the wall of an artery. Often this wall is weakened by disease, injury or an abnormality present at birth. Aneurysms are often caused or made worse by high blood pressure. They aren't always life-threatening, but serious consequences—such as a hemorrhagic stroke-can result if one bursts in the brain. Aneurysm can occur in the aorta, particularly in the abdominal aorta. Large aneurysms may require surgery to prevent rupture as was done to vice-president Cheney in September 2005.

Angina Pectoris: Angina is a characteristic type of chest pain due to reduced blood supply to the heart. It is described by some patients as a "crushing of the chest" and often radiates to the left arm or jaw. **See Stable and Unstable Angina.**

Angiogram: See Coronary Angiogram.

Angioplasty: See Coronary Angioplasty.

Angiotensin Converting Enzyme (ACE) Inhibitors: These medications prevent the conversion of angiotensin I to angiotensin II, a powerful agent that causes arteries to constrict. Angiotensin II is implicated in hypertension and heart disease. It is used for treatment of patients with diabetes and kidney disease, as well as, for some heart attack survivors.

Angiotensin II Receptor Blockers (ARBs): This medication block the action of angiotensin II. It is as effective as ACE inhibitors and may have fewer adverse effects, such as coughing

AED: AEDs (automatic external defibrillators) are usually placed in public places, air planes and offices. These can be used by people without training because AEDs provides simple instructions to carry out the necessary steps

Automatic Implantable Cardioverter Defibrillator (AICD): These devices are implanted in persons who have had previous cardiac arrest or are at high risk of having one. The device automatically senses cardiac arrest and takes appropriate action. See **Defibrillation**.

Aorta: The largest artery into which the heart pumps the oxygenated blood.

Arrhythmia:- An abnormal rate of muscular contractions in the heart. People usually feel this as skipping, fluttering or racing of heart. Not all arrhythmia is serious.

Arterial spasm: A condition in which the diameter of the artery is temporarily reduced, limiting the blood supply. In the olden days, arterial spasm was thought to be an important cause of heart-attack. Recent studies suggest that it plays only a minor role.

Artery - A blood vessel that supplies oxygenated blood from the heart to different parts of the body.

Atherectomy: A procedure to improve blood supply to the heart without surgery. During this procedure, a catheter with a special grinding device is used to **clear away the plaque** in the blocked artery.

Atherogenic Lipid Profile: A combination of high triglycerides, low HDL, and elevated non-HDL cholesterol. This condition is common among Indians and is associated with a high risk of heart disease.

Antiatherogenic Lipid Profile: A lipid profile in which the HDL level is high and triglyceride level is low. This pattern is associated with a low risk of heart disease and is particularly common among blacks, Japanese and Chinese.

Atrial fibrillation: A condition where the upper chamber of heart quivers in an uncoordinated, uncontrolled manner. This results in incomplete emptying of this chamber predisposing to stasis (stagnation of blood without circulation) and blood clot formation. This is common in the elderly and is an important cause of stroke.

Body Mass Index (BMI): The ratio of body weight in kilograms divided by height in meters squared. This is the yardstick to categorize people as overweight (BMI above 25) or obese (BMI above 30)

Blood Pressure (systolic, diastolic): The force of blood pressing against artery walls. Systolic blood pressure is the blood pressure when the heart pumps blood into the artery (normally below 120 mm Hg) and diastolic blood pressure is the one between heart beats (normally below 80 mm Hg).

Bypass Surgery: See **Coronary Bypass Surgery.**

Cardiovascular Disease (CVD): Diseases of the heart and blood vessels (cardio= heart, vascular = blood vessel). Common CVD conditions include hypertension, coronary artery disease, peripheral vascular disease and cerebro-vascular disease.

Coronary Artery Revascularization Procedure (CARP): These are procedures to mechanically relieve the block in the coronary arteries and improve the blood supply to the heart muscle. These procedures include **coronary angioplasty, stents** and **by-pass surgery.**

Cardiac Arrest: The sudden, abrupt loss of heart function. It is also called sudden cardiac arrest or unexpected cardiac arrest. The person usually dies in the absence of appropriate treatment. President Eisenhower is reported to have had 14 cardiac arrest in the last 14 years of his life (and 7 heart attacks). See **Sudden Death/ Ventricular Fibrillation.**

Cardiac Catheterization: A very small tube (catheter) is inserted into a blood vessel in your groin or arm. This is the first step in performing a coronary angiogram, angioplasty or stent.

Cerebrovascular disease (CBVD): The disease of the brain and its blood vessels (cerebro=brain, vascular=blood vessel). Stroke is one of its most common complications.

Cholesterol : A soft, waxy substance found in the bloodstream and every cell of the human body. A high blood level of cholesterol is primarily responsible for plaque build-up and heart attack. Total cholesterol consists of bad cholesterol (LDL) and good cholesterol (HDL).

Coronary Artery Disease (CAD): The diseases of the coronary artery that supplies blood to the heart muscles. In this book, this term is synonymous with heart disease.

Coronary Angiogram: In simple terms, an x-ray of the coronary arteries, in which a dye is injected into the artery through a catheter, to see if any are narrowed or blocked with plaque.

Coronary Angioplasty (balloon angioplasty): A procedure that allows opening of the narrowed coronary arteries without surgery. Angioplasty, together with stenting, is called **Percutaneous Coronary Interventions (PCI).** See also **Cardiac catheterization.**

Coronary Bypass Surgery (CABG or "Cabbage"): This surgery reroutes, or "bypasses," blood flow around clogged arteries to restore blood supply to areas of heart muscle that do not receive an adequate supply (because of narrowed or blocked coronary arteries). In this procedure, a blood vessel is taken from another part of the body (usually the leg) and attached above and below the narrowed segment of the coronary artery.

Coronary Event: Any significant occurrence related to heart disease, such as a heart attack, death, coronary angioplasty/stent or bypass surgery. See also **MACE.**

Coronary Heart Disease (CHD): See **Coronary Artery Disease.**

Coronary Occlusion: Complete blockage of the artery, usually from a blood clot on a partially narrowed artery.

Coronary Stent: This is a wire mesh tube that is used to prop open an artery that has recently been dilated using angioplasty.

Coronary Thrombosis: The medical term for a blood clot in the coronary artery. It occurs usually from a rupture of an unstable or vulnerable plaque.

C-reactive Protein: A protein in the blood associated with inflammation as well as obesity. An elevated level of CRP is a strong predictor of heart attack and diabetes.

Defibrillation: A process in which an electronic device gives an electric shock to the heart. This helps reestablish normal cardiac rhythms in a heart having ventricular fibrillation, a dangerous arrhythmia that causes cardiac arrest.

Defibrillator: An electronic device used in defibrillation in patients suffering from a cardiac arrest due to ventricular fibrillation. See also **AICD.**

Diabetes Mellitus: Medical term for diabetes—a disease characterized by abnormal levels of lipids, and blood sugar. It is associated with a very high risk of heart attack.

Diuretic: This medication is commonly know as "water pill" and is used for controlling blood pressure. This medication helps eliminate excess water from the body, thereby reducing blood pressure.

Dyslipidemia: This is a medical term that includes any abnormalities involving cholesterol, triglycerides, HDL, and lipoprotein(a). This is a term preferable to hyperlipidemia or high cholesterol since low HDL is covered under dyslipidemia.

Electron-Beam Computed Tomography (EBCT): Commonly known as heart scan, this test detects calcified coronary plaque. It does not show non-calcified plaque or the severity of arterial blockage.

Ejection Fraction: The ejection fraction is the fraction of the blood that is pumped out of the heart with each heart beat. This is an important measure of the pumping ability of the heart muscle (left ventricle). The normal ejection fraction is more than 55% in healthy people. The ejection fraction is reduced after a heart-attack proportional to its severity.

Electrocardiography (ECG, EKG): This is a recording of the electrical activity of the heart and the mainstay of the diagnosis of heart attack as well as arrhythmia.

Epidemiology: The study of the causes and prevention of disease in populations, or communities, making it the main source of evidence for public health decision making. Epidemiology is generally consider the basic sicence of the popolation.

Exercise Stress Test: This is usually called a treadmill test since the treadmill is most commonly used equipment for stressing the heart. This test helps determine if you have **ischemia** resulting from severe narrowing of the coronary arteries. Ischemia renders people at risk of heart attack. It also helps doctors determine exercise type and intensity appropriate for a patient. The test is abnormal only when at least two arteries show significant narrowing.

Fats: These are organic compounds that are made up of carbon, hydrogen, and oxygen; they are the most concentrated source of energy in foods. Fats belong to a group of substances called lipids. Fats come in liquid or solid form. All fats are combinations of saturated and unsaturated fatty acids. Fats can be called very saturated or very unsaturated depending on their proportions. Fat is an important energy source and aids in several important cell functions, including the production of steroids and sex hormones. See **MUFA, PUFA and SAFA.**

High Density Lipoprotein (HDL): This is the good cholesterol that protects against heart disease. A low level of HDL confers a high risk of heart disease, even when cholesterol level is normal. See **Cholesterol.**

Homocysteine: This is an amino acid in the blood. An excess level is associated with a heart attack, stroke, and death at a young age.

Hyperglycemia and Hypoglycemia: These are medical terms for high and low blood sugar respectively. Both these conditions are important in people with diabetes.

Hypertension: This condition refers to high blood pressure (more than 140 mm Hg systolic or more than 90 mm Hg diastolic). See also **Blood Pressure.**

Ischemia: This refers to the muscles like heart that are not getting enough blood supply due to severe narrowing of arteries.

Intravascular Ultrasound (IVUS): This is a method of visualizing the plaque in the arteries by using ultrasound.

Low Density Lipoprotein (LDL) Cholesterol: This is principal dangerous cholesterol that is involved in plaque formation leading to hear attack. The optimal level has been recently reduced to 40 mg/dL that corresponding to a total cholesterol level of 110 to 120 mg/dL. **See also Cholesterol.**

LDL Apheresis: This is a dialysis like treatment to remove LDL and lipoprotein(a) in people with familial hypercholesterolemia. In chilidren with very high colesterol, this is often combined with maximum aggressive triple medical therapy to delay bypass surgery and valve replacement to an age past adolescence.

Left Ventricular Hypertrophy (LVH): It is the enlargement and thickening of the left ventricle, the principal pumping chamber of the heart. This is a dreaded complication of persons with uncontrolled hypertension leading to heart failure and sudden death.

Lipids: In this book, lipids refer to cholesterol and triglycerides found in blood. See also **Fats.**

Lipoproteins: These are particles containing lipids and proteins. Four important lipoproteins are LDL, HDL, VLDL and lipoprotein(a).

Lipoprotein(a): Lipoprotein(a) is a genetic variant of

LDL (bad cholesterol) with an abnormal protein called apo(a) attached to it. Lipoprotein(a) is one of the most common and important emerging risk factor for premature heart disease among Indians.

Major Acute Cardiac Events (MACE): Significant cardiac events include heart attack, coronary angioplasty/ stent, bypass surgery and / or cardiac death. I refer to these as **coronary events** in this book.

Meta-analysis: Meta-analysis refers to an exhaustive and systemic analysis of all the published data on the subject, usually 20-100 studies involving several hundred thousand patients.

Myocardial Perfusion Imaging (MPI): This technique allows physicians to obtain very clear images of the heart and locate areas of the heart muscle that do not receive adequate blood supply due to narrowing of the coronary arteries. MPI techniques include stress echocardiogram and nuclear perfusion imaging. To obtain nuclear images, tiny amounts of radioactive materials (called "tracers") are introduced into the person's body. The tracers emit a certain type of energy called gamma rays, which are detected by machines. Commonly used tracers include Thallium and Myoview.

Monounsaturated Fatty Acids (MUFA): These are good fats that lower LDL and increase HDL. Virgin olive oil, canola oil and nuts are good sources of MUFA.

National Cholesterol Education Program (NCEP): The NCEP was created in 1985 by the National Heart, Lung, and Blood Institute (NHLBI), to educate professionals and the public about the risk of high cholesterol and the benefits of lowering it.

National Heart, Lung, and Blood Institute (NHLBI): This is an independent scientific body that distributes government grants for cardiovascular research. It also supports educational efforts to teach the public about the risk factors. NHLBI-supported activities include

Oxidation: The removal of an electron from a molecule. Oxidation of LDL is a crucial step in the development of atherosclerosis or plaque build-up that leads to heart attack.

Percutaneous Coronary Interventions (PCI): See **Coronary Angioplasty and stent.**

Peripheral Vascular Disease (PVD): Also known as PAD (Peripheral Artery Disease). This is a disease of the blood vessels characterized by hardening and narrowing of the arteries that supply the legs and feet. Persons with PVD often have far advanced heart disease and often die from that.

Plant Sterols: These are plant products which retard the absorption of dietary cholesterol. It is used to lower the cholesterol as an adjunct to medication.

Polyunsaturated Fatty Acids (PUFA): This is healthy fat that lowers LDL but may also lower HDL. The recommended maximum is less than 10% of total calories consumed. Most vegetable oils are rich in PUFA. See **Fats.**

Prognosis: This is a medical term that reflects the likely outcome or course of a disease including the chance of recovery, recurrence or death.

Proportionate Mortality Ratio (PMR): It is a measure of the proportion of deaths due to a given disease compared to death from all causes.

Restenosis: This refers to recurrence of narrowing of coronary arteries following procedures such as angioplasty, stent or bypass surgery. This often leads to repeat procedures. Low HDL and high lipoprotein(a) are important contributors to restenosis. See **Stenosis.**

Saturated Fatty Acids (SAFA): These are dangerous fats that raise the LDL. Common sources of SAFA include butter, ghee and fat cuts of meats. See **also Fats.**

Sick sinus syndrome (SSS): The sick sinus syndrome is a problem with the heart's natural pacemaker, the sinus node, which is located at the top of the right atrium. The sinus node normally produces electrical impulses that cause the heart to beat regularly (60 to 100 beats per minute). The SSS causes the heart to beat too fast or too slow and sometimes alternate between beating too fast and too slow. Sometimes there may be prolonged pauses between heart beats, when the patient experiences dizziness and sometimes syncope (fainting). The fast rates are treated with medications, whereas, the slow rates a treated with a pacemaker. Sick sinus has no correlation with heart attack, but high correlation with stroke (atrial fibrillation).

Stable Angina: See **Angina Pectoris.**

Standardized Mortality Rate: The number of deaths occurring per 100,000 population per year. The 2005 American heart Association statistics use a standard population (2000), so that these rates aren't affected by changes or differences in the age composition of the population. The **Age-Adjusted death rates** are calculated in accordance with a standard age structure to minimize the effects of age differences, when the rates are compared between populations or over time.

Standardized Mortality Ratio (SMR): This allows a comparison of mortality rates among different populations. An SMR of 100 implies that the rates are the same for the population of interest and the standard population. An SMR more than 164 in Indians implies that the rate is 64% higher than the general population.

Stenosis: This refers to constriction or narrowing of an artery by buildup of fat, cholesterol and other substances over time. See **also Restenosis.**

Stroke: This event occurs when blood flow to the brain is suddenly blocked. The corresponding part of the brain could die if blood circulation is not restored. Paralysis and resulting disability is the major complication, although death can also occur after a stroke.

Sudden Death: This is death occurring without symptoms or within one hour of chest pain or heart attack. Sudden death may the first and only symptom in one-third of patients with heart disease. See **Cardiac Arrest.**

Thrombosis: See **Coronary Thrombosis.**

Transient Ischemic Attack (TIA): This is commonly known as "a mini-stroke." This is usually a warning of impending stroke. In this condition, there is a temporary blockage in the artery, interrupting the blood supply to the brain and resulting in symptoms. The difference between TIA and stroke is that all symptoms disappear within a few minutes to a few hours in TIA, whereas, the symptoms and the disability persist after a stroke. The short-term risk of stroke after TIA is about 10 to 20% in the first three months with much of the risk front-loaded in the first week.

Thallium (Myoview) test: See **Myocardial Perfusion Imaging.**

Trans fats: This is the most dangerous and deadly form of fats that increase LDL and lower HDL. Common sources of trans fats include fried foods and commercial baked products such as samosa and donut. See **Fats.**

Triglycerides: These are the fat molecules in blood. A high level of triglycerides is associated with blood clots and heart attacks. See **Cholesterol.**

Unstable Angina: This condition refers to severe chest pain from poor blood supply to the heart that occurs without physical activity. Unstable angina usually results in heart attack in the absence of appropriate treatment. See also **Angina Pectoris.**

Ventricular Fibrillation: This is the most common form of cardiac arrest. This leads to sudden death in the absence of defibrillation within 5 to 10 minutes. See **also Defibrillation.**

Very Low Density Lipoprotein (VLDL): Forms of lipoprotein with large amounts of triglycerides. VLDL cholesterol accounts for the cholesterol that is not indicated by LDL or HDL. For practical purposes, VLDL is calculated as 20% of the triglycerides.

BIBLIOGRAPHY

Chapter I: Understanding the basics of heart disease

1. American Heart Association. *Heart Disease and Stroke Statistics - 2005 Update.* Dallas, Texas.: ©2005, American Heart Association.
2. Anand S, Yusuf S, Vuksan V, et al. Differences in risk factors, atherosclerosis, and cardiovascular disease between ethnic groups in Canada: the Study of Health Assessment and Risk in Ethnic groups (SHARE). *Lancet* 2000;356:279-284.
3. Bahl VK, Prabhakaran D, Karthikeyan G. Coronary artery disease in Indians. *Indian Heart J* 2001;53:707-713.
4. Balarajan R. Ethnic differences in mortality from ischaemic heart disease and cerebrovascular disease in England and Wales. *Bmj* 1991;302:560-4.
5. Balrajan R. *Health Trends.* 1996; 28:45-51.
6. Bhopal R, Fischbacher C, Vartiainen E, Unwin N, White M, Alberti G. Predicted and observed cardiovascular disease in South Asians: application of FINRISK, Framingham and SCORE models to Newcastle Heart Project data. *J Public Health (Oxf)* 2005;27:93-100.
7. Bhopal R, Unwin N, WhiteM, et al. Heterogeneity of coronary heart disease risk factors in Indian, Pakistani, Bangladeshi, and European origin populations: cross sectional study. *BMJ* 1999;319:215-220.
8. Bittl JA. Advances in coronary angioplasty. *N Engl J Med* 1996;335:1290- 302.
9. Chadha SL, Radhakrishan S, Ramachandran K. Epidemiological study of coronary heart disease in urban population of New Delhi. *Ind J Med Res* 1990;92 (B):424-430.
10. Danarag TJ, Acker M, Danaraj W, Ong W, Yam T. Ethnic group differences in coronary heart disease in Singapore: an analysis of necropsy records. *Am Heart J.* 1959;58:516-526.
11. Davies MJ. The pathophysiology of acute coronary syndromes. *Heart* 2000;83:361-6.
12. Decline in deaths from heart disease and stroke--United States, 1900-1999. *Mortality and morbidity Weekly review* 1999: 48:64.
13. Enas EA, Garg A, Davidson MA, Nair VM, Huet BA, Yusuf S. Coronary heart disease and its risk factors in first-generation immigrant Asian Indians to the United States of America. *Indian Heart J* 1996;48:343-353.
14. Enas EA, Jacob S. Decline of CAD in developed countries: Lessons for India. In: Sethi K, ed. Coronary Artery Disease in Indians - A Global Perspective. *Mumbai: Cardiological Society of India,* 1998:98 -113.
15. Enas EA, Mehta J. Malignant coronary artery disease in young Asian Indians: Thoughts on pathogenesis, prevention, and treatment. *Clin Cardiol* 1995; 18:131-135.
16. Enas EA, Senthilkumar A, Vinod C, Puthumans N. Dyslipidemia among Indo-Asians: Strategies for identification and management. *Brit J Diabetes and Vascular Disease* 2005;5:81-90.
17. Enas EA, Senthilkumar A. Coronary artery disease in Asian Indians: An update and review. In: Gundu HR Rao, Thanikachalam S, eds. Coronary Artery Disease: Risk promoters, pathophysiology, and prevention. *New Delhi: Jaypee,* 2005:21-57.
18. Enas EA, Yusuf S, Mehta J. Meeting of International Working Group on coronary artery disease in South Asians. *Indian Heart J.* 1996;48:727-732.
19. Enas EA, Yusuf S, Mehta J. Prevalence of coronary artery disease in Asian Indians. *Am J Cardiol* 1992;70:945 - 949.
20. Enas EA. Arresting and reversing the epidemic of CAD among Indians. In: Kumar A, ed. Current Perspectives in Cardiology. *Chennai: Cardiological Society of India,* 2000:109-128.
21. Enas EA. Coronary artery disease epidemic in Indians: A cause for alarm and call for action. *J Indian Med Assoc* 2000;98:694-5, 697-702.
22. Enas EA. Why is there an epidemic of malignant CAD in young Indians? *Asian J Clin Cardiol* 1998;1:43-59.
23. Glagov S, Weisenberg E, Zarins C, Stankunavicius R, Kolettis G. Compensatory enlargement of human atherosclerotic coronary arteries. *N Engl J Med* 1987;316:1371 - 1375.
24. Glagov S, Bassiouny HS, Sakaguchi Y, Goudet CA, Vito RP. Mechanical determinants of plaque modeling, remodeling and disruption. *Atherosclerosis* 1997;131 Suppl:S13-4.
25. Gupta R, Gupta VP. Meta-analysis of coronary heart disease prevalence in India. *Indian Heart J* 1996;48:241-245.
26. Herrmann HC. Prevention of cardiovascular events after percutaneous coronary intervention. *N Engl J Med* 2004;350:2708-10.
27. Hughes LO, Raval U, Raftery E. First myocardial infarctions in Asian and White men. *BMJ* 1989;298:1345-1350.
28. Ismail J, Jafar TH, Jafary FH, WhiteF, Faruqui AM, Chaturvedi N. Risk factors for non-fatal myocardial infarction in young South Asian adults. *Heart* 2004;90:259-63.
29. Kaimkhani Z, Ali M, Faruqui AM. Coronary artery diameter in a cohort of adult Pakistani population. *J Pak Med Assoc* 2004; 54:258-61.
30. Klatsky AL, Tekawa I, Armstrong MA, Sidney S. The risk of hospitalization for ischemic heart disease among Asian Americans in northern California. *Am J Public Health.* 1994;84:1672-1675.
31. Krishnaswami S. Prevalence of coronary artery disease in India. *Indian Heart J* 2002;54:103.
32. Lange RA, Hillis LD. Reperfusion therapy in acute myocardial infarction. *N Engl J Med* 2002;346:954-5.
33. Libby P. Current concepts of the pathogenesis of the acute coronary syndromes. *Circulation* 2001;104:365-372.
34. Libby P. Molecular bases of the acute coronary syndromes. *Circulation* 1995;91:2844-50.
35. Libby P. Vascular biology of atherosclerosis: overview and state of the art. *Am J Cardiol* 2003;91:3A-6A.
36. Lowry P J, Lamb P, Watson RD, et al. Influence of racial origin on admission rates of patients with suspected myocardial infarction in Birmingham. *Br Heart J.* 1991;66(1):29-35.
37. Lytle BW. Prolonging patency--choosing coronary bypass grafts. *N Engl J Med* 2004;351:2262-4.
38. Mak KH, Chia KS, Kark JD, et al. Ethnic differences in acute myocardial infarction in Singapore. *Eur Heart J* 2003;24:151-60.
39. Mammi MV, Pavithran K, Abdu Rahiman P, Pisharody R, Sugathan K. Acute myocardial infarction in north Kerala--a 20 year hospital based study. *Indian Heart J* 1991;43:93-6.
40. Mohan V, Deepa R, Shanthi Rani S, Premalatha G. Prevalence of coronary artery disease and its relationship to lipids in a selected population in South India. The Chennai Urban Population Study (CUPS No. 5). *J Am Coll Cardiol* 2001;38:682-687.
41. Prabhakaran D, Shah P, Chaturvedi V, Ramakrishnan L, Manhapra A, Reddy KS. Cardiovascular risk factor prevalence among men in a large industry of northern India. *Natl Med J India* 2005;18:59-65.
42. Raman Kutty V, Balakrishnan K, Jayasree A, et al. Prevalence of coronary heart disease in the rural population of Thiruvananthapuram district, Kerala, India. *Int J Cardiol* 1993;39:59-70.
43. Reddy KS. Rising burden of cardiovascular diseases in India. In: Sethi KK, ed. Coronary Artery Disease in Indians: A Global Perspective. Mumbai: *Cardiological Society of India,* 1998:63-72.
44. Sharma SN, Kaul U, Wasir HS, et al. Coronary arteriographic profile in young and old Indian patients with ischaemic heart disease: A comparative study. *Indian Heart J* 1990;42:365-369.
45. Strike PC, Steptoe A. Behavioral and emotional triggers of acute coronary syndromes: a systematic review and critique. *Psychosom Med* 2005;67:17986.
46. Tso DK, Moe G. Cardiovascular disease in Chinese Canadians: a case-mix study from an urban tertiary care cardiology clinic. *Can J Cardiol* 2002;18:861-9.
47. Uddin SN, Siddiqui NI, Bagum F, Malik F, Rahman S, Ali MS. Coronary artery disease in young adults - angiographic profile. *Mymensingh Med J* 2004;13:11-5.
48. Venketasubramanian N, Tan LC, Sahadevan S, et al. Prevalence of stroke among Chinese, Malay, and Indian Singaporeans: a community-based tri-racial cross-sectional survey. *Stroke* 2005;36:551-6.
49. Wright DJ, Roberts AP. Which doctors die first? Analysis of BMJ obituary columns. *Bmj* 1996;313:1581-2.
50. Yusuf S, Reddy S, Ounpuu S, Anand S. Global burden of cardiovascular diseases: Part II: variations in cardiovascular disease by specific ethnic groups and geographic regions and prevention strategies. *Circulation* 2001;104:2855-2864. 70.

Chapter II: Heart disease far more predictable than you think

1. Aarabi M, Jackson PR. Predicting coronary risk in UK South Asians: an adjustment method for Framingham-based tools. *Eur J Cardiovasc Prev Rehabil* 2005;12:46-51.
2. Anjana M, Sandeep S, Deepa R, Vimaleswaran KS, Farooq S, Mohan V. Visceral and central abdominal fat and anthropometry in relation to diabetes in Asian Indians. *Diabetes Care* 2004;27:2948-53.
3. Barbagallo CM, Averna MR, Frada G, Noto D, Cavera G, Notarbartolo A. Lipoprotein profile and high-density lipoproteins: subfractions distribution in centenarians. *Gerontology* 1998;44:106-10.
4. Barzilai N, Atzmon G, Schechter C, et al. Unique lipoprotein phenotype and genotype associated with exceptional longevity. *Jama* 2003;290:2030-40.
5. Bersot TP, Pepin GM, Mahley RW. Risk determination of dyslipidemia in

populations characterized by low levels of high-density lipoprotein choles-terol. *Am Heart J* 2003;146:1052-9.

6. Bhopal R, Unwin N, WhiteM, et al. Heterogeneity of coronary heart disease risk factors in Indian, Pakistani, Bangladeshi, and European origin popula-tions: cross sectional study. *BMJ* 1999;319:215-220.

7. Boizel R, Benhamou PY, Lardy B, Laporte F, Foulon T, Halimi S. Ratio of triglycerides to HDL cholesterol is an indicator of LDL particle size in patients with type 2 diabetes and normal HDL cholesterol levels. *Diabetes Care* 2000;23:1679-1685.

8. Cappuccio FP, Oakeshott P, Strazzullo P, Kerry SM. Application of Framingham risk estimates to ethnic minorities in United Kingdom and impli-cations for primary prevention of heart disease in general practice: cross sec-tional population based study. *Bmj* 2002;325:1271.

9. Castelli WP, Garrison RJ, Wilson PW, Abbott RD, Kalousdian S, Kannel WB. Incidence of coronary heart disease and lipoprotein cholesterol levels. The Framingham Study. *Jama* 1986;256:2835-8.

10. Chadha S L, Tandon R, Shekhawat S, Gopinath N. An epidemiological stud od pressure in school children (5-14 years) in Delhi. *Indian Heart J* 1999;51:178-82.

11. AV, Bakris GL, Black HR, et al. The Seventh Report of the Joint National Committee on Prevention, Detection, Evaluation, and Treatment of High Blood Pressure: the JNC 7 report. *Jama* 2003;289:2560-72.

12. Conroy RM, Pyorala K, Fitzgerald AP, et al. Estimation of ten-year risk of fatal cardiovascular disease in Europe: the SCORE project. *Eur Heart J* 2003;24:987-1003.

13. Coutinho M, Gerstein HC, Wang Y, Yusuf S. The relationship between glu-cose and incident cardiovascular events: A metaregression analysis of pub-lished data from 20 studies of 95,783 individuals followed for 12.4 years. *Diabetes Care* 1999;22:233-240.

14. D'Agostino RB Sr, Grundy S, Sullivan LM, Wilson P. Validation of the Framingham coronary heart disease prediction scores: results of a multiple ethnic groups investigation. *Jama* 2001;286:180-187.

15. Drexel H, Aczel S, Marte T, et al. Is atherosclerosis in diabetes and impaired fasting glucose driven by elevated LDL cholesterol or by decreased HDL cho-lesterol? *Diabetes Care* 2005;28:101-7.

16. Empana JP, Ducimetiere P, Arveiler D, et al. Are the Framingham and PRO-CAM coronary heart disease risk functions applicable to different European populations? The PRIME Study. *Eur Heart J* 2003;24:1903-11.

17. Gaziano JM, Hennekens CH, O'Donnell CJ, Breslow JL, Buring JE. Fasting triglycerides, high-density lipoprotein, and risk of myocardial infarction. *Circulation* 1997;96:2520-5.

18. Gaziano JM, Sesso HD, Breslow JL, Hennekens CH, Buring JE. Relation between systemic hypertension and blood lipids on the risk of myocardial infarction. *Am J Cardiol* 1999;84:768-73.

19. Gimeno-Orna JA, Faure-Nogueras E, Sancho-Serrano MA. Usefulness of total cholesterol/HDL-cholesterol ratio in the management of diabetic dyslipi-daemia. *Diabet Med* 2005;22:26-31.

20. Grundy SM, Cleeman JI, Merz CN, et al. Implications of recent clinical trials for the National Cholesterol Education Program Adult Treatment Panel III guidelines. *Circulation* 2004;110:227-39.

21. Grundy SM. Age as a risk factor: you are as old as your arteries . *Am J Cardiol* 1999;83:1455-7, A7.

22. Gupta R, Gupta KD. Total cholesterol and mortality in patients with pre-exist-ing coronary artery disease. *Natl Med J India* 1992;5:111-4.

23. Gupta R. Trends in hypertension epidemiology in India. *J Hum Hypertens* 2004;18:73-8.

24. Hawkes K. Grandmothers and the evolution of human longevity. *Am J Hum Biol* 2003;15:380-400.

25. Heartstats.org

26. Hense HW, Schulte H, Lowel H, Assmann G, Keil U. Framingham risk func-tion overestimates risk of coronary heart disease in men and women from Germany--results from the MONICA Augsburg and the PROCAM cohorts. *Eur Heart J* 2003;24:937-45.

27. Hong CY, Chia KS, Hughes K, Ling SL. Ethnic differences among Chinese, Malay and Indian patients with type 2 diabetes mellitus in Singapore. *Singapore Med J* 2004;45:154-60.

28. Hu FB, Stampfer MJ, Haffner SM, Solomon CG, Willett WC, Manson JE. Elevated risk of cardiovascular disease prior to clinical diagnosis of type 2 diabetes. *Diabetes Care* 2002;25:1129-34.

29. Hu FB, Stampfer MJ, Solomon CG, et al. The impact of diabetes mellitus on mortality from all causes and coronary heart disease in women: 20 years of follow-up. *Arch Intern Med* 2001;161:1717-1723.

30. Hughes LO, Wojciechowski AP, Raftery EB. Relationship between plasma cho-lesterol and coronary artery disease in Asians. *Atherosclerosis* 1990;83:15-20.

31. Joseph A, Kutty VR, Soman CR. High risk for coronary heart disease in Thiruvananthapuram City: A study of serum lipids and other risk factors. *Indian Heart J* 2000;52:29-35.

32. Juutilainen A, Kortelainen S, Lehto S, Ronnemaa T, Pyorala K, Laakso M. Gender difference in the impact of type 2 diabetes on coronary heart disease risk. *Diabetes Care* 2004;27:2898-904.

33. Liu JL, Hong Y, D'Agostino RB, Sr., et al. Predictive value for the Chinese population of the Framingham CHD risk assessment tool compared with the Chinese Multi-Provincial Cohort Study. *Jama* 2004;291:2591-9.

34. Lloyd-Jones DM, Wilson PW, Larson MG, et al. Framingham risk score and prediction of lifetime risk for coronary heart disease. *Am J Cardiol* 2004;94:20-4.

35. Makinen J, Jarvisalo MJ, Pollanen P, et al. Increased carotid atherosclerosis in andropausal middle-aged men. *J Am Coll Cardiol* 2005;45:1603-8.

36. Menotti A, Lanti M, Puddu PE, Kromhout D. Coronary heart disease inci-dence in northern and southern European populations: A reanalysis of the Seven Countries Study for a European coronary risk chart. *Heart* 2000;84:238-244.

37. Miller M, Kwiterovich PO, Jr. Isolated low HDL-cholesterol as an important risk factor for coronary heart disease. *Eur Heart J* 1990;11 Suppl H:9-14.

38. Mohan V, Deepa R, Premlatha G, Sastry N, Revathi S. Hypercholesterolemia, not hypertriglyceridemia is associated with coronary heart disease in normals and diabetic subjects - a population-based study in Chennai. *Indian Heart J* 1997;49:618.

39. Mohan V, Deepa R, Shanthi Rani S, Premalatha G. Prevalence of coronary artery disease and its relationship to lipids in a selected population in South India. The Chennai Urban Population Study (CUPS No. 5). *J Am Coll Cardiol* 2001;38:682-687.

40. Nasir K, Michos ED, Rumberger JA, et al. Coronary artery calcification and family history of premature coronary heart disease: sibling history is more strongly associated than parental history. *Circulation* 2004;110:2150-6.

41. NCEP III. Third Report of the National Cholesterol Education Program (NCEP) Adult Treatment Panel III. *National Institute of Health*, 2002.

42. Qiao Q, Hu G, Tuomilehto J, et al. Age- and sex-specific prevalence of dia-betes and impaired glucose regulation in 11 Asian cohorts. *Diabetes Care* 2003;26:1770-80.

43. Quirke TP, Gill PS, Mant JW, Allan TF. The applicability of the Framingham coronary heart disease prediction function to black and minority ethnic groups in the UK. *Heart* 2003;89:785-6.

44. Ramachandran A, Snehalatha C, Vijay V. Temporal changes in prevalence of type 2 diabetes and impaired glucose tolerance in urban southern India. *Diabetes Res Clin Pract* 2002;58:55-60.

45. Ramachandran A, Snehalatha C, Kapur A, et al. High prevalence of diabetes and impaired glucose tolerance in India: National Urban Diabetes Survey. *Diabetologia* 2001;44:1094-1101.

46. Raman Kutty V, Joseph A, Soman CR. High prevalence of type 2 diabetes in an urban settlement in Kerala, India. *Ethn Health* 1999;4:231-9.

47. Ridker PM, Rifai N, Cook NR, Bradwin G, Buring JE. Non-HDL cholesterol, apolipoproteins A-I and B100, standard lipid measures, lipid ratios, and CRP as risk factors for cardiovascular disease in women. *Jama* 2005;294:326-33.

48. Sharrett AR, Ballantyne CM, Coady SA, et al. Coronary heart disease predic-tion from lipoprotein cholesterol levels, triglycerides,lipoprotein(a), apolipoproteins A-I and B, and HDL density subfractions: The Atherosclerosis Risk in Communities (ARIC) Study. *Circulation* 2001;104:1108-13.

49. Stamler J, Daviglus ML, Garside DB, Dyer AR, Greenland P, Neaton JD. Relationship of baseline serum cholesterol levels in three large cohorts of younger men to long-term coronary, cardiovascular, and all-cause mortality and to longevity. *JAMA* 2000;284:311-318.

50. Strandberg TE, Strandberg A, Rantanen K, Salomaa VV, Pitkala K, Miettinen TA. Low cholesterol, mortality, and quality of life in old age during a 39-year follow-up. *J Am Coll Cardiol* 2004;44:1002-8.

51. Turner RC, Millns H, Neil HA, et al. Risk factors for coronary artery disease in non-insulin dependent diabetes mellitus: United Kingdom Prospective Diabetes Study (UKPDS: 23). *Bmj* 1998;316:823-828.

52. van den Hoogen PC, Feskens E, Nagelkerke N, Menotti A, Nissinen A, Kromhout D. The relation between blood pressure and mortality due to coro-nary heart disease among men in different parts of the world. Seven Countries Study Research Group. *N Engl J Med* 2000;342:1-8.

53. Verschuren WMM, Jacobs D, Bloemberg B, et al. Serum total cholesterol and long-term coronary heart disease mortality in different cultures: Twenty-five year follow-up of the Seven Countries Study. *JAMA* 1995;274:131-136.

54. Wannamethee SG, Shaper AG, Lennon L. Cardiovascular disease incidence and mortality in older men with diabetes and in men with coronary heart dis-ease. *Heart* 2004;90:1398-403.

55. Whitmer RA, Sidney S, Selby J, Johnston SC, Yaffe K. Midlife cardiovascular risk factors and risk of dementia in late life. *Neurology* 2005;64:277-81.
56. Wild S, Roglic G, Green A, Sicree R, King H. Global prevalence of diabetes: estimates for the year 2000 and projections for 2030. *Diabetes Care* 2004;27:1047-53.
57. Woods SE, Smith JM, Sohail S, Sarah A, Engle A. The influence of type 2 diabetes mellitus in patients undergoing coronary artery bypass graft surgery: an 8-year prospective cohort study. *Chest* 2004;126:1789-95.
58. WWW. Heartstat.org
59. Yan LL, Liu K, Matthews KA, Daviglus ML, Ferguson TF, Kiefe CI. Psychosocial factors and risk of hypertension: the Coronary Artery Risk Development in Young Adults (CARDIA) study. *Jama* 2003;290:2138-48.
60. Yusuf S, Hawken S, Ounpuu S, et al. Effect of potentially modifiable risk factors associated with myocardial infarction in 52 countries (the INTERHEART study): case-control study. *Lancet* 2004;364:937-52.

Chapter III: Heart disease: advanced concepts

1. Alexander CM, Landsman PB, Teutsch SM, Haffner SM. NCEP-defined metabolic syndrome, diabetes, and prevalence of coronary heart disease among NHANES III participants age 50 years and older. *Diabetes* 2003;52:1210-4.
2. Anand S, Enas EA, Pogue J, Haffner S, Pearson T, Yusuf S. Elevated lipoprotein(a) levels in South Asians in North America. *Metabolism* 1998;47:182184.
3. Anand S, Yusuf S, Vuksan V, et al. Differences in risk factors, atherosclerosis, and cardiovascular disease between ethnic groups in Canada: the Study of Health Assessment and Risk in Ethnic groups (SHARE). *Lancet* 2000;356:279-284.
4. Anand SS, Razak F, Yi Q, et al. C-reactive protein as a screening test for cardiovascular risk in a multiethnic population. *Arterioscler Thromb Vasc Biol* 2004;24:1509-15.
5. Assmann G, Schulte H, von Eckardstein A. Hypertriglyceridemia and elevated lipoprotein(a) are risk factors for major coronary events in middle-aged men. *Am J Cardiol* 1996;77:1179-1184.
6. Berg K, Dahlen G, Christophersen B, Cook T, Kjekshus J, Pedersen T. Lipoprotein(a) lipoprotein level predicts survival and major coronary events in the Scandinavian Simvastatin Survival Study. *Clin Genet* 1997;52:254-261.
7. Blair SN, Kampert JB, Kohl HW, 3rd, et al. Influences of cardiorespiratory fitness and other precursors on cardiovascular disease and all-cause mortality in men and women. *Jama* 1996;276:205-10.
8. Bostom AG, Cupples LA, Jenner JL, et al. Elevated plasma lipoprotein(a) and coronary heart disease in men aged 55 years and younger. A prospective study. *Jama* 1996;276:544-548.
9. Buchwald H, Avidor Y, Braunwald E, et al. Bariatric surgery: a systematic review and meta-analysis. *Jama* 2004;292:1724-37.
10. Budde T, Fechtrup C, Bosenberg E, et al. Plasma Lipoprotein(a) levels correlate with number, severity, and length- extension of coronary lesions in male patients undergoing coronary arteriography for clinically suspected coronary atherosclerosis. *Arterioscler Thromb* 1994;14:1730-6.
11. Chambers JC, Eda S, Bassett P, et al. C-reactive protein, insulin resistance, central obesity, and coronary heart disease risk in Indian Asians from the United Kingdom compared with European whites. *Circulation* 2001;104:145150.
12. Chambers JC, Obeid OA, Refsum H, et al. Plasma homocysteine concentrations and risk of coronary heart disease in UK Indian Asian and European men. *Lancet* 2000;355:523-527.
13. Chandalia M, Abate N, Cabo-Chan AV, Jr., Devaraj S, Jialal I, Grundy SM. Hyperhomocysteinemia in Asian Indians living in the United States. *J Clin Endocrinol Metab* 2003;88:1089-95.
14. Chandalia M, Cabo-Chan AV, Jr., Devaraj S, Jialal I, Grundy SM, Abate N. Elevated plasma high-sensitivity C-reactive protein concentrations in Asian Indians living in the United States. *J Clin Endocrinol Metab* 2003;88:3773-6.
15. Christopher R, Kailasanatha KM, Nagaraja D, Tripathi M. Case-control study of serum lipoprotein(a) and apolipoproteins A-I and B in stroke in the young. *Acta Neurol Scand* 1996;94:127-30.
16. Conus F, Allison DB, Rabasa-Lhoret R, et al. Metabolic and behavioral characteristics of metabolically obese but normal-weight women. *J Clin Endocrinol Metab* 2004;89:5013-20.
17. Coutinho M, Gerstein HC, Wang Y, Yusuf S. The relationship between glucose and incident cardiovascular events: A metaregression analysis of published data from 20 studies of 95,783 individuals followed for 12.4 years. *Diabetes Care* 1999;22:233-240.
18. Deurenberg P, Deurenberg-Yap M, Guricci S. Asians are different from Caucasians and from each other in their body mass index/body fat per cent relationship. *Obes Rev* 2002;3:141-6.
19. Deurenberg-Yap M, Chew SK, Deurenberg P. Elevated body fat percentage and cardiovascular risks at low body mass index levels among Singaporean Chinese, Malays and Indians. *Obes Rev* 2002;3:209-15.
20. Enas EA, Dhawan J, Petkar S. Coronary artery disease in Asian Indians: Lessons learned so far and the role of Lp(a). *Indian Heart J* 1997;49:25-34.
21. Enas EA. Dyslipidemia among Indo-Asians: Stratgies for identification and management. *Brit J of Diabetes and Vascular Dis* 2005;5:81-90.
22. Foody JM, Milberg JA, Robinson K, Pearce GL, Jacobsen DW, Sprecher DL. Homocysteine and lipoprotein(a) interact to increase CAD risk in young men and women. *Arterioscler Thromb Vasc Biol* 2000;20:493-9.
23. Forouhi NG, Sattar N, McKeigue PM. Relation of C-reactive protein to body fat distribution and features of the metabolic syndrome in Europeans and South Asians. *Int J Obes Relat Metab Disord* 2001;25:1327-31.
24. Gambhir JK, Kaur H, Gambhir DS, Prabhu KM. Lipoprotein(a) as an independent risk factor for coronary artery disease in patients below 40 years of age. *Indian Heart J* 2000;52:411-415.
25. Goel MS, McCarthy EP, Phillips RS, Wee CC. Obesity among US immigrant subgroups by duration of residence. *Jama* 2004;292:2860-7.
26. Grundy SM, Hansen B, Smith SC, Jr., Cleeman JI, Kahn RA. Clinical management of metabolic syndrome: report of the American Heart Association/National Heart, Lung, and Blood Institute/American Diabetes Association conference on scientific issues related to management. *Circulation* 2004;109:551-6.
27. Gupta R, Kastia S, Rastogi S, Kaul V, Nagar R, Enas EA. Lipoprotein(a) in coronary heart disease: A case-control study. *Indian Heart J* 2000;52:407-410.
28. Gupta R, Vasisht S, Bahl VK, Wasir HS. Correlation of lipoprotein(a) to angiographically defined coronary artery disease in Indians. *Int J Cardiol* 1996;57:265-270.
29. Heartstat.org
30. Hebert PR, Rich-Edwards JW, Manson JE, et al. Height and incidence of cardiovascular disease in male physicians. *Circulation* 1993;88:1437-43.
31. Hoogeveen RC, Gambhir JK, Gambhir DS, et al. Evaluation of Lp[a] and other independent risk factors for CHD in Asian Indians and their USA counterparts. *J Lipid Res* 2001;42:631-638.
32. Hopkins PN, Wu LL, Hunt SC, James BC, Vincent GM, Williams RR. Lipoprotein(a) interactions with lipid and nonlipid risk factors in early familial coronary artery disease. *Arterioscler Thromb Vasc Biol* 1997;17:2783-92.
33. Isomaa B, Almgren P, Tuomi T, et al. Cardiovascular morbidity and mortality associated with the metabolic syndrome. *Diabetes Care* 2001;24:683-689.
34. Isser HS, Puri VK, Narain VS, Saran RK, Dwivedi SK, Singh S. Lipoprotein (a) and lipid levels in young patients with myocardial infarction and their first-degree relatives. *Indian Heart J* 2001;53:463-6.
35. Katzmarzyk PT, Church TS, Blair SN. Cardiorespiratory fitness attenuates the effects of the metabolic syndrome on all-cause and cardiovascular disease mortality in men. *Arch Intern Med* 2004;164:1092-7.
36. Khaw KT, Wareham N, Bingham S, Luben R, Welch A, Day N. Association of hemoglobin A1c with cardiovascular disease and mortality in adults: the European prospective investigation into cancer in Norfolk. *Ann Intern Med* 2004;141:413-20.
37. Kip KE, Marroquin OC, Kelley DE, et al. Clinical importance of obesity versus the metabolic syndrome in cardiovascular risk in women: a report from the Women's Ischemia Syndrome Evaluation (WISE) study. *Circulation* 2004;109:706-13.
38. Knox SS, Weidner G, Adelman A, Stoney CM, Ellison RC. Hostility and physiological risk in the National Heart, Lung, and Blood Institute Family Heart Study. *Arch Intern Med* 2004;164:2442-7.
39. Larsson B, Bengtsson C, Bjorntorp P, et al. Is abdominal body fat distribution a major explanation for the sex difference in the incidence of myocardial infarction? The study of men born in 1913 and the study of women, Goteborg, Sweden. *Am J Epidemiol* 1992;135:266-73.
40. Lavie CJ, Milani RV. Prevalence of hostility in young coronary artery disease patients and effects of cardiac rehabilitation and exercise training. *Mayo Clin Proc* 2005;80:335-42.
41. Lee CD, Blair SN, Jackson AS. Cardiorespiratory fitness, body composition, and all-cause and cardiovascular disease mortality in men. *Am J Clin Nutr* 1999;69:373-80.
42. Lemieux I, Pascot A, Couillard C, et al. Hypertriglyceridemic waist: A marker of the atherogenic metabolic triad (hyperinsulinemia; hyperapolipoprotein B; small, dense LDL) in men? *Circulation* 2000;102:179-184.
43. Lissner L, Bjorkelund C, Heitmann BL, Seidell JC, Bengtsson C. Larger hip circumference independently predicts health and longevity in a Swedish female cohort. *Obes Res* 2001;9:644-6.
44. Low PS, Heng CK, Saha N, Tay JS. Racial variation of cord plasma lipoprotein(a) levels in relation to coronary risk level: a study in three ethnic groups

in Singapore. *Pediatr Res* 1996;40:718-22.

45. Malik S, Wong ND, Franklin S, et al. Impact of the metabolic syndrome on mortality from coronary heart disease, cardiovascular disease, and all causes in United States adults. *Circulation* 2004;110:1245-50.

46. Matthews KA, Gump BB, Harris KF, Haney TL, Barefoot JC. Hostile behaviors predict cardiovascular mortality among men enrolled in the multiple risk factor intervention trial. *Circulation* 2004;109:66-70.

47. McCully KS. Homocysteine, vitamins, and prevention of vascular disease. *Mil Med* 2004;169:325-9.

48. Misra A. C-reactive protein in young individuals: problems and implications for Asian Indians. *Nutrition* 2004;20:478-81.

49. Mohan V, Deepa R, Haranath SP, et al. Lipoprotein(a) is an independent risk factor for coronary artery disease in NIDDM patients in South India. *Diabetes Care* 1998;21:1819-23.

50. Nishtar S, Wierzbicki AS, Lumb PJ, et al. Waist-hip ratio and low HDL predict the risk of coronary artery disease in Pakistanis. *Curr Med Res Opin* 2004;20:55-62.

51. Nissen SE, Tuzcu EM, Schoenhagen P, et al. Statin therapy, LDL cholesterol, C-reactive protein, and coronary artery disease. *N Engl J Med* 2005;352:2938.

52. Nygard O, Nordrehaug JE, Refsum H, Ueland PM, Farstad M, Vollset SE. Plasma homocysteine levels and mortality in patients with coronary artery disease. *N Engl J Med* 1997;337:230-6.

53. O'Callaghan P, Meleady R, Fitzgerald T, Graham I. Smoking and plasma homocysteine. *Eur Heart J* 2002;23:1580-6.

54. Pereira MA, Kartashov AI, Ebbeling CB, et al. Fast-food habits, weight gain, and insulin resistance (the CARDIA study): 15-year prospective analysis. *Lancet* 2005;365:36-42.

55. Refsum H, Yajnik CS, Gadkari M, et al. Hyperhomocysteinemia and elevated methylmalonic acid indicate a high prevalence of cobalamin deficiency in Asian Indians. *Am J Clin Nutr* 2001;74:233-41.

56. Ridker PM, Cannon CP, Morrow D, et al. C-reactive protein levels and outcomes after statin therapy. *N Engl J Med* 2005;352:20-8.

57. Rifai N, Ma J, Sacks FM, et al. Apolipoprotein(a) size and lipoprotein(a) concentration and future risk of angina pectoris with evidence of severe coronary atherosclerosis in men: The Physicians' Health Study. *Clin Chem* 2004;50:1364-71.

58. Rosengren A, Hawken S, Ounpuu S, et al. Association of psychosocial risk factors with risk of acute myocardial infarction in 11119 cases and 13648 controls from 52 countries (the INTERHEART study): case-control study. *Lancet* 2004;364:953-62.

59. Roumeguere T, Wespes E, Carpentier Y, Hoffmann P, Schulman CC. Erectile dysfunction is associated with a high prevalence of hyperlipidemia and coronary heart disease risk. *Eur Urol* 2003;44:355-9.

60. Rozanski A, Blumenthal JA, Davidson KW, Saab PG, Kubzansky L. The epidemiology, pathophysiology, and management of psychosocial risk factors in cardiac practice: the emerging field of behavioral cardiology. *J Am Coll Cardiol* 2005;45:637-51.

61. Sattar N, Gaw A, Scherbakova O, et al. Metabolic syndrome with and without C-reactive protein as a predictor of coronary heart disease and diabetes in the West of Scotland Coronary Prevention Study. *Circulation* 2003;108:414-9.

62. Seidell JC, Han TS, Feskens EJ, Lean ME. Narrow hips and broad waist circumferences independently contribute to increased risk of non-insulin-dependent diabetes mellitus. *J Intern Med* 1997;242:401-6.

63. Snijder MB, Dekker JM, Visser M, et al. Trunk fat and leg fat have independent and opposite associations with fasting and postload glucose levels: the Hoorn study. *Diabetes Care* 2004;27:372-7.

64. St-Onge MP, Janssen I, Heymsfield SB. Metabolic Syndrome in Normal-Weight Americans: New definition of the metabolically obese, normal-weight individual. *Diabetes Care* 2004;27:2222-8.

65. St-Pierre J, Lemieux I, Vohl MC, et al. Contribution of abdominal obesity and hypertriglyceridemia to impaired fasting glucose and coronary artery disease. *Am J Cardiol* 2002;90:15-8.

66. Tan CE, Ma S, Wai D, Chew SK, Tai ES. Can we apply the National Cholesterol Education Program Adult Treatment Panel definition of the metabolic syndrome to Asians? *Diabetes Care* 2004;27:1182-6.

67. Van Gaal LF, Rissanen AM, Scheen AJ, Ziegler O, Rossner S. Effects of the cannabinoid-1 receptor blocker rimonabant on weight reduction and cardiovascular risk factors in overweight patients: 1-year experience from the RIO-Europe study. *Lancet* 2005;365:1389-97.

68. Velmurugan K, Deepa R, Ravikumar R, et al. Relationship of lipoprotein(a) with intimal medial thickness of the carotid artery in Type 2 diabetic patients in south India. *Diabet Med* 2003;20:455-61.

69. Wang Y, Rimm EB, Stampfer MJ, Willett WC, Hu FB. Comparison of abdominal adiposity and overall obesity in predicting risk of type 2 diabetes among

men. *Am J Clin Nutr* 2005;81:555-63.

70. Whincup PH, Gilg JA, Papacosta O, et al. Early evidence of ethnic differences in cardiovascular risk: cross sectional comparison of British South Asian and white children. *Bmj* 2002;324:635.

71. Wong ND, Pio JR, Franklin SS, L'Italien GJ, Kamath TV, Williams GR. Preventing coronary events by optimal control of blood pressure and lipids in patients with the metabolic syndrome. *Am J Cardiol* 2003;91:1421-6.

72. WWW. Heartstat.org .

73. Zairis MN, Ambrose JA, Manousakis SJ, et al. The impact of plasma levels of C-reactive protein, lipoprotein (a) and homocysteine on the long-term prognosis after successful coronary stenting. The global evaluation of new events and restenosis after stent implantation study. *J Am Coll Cardiol* 2002;40:1375.

74. Zhu S, Wang Z, Heshka S, Heo M, Faith MS, Heymsfield SB. Waist circumference and obesity-associated risk factors among whites in the third National Health and Nutrition Examination Survey: clinical action thresholds. *Am J Clin Nutr* 2002;76:743-9.

Chapter IV: Heart disease among Particular populations

1. Aarabi M, Jackson PR. Predicting coronary risk in UK South Asians: an adjustment method for Framingham-based tools. *Eur J Cardiovasc Prev Rehabil* 2005;12:46-51.

2. Benfante R. Studies of cardiovascular disease and cause-specific mortality trends in Japanese-American men living in Hawaii and risk factor comparisons with other Japanese populations in the Pacific region: a review. *Hum Biol* 1992;64:791-805.

3. Berenson GS, Srinivasan SR, Bao W, Newman WP, 3rd, Tracy RE, Wattigney WA. Association between multiple cardiovascular risk factors and atherosclerosis in children and young adults. The Bogalusa Heart Study. *N Engl J Med* 1998;338:1650-6.

4. Bhopal R, Fischbacher C, Vartiainen E, Unwin N, WhiteM, Alberti G. Predicted and observed cardiovascular disease in South Asians: application of FINRISK, Framingham and SCORE models to Newcastle Heart Project data. *J Public Health (Oxf)* 2005;27:93-100.

5. Bierman EL. George Lyman Duff Memorial Lecture. Atherogenesis in diabetes. *Arterioscler Thromb* 1992;12:647-56.

6. Chadha S L, Tandon R, Shekhawat S, Gopinath N. An epidemiological study of blood pressure in school children (5-14 years) in Delhi. *Indian Heart J* 1999;51:178-82.

7. Chaturvedi N, Jarrett J, Morrish N, Keen H, Fuller JH. Differences in mortality and morbidity in African Caribbean and European people with non-insulin dependent diabetes mellitus: results of 20 year follow up of a London cohort of a multinational study. *Bmj* 1996;313:848-52.

8. Cheng TO. A preventable epidemic of coronary heart disease in modern China. *Eur J Cardiovasc Prev Rehabil* 2005;12:1-4.

9. Cuasay LC, Lee ES, Orlander PP, Steffen-Batey L, Hanis CL. Prevalence and determinants of type 2 diabetes among Filipino-Americans in the Houston, Texas metropolitan statistical area. *Diabetes Care* 2001;24:2054-8.

10. Daviglus ML, Stamler J, Pirzada A, et al. Favorable cardiovascular risk profile in young women and long-term risk of cardiovascular and all-cause mortality. *Jama* 2004;292:1588-92.

11. de Ferranti SD, Gauvreau K, Ludwig DS, Neufeld EJ, Newburger JW, Rifai N. Prevalence of the Metabolic Syndrome in American Adolescents: Findings From the Third National Health and Nutrition Examination Survey. *Circulation* 2004;110:2494-2497.

12. Eaton CB, Schaad DC, Rybicki B, et al. Risk factors for cardiovascular disease in U.S. medical students: the Preventive Cardiology Academic Award Collaborative Data Project. *Am J Prev Med* 1990;6:14-22.

13. Empana JP, Ducimetiere P, Arveiler D, et al. Are the Framingham and PRO-CAM coronary heart disease risk functions applicable to different European populations? The PRIME Study. *Eur Heart J* 2003;24:1903-11.

14. Enas EA, Dhawan J, Petkar S. Coronary artery disease in Asian Indians: Lessons learned so far and the role of Lp(a). *Indian Heart J* 1997;49:25-34.

15. Enas EA, Senthilkumar A, Juturu V, Gupta R. Coronary artery disease in women. *Indian Heart J* 2001;53:282-292.

16. Enas EA, Senthilkumar A. Conquering the epidemic of coronary artery disease among Indians: Crucial role of cardiologists. *Cardiology Today* 2001;5:282-294.

17. Enas EA. Arresting and reversing the epidemic of CAD among Indians. In: Kumar A, ed. Current Perspectives in Cardiology. Chennai: *Cardiological Society of India*, 2000:109-128.

18. Enas EA. Coronary artery disease epidemic in Indians: A cause for alarm and call for action. *J Indian Med Assoc* 2000;98:694-5, 697-702.

19. Enas EA. High rates of CAD in Asian Indians in the United States despite intense modification of lifestyle: What next? *Current Science*

1998;74:10811086.
20. Enas EA. The essence and nonsense of stress:The straw that breaks the camel's back. *AAPI Journal* 1996;8:47-48.
21. Enas EA. Why is there an epidemic of malignant CAD in young Indians? *Asian J Clin Cardiol* 1998;1:43-59.
22. Enos WF, Holmes RH, Beyer J. Landmark article, July 18, 1953: Coronary disease among United States soldiers killed in action in Korea. Preliminary report. By William F. Enos, Robert H. Holmes and James Beyer. *Jama* 1986;256:2859-62.
23. Gillum RF, Mussolino ME, Madans JH. Coronary heart disease incidence and survival in African-American women and men. The NHANES I Epidemiologic Follow-up Study. *Ann Intern Med* 1997;127:111-8.
24. Gu D, Reynolds K, Wu X, et al. Prevalence of the metabolic syndrome and overweight among adults in China. *Lancet* 2005;365:1398-405.
25. Harland JO, Unwin N, Bhopal RS, et al. Low levels of cardiovascular risk factors and coronary heart disease in a UK Chinese population. *J Epidemiol Community Health* 1997;51:636-42.
26. Hopkins PN, Wu LL, Hunt SC, James BC, Vincent GM, Williams RR. Lipoprotein(a) interactions with lipid and nonlipid risk factors in early familial coronary artery disease. *Arterioscler Thromb Vasc Biol* 1997;17:2783-92.
27. Hu G, Jousilahti P, Qiao Q, Peltonen M, Katoh S, Tuomilehto J. The gender-specific impact of diabetes and myocardial infarction at baseline and during follow-up on mortality from all causes and coronary heart disease. *J Am Coll Cardiol* 2005;45:1413-8.
28. Hughes K. Trends in mortality from ischaemic heart disease in Singapore, 1959 to 1983. *Int J Epidemiol* 1986;15:44-50.
29. Jha P, Enas E, Yusuf S. Coronary artery disease in Asian Indians: Prevalence and risk factors. *Asian Am Pac Isl J Health* 1993;1:163-175.
30. Juutilainen A, Kortelainen S, Lehto S, Ronnemaa T, Pyorala K, Laakso M. Gender difference in the impact of type 2 diabetes on coronary heart disease risk. *Diabetes Care* 2004;27:2898-904.
31. Law CM, Shiell AW, Newsome CA, et al. Fetal, infant, and childhood growth and adult blood pressure: a longitudinal study from birth to 22 years of age. *Circulation* 2002;105:1088-92.
32. Lee J, Heng D, Chia KS, Chew SK, Tan BY, Hughes K. Risk factors and incident coronary heart disease in Chinese, Malay and Asian Indian males: the Singapore Cardiovascular Cohort Study. *Int J Epidemiol* 2001;30:983-988.
33. Ludwig DS, Ebbeling CB. Type 2 diabetes mellitus in children: primary care and public health considerations. *Jama* 2001;286:1427-30.
34. McGill HC Jr, McMahan CA, Malcom GT, Oalmann MC, Strong JP. Effects of serum lipoproteins and smoking on atherosclerosis in young men and women. The PDAY Research Group. Pathobiological Determinants of Atherosclerosis in Youth. *Arterioscler Thromb Vasc Biol* 1997;17:95-106.
35. Menotti A, Lanti M, Puddu PE, Kromhout D. Coronary heart disease incidence in northern and southern European populations: A reanalysis of the Seven Countries Study for a European coronary risk chart. *Heart* 2000;84:238-244.
36. Mosca L, Appel LJ, Benjamin EJ, et al. Evidence-based guidelines for cardiovascular disease prevention in women. *Circulation* 2004;109:672-93.
37. Napoli C, Glass CK, Witztum JL, Deutsch R, D'Armiento FP, Palinski W. Influence of maternal hypercholesterolaemia during pregnancy on progression of early atherosclerotic lesions in childhood: Fate of Early Lesions in Children (FELIC) study. *Lancet* 1999;354:1234-41.
38. Nishtar S, Wierzbicki AS, Lumb PJ, et al. Waist-hip ratio and low HDL predict the risk of coronary artery disease in Pakistanis. *Curr Med Res Opin* 2004;20:55-62.
39. Okelo S, Taylor AL, Wright JT, Jr., Gordon N, Mohan G, Lesnefsky E. Race and the decision to refer for coronary revascularization: the effect of physician awareness of patient ethnicity. *J Am Coll Cardiol* 2001;38:698-704.
40. Orth-Gomer K, Mittleman MA, Schenck-Gustafsson K, et al. Lipoprotein(a) as a determinant of coronary heart disease in young women. *Circulation* 1997;95:329-34.
41. Palaniappan L, Anthony MN, Mahesh C, et al. Cardiovascular risk factors in ethnic minority women aged less-than-or- equal30 years. *Am J Cardiol* 2002;89:524-529.
42. Palaniappan L, Wang Y, Fortmann SP. Coronary heart disease mortality for six ethnic groups in California, 1990-2000. *Ann Epidemiol* 2004;14:499-506.
43. Parodi PW. The French paradox unmasked: the role of folate. *Med Hypotheses* 1997;49:313-8.
44. Ramachandran A, Snehalatha C, Satyavani K, Sivasankari S, Vijay V. Type 2 diabetes in Asian-Indian urban children. *Diabetes Care* 2003;26:1022-5.
45. Reaven PD, Sacks J. Reduced coronary artery and abdominal aortic calcification in Hispanics with type 2 diabetes. *Diabetes Care* 2004;27:1115-20.
46. Reddy KS, Prabhakaran D, Shah P, Shah B. Differences in body mass index

and waist: hip ratios in North Indian rural and urban populations. *Obes Rev* 2002;3:197-202.
47. Ridker PM, Cook NR, Lee IM, et al. A randomized trial of low-dose aspirin in the primary prevention of cardiovascular disease in women. *N Engl J Med* 2005;352:1293-304.
48. Rozin P, Kabnick K, Pete E, Fischler C, Shields C. The ecology of eating: smaller portion sizes in France Than in the United States help explain the French paradox. *Psychol Sci* 2003;14:450-4.
49. Solymoss BC, Marcil M, Wesolowska E, Gilfix BM, Lesperance J, Campeau L. Relation of coronary artery disease in women 60 years of age to the combined elevation of serum lipoprotein (a) and total cholesterol to high-density cholesterol ratio. *Am J Cardiol* 1993;72:1215-1219.
50. Troxel WM, Matthews KA, Gallo LC, Kuller LH. Marital quality and occurrence of the metabolic syndrome in women. *Arch Intern Med* 2005;165:10227.
51. Turhan H, Yasar AS, Basar N, Bicer A, Erbay AR, Yetkin E. High prevalence of metabolic syndrome among young women with premature coronary artery disease. *Coron Artery Dis* 2005;16:37-40.
52. Tuzcu EM, Kapadia SR, Tutar E, et al. High prevalence of coronary atherosclerosis in asymptomatic teenagers and young adults: evidence from intravascular ultrasound. *Circulation* 2001;103:2705-2710.
53. Ueshima H, Okayama A, Saitoh S, et al. Differences in cardiovascular disease risk factors between Japanese in Japan and Japanese-Americans in Hawaii: the INTERLIPID study. *J Hum Hypertens* 2003;17:631-9.
54. van den Hoogen PC, Feskens E, Nagelkerke N, Menotti A, Nissinen A, Kromhout D. The relation between blood pressure and mortality due to coronary heart disease among men in different parts of the world. Seven Countries Study Research Group. *N Engl J Med* 2000;342:1-8.
55. Van Horn L, Greenland P. Prevention of coronary artery disease is a pediatric problem. *JAMA* 1997;287:1779 - 1780.
56. Weinstein AR, Sesso HD, Lee IM, et al. Relationship of physical activity vs body mass index with type 2 diabetes in women. *Jama* 2004;292:1188-94.
57. Wessel TR, Arant CB, Olson MB, et al. Relationship of physical fitness vs body mass index with coronary artery disease and cardiovascular events in women. *Jama* 2004;292:1179-87.
58. Wiegman A, Hutten BA, de Groot E, et al. Efficacy and safety of statin therapy in children with familial hypercholesterolemia: a randomized controlled trial. *Jama* 2004;292:331-7.

Chapter V: Practical steps for preventing heart disease

1. Anthony Robbins, Awaken the Giant Within, *Simon & Schuster*, 1992.
2. Bazzano LA, He J, Ogden LG, et al. Fruit and vegetable intake and risk of cardiovascular disease in US adults: the first National Health and Nutrition Examination Survey Epidemiologic Follow-up Study. *Am J Clin Nutr* 2002;76:93-9.
3. Benjamin EJ, Sidney S. 33rd Bethesda Conference. Preventive Cardiology: How can we do better. *J Am Cardiol* 2002;40:585-603.
4. Boyer J, Liu RH. Apple phytochemicals and their health benefits. *Nutr J* 2004;3:5.
5. Bucher HC, Hengstler P, Schindler C, Meier G. N-3 polyunsaturated fatty acids in coronary heart disease: a meta-analysis of randomized controlled trials. *Am J Med* 2002;112:298-304.
6. Chu YF, Sun J, Wu X, Liu RH. Antioxidant and antiproliferative activities of common vegetables. *J Agric Food Chem* 2002;50:6910-6.
7. Connor SL, Connor WE. Are fish oils beneficial in the prevention and treatment of coronary artery disease? *Am J Clin Nutr* 1997;66:1020S-1031S.
8. Dowse GK, Gareeboo H, Alberti KG, et al. Changes in population cholesterol concentrations and other cardiovascular risk factor levels after five years of the non- communicable disease intervention programme in Mauritius. Mauritius Non- communicable Disease Study Group. *Bmj* 1995;311:1255-9.
9. Enas A Enas, A Senthilkumar, Hancy Chennikkara, Marc A Bjurlin," Prudent Diet and Preventive Nutrition from Pediatrics to Geriatrics: Current Knowledge and Practical Recommendations", *Indian Heart Journal July - August*, 2003;55(4) 310-338 (A free PDF copy of this article can be downloaded from July 2003 archives of the Indian Heart Journal http://indian-heartjournal.com/).
10. Enas EA. Cooking oil, cholesterol and coronary artery disease. *Indian Heart J* 1996;48:423-428.
11. Enas EA. Management of coronary risk factors: Role of lifestyle modification. *Cardiology Today* 1998;2:17-29.
12. Fung TT, Hu FB, Pereira MA, et al. Whole-grain intake and the risk of type 2 diabetes: a prospective study in men. *Am J Clin Nutr* 2002;76:535-40.
13. Garcia Rodriguez LA, Hernandez-Diaz S, de Abajo FJ. Association between aspirin and upper gastrointestinal complications: systematic review of epi-

demiologic studies. *Br J Clin Pharmacol* 2001;52:563-71.

14. Gross LS, Li L, Ford ES, Liu S. Increased consumption of refined carbohydrates and the epidemic of type 2 diabetes in the United States: an ecologic assessment. *Am J Clin Nutr* 2004;79:774-9.

15. Grundy SM, Balady G, Criqui M, et al. Primary prevention of coronary heart disease: guidance from Framingham: A statement for healthcare professionals from the AHA Task Force on Risk Reduction. American Heart Association. *Circulation* 1998;97:1876-87.

16. Grundy SM. Primary prevention of coronary heart disease: Integrating risk assessment with intervention. *Circulation* 1999;100:988-998.

17. Harris WS, Park Y, Isley WL. Cardiovascular disease and long-chain omega-3 fatty acids. *Curr Opin Lipidol* 2003;14:9-14.

18. Haskell WL, Sims C, Myll J, Bortz WM, St Goar FG, Alderman EL. Coronary artery size and dilating capacity in ultradistance runners. *Circulation* 1993;87:1076-82.

19. Heber D, Bowerman S. Applying science to changing dietary patterns. *J Nutr* 2001;131:3078S-81S.

20. Howard M. Shapiro, Picture Perfect Weight Loss, *Rodale,* 2000.

21. Hu FB, Bronner L, Willett WC, et al. Fish and omega-3 fatty acid intake and risk of coronary heart disease in women. *Jama* 2002;287:1815-21.

22. Hu FB, Stampfer M, Manson J, et al. Frequent nut consumption and risk of coronary heart disease in women: Prospective cohort study. *BMJ* 1998;317:1341-1345.

23. Is organic food healthier? To date, there's no convincing evidence that organic foods are safer or more nutritious than conventionally produced foods. *Health News* 2004;10:3.

24. Jacobs DR Jr, Steffen LM. Nutrients, foods, and dietary patterns as exposures in research: a framework for food synergy. *Am J Clin Nutr* 2003;78:508S513S.

25. Katan MB, Zock PL, Mensink RP. Dietary oils, serum lipoproteins, and coronary heart disease. *Am J Clin Nutr* 1995;61:1368S-1373S.

26. Klatsky AL, Armstrong MA, Friedman GD. Red wine, white wine, liquor, beer, and risk for coronary artery disease hospitalization. *Am J Cardiol* 1997;80:416-20.

27. Klein S, Sheard NF, Pi-Sunyer X, et al. Weight management through lifestyle modification for the prevention and management of type 2 diabetes: rationale and strategies: a statement of the American Diabetes Association, the North American Association for the Study of Obesity, and the American Society for Clinical Nutrition.. *Diabetes Care* 2004;27:2067-73.

28. Kris-Etherton PM, Harris WS, Appel LJ. Omega-3 fatty acids and cardiovascular disease: new recommendations from the American Heart Association. *Arterioscler Thromb Vasc Biol* 2003;23:151-2.

29. Lazarus SA, Garg ML. Tomato extract inhibits human platelet aggregation in vitro without increasing basal cAMP levels. *Int J Food Sci Nutr* 2004;55:24956.

30. Manson JE, Tosteson H, Ridker P, et al. The primary prevention of myocardial infarction. *N Eng J Med* 1992;326:1406 - 1416.

31. Mendis S, Samarajeewa U, Thattil RO. Coconut fat and serum lipoproteins: effects of partial replacement with unsaturated fats. *Br J Nutr* 2001;85:583589.

32. Merchant AT, Anand SS, Vuksan V, et al. Protein intake is inversely associated with abdominal obesity in a multi-ethnic population. *J Nutr* 2005;135:1196-201.

33. Mora S, Redberg RF, Cui Y, et al. Ability of exercise testing to predict cardiovascular and all-cause death in asymptomatic women: a 20-year follow-up of the lipid research clinics prevalence study. *Jama* 2003;290:1600-7.

34. Ng TK, Hassan K, Lim JB, Lye MS, Ishak R. Nonhypercholesterolemic effects of a palm-oil diet in Malaysian volunteers. *Am J Clin Nutr* 1991;53:1015S-1020S.

35. Parikh P, McDaniel MC, Ashen MD, et al. Diets and cardiovascular disease: an evidence-based assessment. *J Am Coll Cardiol* 2005;45:1379-87.

36. Reddy KS, Katan MB. Diet, nutrition and the prevention of hypertension and cardiovascular diseases. *Public Health Nutr* 2004;7:167.

37. Reiser R, Probstfield JL, Silvers A, et al. Plasma lipid and lipoprotein response of humans to beef fat, coconut oil and safflower oil. *Am J Clin Nutr* 1985;42:190-7.

38. Richard N. Bolles, What Color is Your Parachute, *Ten Speed Press,* 1999.

39. Salmeron J, Manson JE, Stampfer MJ, Colditz GA, Wing AL, Willett WC. Dietary fiber, glycemic load, and risk of non-insulin-dependent diabetes mellitus in women. *Jama* 1997;277:472-7.

40. Spiller GA, Jenkins DJ, Cragen LN, et al. Effect of a diet high in monounsaturated fat from almonds on plasma cholesterol and lipoproteins. *J Am Coll Nutr* 1992;11:126-30.

41. Thompson PD, Buchner D, Pina IL, et al. Exercise and physical activity in the prevention and treatment of atherosclerotic cardiovascular disease: a statement from the Council on Clinical Cardiology (Subcommittee on Exercise, Rehabilitation, and Prevention) and the Council on Nutrition, Physical Activity, and Metabolism (Subcommittee on Physical Activity). *Circulation* 2003;107:3109-16.

42. Walter C. Willet, Eat, Drink and Be Healthy, *Simon & Schuster,* 2001.

Chapter VI: Controlling hypertension, dyslipidemia, and diabetes

1. Appel LJ. Lifestyle modification as a means to prevent and treat high blood pressure. *J Am Soc Nephrol* 2003;14:S99-S102.

2. Aronson D, Sella R, Sheikh-Ahmad M, et al. The association between cardiorespiratory fitness and C-reactive protein in subjects with the metabolic syndrome. *J Am Coll Cardiol* 2004;44:2003-7.

3. Asztalos BF, Batista M, Horvath KV, et al. Change in {alpha}1 HDL Concentration Predicts Progression in Coronary Artery Stenosis. *Arterioscler Thromb Vasc Biol* 2003;23:847-852.

4. Asztalos BF, Horvath KV, McNamara JR, Roheim PS, Rubinstein JJ, Schaefer EJ. Comparing the effects of five different statins on the HDL subpopulation profiles of coronary heart disease patients. *Atherosclerosis* 2002;164:361-9.

5. Berg K, Dahlen G, Christophersen B, Cook T, Kjekshus J, Pedersen T. Lipoprotein(a) lipoprotein level predicts survival and major coronary events in the Scandinavian Simvastatin Survival Study. *Clin Genet* 1997;52:254-261.

6. Blair SN, Church TS. The fitness, obesity, and health equation: is physical activity the common denominator? *Jama* 2004;292:1232-4.

7. Buchwald H, Avidor Y, Braunwald E, et al. Bariatric surgery: a systematic review and meta-analysis. *Jama* 2004;292:1724-37.

8. Cheung MC, Zhao XQ, Chait A, Albers JJ, Brown BG. Antioxidant supplements block the response of HDL to simvastatin-niacin therapy in patients with coronary artery disease and low HDL. *Arterioscler Thromb Vasc Biol* 2001;21:1320-1326.

9. Chobanian AV, Bakris GL, Black HR, et al. The Seventh Report of the Joint National Committee on Prevention, Detection, Evaluation, and Treatment of High Blood Pressure: the JNC 7 report. *Jama* 2003;289:2560-72.

10. Daida GH, Lee YJ, Yokoi H, et al. Prevention of restenosis after percutaneous transluminal coronary angioplasty by reducing lipoprotein (a) levels with low-density lipoprotein apheresis. Low-Density Lipoprotein Apheresis Angioplasty Restenosis Trial (L-ART) Group. *Am J Cardiol* 1994;73:1037-40.

11. Dansinger ML, Gleason JA, Griffith JL, Selker HP, Schaefer EJ. Comparison of the Atkins, Ornish, Weight Watchers, and Zone diets for weight loss and heart disease risk reduction: a randomized trial. *Jama* 2005;293:43-53.

12. Enas EA, Senthilkumar A, Chennikkara H, Bjurlin MA. Prudent diet and preventive nutrition from pediatrics to geriatrics: current knowledge and practical recommendations. *Indian Heart J* 2003;55:310-38.

13. Enas EA. Dyslipidemia among Indo-Asians: Strategies for identification and management. *Brit J of Diabetes and Vascular Dis* 2005;5:81-90.

14. Frost G, Leeds AA, Dore CJ, Madeiros S, Brading S, Dornhorst A. Glycaemic index as a determinant of serum HDL-cholesterol concentration. *Lancet* 1999;353:1045-8.

15. Gaziano JM, Sesso HD, Breslow JL, Hennekens CH, Buring JE. Relation between systemic hypertension and blood lipids on the risk of myocardial infarction. *Am J Cardiol* 1999;84:768-73.

16. Goldberg RB, Kendall DM, Deeg MA, et al. A comparison of lipid and glycemic effects of pioglitazone and rosiglitazone in patients with type 2 diabetes and dyslipidemia. *Diabetes Care* 2005;28:1547-54.

17. Gordon N F, Salmon RD, Franklin BA, et al. Effectiveness of therapeutic lifestyle changes in patients with hypertension, hyperlipidemia, and/or hyperglycemia. *Am J Cardiol* 2004;94:1558-61.

18. Graham DJ, Staffa JA, Shatin D, et al. Incidence of hospitalized rhabdomyolysis in patients treated with lipid-lowering drugs. *Jama* 2004;292:2585-90.

19. Grundy SM, Cleeman JI, Merz CN, et al. Implications of recent clinical trials for the National Cholesterol Education Program Adult Treatment Panel III guidelines. *Circulation* 2004;110:227-39.

20. Grundy SM, Vega GL, McGovern ME, et al. Efficacy, safety, and tolerability of once-daily niacin for the treatment of dyslipidemia associated with type 2 diabetes: results of the assessment of diabetes control and evaluation of the efficacy of niaspan trial. *Arch Intern Med* 2002;162:1568-76.

21. Grundy SM. Primary prevention of coronary heart disease: Integrating risk assessment with intervention. *Circulation* 1999;100:988-998. 1.

22. Haffner SM. Dyslipidemia management in adults with diabetes. *Diabetes Care* 2004;27 Suppl 1:S68-71

23. Harris WS, Ginsberg HN, Arunakul N, et al. Safety and efficacy of Omacor in severe hypertriglyceridemia. *J Cardiovasc Risk* 1997;4:385-91.

24. Hartung GH, Foreyt JP, Mitchell RE, Vlasek I, Gotto AM, Jr. Relation of diet to high-density-lipoprotein cholesterol in middle-aged marathon runners, jog-

gers, and inactive men. *N Engl J Med* 1980;302:357-61.

25. Impact of Intensive Lifestyle and Metformin Therapy on Cardiovascular Disease Risk Factors in the Diabetes Prevention Program. *Diabetes Care* 2005;28:888-894.

26. Jenkins DJ, Kendall CW, Marchie A, et al. Direct comparison of a dietary portfolio of cholesterol-lowering foods with a statin in hypercholesterolemic participants. *Am J Clin Nutr* 2005;81:380-7.

27. Jenkins DJ, Kendall CW, Marchie A, et al. Dose response of almonds on coronary heart disease risk factors: blood lipids, oxidized low-density lipoproteins, lipoprotein(a), homocysteine, and pulmonary nitric oxide: a randomized, controlled, crossover trial. *Circulation* 2002;106:1327-32.

28. Jiang R, Schulze MB, Li T, et al. Non-HDL cholesterol and apolipoprotein B predict cardiovascular disease events among men with type 2 diabetes. *Diabetes Care* 2004;27:1991-7.

29. Katzmarzyk PT, Church TS, Blair SN. Cardiorespiratory fitness attenuates the effects of the metabolic syndrome on all-cause and cardiovascular disease mortality in men. *Arch Intern Med* 2004;164:1092-7.

30. Khanal S, Obeidat O, Lu M, et al. Dyslipidemia in patients with angiographically confirmed coronary artery disease--an opportunity for improvement. *Clin Cardiol* 2004;27:577-80.

31. Khaw KT, Wareham N, Bingham S, Luben R, Welch A, Day N. Association of hemoglobin A1c with cardiovascular disease and mortality in adults: the European prospective investigation into cancer in Norfolk. *Ann Intern Med* 2004;141:413-20.

32. Klein S, Burke LE, Bray GA, et al. Clinical implications of obesity with specific focus on cardiovascular disease: a statement for professionals from the American Heart Association Council on Nutrition, Physical Activity, and Metabolism: endorsed by the American College of Cardiology Foundation. *Circulation* 2004;110:2952-67.

33. Kris-Etherton PM, Zhao G, Binkoski AE, Coval SM, Etherton TD. The effects of nuts on coronary heart disease risk. *Nutr Rev* 2001;59:103-11.

34. Langenfeld MR, Forst T, Hohberg C, et al. Pioglitazone decreases carotid intima-media thickness independently of glycemic control in patients with type 2 diabetes mellitus: results from a controlled randomized study. *Circulation* 2005;111:2525-31.

35. Law MR, Wald NJ, Thompson SG. By how much and how quickly does reduction in serum cholesterol concentration lower risk of ischaemic heart disease? *BMJ* 1994;308:367-372.

36. Lewington S, Clarke R, Qizilbash N, Peto R, Collins R. Age-specific relevance of usual blood pressure to vascular mortality: a meta-analysis of individual data for one million adults in 61 prospective studies. *Lancet* 2002;360:1903-13.

37. Lu W, Resnick HE, Jablonski KA, et al. Non-HDL Cholesterol as a Predictor of Cardiovascular Disease in Type 2 Diabetes: The Strong Heart Study. *Diabetes Care* 2003;26:16-23.

38. Luc G, Bard JM, Ferrieres J, et al. Value of HDL cholesterol, apolipoprotein A-I, lipoprotein A-I, and lipoprotein A-I/A-II in prediction of coronary heart disease: the PRIME Study. Prospective Epidemiological Study of Myocardial Infarction. *Arterioscler Thromb Vasc Biol* 2002;22:1155-61.

39. Lungershausen Y K, Abbey M, Nestel PJ, Howe PR. Reduction of blood pressure and plasma triglycerides by omega-3 fatty acids in treated hypertensives. *J Hypertens* 1994;12:1041-5.

40. McLaughlin T, Abbasi F, Cheal K, Chu J, Lamendola C, Reaven G. Use of metabolic markers to identify overweight individuals who are insulin resistant. *Ann Intern Med* 2003;139:802-9.

41. Mensink RP, Zock PL, Kester AD, Katan MB. Effects of dietary fatty acids and carbohydrates on the ratio of serum total to HDL cholesterol and on serum lipids and apolipoproteins: a meta-analysis of 60 controlled trials. *Am J Clin Nutr* 2003;77:1146-55.

42. Mosca L, Merz NB, Blumenthal RS, et al. Opportunity for intervention to achieve american heart association guidelines for optimal lipid levels in high-risk women in a managed care setting. *Circulation* 2005;111:488-93.

43. NCEP III. Third Report of the National Cholesterol Education Program(NCEP) Adult Treatment Panel III. *National Institute of Health,* 2002.

44. Pan J, Van JT, Chan E, Kesala RL, Lin M, Charles MA. Extended-release niacin treatment of the atherogenic lipid profile and lipoprotein(a) in diabetes. *Metabolism* 2002;51:1120-7.

45. Parikh P, McDaniel MC, Ashen MD, et al. Diets and cardiovascular disease: an evidence-based assessment. *J Am Coll Cardiol* 2005;45:1379-87.

46. Pfutzner A, Marx N, Lubben G, et al. Improvement of cardiovascular risk markers by pioglitazone is independent from glycemic control: results from the pioneer study. *J Am Coll Cardiol* 2005;45:1925-31.

47. Ratner R, Goldberg R, Haffner S, et al. Impact of intensive lifestyle and metformin therapy on cardiovascular disease risk factors in the diabetes prevention program. *Diabetes Care* 2005;28:888-94.

48. Reddy KS, Katan MB. Diet, nutrition and the prevention of hypertension and cardiovascular diseases. *Public Health Nutr* 2004;7:167-86.

49. Rifai N, Ma J, Sacks FM, et al. Apolipoprotein(a) size and lipoprotein(a) concentration and future risk of angina pectoris with evidence of severe coronary atherosclerosis in men: The Physicians' Health Study. *Clin Chem* 2004;50:1364-71.

50. Schernthaner G, Matthews DR, Charbonnel B, Hanefeld M, Brunetti P. Efficacy and safety of pioglitazone versus metformin in patients with type 2 diabetes mellitus: a double-blind, randomized trial. *J Clin Endocrinol Metab* 2004;89:6068-76.

51. Shishehbor MH, Hoogwerf BJ, Lauer MS. Association of triglyceride-to-HDL cholesterol ratio with heart rate recovery. *Diabetes Care* 2004;27:936-41.

52. Shlipak MG, Simon JA, Vittinghoff E, et al. Estrogen and progestin, lipoprotein(a), and the risk of recurrent coronary heart disease events after menopause. *JAMA* 2000;283:1845-1852.

53. Snow V, Barry P, Fitterman N, Qaseem A, Weiss K. Pharmacologic and surgical management of obesity in primary care: a clinical practice guideline from the American College of Physicians. *Ann Intern Med* 2005;142:525-31.

54. Standards of Medical Care in Diabetes. *Diabetes Care* 2005;28:S4-S36.

55. Szapary PO, Wolfe ML, Bloedon LT, et al. Guggulipid for the treatment of hypercholesterolemia: a randomized controlled trial. *Jama* 2003;290:765-72.

56. Van Gaal LF, Rissanen AM, Scheen AJ, Ziegler O, Rossner S. Effects of the cannabinoid-1 receptor blocker rimonabant on weight reduction and cardiovascular risk factors in overweight patients: 1-year experience from the RIO-Europe study. *Lancet* 2005;365:1389-97.

57. Whelton PK, He J, Appel LJ, et al. Primary prevention of hypertension: clinical and public health advisory from The National High Blood Pressure Education Program. *Jama* 2002;288:1882-8.

58. Winkler K, Konrad T, Fullert S, et al. Pioglitazone reduces atherogenic dense LDL particles in nondiabetic patients with arterial hypertension: a double-blind, placebo-controlled study. *Diabetes Care* 2003;26:2588-94.

59. Wong ND, Pio JR, Franklin SS, L'Italien GJ, Kamath TV, Williams GR. Preventing coronary events by optimal control of blood pressure and lipids in patients with the metabolic syndrome. *Am J Cardiol* 2003;91:1421-6.

60. Yamamoto A, Temba H, Horibe H, et al. Life style and cardiovascular risk factors in the Japanese population--from an epidemiological survey on serum lipid levels in Japan 1990 part 1: influence of life style and excess body weight on HDL-cholesterol and other lipid parameters in men. *J Atheroscler Thromb* 2003;10:165-75.

Chapter VII

1. Aarabi M, Jackson PR. Predicting coronary risk in UK South Asians: an adjustment method for Framingham-based tools. *Eur J Cardiovasc Prev Rehabil* 2005;12:46-51.

2. Abate N, Garg A, Enas EA. Physico-chemical properties of low density lipoproteins in normolipidemic Asian Indian men. *Horm Metab Res* 1995;27:326-331.

3. Ambrose JA, Fuster V. The risk of coronary occlusion is not proportional to the prior severity of coronary stenoses. *Heart* 1998;79:3-4.

4. Anand K, Chowdhury D, Singh KB, Pandav CS, Kapoor SK. Estimation of mortality and morbidity due to strokes in India. *Neuroepidemiology* 2001;20:208-11.

5. Ballantyne CM, Hoogeveen RC, Bang H, et al. Lipoprotein-associated phospholipase A2, high-sensitivity C-reactive protein, and risk for incident coronary heart disease in middle-aged men and women in the Atherosclerosis Risk in Communities (ARIC) study. *Circulation* 2004;109:837-42.

6. Bhalodkar NC, Blum S, Rana T, et al. Comparison of levels of large and small high-density lipoprotein cholesterol in Asian Indian men compared with Caucasian men in the Framingham Offspring Study. *Am J Cardiol* 2004;94:1561-3.

7. Bhalodkar NC, Blum S, Rana T, Bhalodkar A, Kitchappa R, Enas EA. Effect of leisure time exercise on high-density lipoprotein cholesterol, its subclasses, and size in asian indians. *Am J Cardiol* 2005;96:98-100.

8. Bittl JA. Advances in coronary angioplasty. *N Engl J Med* 1996;335:1290302.

9. Blake GJ, Otvos JD, Rifai N, Ridker PM. Low-density lipoprotein particle concentration and size as determined by nuclear magnetic resonance spectroscopy as predictors of cardiovascular disease in women. *Circulation* 2002;106:1930-7.

10. Blankenhorn DH, Selzer RH, Crawford DW, et al. Beneficial effects of colestipol-niacin therapy on the common carotid artery. Two- and four-year reduction of intima-media thickness measured by ultrasound. *Circulation* 1993;88:20-8.

11. Blumenthal JA, Sherwood A, Babyak MA, et al. Effects of exercise and stress management training on markers of cardiovascular risk in patients with ischemic heart disease: a randomized controlled trial. *Jama* 2005;293:1626-34.

12. Brown BG, Albers JJ, Fisher LD, et al. Regression of coronary artery disease as a result of intensive lipid- lowering therapy in men with high levels of apolipoprotein B. *N Engl J Med* 1990;323:1289-98.

13. Budoff MJ. Noninvasive coronary angiography using computed tomography. *Expert Rev Cardiovasc Ther* 2005;3:123-32.

14. Carrozza JP Jr, Sellke FW. A 69-year-old woman with left main coronary artery disease. *Jama* 2004;292:2506-14.

15. Criqui MH, Denenberg JO, Langer RD, Fronek A. The epidemiology of peripheral arterial disease: importance of identifying the population at risk. *Vasc Med* 1997;2:221-6.

16. Cromwell WC, Otvos JD. Low-density Lipoprotein Particle Number and Risk for Cardiovascular Disease. *Curr Atheroscler Rep* 2004;6:381-7.

17. Dagenais GR, Yi Q, Mann JF, Bosch J, Pogue J, Yusuf S. Prognostic impact of body weight and abdominal obesity in women and men with cardiovascular disease. *Am Heart J* 2005;149:54-60.

18. Daida GH, Lee YJ, Yokoi H, et al. Prevention of restenosis after percutaneous transluminal coronary angioplasty by reducing lipoprotein (a) levels with low-density lipoprotein apheresis. Low-Density Lipoprotein Apheresis Angioplasty Restenosis Trial (L-ART) Group. *Am J Cardiol* 1994;73:1037-40.

19. Daviglus ML, Liu K, Pirzada A, et al. Favorable cardiovascular risk profile in middle age and health-related quality of life in older age. *Arch Intern Med* 2003;163:2460-8.

20. De Luca G, Suryapranata H, Ottervanger JP, Antman EM. Time delay to treatment and mortality in primary angioplasty for acute myocardial infarction: every minute of delay counts. *Circulation* 2004;109:1223-5.

21. Diaz A, Bourassa MG, Guertin MC, Tardif JC. Long-term prognostic value of resting heart rate in patients with suspected or proven coronary artery disease. *Eur Heart* J 2005;26:967-74.

22. Fishbein MC, Siegel RJ. How big are coronary atherosclerotic plaques that rupture? *Circulation* 1996;94:2662-6.

23. Greenland P, LaBree L, Azen SP, Doherty TM, Detrano RC. Coronary artery calcium score combined with Framingham score for risk prediction in asymptomatic individuals. *Jama* 2004;291:210-5.

24. Grundy SM, D'Agostino Sr RB, Mosca L, et al. Cardiovascular risk assessment based on US cohort studies: findings from a National Heart, Lung, and Blood institute workshop. *Circulation* 2001;104:491-496.

25. Grundy SM, Pasternak R, Greenland P, Smith S, Jr., Fuster V. Assessment of cardiovascular risk by use of multiple-risk-factor assessment equations: A statement for healthcare professionals from the American Heart Association and the American College of Cardiology. *Circulation* 1999;100:1481-1492.

26. Grundy SM. Coronary plaque as a replacement for age as a risk factor in global risk assessment. *Am J Cardiol* 2001;88:8E-11E.

27. Hambrecht R, Walther C, Mobius-Winkler S, et al. Percutaneous coronary angioplasty compared with exercise training in patients with stable coronary artery disease: a randomized trial. *Circulation* 2004;109:1371-8.

28. Katritsis DG, Ioannidis JP. Percutaneous coronary intervention versus conservative therapy in nonacute coronary artery disease: a meta-analysis. *Circulation* 2005;111:2906-12.

29. Khanal S, Obeidat O, Lu M, et al. Dyslipidemia in patients with angiographically confirmed coronary artery disease--an opportunity for improvement. Clin Cardiol 2004;27:577-80.

30. Kong DF, Eisenstein EL, Sketch MH, Jr., et al. Economic impact of drug-eluting stents on hospital systems: a disease-state model. *Am Heart J* 2004;147:449-56.

31. Kuettner A, Beck T, Drosch T, et al. Diagnostic accuracy of noninvasive coronary imaging using 16-detector slice spiral computed tomography with 188 ms temporal resolution. *J Am Coll Cardiol* 2005;45:123-7.

32. Kulkarni KR, Marcovina SM, Krauss RM, Garber DW, Glasscock AM, Segrest JP. Quantification of HDL2 and HDL3 cholesterol by the Vertical Auto Profile-II (VAP-II) methodology. *J Lipid Res* 1997;38:2353-64.

33. Kullo IJ, Gau GT, Tajik AJ. Novel risk factors for atherosclerosis. *Mayo Clin Proc* 2000;75:369-80.

34. Little WC, Constantinescu M, Applegate RJ, et al. Can coronary angiography predict the site of a subsequent myocardial infarction in patients with mild-to-moderate coronary artery disease? *Circulation* 1988;78:1157-1166.

35. Malik S, Wong ND, Franklin SS, et al. Impact of the metabolic syndrome on mortality from coronary heart disease, cardiovascular disease, and all causes in United States adults. *Circulation* 2004;110:1245-50.

36. Marcovina SM, Koschinsky ML, Albers JJ, Skarlatos S. Report of the National Heart, Lung, and Blood Institute Workshop on Lipoprotein(a) and Cardiovascular Disease: recent advances and future directions. *Clin Chem* 2003;49:1785-96.

37. Myers J, Prakash M, Froelicher V, Do D, Partington S, Atwood JE. Exercise capacity and mortality among men referred for exercise testing. *N Engl J Med* 2002;346:793-801.

38. Natarajan S, Glick H, Criqui M, Horowitz D, Lipsitz SR, Kinosian B. Cholesterol measures to identify and treat individuals at risk for coronary heart disease. *Am J Prev Med* 2003;25:50-7.

39. Ndrepepa G, Mehilli J, Bollwein H, Pache J, Schomig A, Kastrati A. Sex-associated differences in clinical outcomes after coronary stenting in patients with diabetes mellitus. *Am J Med* 2004;117:830-6.

40. Nissen SE, Tuzcu EM, Schoenhagen P, et al. Effect of intensive compared with moderate lipid-lowering therapy on progression of coronary atherosclerosis: a randomized controlled trial. *Jama* 2004;291:1071-80.

41. Nissen SE. Application of intravascular ultrasound to characterize coronary artery disease and assess the progression or regression of atherosclerosis. *Am J Cardiol* 2002;89:24B-31B.

42. O'Connor NJ, Morton JR, Birkmeyer JD, Olmstead EM, O'Connor GT. Effect of coronary artery diameter in patients undergoing coronary bypass surgery. Northern New England Cardiovascular Disease Study Group. *Circulation* 1996;93:652-655.

43. Pletcher MJ, Tice JA, Pignone M, Browner WS. Using the coronary artery calcium score to predict coronary heart disease events: a systematic review and meta-analysis. *Arch Intern Med* 2004;164:1285-92.

44. Qureshi MA, Safian RD, Grines CL, et al. Simplified scoring system for predicting mortality after percutaneous coronary intervention. *J Am Coll Cardiol* 2003;42:1890-5.

45. Rajagopalan N, Miller TD, Hodge DO, Frye RL, Gibbons RJ. Identifying high-risk asymptomatic diabetic patients who are candidates for screening stress single-photon emission computed tomography imaging. *J Am Coll Cardiol* 2005;45:43-9.

46. Ridker PM, Rifai N, Cook NR, Bradwin G, Buring JE. Non-HDL cholesterol, apolipoproteins A-I and B100, standard lipid measures, lipid ratios, and CRP as risk factors for cardiovascular disease in women. *Jama* 2005;294:326-33.

47. Seman J, DeLuca C, Jenner JL, et al. Lipoprotein(a)-cholesterol and coronary heart disease in the Framingham Heart Study. *Clin Chem* 1999;45:1039-46.

48. Shah PK, Amin J. Low high density lipoprotein level is associated with increased restenosis rate after coronary angioplasty. *Circulation* 1992;85:1279-85.

49. Spertus JA, Salisbury AC, Jones PG, Conaway DG, Thompson RC. Predictors of quality-of-life benefit after percutaneous coronary intervention. *Circulation* 2004;110:3789-94.

50. Stamler J, Stamler R, Neaton JD, et al. Low risk-factor profile and long-term cardiovascular and noncardiovascular mortality and life expectancy: Findings for 5 large cohorts of young adult and middle-aged men and women. *JAMA* 1999;282:2012-2018.

51. Superko HR, Enas EA, Kotha P, Bhat NK, Garrett B. High-density lipoprotein subclass distribution in individuals of Asian Indian descent: the National Asian Indian Heart Disease Project. *Prev Cardiol* 2005;8:81-6.

52. Superko HR, Krauss RM. Coronary artery disease regression. Convincing evidence for the benefit of aggressive lipoprotein management. *Circulation* 1994;90:1056-69.

53. Taylor AJ, Sullenberger LE, Lee HJ, Lee JK, Grace KA. Arterial Biology for the Investigation of the Treatment Effects of Reducing Cholesterol (ARBITER) 2: A Double-Blind, Placebo-Controlled Study of Extended-Release Niacin on Atherosclerosis Progression in Secondary Prevention Patients Treated With Statins. *Circulation* 2004;110:3512-7.

54. Weintraub WS, Jones EL, Craver JM, Grosswald R, Guyton RA. In-hospital and long-term outcome after reoperative coronary artery bypass graft surgery. *Circulation* 1995;92:II50-7.

55. Weintraub WS, Veledar E, Thompson T, Burnette J, Jurkovitz C, Mahoney E. Percutaneous coronary intervention outcomes in octogenarians during the stent era (National Cardiovascular Network). *Am J Cardiol* 2001;88:1407-10,A6.

56. Whitaker RC, Wright JA, Pepe MS, Seidel KD, Dietz WH. Predicting obesity in young adulthood from childhood and parental obesity. *N Engl J Med* 1997;337:869-73.

57. Williams PT, Superko HR, Haskell WL, et al. Smallest LDL particles are most strongly related to coronary disease progression in men. *Arterioscler Thromb Vasc Biol* 2003;23:314-21.

58. Witte DR, Taskinen MR, Perttunen-Nio H, Van Tol A, Livingstone S, Colhoun HM. Study of agreement between LDL size as measured by nuclear magnetic resonance and gradient gel electrophoresis. *J Lipid Res* 2004;45:1069-76.

59. Yamamoto H, Imazu M, Yamabe T, Ueda H, Hattori Y, Yamakido M. Risk factors for restenosis after percutaneous transluminal coronary angioplasty:

role of lipoprotein (a). *Am Heart J* 1995;130:1168-73.

Chapter VIII: Cardiovascular medications and devices

1. Abebe W. Herbal medication: potential for adverse interactions with analgesic drugs. *J Clin Pharm Ther* 2002;27:391-401.
2. Awang DV, Fugh-Berman A. Herbal interactions with cardiovascular drugs. *J Cardiovasc Nurs* 2002;16:64-70.
3. Bays HE, Dujovne CA, McGovern ME, et al. Comparison of once-daily, niacin extended-release/lovastatin with standard doses of atorvastatin and simvastatin (the ADvicor Versus Other Cholesterol-Modulating Agents Trial Evaluation [ADVOCATE]). Am J Cardiol 2003;91:667-72. Kashyap ML, McGovern ME, Berra K, et al. Long-term safety and efficacy of a once-daily niacin/lovastatin formulation for patients with dyslipidemia. *Am J Cardiol* 2002;89:672-8.
4. Brown BG, Zhao XQ, Chait A, et al. Simvastatin and niacin, antioxidant vitamins, or the combination for the prevention of coronary disease. *N Engl J Med* 2001;345:1583-92.
5. Canner PL, Berge KG, Wenger NK, et al. Fifteen year mortality in Coronary Drug Project patients: long-term benefit with niacin. *J Am Coll Cardiol* 1986;8:1245-55.
6. Canner PL, Furberg CD, Terrin ML, McGovern ME. Benefits of niacin by glycemic status in patients with healed myocardial infarction (from the Coronary Drug Project). *Am J Cardiol* 2005;95:254-7.
7. Cannon CP, Braunwald E, McCabe CH, et al. Comparison of Intensive and Moderate Lipid Lowering with Statins after Acute Coronary Syndromes. *N Engl J Med* 2004.
8. Chan KA, Truman A, Gurwitz JH, et al. A cohort study of the incidence of serious acute liver injury in diabetic patients treated with hypoglycemic agents. *Arch Intern Med* 2003;163:728-34.
9. Dujovne CA. Side effects of statins: hepatitis versus "transaminitis"-myositis versus "CPKitis". *Am J Cardiol* 2002;89:1411-3.
10. Elam MB, Hunninghake DB, Davis KB, et al. Effect of niacin on lipid and lipoprotein levels and glycemic control in patients with diabetes and peripheral arterial disease: the ADMIT study: A randomized trial. Arterial Disease Multiple Intervention Trial. *Jama* 2000;284:1263-70.
11. Enas EA. Dyslipidemia among Indo-Asians: Strategies for identification and management. *Brit J of Diabetes and Vascular Dis* 2005;5:81-90.
12. Estes JD, Stolpman D, Olyaei A, et al. High prevalence of potentially hepatotoxic herbal supplement use in patients with fulminant hepatic failure. *Arch Surg* 2003;138:852-8.
13. Goldberg AC. A meta-analysis of randomized controlled studies on the effects of extended-release niacin in women. *Am J Cardiol* 2004;94:121-4.
14. Graham DJ, Staffa JA, Shatin D, et al. Incidence of hospitalized rhabdomyolysis in patients treated with lipid-lowering drugs. *Jama* 2004;292:2585-90.
15. Grundy SM, Cleeman JI, Merz CN, et al. Implications of recent clinical trials for the National Cholesterol Education Program Adult Treatment Panel III guidelines. *Circulation* 2004;110:227-39.
16. Grundy SM, Vega GL, McGovern ME, et al. Efficacy, safety, and tolerability of once-daily niacin for the treatment of dyslipidemia associated with type 2 diabetes: results of the assessment of diabetes control and evaluation of the efficacy of niaspan trial. *Arch Intern Med* 2002;162:1568-76.
17. Grundy SM, Vega GL, Yuan Z, Battisti WP, Brady WE, Palmisano J. Effectiveness and tolerability of simvastatin plus fenofibrate for combined hyperlipidemia (the SAFARI trial). *Am J Cardiol* 2005;95:462-8.
18. Hayden M, Pignone M, Phillips C, Mulrow C. Aspirin for the primary prevention of cardiovascular events: a summary of the evidence for the U.S. Preventive Services Task Force. *Ann Intern Med* 2002;136:161-72.
19. Hu Z, Yang X, Ho PC, et al. Herb-drug interactions: a literature review. *Drugs* 2005;65:1239-82.
20. Hunninghake DB, McGovern ME, Koren M, et al. A dose-ranging study of a new, once-daily, dual-component drug product containing niacin extended-release and lovastatin. *Clin Cardiol* 2003;26:112-8.
21. Jacobson TA. Comparative pharmacokinetic interaction profiles of pravastatin, simvastatin, and atorvastatin when coadministered with cytochrome P450 inhibitors. *Am J Cardiol* 2004;94:1140-6.
22. Jones PH. Statins as the cornerstone of drug therapy for dyslipidemia: monotherapy and combination therapy options. *Am Heart J* 2004;148:S9-13.
23. Kashyap ML, McGovern ME, Berra K, et al. Long-term safety and efficacy of a once-daily niacin/lovastatin formulation for patients with dyslipidemia. *Am J Cardiol* 2002;89:672-8.
24. Kuo PI, Severino R, Pashkow FJ. Mortality rates and hemorrhagic complications in asian-pacific islanders during treatment of acute myocardial infarction. *Am J Cardiol* 2004;94:644-6, A9.
25. LaRosa JC, Grundy SM, Waters DD, et al. Intensive lipid lowering with atorvastatin in patients with stable coronary disease. *N Engl J Med* 2005;352:1425-35.
26. Lead poisoning associated with ayurvedic medications--five states, 2000-2003. *MMWR Morb Mortal Wkly* Rep 2004;53:582-4.
27. Lonn E, Bosch J, Yusuf S, et al. Effects of long-term vitamin E supplementation on cardiovascular events and cancer: a randomized controlled trial. *Jama* 2005;293:1338-47.
28. Meyers CD, Carr MC, Park S, Brunzell JD. Varying cost and free nicotinic acid content in over-the-counter niacin preparations for dyslipidemia. *Ann Intern Med* 2003;139:996-1002.
29. Miller ER 3rd, Pastor-Barriuso R, Dalal D, Riemersma RA, Appel LJ, Guallar E. Meta-analysis: high-dosage vitamin E supplementation may increase all-cause mortality. *Ann Intern Med* 2005;142:37-46.
30. Miller KL, Liebowitz RS, Newby LK. Complementary and alternative medicine in cardiovascular disease: a review of biologically based approaches. *Am Heart J* 2004;147:401-11.
31. Morgan J, Carey C, Lincoff A, Capuzzi D. High-density Lipoprotein Subfractions and Risk of Coronary Artery Disease. *Curr Atheroscler Rep* 2004;6:359-65.
32. Morgan JM, Capuzzi DM, Baksh RI, et al. Effects of extended-release niacin on lipoprotein subclass distribution. *Am J Cardiol* 2003;91:1432-6.
33. Mulrow C, Pignone M. An editorial update: should she take aspirin? *Ann Intern Med* 2005;142:942-3.
34. NCEP III. Third Report of the National Cholesterol Education Program(NCEP) Adult Treatment Panel III. *National Institute of Health,* 2002.
35. Nissen SE, Tuzcu EM, Schoenhagen P, et al. Effect of intensive compared with moderate lipid-lowering therapy on progression of coronary atherosclerosis: a randomized controlled trial. *Jama* 2004;291:1071-80.
36. Omar MA, Wilson JP. FDA adverse event reports on statin-associated rhabdomyolysis. *Ann Pharmacother* 2002;36:288-95.
37. Pan J, Van JT, Chan E, Kesala RL, Lin M, Charles MA. Extended-release niacin treatment of the atherogenic lipid profile and lipoprotein(a) in diabetes. *Metabolism* 2002;51:1120-7.
38. Roberts WC. The rule of 5 and the rule of 7 in lipid-lowering by statin drugs. *Am J Cardiol* 1997;80:106-107.
39. Roberts WC. Two more drugs for dyslipidemia. Am J Cardiol 2004;93:80911.
40. Saper RB, Kales SN, Paquin J, et al. Heavy metal content of ayurvedic herbal medicine products. *Jama* 2004;292:2868-73.
41. Sibley C, McGann S, Stone NJ. Long-term survival of childhood coronary artery disease in a patient severely affected with familial hypercholesterolemia. *Am J Cardiol* 2004;94:699-700.
42. Stein EA, Lane M, Laskarzewski P. Comparison of statins in hypertriglyceridemia. *Am J Cardiol* 1998;81:66B-69B.
43. Superko HR, McGovern ME, Raul E, Garrett B. Differential effect of two nicotinic acid preparations on low-density lipoprotein subclass distribution in patients classified as low-density lipoprotein pattern A, B, or I. *Am J Cardiol* 2004;94:588-94.
44. Taylor AJ, Sullenberger LE, Lee HJ, Lee JK, Grace KA. Arterial Biology for the Investigation of the Treatment Effects of Reducing Cholesterol (ARBITER) 2: A Double-Blind, Placebo-Controlled Study of Extended-Release Niacin on Atherosclerosis Progression in Secondary Prevention Patients Treated With Statins. *Circulation* 2004;110:3512-7.
45. Wald NJ, Law MR. A strategy to reduce cardiovascular disease by more than 80%. *Bmj* 2003;326:1419.
46. Wolfe M L, Vartanian SF, Ross JL, et al. Safety and effectiveness of Niaspan when added sequentially to a statin for treatment of dyslipidemia. *Am J Cardiol* 2001;87:476-479.
47. Wong ND, Pio JR, Franklin SS, L'Italien GJ, Kamath TV, Williams GR. Preventing coronary events by optimal control of blood pressure and lipids in patients with the metabolic syndrome. *Am J Cardiol* 2003;91:1421-6.

An extended list of references will be included in the professional edition. These references are also available for purchase, prior to the publication of the professional edition.

INDEX

Quick Order Form

Fax orders: **630-961-9554**

Email orders: book@cadiresearch.com

Postal orders: Advanced Heart & Lipid Clinic
              4121 Fairview Ave # 103, Downers Grove, IL 60515, USA

Save $30! Order your own copy today

" How to Beat the Heart Disease Epidemic among South Asians: A prevention and management guide for Asian Indians and their doctors" by Dr. Enas A. Enas at the pre-publication price of $29.95 (List price $59.95)

Discount valid through December 31st, 2005

☐ Yes, I want _____ copies of "Beat the Heart Disease Epidemic among Asian Indians" at $29.99 each ($59.95 after December 31st 2005)
☐ Yes, I am interested in having Dr. Enas and Dr. Kannan give a seminar to my company, association, school, or organization. Please contact me.

Include $6.95 US shipping and handling for one book and $2.95 for each additional book.
Bulk orders welcome! Send an email to book@cadiresearch.com
Contact us for International orders.

Payment must accompany order.
My check or money order (payable in US Dollars in a US Bank to Advance Heart Lipid Clinic)
for $ _____ is enclosed

Please charge my ☐ Visa ☐ Mastercard ☐ American Express

Name _____

Organization_____

Address_____

City/State/Zip_____

Phone_____Email_____

Card #_____

Exp. Date_____Signature_____